Public Health Law

Power, Duty, Restraint

Revised and Expanded Second Edition

Lawrence O. Gostin

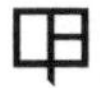

UNIVERSITY OF CALIFORNIA PRESS
Berkeley · Los Angeles · London

THE MILBANK MEMORIAL FUND
New York

University of California Press, one of the most distinguished university presses in the United States, enriches lives around the world by advancing scholarship in the humanities, social sciences, and natural sciences. Its activities are supported by the UC Press Foundation and by philanthropic contributions from individuals and institutions. For more information, visit www.ucpress.edu.

The Milbank Memorial Fund is an endowed operating foundation that engages in nonpartisan analysis, study, research, and communication on significant issues in health policy. In the Fund's own publications, in reports or books it publishes with other organizations, and in articles it commissions for publication by other organizations, the Fund endeavors to maintain the highest standards for accuracy and fairness. Statements by individual authors, however, do not necessarily reflect opinions or factual determinations of the Fund. For more information, visit www.milbank.org.

University of California Press
Berkeley and Los Angeles, California

University of California Press, Ltd.
London, England

Library of Congress Cataloging-in-Publication Data

Gostin, Larry O. (Larry Ogalthorpe)
Public health law : power, duty, restraint / Lawrence O. Gostin. — 2nd ed.
p. cm.
Includes bibliographical references and index.
ISBN-13: 978-0-520-25376-6 (pbk. : alk. paper)
1. Public health laws—United States. I. Title.

KF3775.G67 2008
344.7304—dc22 2007004267

Manufactured in the United States of America

16 15 14 13 12 11 10 09 08
10 9 8 7 6 5 4 3 2 1

The paper used in this publication meets the minimum requirements of ANSI/ASTM Z39.48-1992 (R 1997) *(Permanence of Paper)*.

Public Health Law

CALIFORNIA/MILBANK BOOKS ON HEALTH AND THE PUBLIC

1. *The Corporate Practice of Medicine: Competition and Innovation in Health Care,* by James C. Robinson
2. *Experiencing Politics: A Legislator's Stories of Government and Health Care,* by John E. McDonough
3. *Public Health Law: Power, Duty, Restraint,* by Lawrence O. Gostin
4. *Public Health Law and Ethics: A Reader,* edited by Lawrence O. Gostin
5. *Big Doctoring in America: Profiles in Primary Care,* by Fitzhugh Mullan, M.D.
6. *Deceit and Denial: The Deadly Politics of Industrial Pollution,* by Gerald Markowitz and David Rosner
7. *Death Is That Man Taking Names: Intersections of American Medicine, Law, and Culture,* by Robert A. Burt
8. *When Walking Fails: Mobility Problems of Adults with Chronic Conditions,* by Lisa I. Iezzoni
9. *What Price Better Health? Hazards of the Research Imperative,* by Daniel Callahan
10. *Sick to Death and Not Going to Take It Anymore! Reforming Health Care for the Last Years of Life,* by Joanne Lynn
11. *The Employee Retirement Income Security Act of 1974: A Political History,* by James A. Wooten
12. *Evidence-Based Medicine and the Search for a Science of Clinical Care,* by Jeanne Daly
13. *Disease and Democracy: The Industrialized World Faces AIDS,* by Peter Baldwin
14. *Medicare Matters: What Geriatric Medicine Can Teach American Health Care,* by Christine K. Cassel
15. *Are We Ready? Public Health since 9/11,* by David Rosner and Gerald Markowitz
16. *State of Immunity: The Politics of Vaccination in Twentieth-Century America,* by James Colgrove
17. *Low Income, Social Growth, and Good Health: A History of Twelve Countries,* by James C. Riley
18. *Searching Eyes: Privacy, the State, and Disease Surveillance in America,* by Amy L. Fairchild, Ronald Bayer, and James Colgrove

Contents

Illustrations

PHOTOGRAPHS

FIGURES

Tables

Boxes

Foreword

The Milbank Memorial Fund is an endowed operating foundation that works to improve health by helping decision makers in the public and private sectors acquire and use the best available evidence to inform policy for health care and population health. The Fund has engaged in nonpartisan analysis, research, and communication about significant issues in health policy since its inception in 1905.

Public Health Law: Power, Duty, Restraint was the third of what are now nineteen California/Milbank Books on Health and the Public. The publishing partnership between the Fund and the University of California Press encourages the synthesis and communication of findings from research and experience, which could contribute to more effective health policy.

Larry Gostin offers fresh information and analysis in every chapter of this second edition. Perhaps most important, he describes increased attention to the strengths and weaknesses of public health law as a result of events since its initial publication.

The first edition appeared a year before the first of a series of challenges to public health, each of which has stimulated changes in law and regulation as well as the allocation of new resources by government at every level. These challenges include the events of September 11, 2001, the twenty-two cases of anthrax in the next several months, the SARS epidemic, the increased risk of a pandemic of avian flu, hurricanes Katrina and Rita, and, as this edition went to press, news that public health regulations could not prevent a willful Atlanta lawyer with tuberculosis from risking the health of people on several airplanes and two continents.

During the past seven years, moreover, the field of public health law has expanded in size and scope. For the first time in over a century, public health law is increasingly recognized as one of the professions of public health, as essential as medicine, the laboratory sciences, and epidemiology. This book has contributed to the growth of the field as a text in many schools of law and public health and as the source of numerous citations in articles and books.

Gostin has been a leader in studying, interpreting, and teaching public health law—as well as in drafting it—for three decades. In writing and then revising this book, he says, "I aspire to create a record of the field of public health law at the turn of the millennium." He has achieved that aspiration.

Daniel M. Fox
President Emeritus

Carmen Hooker Odom
President

Samuel L. Milbank
Chairman

Preface to the Second Edition

Good health is fundamentally important because it is essential to happiness, livelihood, political participation, and many of the other elements necessary for a life full of contentment and achievement. Certainly, health is not the only important social value, and on occasion, public health aspirations have to yield to other values. Additionally, elected officials are not obligated to spend inordinate amounts of tax dollars on a single public good, such as health, when there are many competing political claims for limited resources. Nevertheless, I think it is important that any book purporting to examine carefully the interface between law and health begin by emphasizing the powerful collective benefits afforded by ensuring the conditions for a healthy population.

Libraries throughout the United States and other highly developed countries are replete with books on the general subject of law and health. Why then offer a book on public health law? The reason is that the vast majority of these books are concerned principally with medicine and personal health care services—clinical decision making, delivery, organization, and finance. Personal medical services are an important part of what makes a community healthy. Yet medicine is only one contributor to health, and probably a relatively small one at that. Virtually all national health expenditures (excluding environmental funding) are devoted to medical care; only a tiny fraction is allocated to population-based public health initiatives. I am delighted to note, however, that since the last edition of this book, scholarly attention to the field of public health law has surged. The modern interest in population health has focused on potentially catastrophic threats to the public's health, including bioterrorism (e.g., anthrax and smallpox), emerging infectious diseases (e.g., SARS, pandemic influenza), and chronic diseases caused by human behavior (e.g., tobacco, high-calorie diet, and sedentary lifestyle). This extensively revised second edition focuses on contemporary issues of great importance, including security, preparedness, obesity, and global health.

In this book, I offer a systematic definition and theory of public health law. The definition is based on a broad notion of the government's inherent responsibility to advance the population's health and well-being:

> Public health law is the study of the legal powers and duties of the state, in collaboration with its partners (e.g., health care, business, the community, the media, and academe), to ensure the conditions for people to be healthy (to identify, prevent, and ameliorate risks to health in the population), and of the limitations on the power of the state to constrain for the common good the autonomy, privacy, liberty, proprietary, or other legally protected interests of individuals. The prime objective of public health law is to pursue the highest possible level of physical and mental health in the population, consistent with the values of social justice.

I explain why public health law is a coherent field, distinct from other intellectual activities at the intersection of law and health. In particular, I offer five characteristics that distinguish public health law from the vast literature on law and medicine (see figure 1):

- Government's responsibility to advance the public's health
- Coercion and limits on state power
- Government's partners in the public health system
- The population perspective
- Communities and civic participation
- The prevention orientation
- Social justice

This book, therefore, is about the complex problems that arise when government regulates to prevent injury and disease or to promote the public's health. The government possesses the authority and responsibility to persuade, create incentives, or even compel individuals and businesses to conform to health and safety standards for the collective good. This power and obligation forms the essence of what we call public health law.

In addition to offering a definition and theory, I examine the analyt-

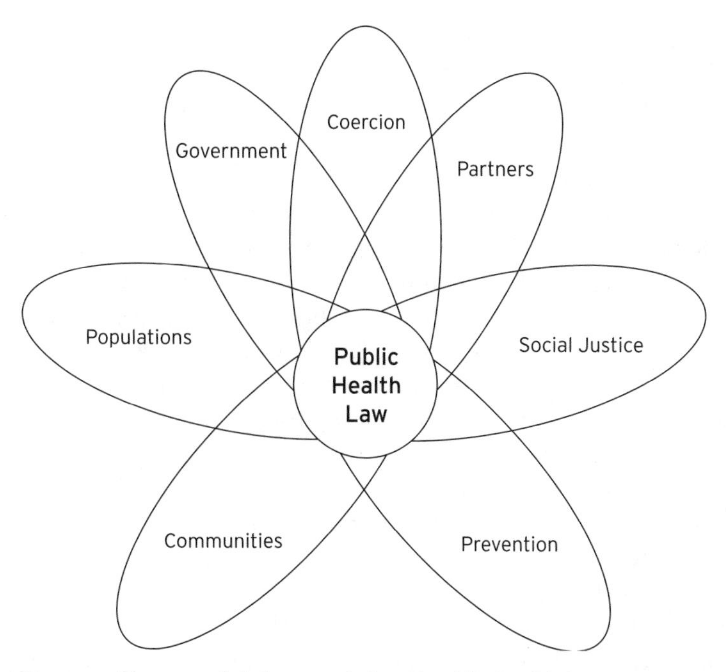

Figure 1. The essential characteristics of public health law.

ical methods and tools of public health law, principally constitutional law, which empowers government to act for the community's health and limits that power; statutory and administrative law, which provides the vast regulatory structure at the federal, state, and local levels for responding to health threats; tort law, which affords a civil remedy against individuals and businesses whose unreasonably risky conduct causes injury or disease; and international law, which guides and binds nation-states and other entities in activities, relations, and transactions that transcend national borders.

Accordingly, much of the book discusses the extensive body of legal doctrine that informs the field of public health law. A book on public health law intended for a broad audience cannot consider all the nuances and complexities of legal doctrine. For the sake of succinctness and clarity, the text sometimes may imply that the law is more monolithic and predictable than it really is. Subsequent chapters present some of the subtleties of the law as applied to particular problems in public health. Nevertheless, a much more careful examination of statutes, administrative rules, and policies is essential in resolving specific legal problems facing public health authorities.

I often return to two themes in this book: the trade-offs between public goods and private rights, and the dilemma of whether to use coercive or voluntary public health measures. As to the first theme, I emphasize the collective goods that are achieved, or achievable, through legal and regulatory approaches. Seen in this way, the law is a potent tool for the realization of healthier and safer populations. At the same time, I closely examine the complexity of, and conundrums posed by, public health regulation. Though public health regulation is intended to achieve public goods, it often does so at the expense of private rights and interests. Consequently, in thinking about public health regulation, we have to take a hard look at the trade-offs—between the common welfare, on the one hand, and the personal burdens and economic interests of individuals and businesses, on the other.

Characterizing these trade-offs between collective goods and individual rights is only one of several possible ways to conceptualize the problem. Another way would be to characterize the trade-off as between two collective goods: the good of public health and the good of limited government. After all, society gains a great deal of benefit from the protection of individual liberties through a constitutional system of limited governmental interference. Still, an analysis of collective goods versus individual rights captures at least one important way of thinking about public health.

Another problem with characterizing public health law as a series of trade-offs between private rights and public goods is that often the most effective public health policy is to enhance private rights to attain public goods. My friend the late Jonathan Mann was particularly eloquent in urging the conclusion that public health and human rights are synergistic; preserving and promoting individual rights most often advances human well-being. Certainly, coercive policies may have unintended effects on group behaviors (e.g., driving people away from health care services). Furthermore, antidiscrimination, privacy, and other legal safeguards have public health, as well as intrinsic, value. Nevertheless, sometimes public health officials confront hard choices between public goods and private rights, and many of the chapters in this book explore these complex choices.

The trade-offs between individual and population-based perspectives lead to a second, related theme. Public health scholars and practitioners, for as long as people have organized societies to defend their health and security, have grappled with the decision of whether to use voluntary or coercive approaches in achieving collective benefits. Is it always, or almost always, better to persuade individuals to change their behavior, to provide the means for behavioral change, and to restructure environments to promote the public's health? Alternatively, should public health authorities resort to compulsion of individuals and businesses? And, if compulsion is warranted, under what circumstances should public health authorities wield their power? In this book, I propose a systematic evaluation of public health regulation that helps balance private rights and public goods. The model I propose is intended to assess the circumstances when government rightfully should be able to demand conformance with public standards.

In writing this book, I learned a great deal about myself. I come from a strong civil liberties background. A young Fulbright scholar at the Universities of Oxford and London in the mid-1970s, I went on to become the legal director of the National Association of Mental Health (MIND) (where I brought a series of landmark cases before the European Court of Human Rights) and, later, the head of the National Council of Civil Liberties (the U.K. equivalent of the American Civil Liberties Union). After returning to the United States in the late 1980s, I served on the ACLU's National Board of Directors and National Executive Committee, and in the early 1990s, I chaired its Privacy Committee. During all those years, I subscribed to the dominant liberal position that individual freedom is by far the preferred value to guide ethical and legal analysis in matters of physical and mental health.

My devotion to civil liberties was particularly strained by events surrounding September 11 and the anthrax attacks, only a year after the first edition of this book was published. The CDC asked the Center for Law and the Public's Health to draft the Model State Emergency Health Powers Act (MSEHPA). Although the act was a great success, having been adopted in whole or part in the majority of states, it was also a lesson in civics. The MSEHPA, in an era of deep concern about terrorism and civil liberties, became a lightning rod for debates about public health preparedness and conformance with the rule of law.

Despite my background as a civil libertarian, in this book I question the primacy of individual freedom (and the associated concepts of autonomy, privacy, and liberty) as the prevailing social norm. Freedom is a powerful and important idea, but I think scholars have given insufficient attention to equally strong values that are captured by the notions of partnership, citizenship, and community. As members of a society in which we all share a common bond, our responsibility is not simply to defend our own right to be free from economic or personal restraint. We also have an obligation to protect and defend the community as a whole against threats to health, safety, and security. Each member of society owes a duty—one to another—to promote the common good. And each member benefits from participating in a well-regulated society that reduces risks that are common to all.

In summary, this book offers a theory and definition of public health law, an examination of its principal analytical methods, and an exploration of its dominant themes, such as the trade-offs between individual rights and public benefits and between voluntary and coercive public health approaches. In this book, I aspire to create a record of the field of public health law at the turn of the millennium. The transition from the nineteenth to the twentieth century marked, perhaps, the golden age of public health, and several influential treatises were written on public health law. I learned a great deal from these works, and I hope that scholars in future generations may benefit from observing the field of public health law through the lens of this book. Although, to be sure, it falls far short of the task required to resolve the profoundly complicated problems that have long perplexed scholars of public health law, the book at least tries to provide an honest account of the doctrine and the controversies facing the field at this time in history. And the modern age is a profoundly important time for the field, as it struggles with major health threats ranging from emerging infectious diseases (e.g., SARS and pandemic influenza) and bioterrorism (e.g., anthrax and smallpox) to natural disasters (e.g., the Gulf Coast hurricanes and the Asian tsunamis) and chronic diseases caused by overweight and obesity.

I have in mind diverse audiences for this book. Most important, it is designed for scholars and practitioners in public health generally and public health law particularly. It is intended to be useful for legislators as well as officials in the executive and judicial branches at the federal, state, and local levels. I have also designed this book for teachers and students of public health law and hope that it provides a useful and systematic method of instruction for courses in schools of law, public health, medicine, health administration, and other fields. I am gratified that the first edition of this book found its way into courses in major universities in the United States and abroad. For pedagogic purposes, *Public Health Law and Ethics: A Reader,* comprising the major scholarly articles and judicial cases in the field, accompanies this book. This reader will be updated on the Internet periodically to ensure its timeliness: www.oneillinstitute.org/reader. I welcome the guidance of my colleagues in making the book and supplemental readings clearer and more informative.

I hope that the informed lay public will also read this book. Public health law fundamentally concerns the relationships among political representatives and their constituents. As such, the field is one that every informed citizen should study and understand. The subject is fascinating and nuanced, taking the reader into constitutional history and design, theories of democracy and political participation, and the rights and obligations of individuals and businesses.

ORGANIZATION OF THE BOOK

The book is organized into four major parts:

- Conceptual Foundations of Public Health Law
- Law and the Public's Health
- Public Health and Civil Liberties in Conflict
- The Future of the Public's Health

This expanded second edition contains a great deal of new material, including chapters on administrative law and regulation, global health law, and obesity. The second edition also contains new boxed text, which focuses on major contemporary problems, such as biosecurity, emerging infectious diseases, and diabetes.

Part 1 covers the conceptual foundations of public health law in two chapters—one developing a theory and definition of the field and the other offering a systematic evaluation of public health regulation. The first chapter characterizes the field, while the second carefully examines the critical idea of risk regulation.

Part 2 comprises five chapters that cover the major legal disciplines relevant to public health: constitutional law, administrative law, tort law, and global health law. These chapters contain considerable discussion of legal doctrine that may be at once insufficiently detailed for legal scholars and overly pedantic for students of public health. Despite the unavoidable difficulties of addressing multiple audiences, I felt it important to develop a common understanding of the constitutional basis for the exercise of public health powers and the limits on those powers. I also felt it was important to explain how public health agency law, tort law, and international law powerfully influence public and private activities that affect, for good or bad, the public's health and safety.

Part 3, consisting of five chapters, explores the major substantive areas of public health practice as well as conflicts with individual rights and interests—both personal and economic. By constructing the chapters in this way, I was able both to explain doctrinal areas in public health law and to show their effects on individuals and businesses. This method of development also allowed me to investigate the paradoxes of public health law (e.g., the fact that regulation has a beneficial effect on the population's health but often an adverse effect on personal and economic interests). I do not cover the full range of public health practice, but I do attempt to provide a representative survey: surveillance and public health research, health communication and behavior, medical countermeasures, public health strategies, and commercial regulation.

Part 4, consisting of only one chapter, envisions the future of the public's health. In this chapter, I return to some of the important themes presented in this book and demonstrate the strong connections between politics and public health. The book concludes with a case study on one of the most fascinating contemporary problems at the interface of law and the public's health: chronic diseases caused by overweight and obesity. Through this case study, I demonstrate how law can be used as a tool to improve the public's health, but in a way that goes to the heart of the field's political credibility and legitimacy.

CONVENTIONS

This book was written for scholars and practitioners in both law and public health. In an attempt to make this material as widely accessible as possible, a modified version of *The Chicago Manual of Style* (15th edition rev.) was used for the bibliography and endnotes. *The Bluebook: A Uniform System of Citation* (18th edition) was used for judicial cases as well as statutes and regulations.

Acknowledgments

I am indebted to many people for their vital contributions to this book. First, I would like to thank Daniel M. Fox, president of the Milbank Memorial Fund, and Lynne Withey, director of the University of California Press, who supported, organized, and persistently encouraged this enterprise from its very beginnings.

My academic institutions, Georgetown University Law Center and the Johns Hopkins Bloomberg School of Public Health, and the Center for Law and the Public's Health, have been intellectual homes for this project, and many other related projects, on public health law. My valued colleagues within the Center have been close collaborators with me in exploring the field of public health law and ethics for many years, including Scott Burris, David Fidler, Lance Gable, Kristine Gebbie, James Hodge, Peter Jacobson, Lesley Stone, Stephen Teret, and Jon Vernick.

The field of health law has blossomed since the first edition of this book, culminating in a generous gift given to Georgetown University in 2006 to establish the Linda D. and Timothy J. O'Neill Institute for National and Global Health Law. I am deeply grateful to Tim and Linda O'Neill for having the confidence in Georgetown to establish the Institute, and to Dean T. Alexander Aleinikoff, Kevin Conry, Dean Bette Keltner, and the faculty and staff at Georgetown University Law Center for their enthusiasm for this project.

I had exceptional editorial and research assistance at Georgetown. Zinta Saulkalns and Simona Martinez-McConnell spent endless hours reading and editing the manuscript and graphics in this book. My research team at Georgetown Law Center was equally important. Among the students participating in the research team over several years were Shira Epstein, Anna Dolinsky, Alice Brown, Mikhel Schecter, Lauren Dunning, Auburn Daily, Joanne Chan, Katie Fink, John McArter, Lizzy Pike, Courtney Roberts, Samantha Stokes, Melissa Ann Higdon, Kimberley Bassett, and Kate Cherry. I want to especially thank a few students and fellows: Deborah Rubbens, Peter Currie, John Kraemer, Emily Hughes, Katrina Pagonis, Karen Sokol, Oscar Cabrera, and Michael Gottlieb, for exceptional scholarly work. I also want to thank Stephen Barbour and Micah Thorner, whose organizational skills and dedication were invaluable resources.

Beyond all, I can never repay the debt that I owe to Benjamin Berkman, Sloan Fellow at Georgetown University Law Center. Ben was a constant guide and partner in this manuscript. He worked with me with great skill, dedication, and selflessness on every aspect of this scholarly project.

Outside my own academic institutions I have found close colleagues and friends with whom to share enduring interests in public health law and ethics. Among my closest colleagues, whose work always inspires me, are Ronald Bayer (Columbia), Richard J. Bonnie (Virginia), Allan M. Brandt (Harvard), James Curran (Emory), the late William Curran (Harvard), Nancy Neveloff Dubler (Albert Einstein), Frank Grad (Columbia), the Hon. Justice Michael Kirby (High Court of Australia), Howard Markel (Michigan), Michelle Mello (Harvard), Wendy Parmet (Northeastern), Sara Rosenbaum (George Washington), and Mark Rothstein (Louisville). Peter Jacobson (Michigan) and Daniel Strouse (Arizona State) test-piloted the first edition of this book with their students and have given me useful feedback over the past five years. Several close colleagues reviewed the current edition: David Fidler, Dan Fox, Peter Jacobson, Gene Matthews, Wendy Parmet, and Mark Rothstein. I have learned a great deal from all these colleagues and many more too numerous to mention.

I have been fortunate to work with many of the major public health organizations in the United States and globally. These organizations, and the people with whom I have worked, have contributed a great deal to my development as a public health law scholar. In the United States, I have been associated with the following agencies, boards, and committees: CDC's Public Health Law Program (Richard Goodman and Anthony Moulton) and Office of the General Counsel (Paula Cocher, Gene W. Matthews, and Verla S. Neslund); Institute of Medicine (Harvey Fineberg,

Rose Martinez, Andrew Pope, Hugh Tilson, Kathleen Stratton, and Ken Warner); the Council of State and Territorial Epidemiologists (Guthrie Birkhead, John Middaugh, and Michael Osterholm); and the Turning Point Project, Robert Wood Johnson Foundation (including Bobbie Berkowitz, Deborah Erickson, and Jack Thompson).

Internationally, I have had the opportunity to collaborate with the following organizations: the Joint United Nations Programme on AIDS (previously WHO's Global Programme on AIDS) (the late Jonathan Mann, Daniel Tarantola, Peter Piot, Susan Timberlake, and Helen Wachirs); and the World Health Organization (including Sev Fluss, Alexander Capron, and Genevieve Pinet).

I thank, most of all, the people who mean the most to me and to whom this book is dedicated: my family, Jean, Bryn, and Kieran. In addition to providing the kind of support that only a lifetime of love can assure, my wife Jean worked on the graphics, which are so helpful in clarifying and visualizing the intellectual ideas presented in this book.

Lawrence O. Gostin
Associate Dean
Linda and Timothy O'Neill Professor of Global Health Law
Faculty Director, O'Neill Institute for National and Global Health Law
Georgetown University Law Center
Washington, D.C.
March 2008

PART ONE

Conceptual Foundations of Public Health Law

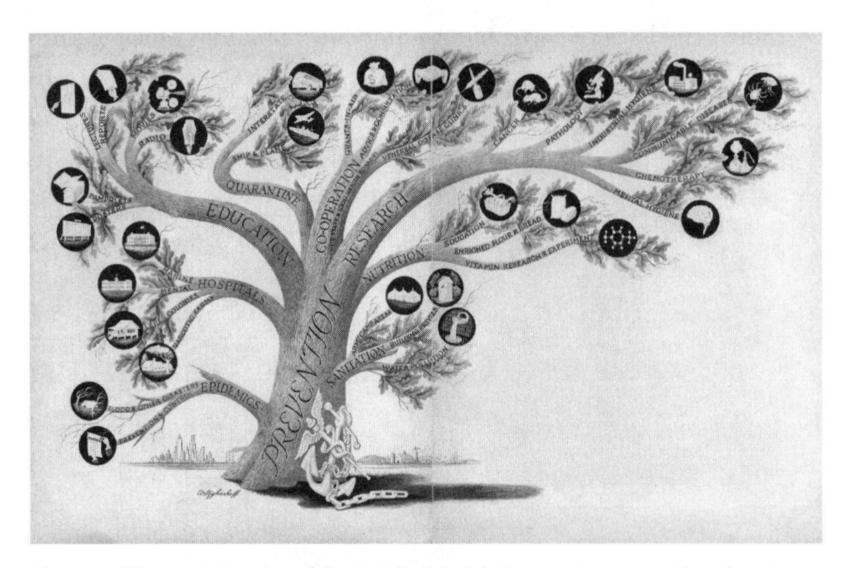

Photo 1. The varied tasks of the Public Health Service in 1941. This drawing of a public health tree depicting the varied tasks of the Public Health Service appeared in *Fortune* magazine in 1941. A 1798 law for the care of sick and disabled seamen created the Marine Hospital Service, the forerunner of the Public Health Service, and provided the federal government with a major role in the public's health.

CHAPTER 1

A Theory and Definition of Public Health Law

> [Public health law] should not be confused with medical jurisprudence, which is concerned only in the legal aspects of the application of medical and surgical knowledge to individuals. . . . [P]ublic health is not a branch of medicine, but a science in itself, to which, however, preventive medicine is an important contributor. Public health law is that branch of jurisprudence which treats of the application of common and statutory law to the principles of hygiene and sanitary science.
>
> James A. Tobey (1926)

The literature, both academic and judicial, on the intersection of law and health is pervasive. The subject of law and health is widely taught (in schools of law, medicine, public health, and health administration), practiced (by "health lawyers"), and analyzed (by scholars in the related fields of health law, bioethics, and health policy).[1] The fields that characterize these branches of study are called health law, health care law, law and medicine, forensic medicine, and public health law. Do these names imply different disciplines, each with a coherent theory, structure, and method that sets it apart? Notably absent from the extant literature is a theory of the discipline of public health law, an exploration of its doctrinal boundaries, and an assessment of its analytical methodology.[2]

Public health law shares conceptual terrain with the field of law and medicine, or health care law, but remains a distinct discipline. My claim is not that public health law is contained within a tidy doctrinal package; its boundaries are blurred and overlap other paths of study within law and health. Nor is public health law easy to define and characterize; the field is as complex and confused as public health itself. Rather, I posit, public health law is susceptible to theoretical and practical differentiation from other disciplines at the nexus of law and health.

Public health law can be defined, its boundaries circumscribed, and its analytical methods detailed in ways that distinguish it as a discrete discipline—just as the disciplines of medicine and public health can be demarcated.[3] With this book I hope to provide a fuller understanding of the varied roles of law in advancing the public's health. The core idea I propose is that law can be an essential tool for creating conditions to enable people to lead healthier and safer lives.

In this opening chapter, I offer a theory and definition of public health law, an examination of its core values, an assessment of state statutes in establishing the legal foundations of public health agencies, a categorization of the various models through which law acts as a tool to advance the public's health, and, finally, a description of the current debate over the legitimate scope of public health. These are the questions I will pursue: What is public health law and what are its doctrinal boundaries? Why should population health be a salient public value? What are the legal foundations of governmental public health? How can law be effective in reducing illness and premature death? And what are the political conflicts faced by public health in the early twenty-first century?

PUBLIC HEALTH LAW: A DEFINITION AND CORE VALUES

My definition of public health law follows, and the remainder of this chapter offers a justification as well as an expansion of the ideas presented:

> Public health law is the study of the legal powers and duties of the state, in collaboration with its partners (e.g., health care, business, the community, the media, and academe), to ensure the conditions for people to be healthy (to identify, prevent, and ameliorate risks to health in the population), and of the limitations on the power of the state to constrain for the common good the autonomy, privacy, liberty, proprietary, and other legally protected interests of individuals. The prime objective of public health law is to pursue the highest possible level of physical and mental health in the population, consistent with the values of social justice.

Several themes emerge from this definition: (1) government power and duty, (2) coercion and limits on state power, (3) government's partners

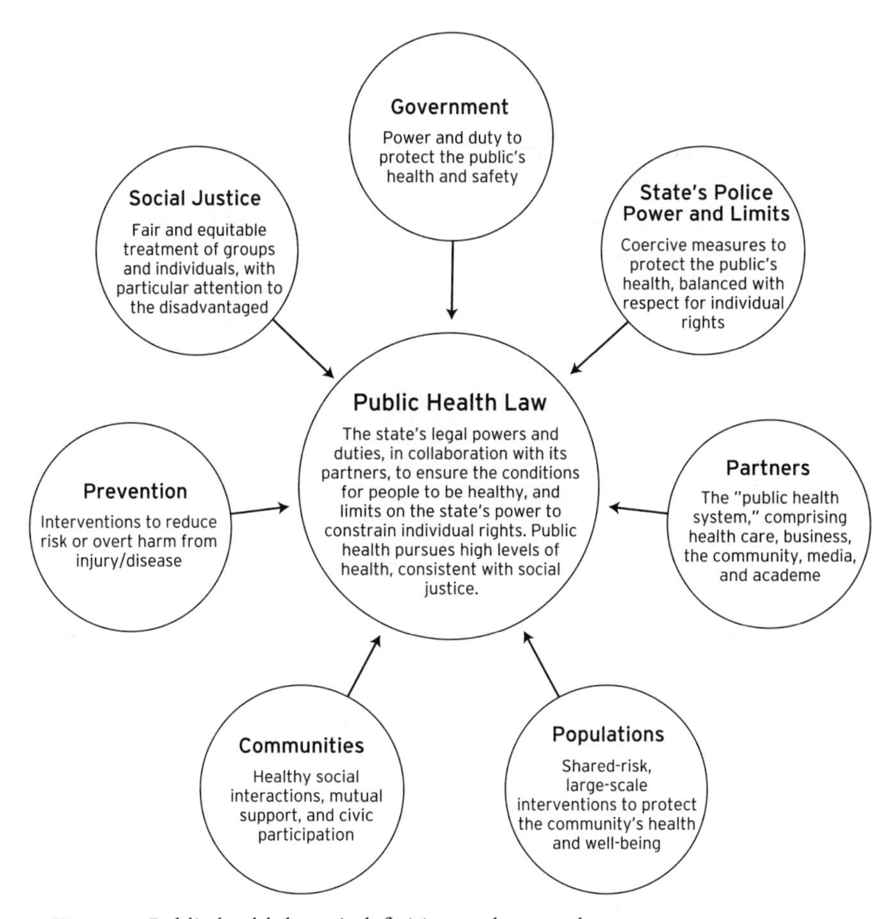

Figure 2. Public health law: A definition and core values.

in the "public health system," (4) the population focus, (5) communities and civic participation, (6) the prevention orientation, and (7) social justice (see figure 2).

Government Power and Duty: Health as a Salient Value

Why does government have the power and duty to safeguard the public's health? To understand the state's obligations, it will be helpful first to explore the meaning of the concepts of "public health" and the "common good." I will then offer a theory as to why health should be a salient value of government.

THE "PUBLIC'S" HEALTH

The word *public* in public health has two overlapping meanings—one that refers to the entity that takes primary responsibility for the public's health, and another that indicates who has a legitimate expectation of receiving the benefits.

The government has primary responsibility for the public's health. The government is the public entity that acts on behalf of the people and gains its legitimacy through a political process. A characteristic form of "public" or state action occurs when a democratically elected government exercises powers or duties to protect or promote the population's health.

The population as a whole has a legitimate expectation of benefiting from public health services. The population elects the government and holds the state accountable for a meaningful level of health protection. Public health should possess broad appeal to the electorate because it is a universal aspiration. What best serves the population, of course, may not always be in the interests of all its members, making public health highly political. What constitutes "enough" health? What kinds of services are necessary? How will services be paid for and distributed? These remain political questions. Democratic governments will never devote unlimited resources to public health. Core public health functions compete for scarce resources with other demands for services, and resources are allocated through a prescribed political process. In this sense, Dan Beauchamp is instructive in suggesting that a healthy republic is not achieved solely through a strong sense of communal welfare, but is also the result of a vigorous and expanded democratic discussion about the population's health.[4]

"THE COMMON" AND "THE GOOD"

If individual interests are to give way to communal interests in healthy populations, it is important to understand the value of "the common" and "the good." The field of public health would profit from a vibrant conception of "the common" that sees the public interest as more than the aggregation of individual interests. A nonaggregative understanding of public goods recognizes that everyone benefits from living in a society that regulates the risks shared by all.[5] Laws designed to promote the common good may sometimes constrain individual actions (smoking in public places, riding a motorcycle without a helmet, etc.). As members of society, we have common goals that go beyond our narrow interests. Individuals have a stake in healthy and secure communities where they can live in peace and well-being. An unhealthy or insecure community may produce harms common to all, such as increased crime and violence, impaired social relationships, and a less productive workforce. Consequently, people may have to forgo some self-interest in exchange for the protection and satisfaction gained from sustaining healthier and safer communities.

We also need to better understand the concept of "the good." In medicine, the meaning of "the good" is defined purely in terms of the individual's wants and needs. It is the patient, not the physician or family, who decides the appropriate course of action. In public health, the meaning of "the good" is far less clear. Who decides which value is more important—freedom or health? One strategy for public health decision making would be to allow people to decide for themselves, but this would thwart many public health initiatives. For example, if individuals could decide whether to acquiesce to a vaccination or permit reporting of personal information to the health department, it would result in a "tragedy of the commons."[6]

The public health community takes it as an act of faith that health must be society's overarching value. Yet politicians do not always see it that way, expressing preferences, say, for highways, energy, and the military. The lack of political commitment to population health can be seen in relatively low public health expenditures.[7] Public health professionals often distrust and shun politicians rather than engage them in dialogue about the importance of population health. What is needed is a clear vision of and rationale for healthy populations as a political priority.

Why should health, as opposed to other communal goods, be a salient value? Two interrelated theories support the role of health as a primary value: (1) *a theory of human functioning*—health is a foundation for personal well-being and the exercise of social and political rights; and (2) *a theory of democracy*—governments are formed primarily to achieve health, safety, and welfare for the population.

HEALTH IS FOUNDATIONAL: A THEORY OF HUMAN FUNCTIONING

Health is foundationally important because of its intrinsic value and singular contribution to human functioning. Health has a special meaning and importance to individuals and the community as a whole.[8] Every person understands, at least intuitively, why health is vital to well-being. Health is necessary for much of the joy, creativity, and productivity that a person derives from life. Individuals with physical and mental health recreate, socialize, work, and engage in family and social activities that bring meaning and happiness to their lives. Certainly, persons with ill health or disability can lead deeply fulfilling lives, but personal health does facilitate many of life's joys and accomplishments. Every person strives for the best physical and mental health achievable, even in the face of existing disease, injury, or disability. The public's health is so instinctively essential that human rights norms embrace health as a basic right.[9]

Perhaps it is not as obvious, however, that health is also essential for the functioning of populations. Without minimum levels of health, people cannot fully engage in social interactions, participate in the political process, exercise rights of citizenship, generate wealth, create art, and provide for the common security. A safe and healthy population builds strong roots for a country's governmental structures, social organizations, cultural endowment, economic prosperity, and national defense. Population health becomes a transcendent value because a certain level of human functioning is a prerequisite for activities that are critical to the public's welfare—social, political, and economic.

Health has an intrinsic and instrumental value for individuals, communities, and nations. People aspire to achieve health because of its importance to a satisfying life, communities promote the health of their neighbors for the mutual benefits of social interactions, and nations build health care and public health infrastructures to cultivate a decent and prosperous civilization.

GOVERNMENT'S OBLIGATION TO PROMOTE HEALTH: A THEORY OF DEMOCRACY

Why does government have an enduring obligation to protect and promote the public's health? Theories of democracy help to explain the government's role in matters of population health. People form governments for their common defense, security, and welfare—goods that can be achieved only through collective action. The first thing that public officials owe to their constituents is protection against natural and man-made hazards. Michael Walzer explains that public health is a classic case of a general communal provision because public funds are expended to benefit all or most of the population without any specific distribution to individuals.[10]

A political community stresses a shared bond among members; organized society safeguards the common goods of health, welfare, and security, while members subordinate themselves to the welfare of the community as a whole.[11] Public health can be achieved only through collective action, not through individual endeavors. Acting alone, individuals cannot ensure even minimum levels of health. Any person of means can procure many of the necessities of life—food, housing, clothing, and even medical care. Yet no single individual or group of individuals can ensure his or her health. Meaningful protection and assurance of the population's health require communal effort. The community as a whole has a stake in environmental protection, hygiene and sanitation, clean air and surface water, uncontaminated food and drinking water, safe roads and products, and control of infectious disease. These collective goods, and many more, are essential conditions for health. Yet these benefits can be secured only through organized action on behalf of the people.

The Power to Coerce and Limits on State Power

> [It is well to cite] the oft quoted aphorism of the Earl of Derby that "sanitary instruction is even more important than sanitary legislation." Sanitarians work toward the ideal that all people will in time know what healthful living is, and that they will in time reach that moral plane when they will practice what they know. While hopeful for the millennium we must work. Law is still necessary. People still incline to acts which are not for their neighbors' good. In our complicated civilization, many restrictions must be placed on individual conduct in order that we may live happily and healthfully one with another.
>
> Charles V. Chapin (1926)

I have suggested that public health law is concerned with governmental responsibilities to the community and the well-being of the population. These ideas encompass what can be regarded as "public" and what constitutes "health" within a political community. Although it may not be obvious, I also suggest that the use of coercion must be part of an informed understanding of public health law, and that state power also must be subject to limits.

Government can do many things to safeguard the public's health and safety that do not require the exercise of compulsory powers, and the state's first recourse should be voluntary measures. Yet government alone is authorized to require conformance with publicly established standards of conduct. Governments are formed not only to attend to the general needs of their constituents, but to insist, through force of law if necessary, that individuals and businesses act in ways that do not place others at unreasonable risk of harm. To defend the common welfare, governments assert their collective power to tax, inspect, regulate, and coerce. Of course, different ideas exist about what compulsory measures are necessary to safeguard the public's health. Reconciling divergent opinions about the desirability of coercion in a given situation (should government resort to force, what kind, and under what circumstances?) is an issue for political resolution. In the next chapter, I propose standards for evaluating public health regulation to help guide policymakers.

THE POWER TO COMPEL INDIVIDUALS AND BUSINESSES FOR THE COMMON GOOD

Protecting and preserving community health is not possible without constraining a wide range of private activities that pose unacceptable risks. Private actors can profit by engaging in practices that damage the rest of society:[12] Individuals derive satisfaction from intimate relationships despite the risks of sexually transmitted infections, industry has incentives to produce goods without consideration of workers' safety or pollution of surrounding areas, and manufacturers find it economical to offer products without regard to high standards of hygiene and safety. In each instance, individuals or organizations act rationally for their own interests, but their actions may adversely affect communal health and safety. Absent governmental authority and willingness to coerce, such threats to the public's health and safety could not easily be reduced.

Although regulation in the name of public health is theoretically intended to safeguard the health and safety of whole populations, it often benefits those most at risk of injury and disease. Everyone gains value from public health regulations, such as food and water standards, but some regulations protect the most vulnerable. For instance, eliminating a toxic waste site, enforcing a building code in a crowded tenement, or closing an unhygienic restaurant holds particular significance for those at immediate risk. Frequently, those at increased risk are particularly vulnerable due to their race, gender, or socioeconomic status.[13]

Perhaps because engaging in risk behavior may promote personal or economic interests, individuals and businesses frequently oppose government regulation. Resistance is sometimes based on philosophical grounds of autonomy, choice, or freedom from government interference. Citizens, and the groups that represent them, claim that regulating self-regarding behaviors, such as the use of seat belts or motorcycle helmets, is not the business of government. Sometimes these arguments extend to activities that harm others, such as unsafe workplace conditions, fuel-inefficient vehicles, or unhygienic restaurants.

Industry often asserts that economic principles militate against state interference. Entrepreneurs tend to accept as a matter of faith that governmental health and safety standards retard economic development and should be avoided. In political arenas, they contest these standards in the name of economic liberty, holding out government taxation and regulation as burdensome and inefficient.

Public health has historically constrained the rights of individuals and businesses so as to protect community interests in health.[14] Whether through the use of reporting requirements affecting privacy, mandatory testing or screening affecting autonomy, environmental standards affecting property, industrial regulation affecting economic freedom, or isolation and quarantine affecting liberty, public health has not shied from controlling individuals and businesses for the aggregate good.

LIMITATIONS ON STATE POWER

Public health powers can legitimately be used to restrict human freedoms and rights to achieve a collective good, but they must be exercised consistently with constitutional and statutory constraints on state action. The inherent prerogative of the state to protect the public's health, safety, and welfare (known as the police powers) is limited by individual rights to autonomy, privacy, liberty, property, and other legally protected interests (see chapter 4). Achieving a just balance between constitutionally protected rights and the powers and duties of the state to defend and advance the public's health poses an enduring problem for public health law.

Any theory of public health law presents a paradox. Government, on the one hand, is compelled by its role as the elected representative of the community to act affirmatively to promote the health of the people. To many, this role requires vigorous measures to control obvious health risks. On the other hand, government cannot unduly assault individuals' rights in the name of the communal good. Health regulation that overreaches, in that it achieves a minimal health benefit with disproportionate human burdens, conflicts with ethical considerations and is not tolerated in a society based on the rule of law. Consequently, scholars and practitioners often perceive a tension between the community's claim to reduce obvious health risks and individuals' claim to be free from government interference. This perceived conflict might be agonizing in some cases and absent in others. Thus, public health law must always pose the questions: Does a coercive intervention truly reduce aggregate health risks, and what, if any, less intrusive interventions might reduce those risks as well or better? Respect for the rights of individuals and fairness toward groups of all races, religions, and cultures remain at the heart of public health law.

It has become fashionable to claim that no real conflict exists between the protection of individual rights and the promotion of population health.[15] According to this view, safeguarding rights is always (or virtually always) consistent with preserving communal health. Indeed, according to this perspective, individual rights and public health are synergistic—the defense of one enhances the value of the other. This rhetorical position serves a purpose but is simplistic. It suggests that a decision to avert a discrete health risk through coercion actually may result in an aggregate increase in injury or disease in the population. The exercise of compulsory powers of isolation or quarantine, for example, may prevent individuals from transmitting a communicable infection, but the social decision to coerce affects group behavior and, ultimately, the population's health. By provoking distrust of or alienation from medical and public health authorities, coercion may shift behaviors to avoidance of testing, counseling, or treatment.

Public health decision making involves complex trade-offs. Will coercive measures to avert a known individual risk be the correct course of action (e.g., isolating a person with tuberculosis who refuses to take the full course of medication), even if doing so may produce a greater aggregate risk? The social calculus is hardly scientific or precise regarding whether compulsion will alter behavior and, if so, in what direction.

Distinct tensions exist in public health law between voluntarism and coercion, civil liberties and public health, and discrete (or individual) health threats and aggregate health outcomes. These competing interests, and the substantive standards and procedural safeguards that circumscribe the lawful exercise of state powers, form the corpus of public health law.

The Public Health System: Partners for Population Health

Although the power and duty to safeguard the public's health historically has been assigned to government through the work of national, state, tribal, and local health agencies, no single agency can ensure the conditions for the public's health. The Institute of Medicine (IOM) views public health agencies as focal institutions at the center of a multisectoral "public health system."[16] Public health agencies can act as a catalyst for action by other government departments (e.g., housing, labor, transportation, and environment). Public health agencies also stimulate, coordinate, and often regulate nongovernmental actors. At the same time, these actors may co-opt agency officials into advocating for their private interests—an idea referred to in the literature as "regulatory capture."[17] The public health system includes many nongovernmental actors, but the IOM focuses on five: health care institutions, the community, businesses, the media, and academe (see figure 3). Although not discussed by the IOM, philanthropic organizations (e.g., Gates Foundation, Rockefeller Foundation, and Kaiser Family Foundation) have far-reaching effects on health policy, service delivery, and research.

Health Care Institutions. Health care is important because personal health is a value in itself and one of the conditions necessary for individual and population health. Public health and health care interact in multiple important ways.[18] Health care institutions collect information and report it to public health agencies, vaccinate populations, diagnose and treat patients with infectious diseases that endanger the public, and provide a range of services to improve community health (e.g., child and maternal health, family planning, and emergency services). However, health care is not fully available to many people. About 15.3 percent of the U.S. population (nearly 45 million people) lacks health insurance, with minorities and the poor disproportionately burdened.[19] Also, health plans do not cover many services for prevention, mental health, substance abuse, and dental health. Health care providers can play an important role in improving health through patient care and investment in promoting the health of the communities they serve.[20]

Community. The term *community* is often imprecise, but includes local entities such as churches, civic organizations, and health advocacy groups, which can contribute to their neighbors' health. Community involvement can effectively promote healthy activities.[21] Community organizations are well positioned to assess needs and inventory resources, formulate collaborative responses, and evaluate outcomes for community health improvements. They can promote healthy lifestyles and facilitate social networks. Communities can also advocate for more government services and help to care for their own members (family, friends, and neighbors).

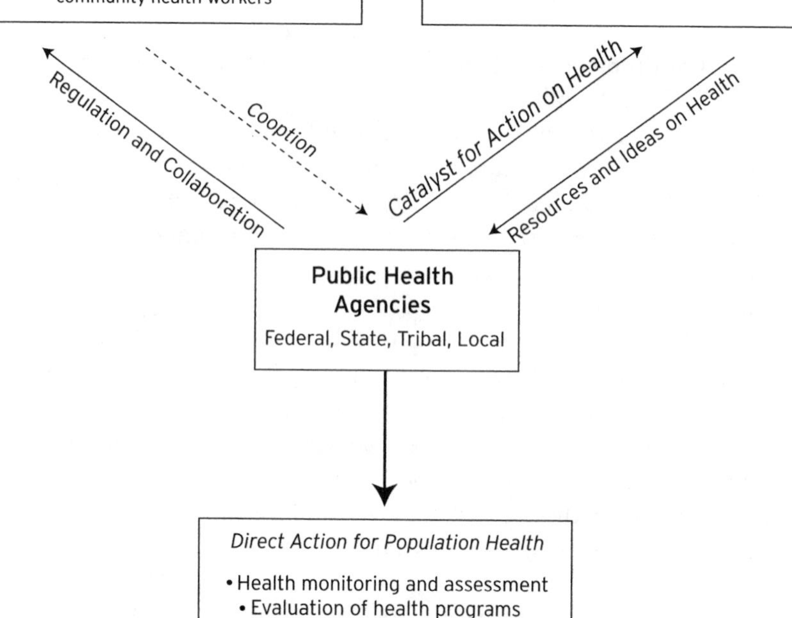

Note: This figure represents the "public health system," consisting of public health agencies and their governmental and nongovernmental partners. Public health agencies take primary responsibility for ensuring the conditions for the public's health. They regulate or collaborate with health care, business, the media, and academe. Sometimes the private sector "co-opts" governmental agencies to act in the interests of private actors. Public health agencies provide a catalyst for other government departments to act on population health. These departments in turn provide resources and ideas to further population health.

Figure 3. The public health system.

Businesses. Businesses play a major role in the health of their employees and the local population through their impact on natural and built environments, workplace conditions, and relationships with communities. They affect worker health (e.g., workplace safety and exposures), economic conditions (e.g., income and quality of life), the natural environment (e.g., emission of toxins or pollutants), and the physical environment (e.g., green spaces). Many businesses also offer health insurance for their workers, demonstrating the close ties between public health, health care, and the private sector.[22] Research demonstrates the cost-effectiveness of prevention and health promotion efforts for an employer's workforce and the value of corporate action in promoting broader community health.[23]

The Media. The news and entertainment media shape public opinion and influence decision making, with potentially critical effects on population health. The media (including television, cinema, and newspapers) help shape popular culture relating to tobacco, food, alcoholic beverages, sex, and illicit drugs. They disseminate information about healthy behaviors and play a particularly crucial role in times of public health emergency. Yet public health activities often attract little media coverage, perhaps because journalists and public health officials do not understand each other's perspectives and methods. Furthermore, the print and broadcast media tend to be much less attentive to diseases that disproportionately burden Blacks relative to Whites.[24] Ongoing dialogue and educational opportunities could improve media coverage of public health and increase airtime for public health messages.

Academe. Academe provides degrees and continuing education to the public health workforce. Academic institutions also foster research into many of the most pressing public health problems, such as obesity, smoking, and HIV/AIDS. However, modifications are needed in curricular and financial incentives to link curricular content and teaching methods more closely to the practice needs of the public health workforce. New investments and academic reorganization can promote community-based prevention research that evaluates the effects of interventions on population health.[25]

Government agencies, therefore, are not only charged with the task of direct action to safeguard the population's health; they also engage with the public and private sectors in partnerships for health. The relationships between public health agencies and their partners are complex, involving a dynamic that ranges from regulation to volunteerism, and from cooperation to cooption. Still, a multisectoral public health system is necessary to ensure favorable conditions for the population's health.

The Population Focus

> Measures to improve public health, relating as they do to such obvious and mundane matters as housing, smoking, and food, may lack the glamour of high-technology medicine, but what they lack in excitement they gain in their potential impact on health, precisely because they deal with the major causes of common disease and disabilities.
>
> Geoffrey Rose (1992)

The crux of public health, as I have sought to demonstrate, is a public or governmental entity that harbors the power and responsibility to assure community well-being. Public health is organized to provide an aggregate benefit to the mental and physical health of all the people in a given community. Classic definitions of public health emphasize this population-based perspective: "'Public health' means the prevailingly healthful or sanitary condition of the general body of people or the community in mass, and the absence of any general or widespread disease or cause of mortality. It is the wholesome sanitary condition of the community at large."[26]

Perhaps the single most important feature of public health is that it strives to improve the functioning and longevity of populations. The field's purpose is to monitor and evaluate health status, as well as to devise strategies and interventions designed to ease the burden of injury, disease, and disability and, more generally, to promote the public's health and safety. Public health interventions reduce mortality and morbidity, thus saving lives and preventing disease on a population level.

Public health differs from medicine, which has the individual patient as its primary focus. The physician diagnoses disease and offers medical treatment to ease symptoms and, where possible, to cure disease. The British epidemiologist Geoffrey Rose compares the scientific methods and objectives of medicine with those of public health. "Why did this patient get this disease at this time?" is a prevailing question in medicine, and it underscores a physician's central concern for sick individuals.[27] Public health, on the other hand, seeks to understand the conditions and causes of ill health (and good health) in the populace as a whole. It seeks to assure a favorable environment in which people can maintain their health. Public health cares about individuals, of course, because of their inherent worth and because a population is healthy only if its constituents (individuals) are relatively free from injury and disease. Indeed, many public health agencies offer medical care for the poor, particularly for conditions that have "spillover" effects for the wider community, such as treatment for sexually transmitted infections (STIs), tuberculosis (TB), and HIV/AIDS. Still, public health's abiding interest is in the well-being and security of populations, not individual patients.

The focus on populations rather than individual patients is grounded not only in theory but in the methods of scientific inquiry and the services offered by public health. The analytical methods and objectives of the primary sciences of public health—epidemiology and biostatistics—are directed toward understanding risk, injury, and disease within populations. Epidemiology, literally translated from Greek, is "the study *(logos)* of what is among *(epi)* the people *(demos)*."[28] Roger Detels notes that "all epidemiologists will agree that epidemiology concerns itself with populations rather than individuals, thereby separating itself from the rest of medicine and constituting the basic science of public health."[29] Epidemiology examines the frequency and distribution of diseases in the population.[30] The population strategy "is the attempt to control the determinants of incidents, to lower the mean level of risk factors, [and] to shift the whole distribution of exposure in a favourable direction."[31] The advantage of a population strategy is that it seeks to reduce underlying causes that make diseases common in populations, creating the potential for reduction in morbidity and premature mortality at the broadest population level.

Communities and Civic Participation

Public health is interested in communities and how they function to protect and promote (or, as is too often the case, endanger) the health of their members. A community has a life in common that stems from such things as a shared history, language, and values. The term *community* can apply to small groups, such as self-help groups, which share a common goal, or to very large groups that, despite the diversity of their members, have common political institutions, symbols, and memories.[32]

Public health officials want to understand what health risks exist among varying populations and, of equal importance, why differences in health risks exist, who engages in risk behavior (e.g., smoking, a high-fat diet, or unsafe sex), and who suffers from high rates of disease (e.g., cancer, heart disease, or diabetes). Public health professionals often observe differences in risk behavior and disease based on race, sex, or socioeconomic status.[33] Understanding the mechanisms and pathways of risk is vital to developing efficacious interventions to improve health within communities.

Beyond understanding the variance of risk within groups, public health encourages individual connectedness to the community. Individuals who feel they belong to a community are more likely to strive for health and security for all members. Viewing health risks as common to the group, rather than specific to individuals, helps foster a sense of collective responsibility for the mutual well-being of *all* individuals. Finding solutions to common problems can forge more cohesive and meaningful community associations.

Finally, many forward thinkers urge greater community involvement in public health decision making so that policy formation becomes a genuinely civic endeavor. Under this view, citizens strive to safeguard their communities through civic participation, open forums, and capacity-building to solve local problems. Public involvement should result in stronger support for health policies and encourage citizens to take a more active role in protecting themselves and the health of their neighbors.[34] Public health authorities, for example, might practice more deliberative forms of democracy, involving closer consultation with consumers and the voluntary organizations that represent them (e.g., town meetings and consumer membership on government advisory committees). This kind of deliberative democracy in public health is increasingly evident in government-community partnerships at the federal, state, and local levels (e.g., AIDS action and breast cancer awareness).

The Prevention Orientation

> It has been shown that external agents have as great an influence on the frequency of sickness as on its fatality; the obvious corollary is that man has as much power to prevent as to cure disease. . . . Yet, medical men, the guardians of public health, never have their attention called to the prevention of sickness; it forms no part of their education. . . . The public do not seek the shield of medical art . . . till the arrows of death already rankle

> in the veins. . . . Public health may be promoted by placing the medical institutions of the country on a liberal scientific basis; by medical societies co-operating to collect statistical observations; and by medical writers renouncing the notion that a science can be founded upon the limited experience of an individual.
>
> William Farr (1837)

> We are moved by sensational images of heroes who leap into action as calamity unfolds before them. But the long, pedestrian slog of prevention is thankless. That is because prevention is nameless and abstract, while a hero's actions are grounded in an easy-to-understand narrative.
>
> Nassim Nicholas Taleb (2005)

The field of public health is often understood to emphasize prevention of injury and disease as opposed to their amelioration or cure. Public health historians tell a classic story of the power of prevention. In September 1854, John Snow wrote, "The most terrible outbreak of cholera which ever occurred in this Kingdom, is probably that which took place in Broad Street, Golden Square [Soho, London], and the adjoining streets, a few weeks ago." Snow, a celebrated epidemiologist, linked the cholera outbreak to a single source of polluted water—the Broad Street pump. He convinced the Board of Guardians of St. James Parish, in whose parish the pump fell, to remove the pump handle as an experiment. Within a week, the outbreak was all but over, with the death toll standing at 616 Sohoites.[35]

Public health prevention may be defined as interventions designed to avert the occurrence of injury or disease. Many of public health's most potent activities are oriented toward prevention: vaccination against infectious diseases, health education to reduce risk behavior, fluoridation to avert dental caries, and seat belts or motorcycle helmets to avoid injuries. Medicine, by contrast, is often focused on the amelioration or cure of injuries or diseases after they have occurred. Physicians usually see patients following an adverse health event, and they target their interventions to reducing the health impact.

Prevention and amelioration, of course, are not mutually exclusive. Medicine is also concerned with prevention, as physicians often counsel patients to avoid risk behaviors such as smoking, consuming high-fat

MISTAKING CAUSE FOR EFFECT.
Boy. "I say, Tommy, I'm blow'd if there isn't a Man a turning on the Cholera."

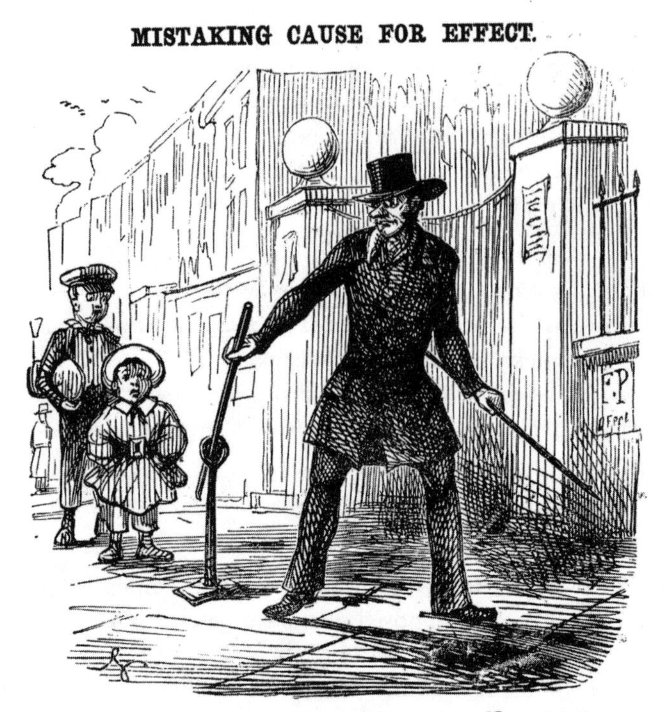

Photo 2. Cholera: The Broad Street pump. In this cartoon, a boy thinks the Water Board man is turning on cholera. In response to the mid-nineteenth-century outbreaks of cholera in Soho, London, John Snow engaged in shoe-leather epidemiology to find the source of the outbreak. He traced the epidemic to a single water pump on Broad Street. Courtesy of The Image Works.

foods, engaging in unprotected sex, or drinking alcoholic beverages to excess. Similarly, public health is concerned with amelioration, as health departments frequently offer health care for the poor. The goals of medicine and public health are especially intertwined in the field of infectious diseases, where medical treatment can reduce contagiousness. The individual benefits from treatment, and society benefits from overall reduced exposure to disease.

A foundational article by Michael McGinnis and William Foege examines the leading causes of death in the United States, revealing different types of thinking in medicine and public health.[36] Medical explanations of death point to discrete pathophysiological conditions, such as cancer, heart disease, cerebrovascular disease, and pulmonary disease.[37] Public health explanations, by contrast, examine the root causes of disease. From this perspective, the leading causes of death are environmental, social, and behavioral factors, such as smoking, alcohol and drug use, diet and activity patterns, sexual behavior, toxic agents, firearms, and motor vehicles. McGinnis and Foege observe that the vast preponderance of government expenditures are devoted to medical treatment of diseases ultimately recorded on death certificates as the nation's leading killers. Only a small fraction of funding is directed to control the root determinants of death and disability. The central message, of course, is that prevention is often more cost-effective than amelioration, and that much of the burden of disease, disability, and premature death can be reduced through prevention.

Social Justice

> The challenge to public health . . . is to overcome inequitable allocation of benefits, the tragedy that would befall us if we made the promise of [science] only for those who could afford it and not for all society. Social evolution . . . will be what we want it to be, and now is the time to make our case. . . . [Public health sciences] offer unbelievable opportunities and unbelievable inequities.
>
> William Foege (2005)

Social justice is viewed as so central to the mission of public health that it has been described as the field's core value: "The historic dream of public health . . . is a dream of social justice."[38] Among the most basic and commonly understood meanings of justice is fair, equitable, and appropriate treatment in light of what is due or owed to individuals and groups.[39]

Social justice captures the twin moral impulses that animate public health: to advance human well-being by improving health and to do so particularly by focusing on the needs of the most disadvantaged.[40] This account of justice has the aim of bringing about the human good of health for all members of the population. An integral part of that aim is the task of identifying and ameliorating patterns of systematic disadvantage that profoundly and pervasively undermine the prospects for well-being of oppressed and subordinated groups—people whose prospects for good health are so limited that their life choices are not even remotely like those of others.[41] These two aspects of justice—health improvement for the population and fair treatment of the disadvantaged—create a richer understanding of public health. Seen through the lens of social justice, the central mission of the public health system is to engage in systematic action to ensure the conditions for improved health for all members of the population, and to redress persistent patterns of systematic disadvantage.

A core insight of social justice is that there are multiple causal pathways to numerous dimensions of disadvantage. The causal pathways to disadvantage include poverty, substandard housing, poor education, unhygienic and polluted environments, and social disintegration. These, and many other causal agents, lead to systematic disadvantage not only in health but also in nearly every aspect of social, economic, and political life. Inequalities of one kind beget other inequalities, and existing inequalities compound, sustain, and reproduce a multitude of deprivations in well-being. Taken in their totality, multiple disadvantages add up to markedly unequal life prospects.

This account of social justice focuses on the totality of social institutions, practices, and policies that both independently and in combination deeply and persistently affect human well-being. It is interventionist, not passive or market-driven, vigorously addressing the determinants of health throughout the lifespan. It recognizes that there are multiple causes of ill and good health, that policies and practices affecting health also affect other valued dimensions of life, and that health is intimately connected to many of the important goods in life. The critical questions at the intersection of public health and justice are what people in society are most vulnerable and at greatest risk, how best to reduce the risk or ameliorate the harm, and how to fairly allocate services and benefits.

Social justice stresses the fair disbursement of common advantages and the sharing of common burdens. Known as distributive justice, this form of justice requires that government act to limit the extent to which the burden of disease falls unfairly upon the least advantaged and to ensure that the burden of the interventions themselves is distributed equitably. Distributive justice also requires fair allocation of public health benefits. This principle might apply, for example, to the fair distribution of vaccines or antiviral medications during a public health emergency, such as a pandemic influenza epidemic.[42]

Social justice demands more than fair distribution of resources. Health hazards threaten the entire population, but the poor and disabled are at heightened risk. For example, during the Gulf Coast hurricanes in 2005, state and federal agencies failed to act expeditiously and with equal concern for all citizens, including the poor and less powerful.[43] Neglecting the needs of the vulnerable predictably harms the whole community by eroding public trust and undermining social cohesion. It signals to those affected and to everyone else that the basic human needs of some matter less than those of others, and it thereby fails to show the respect due to all members of the community. Social justice thus not only encompasses a core commitment to fair distribution of resources, but also calls for policies of action that are consistent with the preservation of human dignity and showing of equal respect for the interests of all members of the community.

These are the quintessential values of public health law—government power and duty, coercion and limits on state power, government's partners in the "public health system," the population focus, communities and civic participation, the prevention orientation, and social justice. To achieve the goals of population health under the rule of law requires sound legal foundations. As the following discussion explains, state statutes establish the infrastructure for public health agencies, ranging from their mission, functions, and powers to their organization and funding.

PUBLIC HEALTH STATUTES: LEGAL FOUNDATIONS OF PUBLIC HEALTH AGENCIES

The field of public health is typically regarded as a positivistic pursuit, and undoubtedly our understanding of the etiology and response to disease is heavily influenced by scientific inquiry. Less well understood is the role of law in public health practice. Law defines the jurisdiction of public health officials and specifies the manner in which they may exercise their authority. State public health statutes create public health agencies, designate their mission and core functions, appropriate their funds, grant their power, and limit their actions to protect a sphere of freedom. They establish boards of health, authorize the collection of health information, and enable monitoring and regulation of dangerous activities. The most important social debates about public health take place in legal forums—legislatures, courts, and administrative agencies—and in the law's language of rights, duties, and justice. It is no exaggeration to say that "the field of public health . . . could not long exist in the manner in which we know it today except for its sound legal basis."[44]

In its influential report *The Future of Public Health,* the IOM agreed that law is essential to population health, but cast serious doubt on the soundness of public health's legal basis. Concluding generally that "this

BOX 1

THE NEED FOR PUBLIC HEALTH LAW REFORM

Scholars have identified deficiencies in many public health law statutes, justifying a political process of modernization.

Problem of Antiquity

The most striking characteristic of state public health law—and the one that underlies many of its defects—is its overall antiquity. Certainly, some statutes are relatively recent in origin. However, much of public health law was framed in the late nineteenth and early to mid-twentieth centuries and contains elements that are forty to one hundred years old. Old public health statutes are often outmoded in ways that directly reduce their effectiveness and conformity with modern standards. These laws often do not reflect contemporary scientific understandings of injury and disease or legal norms for protection of individual rights. Society faces different types of risks today and employs different methods of assessment and intervention. When many of these statutes were written, public health (e.g., epidemiology and biostatistics) and behavioral sciences (e.g., client-centered counseling) were in their infancy. Modern prevention and treatment methods did not exist.

Problem of Multiple Layers of Law

Related to the problem of antiquity is the problem of multiple layers of law. The law in most states consists of successive layers of statutes and amendments, constructed in some cases over one hundred years ago or more in response to existing or perceived health threats. This is particularly troublesome in the area of infectious disease, which forms a substantial part of state health codes. The disparate legal structures of state public health laws can significantly undermine their effectiveness. Because communicable disease laws have been enacted piecemeal in response to specific epidemics, they tell the story of the history of disease control (e.g., smallpox, yellow fever, cholera, tuberculosis, venereal diseases, polio, HIV/AIDS, West Nile virus, and SARS). Laws enacted in such an ad hoc fashion are often inconsistent, redundant, and ambiguous.

Problems of Inconsistency

Public health laws remain fragmented not only within states but also among them. Health codes within the states and territories have evolved independently, leading to profound variation in the structure, substance, and procedures for detecting, controlling, and preventing injury and disease. In fact, statutes and regulations among U.S. jurisdictions vary so significantly in definitions, methods, age, and scope that they defy orderly categorization.[1] There is good reason for wanting greater uniformity among the states in matters of public health: Health threats are rarely confined to single jurisdictions, but pose risks regionally, nationally, or even globally (e.g., air or water pollution, disposal of toxic waste, and the spread of infectious diseases, either naturally or through bioterrorist events). One need only take note of the contemporary outbreaks of West Nile virus, SARS, avian influenza, or Marburg to understand the trans-jurisdictional effects of health threats.

[1] Lawrence O. Gostin, Scott Burris, and Zita Lazzarini, "The Law and the Public's Health: A Study of Infectious Disease Law in the United States," *Columbia Law Review*, 99 (1999): 59-128.

nation has lost sight of its public health goals and has allowed the system of public health activities to fall into disarray,"[45] the IOM put some of the blame on an obsolete and inadequate body of enabling laws and regulations. "Public health law . . . is often outdated and internally inconsistent. This leads to inefficiency and a lack of coordination and may even pose a danger in a crisis."[46] The IOM recommended reform based on the "pioneering work" of the "Turning Point" Model Public Health Act, available on the *Reader* Web site.[47] Problems of antiquity, inconsistency, redundancy, and ambiguity render many statutes ineffective, or even counterproductive, in advancing the population's health (see box 1). These problems exist not only in the United States but in many other countries.[48]

POWER, DUTY, RESTRAINT

The "Turning Point" Model Public Health Act adopts the reform principles characterized in the title of this book: power, duty, and restraint. As the following discussion shows, a modern statute should define the mission and functions of public health agencies, afford a full range of powers, and impose limits on those powers to safeguard personal liberties (see further box 36, p. 438).[49]

Define the Mission and Functions. Broad and well-considered statements of mission and functions are important for organizational, political, and legal reasons (see figures 4 and 5). From an organizational perspective, they establish the purposes or goals of public health agencies, thereby informing and influencing the government's activities. From a political perspective, statements of mission and functions provide a measure of the kinds of activities that are politically sanctioned. When a public health agency is acting under a broad mission and set of core functions, that agency can better justify its decisions to legislators, the governor, and the public. From a legal perspective, courts pay deference to statements of legislative intent and may permit a broad range of activities consistent with the statutory language. Thus, even if the aspirational qualities of mission statements do not produce the desired results, they can help support agency action.

Provide a Full Range of Powers. Although voluntary cooperation is vital to public health officials, they need a full range of powers to ensure compliance with health and safety standards. At present, officials in many states have a sterile choice of either exercising draconian authority, such as deprivation of liberty, or refraining from coercion entirely. The temptation is either to abstain from exercising statutory power completely or to reach for measures that are too restrictive of individual liberty to be

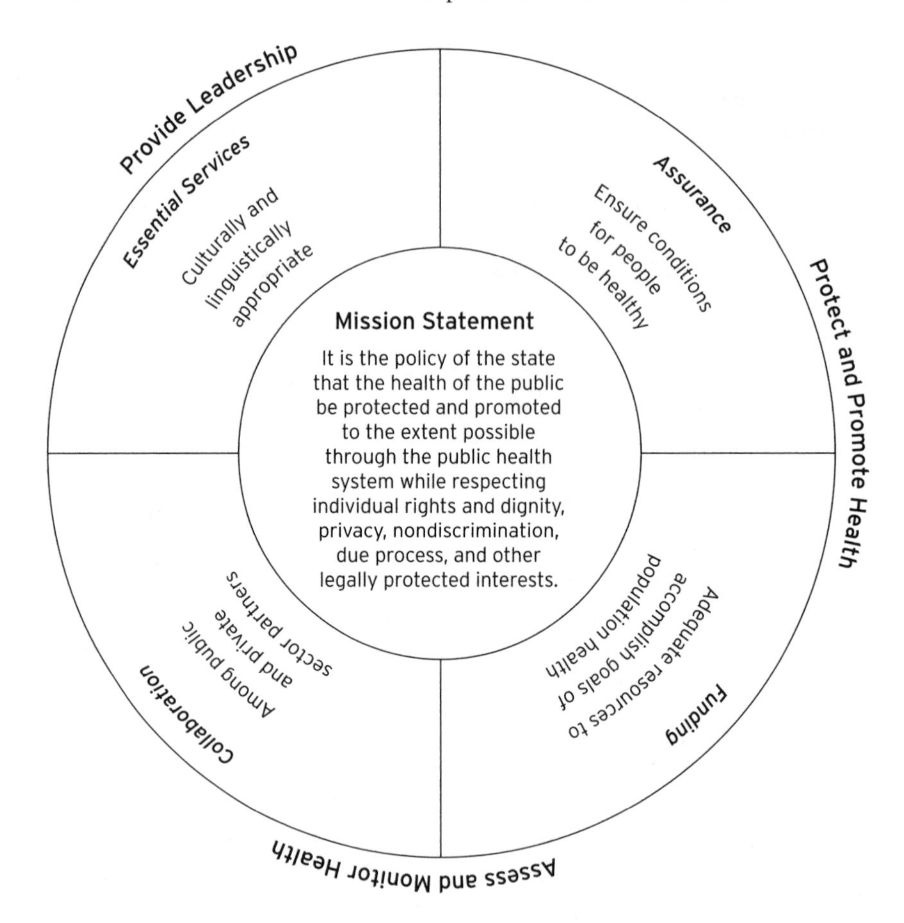

Figure 4. The mission of public health. *Source:* "Turning Point" Model State Public Health Act, September 2003, section II-101, p. 18.

acceptable in a liberal democracy. As a result, authorities may make wrong choices in two opposite directions: failing to react in the face of a real health threat or overreacting by exercising powers that are more intrusive than necessary. Public health officials need a more flexible set of tools, ranging from incentives and minimally coercive interventions to personally restrictive measures.

Impose Limits on Powers. Public health statutes should carefully balance power exercised for the common good with limits on power to protect personal freedom. Restraint on power has both substantive and procedural aspects. Substantively, state statutes should articulate clear criteria for the exercise of public health powers based on objective risk as-

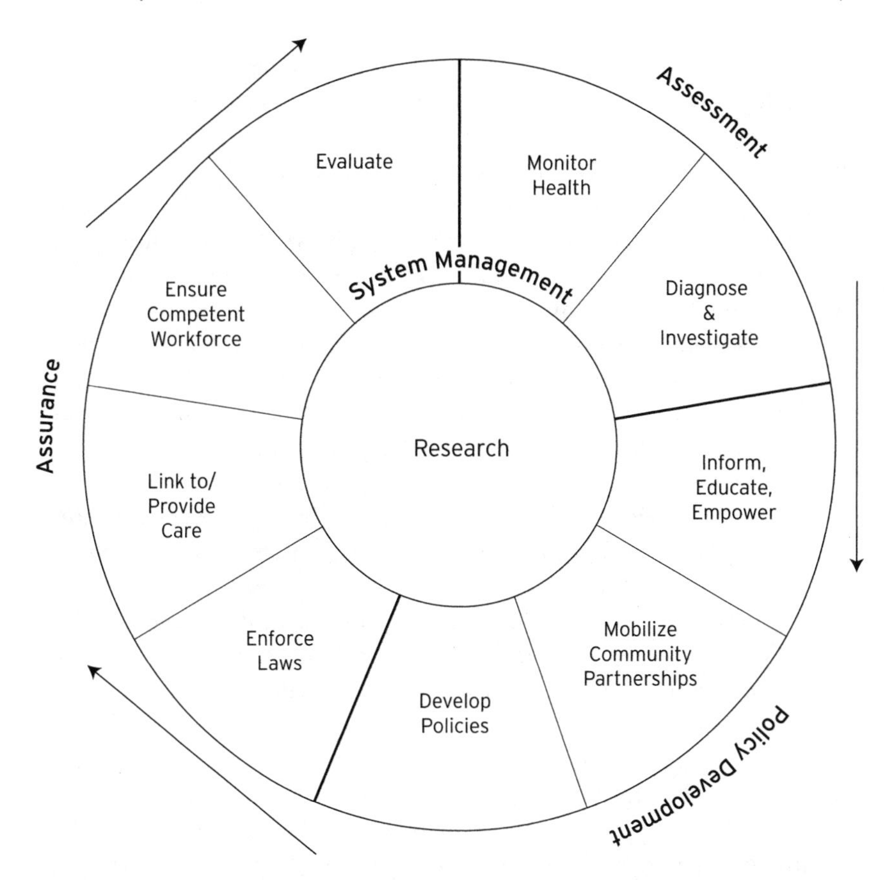

Figure 5. The core functions of public health. *Source*: Public Health Functions Steering Committee, July 1995.

sessments. Although public officials may prefer unfettered discretion, sound standards for action facilitate consistent and informed judgments. Procedurally, public health statutes should require fair processes whenever there is deprivation of a personal, proprietary, or other legally protected interest. Procedural due process, for example, usually should apply to actions that deprive a person of liberty (e.g., isolation or quarantine) or property (e.g., an inspection, license, or nuisance abatement).

THE LAWMAKING PROCESS: BUILDING CONSTITUENCIES AND FORMING PARTNERSHIPS

The methods and goals of public health are often misunderstood and undervalued within government and society. The fact that public health polices the commons and champions population-based risk reduction through behavior change (e.g., smoking cessation, designated drivers, exercise, and diet modification) deprives it of specific beneficiaries who are motivated to form political constituencies. The prevalence of an individualistic market ideology makes it difficult to even speak of public health in the vocabulary of contemporary politics.[50] Public health needs opportunities to draw attention to its resource requirements and its achievements so that it can develop constituencies for programs.

The lawmaking process provides such an opportunity. A bill is the first step toward a coalition. It is an occasion for contact with interest groups and affected communities, some of whom may be motivated to act in support of the bill. Contacts and collaborative efforts also help to establish long-term ties and identify important sources of support for other programs. Moreover, the process of negotiating for support can be a useful and concrete way for health agencies to incorporate the views of those who receive public health services or are subject to regulation.

Legal reform also has the potential to enhance health agencies' relationships with the legislature. Positive lawmaking offers a different sort of contact with legislators than tends to occur in the appropriations process. Public health law reform may offer an occasion to deal with a far greater range of legislators outside the context of contentious budget discussions. The drafting, negotiating, and hearing processes provide a variety of forums for educating lawmakers and their staffs about public health needs and methods and to provide health planners with better information about legislative views and priorities.

Law reform, of course, cannot guarantee better public health. However, by crafting a consistent and uniform approach, carefully delineating the mission and functions of public health agencies, designating a range of flexible powers, and specifying the criteria and procedures for using those powers, the law can become a catalyst, rather than an impediment, to reinvigorating the public health system.

LAW AS A TOOL FOR THE PUBLIC'S HEALTH: MODELS OF LEGAL INTERVENTION

The definition I have proposed and defended does not depict the field of public health law narrowly as a complex set of technical rules buried within state health codes. Rather, public health law should be seen broadly as the authority for and responsibility of organized society to ensure the conditions for the population's health. The law can be empowering, providing innovative solutions to the most implacable health problems. Of the ten great public health achievements in the twentieth century, most were realized, at least in part, through law reform or litigation: vaccinations, safer workplaces, safer and healthier foods, motor vehicle safety, control of infectious diseases, tobacco control, fluoridation of drinking water, family planning, healthier mothers and babies, and the decline in deaths from coronary heart disease and stroke (see figure 6). Consider what role the law might play in addressing the major public health challenges of the twenty-first century, depicted in table 1.

The study of public health law requires, therefore, a detailed understanding of the various legal tools available to prevent injury and disease and to promote the health of the populace.[51] In this section, I offer a taxonomy of the legal tools available to government and private citizens to advance the public's health: taxation and spending, alteration of the informational environment, alteration of the built environment, alteration of the socioeconomic environment, direct regulation, indirect regulation through the tort system, and deregulation (see figure 7). Although in each case the law can be a powerful agent for change, the interventions raise critical social, ethical, or constitutional concerns that warrant careful study. I frame these problems quite simply here but develop the ideas more systematically in the ensuing chapters. What is clear is that public health law is not a scientifically neutral field, but is inextricably bound to politics and society.

Model 1: The Power to Tax and Spend

The power to tax and spend is found in Article I of the U.S. Constitution, providing government with an important regulatory technique.[52] The power to spend supports a broad array of public health services, ranging from education to research. Although funding is far too limited, government spends to establish and maintain a public health infrastructure consisting of a well-trained workforce, electronic information and communications systems, rapid disease surveillance, laboratory capacity, and response capability. In addition to direct funding, government can also set health-related conditions for the receipt of public funds. For example, government can grant funds for highway construction or other public works projects on the condition that the recipients meet designated safety requirements.[53]

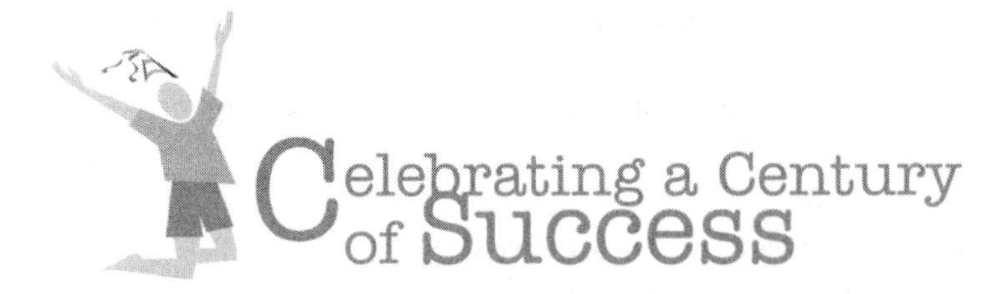

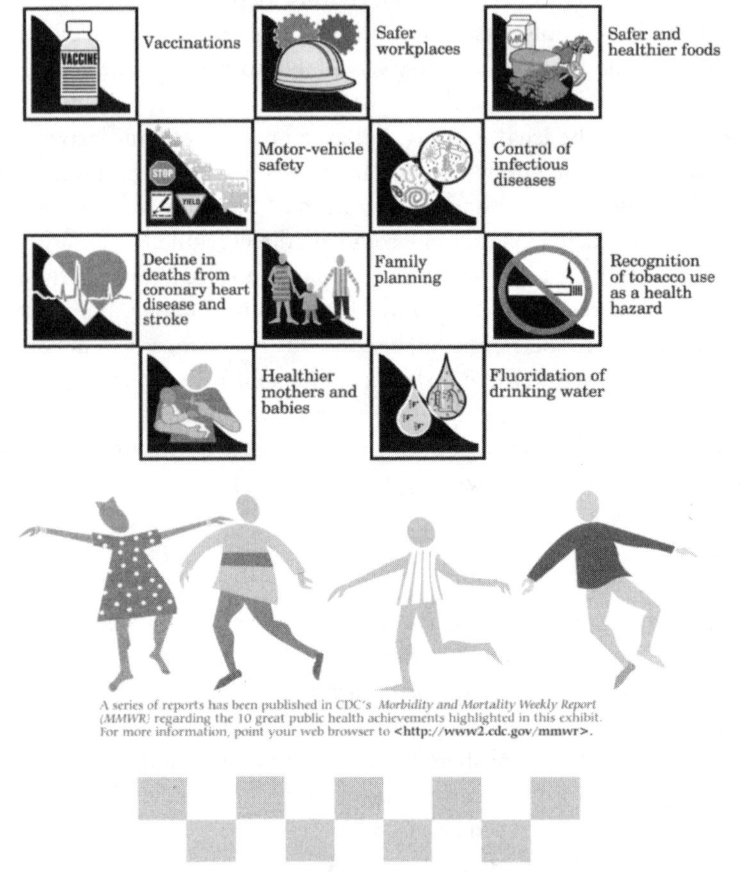

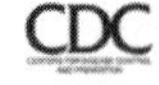

Figure 6. Ten great public health achievements. This illustration by the Centers for Disease Control and Prevention suggests a wide range of modern public health functions. *Source:* Centers for Disease Control and Prevention.

TABLE 1. Current and future public health challenges

To position the nation for the century ahead, we believe that the medical, scientific, and public health communities must do the following:

1. Institute a rational health care system
2. Eliminate health disparities among racial and ethnic groups
3. Focus on children's emotional and intellectual development
4. Achieve a longer "healthspan" for the rapidly growing aging population
5. Integrate physical activity and healthy eating into daily lives
6. Clean up and protect the environment
7. Prepare to respond to emerging infectious diseases
8. Recognize and address the contributions of mental health to overall health and well-being
9. Reduce the toll of violence in society
10. Use new scientific knowledge and technological advances wisely

SOURCE: Jeffrey P. Koplan and David W. Fleming, "Current and Future Public Health Challenges," *JAMA*, 284 (October 4, 2000): 1696–98.

The power to tax provides inducements to engage in beneficial behavior and disincentives to engage in risk activities. Tax relief can be offered for health-producing activities such as medical services, child care, and charitable contributions. At the same time, tax burdens can be placed on the sale of hazardous products, such as cigarettes, alcoholic beverages, and firearms. Of course, taxation can also create perverse incentives, such as tax relief for the purchase of unsafe and fuel-inefficient sport utility vehicles.[54]

Market incentives through the power to tax and spend are more likely than command-and-control regulation to win political acceptance—for example, inducements to avert or clean up dangerous environmental hazards are more acceptable than a compulsory measure. Still, spending and taxing powers are not entirely benign. Taxing and spending can be coercive precisely because the government wields such significant economic power. Economic conservatives, for example, are antagonistic toward proposals to tax high-calorie foods, viewing such proposals as paternalistic and meddlesome. On the other hand, liberals view some taxation as inequitable if rich people benefit while the poor are disadvantaged (e.g., tax breaks for capital gains or offshore tax shelters). Some tax policies serve the rich, the politically connected, or those with special interests (e.g., tax preferences for energy companies or tobacco farmers). Other taxes penalize the poor because they are highly regressive. For example, almost all public health advocates support cigarette taxes, but the individuals who

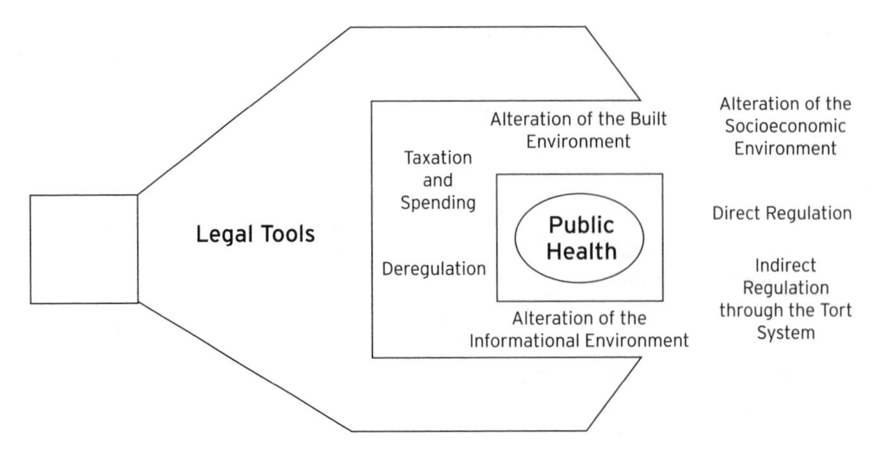

Figure 7. Law as a tool for the public's health: Seven models of legal intervention.

shoulder the principal financial burden are disproportionately indigent and are often members of minority groups[55] (see further chapter 12).

Model 2: The Power to Alter the Informational Environment

The public is bombarded with information that influences life's choices, and this undoubtedly affects health and behavior. The government has several tools at its disposal to alter the informational environment, thereby encouraging people to make more healthful choices about diet, exercise, cigarette smoking, and other behaviors: (1) government, as a health educator, can use communication campaigns as a major public health strategy; (2) government can require businesses to label their products to include instructions for safe use, disclosure of contents or ingredients, and health warnings; and (3) government can limit harmful or misleading information in private marketing by regulating advertising for potentially harmful products, such as cigarettes, firearms, and even dietary supplements.

To many public health advocates, there is nothing inherently wrong with or controversial in ensuring consumers receive full and truthful information. Yet health communication campaigns on topics such as sex, abortion, smoking, or high-fat diets are sometimes highly contested; businesses strongly protest compelled disclosure of certain health risks (e.g., the adverse effects of pharmaceuticals), and the Supreme Court has strongly protected advertising as a First Amendment right.[56] Consequently,

REPORTING
LABORATORY
CLINICS
FOLLOW-UP
EDUCATION
DAILY PRESS
The DUTIES OF THE HEALTH DEPARTMENT IN SYPHILIS CONTROL
U. S. PUBLIC HEALTH SERVICE
Your State and local health departments, in cooperation with voluntary agencies and the physician in private practice, are responsible for the control of syphilis. . . .
You SHOULD SUPPORT THEM

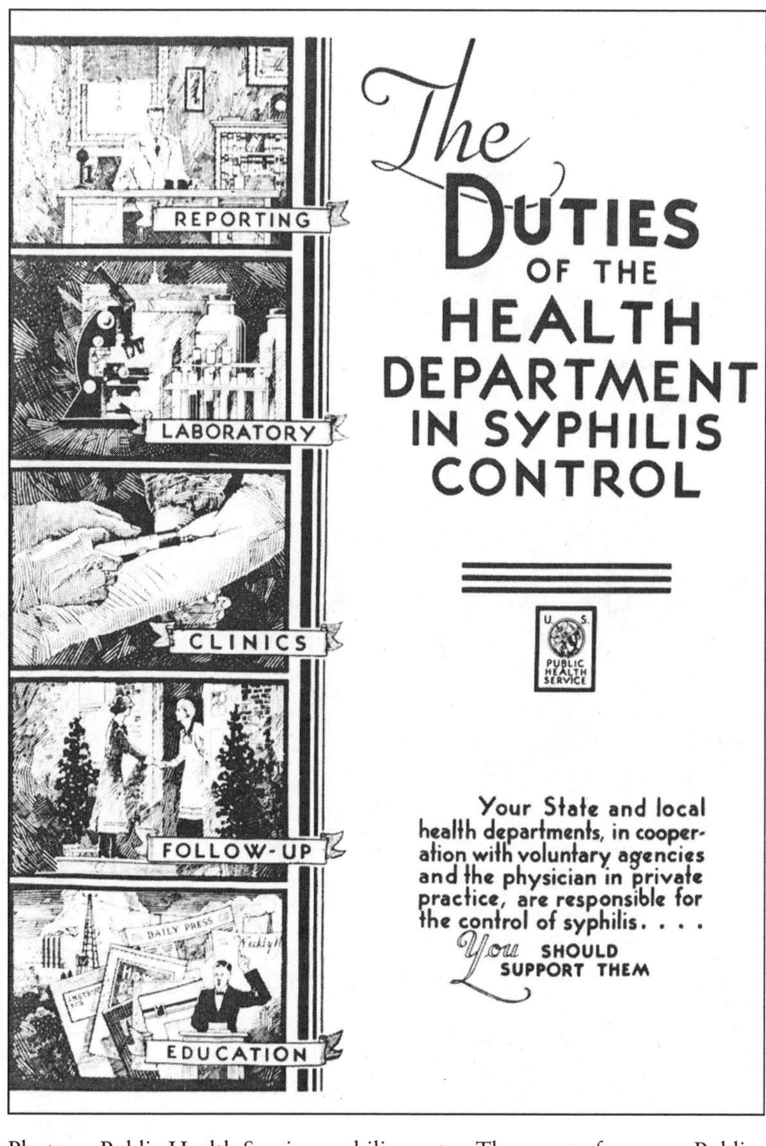

Photo 3. Public Health Service syphilis poster. The cover of a 1940s Public Health Service publication emphasizing the role of state and local governments in planning and conducting campaigns for the diagnosis and treatment of persons with syphilis. This poster illustrates a range of interventions to control syphilis.

there are powerful economic and constitutional interests at stake in any intervention designed to alter the informational environment (see further chapter 9).

Model 3: The Power to Alter the Built Environment

The design of the built or physical environment can hold great potential for addressing the major health threats facing the global community. Public health has a long history of altering the built environment to reduce injury (e.g., workplace safety, traffic calming, and fire codes), infectious diseases (e.g., sanitation, zoning, and housing codes), and environmentally associated harms (e.g., lead paint and toxic emissions). The epidemiological transition from infectious to chronic diseases raises new challenges in the design of neighborhoods to facilitate physical and mental well-being. Although research is limited, we know environments can be designed to promote livable cities and facilitate health-affirming behavior. For example, urban design can be used to encourage more active lifestyles (walking, biking, and playing), improve nutrition (by making healthful foods more accessible and high-calorie foods more avoidable), decrease the use of harmful products (cigarettes and alcoholic beverages), reduce violence (domestic abuse, street crime, and firearm use), and increase social interactions (helping neighbors and building social capital).[57]

Critics offer a stinging assessment of public health efforts to alter the built environment: "The anti-sprawl campaign is about telling [people] how they should live and work, about sacrificing individuals' values to the values of their politically powerful betters. It is coercive, moralistic, nostalgic, [and lacks honesty]."[58] The public health response: "[The] national landscape is largely devoid of places worth caring about. Soulless subdivisions, residential 'communities' utterly lacking in communal life . . . and mile upon mile of clogged collector roads, the only fabric tying our disassociated lives together."[59] Serious disagreement and acrimony apparently exist about the extent to which government should pursue environmental changes in the name of public health. Many of the sharpest disputes focus on modifications to the built environment to reduce obesity, a subject I return to in chapter 13 (see also box 12, p. 213).

Model 4: The Power to Alter the Socioeconomic Environment

There is a social gradient in health that runs from the top to the bottom of society and affects all of us. A

> way to understand this link between status and health is to think of three fundamental human needs: health, autonomy and opportunity for full social participation. All the usual suspects affect health—material conditions, smoking, diet, physical activity and the like—but autonomy and participation are two other crucial influences on health; and the lower the social status, the less autonomy and the less social participation.
>
> Michael Marmot (2005)

A strong and consistent finding of epidemiological research is that socioeconomic status (SES) is correlated with morbidity, mortality, and functioning.[60] SES is a complex phenomenon based on income, education, and occupation. As the epigraph indicates, theorists posit that material disadvantage, diminished control over life's circumstances, and lack of social acceptance all contribute to poor health outcomes.[61] The relationship between SES and health often is referred to as a "gradient" because of the graded and continuous nature of the association; health differences are observed well into the middle ranges of SES.[62] These empirical findings have persisted across time and cultures and remain viable today.[63]

Some researchers go further, concluding that the overall level of economic inequality in a society correlates with (and adversely affects) population health.[64] That is, societies with wide disparities between rich and poor tend to have worse health status than societies with smaller disparities, after controlling for per capita income. These researchers hypothesize that societies with higher degrees of inequality provide less social support and cohesion, making life more stressful and pathogenic. Drawing upon this line of argument, some ethicists contend that "social justice is good for our health."[65]

There is some persuasive anecdotal evidence for this societal inequality theory. The United States ranks twenty-ninth in the world in life expectancy—behind countries with half the income and half the health care expenditures per capita.[66] Among countries with available data, all but four of the twenty-eight preceding the United States have more equal income distributions.[67] The authors of a recent meta-analysis, however, cast doubt on the theory that more equal societies are necessarily healthier, while acknowledging that raising the incomes of the least advantaged will improve their health and thereby increase society-wide health:

> Overall, there seems to be little support for the idea that income inequality is a major, generalizable determinant of population health differences within or between rich countries. Income inequality may, however, directly influence some health outcomes, such as homicide . . . in the United States, but even that is somewhat mixed. Despite little support for a direct effect of income inequality on health per se, reducing income inequality by raising the incomes of the most disadvantaged will improve their health, help reduce health inequalities, and generally improve population health.[68]

Opponents of redistributive policies challenge this last claim, arguing that such policies punish personal accomplishment, thereby discouraging economic growth. Pointing to the correlation between population-wide health and national per capita income, they say redistribution *reduces* population-wide health over the long run by suppressing the growth of per capita income.[69] Redistribution of private wealth, they contend, is a political matter, outside the appropriate scope of the public health enterprise.[70]

The political divide on the role of socioeconomic status in population health may be impossible to bridge. Public health advocates believe a reduction in health disparities is a social imperative, while economic conservatives believe a free-market economy is indispensable to a vibrant and prosperous society. Some commentators go so far as to distinguish between the "old" public health, focused mainly on infectious disease control, and the "new" public health, aimed more broadly at the social and economic determinants of health.[71]

Model 5: Direct Regulation of Persons, Professionals, and Businesses

Government has the power to directly regulate individuals, professionals, and businesses. In a well-regulated society, public health authorities set clear, enforceable rules to protect the health and safety of workers, consumers, and the population at large. Regulation of individual behavior reduces injuries and deaths (e.g., use of seat belts and motorcycle helmets).[72] Licenses and permits enable government to monitor and control the standards and practices of professionals and institutions (e.g., doctors, hospitals, and nursing homes). Finally, inspection and regulation of businesses helps to ensure humane conditions at work, reduce toxic emissions, and improve consumer product safety.

Despite its undoubted value, public health regulation is highly contested terrain. Civil libertarians favor personal freedoms, including autonomy, privacy, and liberty. The fault lines between public health and civil liberties were exposed during the debates about the Model State Emergency Health Powers Act following September 11 and the subsequent anthrax attacks (see box 36, p. 438). Should government act boldly in a public health emergency to quell health threats or should it give precedence to personal rights and liberties?[73] Similar tensions are evident in the area of commercial regulation.[74] Influential economic theories (e.g., laissez-faire) favor open competition and the undeterred entrepreneur. Theorists advocate redressing market failures, such as monopolistic and other anticompetitive practices, rather than restraining free trade. They support relatively unfettered private enterprise and free-market solutions to social problems. Many citizens see a changing role for government from one that actively orders society for the good of the people (what the English call the "nanny state")[75] to one that leaves individuals to make their own personal and economic choices. (For additional discussion of direct regulation of businesses and individuals, see chapters 5, 10, 11, and 12).

Model 6: Indirect Regulation through the Tort System

Attorneys general, public health authorities, and private citizens possess a powerful means of indirect regulation through the tort system. Civil litigation can redress many different kinds of public health harms: environmental damage (e.g., air pollution or groundwater contamination), exposure to toxic substances (e.g., pesticides, radiation, or chemicals), hazardous products (e.g., tobacco or firearms), and defective consumer products (e.g., children's toys, recreational equipment, or household goods). Recently, public health advocates, drawing lessons from successful tobacco strategies, have brought tort actions against firearms manufacturers[76] and fast-food restaurants.[77]

While tort law can be an effective method of advancing the public's health, like any form of regulation, it is not an unmitigated good. The tort system imposes economic and personal burdens on individuals and businesses. Litigation, for example, increases the cost of doing business, thus driving up the price of consumer products. It is important to note that tort actions can deter not only socially harmful activities (e.g., unsafe automobile designs) but also socially beneficial ones (e.g., innovation in vaccine development). It is perhaps for this reason that federal and state legislators have sharply limited tort liability in such controversial areas as consumer protection class actions,[78] medical malpractice lawsuits,[79] and firearm[80] and obesity litigation.[81] Thus, although tort litigation remains a prime strategy for the public health community, it is actively resisted in some political circles (see chapter 6).

Model 7: Deregulation: Laws as a Barrier to Health

Sometimes laws are harmful to the public's health and stand as an obstacle to effective action. In such cases, the best remedy is deregulation. Politicians may urge superficially popular policies that have unintended health consequences. Consider laws that penalize needle exchange programs and pharmacy sales of sterile syringes; that close bathhouses, making it more difficult to reach gay men with condoms and safe sex literature; or that criminalize sex for persons living with HIV/AIDS, thereby potentially driving the epidemic underground.[82]

Deregulation can be controversial because it often involves direct conflict between public health and other social values, such as crime prevention or morality. Drug laws, the closure of bathhouses, and HIV-specific criminal penalties represent society's disapproval of disfavored behaviors. Deregulation becomes a symbol of weakness that is often politically unpopular. Public health advocates may believe passionately in harm-reduction strategies, but the political community may want to use the law to demonstrate social disapproval of certain activities, such as illicit drug use or unprotected sex.[83]

The government, then, has many legal "levers" designed to prevent injury and disease and promote the public's health. Legal interventions can be highly effective and need to be part of the public health officer's arsenal. However, legal interventions can also be controversial, raising important ethical, social, constitutional, and political issues. These conflicts are complex, important, and fascinating for students and scholars of public health law. Much of the remainder of this book examines these difficult problems in more detail.

THE LEGITIMATE SCOPE OF PUBLIC HEALTH AND THE LAW

Public health is purchasable. Within natural limitations, every community can determine its own death rate.

Hermann Biggs (1894)

In this chapter, I have offered a definition of public health law, suggesting that it has several core values: government responsibility for health, state power and restraint, partnerships in the public health system, a population focus, community and civic participation, a prevention orientation, and social justice. I have shown how public health law provides both the foundation for public health agencies and the broader legal tools to advance the population's health. The law creates the mission, functions, funding, and powers of public health agencies, and supplies an array of interventions to ensure conditions in which people can be healthy.

Most public health law and regulation have deep historical roots and strong public support.[84] However, activities at the cutting edge of population health often spark deep social and political dissent. Much of this controversy is about the legitimate scope, or "reach," of public health. The controversy may be informed, in large part, by ideas of individualism, freedom, self-discipline, and personal responsibility that have been foundational in our society.[85] There is a disjunction between the kinds of problems and solutions that are needed on a population level and the way the layperson conceptualizes these problems and their solutions. The lay public conceptualizes health as largely an individual matter rather than a societal issue.

It is not surprising, then, that some prefer a narrow focus on the proximal risk factors for injury and disease.[86] The role of public health agencies, according to this perspective, is to identify risks or harms and intervene to prevent or reduce them. This has been the traditional role of public health: exercising discrete powers such as surveillance (e.g., screening and reporting), injury prevention (e.g., safe consumer products), and infectious disease control (e.g., vaccination, partner notification, and quarantine).

Others prefer a broad focus on the underlying social, economic, and ecological causes of injury and disease. Those favoring this position see public health as an all-embracing enterprise united by the common value of societal well-being.[87] They claim that the jurisdiction of public health reaches "social ills rooted in distal social structures."[88] Ultimately, the field is interested in the equitable distribution of social and economic resources, because social status, race, and wealth are important influences on the health of populations. Similarly, the field is interested in "social capital" because social networks of family and friends, as well as associations with religious and civic organizations, are important factors in public health.[89] (See figure 8 for a depiction of the broad determinants of health.)

For better or worse, the dispute is highly political, with conservative scholars urging limited state action and progressive scholars urging far-reaching policies. The debate is contentious precisely because both sides

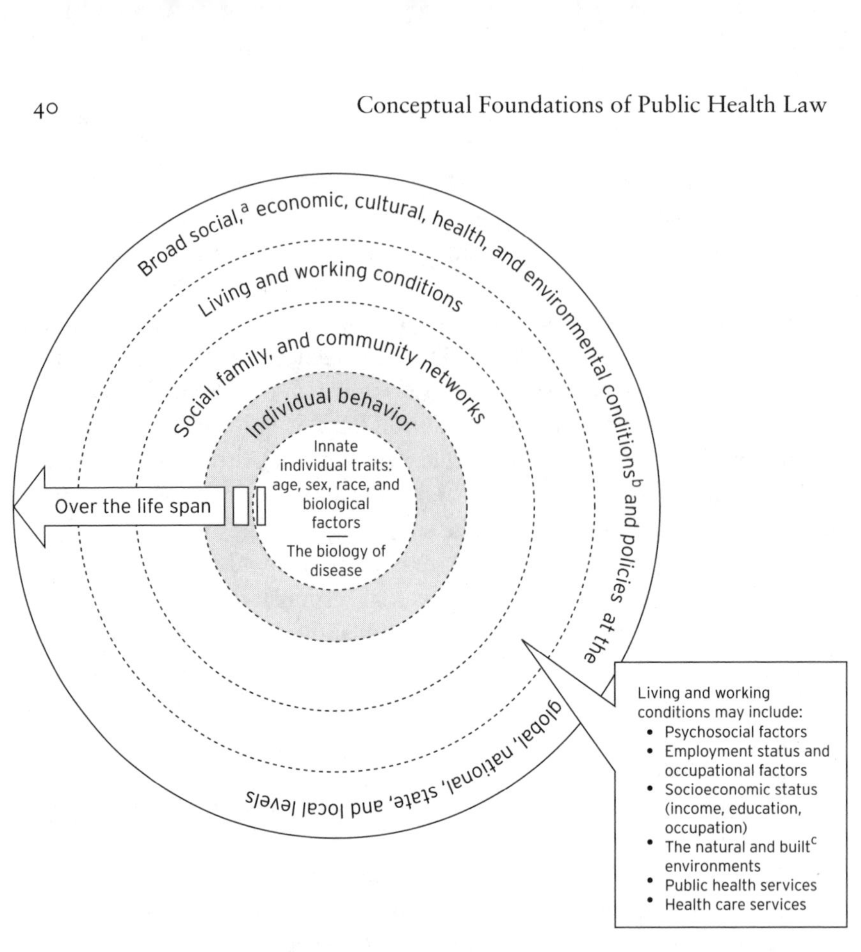

Note: The dotted lines between levels of the model denote interaction effects among the various levels of health determinants.

[a] Social conditions include but are not limited to economic inequality, urbanization, mobility, cultural values, attitudes, and policies related to discrimination and intolerance on the basis of race, gender, and other differences.

[b] Other conditions at the national level might include major sociopolitical shifts, such as recession, war, and governmental collapse.

[c] The built environment includes transportation, water and sanitation, housing, and other dimensions of urban planning.

Figure 8. A guide to thinking about the determinants of population health. *Source:* Reprinted from Institute of Medicine, *The Future of the Public's Health in the Twenty-first Century* (2000), p. 52.

have strong positions. A growing body of evidence demonstrates the value of city planning, building social capital, reducing disparities, and changing aspects of popular culture.[90] Public health agencies must act on the basis of data, and those data are informing officials about the importance of the deep underlying causes of injury and disease.[91]

Yet this all-embracing domain of public health can be troublesome, particularly in a political culture that prizes individual choice and responsibility. Almost everything human beings undertake impacts the public's health, but this does not necessarily justify an overly expansive reach. Public health agencies lack the expertise and resources to tackle problems relating, for example, to culture, housing, and discrimination. This leads inexorably to the problem of garnering political and public support for the public health enterprise. By espousing controversial issues of economic redistribution and social restructuring, the field risks losing its legitimacy. Public health gains credibility from its adherence to science, and if it strays too far into political advocacy, it may lose the appearance of objectivity.

In the end, the field of public health is caught in a dilemma. If it conceives of itself too narrowly, public health will be accused of lacking vision. It will fail to see the root causes of ill health and will fail to utilize the broad range of social, economic, scientific, and behavioral tools necessary to achieve a healthier population. If, however, public health conceives of itself too expansively, it will be accused of overreaching and invading a sphere reserved for politics, not science. The field will lose its ability to explain its mission and functions in comprehensible terms and, consequently, to sell public health in the marketplace of politics and priorities.

The politics of public health are daunting. American culture openly tolerates the expression and enjoyment of wealth and privilege, and it is inclined to treat people's disparate life circumstances as a matter of personal responsibility. Meanwhile, voters have become skeptical of government's ability to ameliorate the harshest consequences of economic and social disadvantage. Polarizing debates about faith and race have supplanted discussions of economic fairness in political campaigns and the public sphere more generally. Political liberalism has been complicit in these trends. Over the past forty years, emphasis has shifted from social obligation and economic fairness to individual freedom, self-reliance, and personal responsibility, thus relocating health from the public sphere to the private realm.[92]

These are the challenges of public health law: Does it act modestly or boldly? Does it choose scientific neutrality or political engagement? Does it leave people alone or change them for their own good? Does it intervene for the common welfare or respect civil liberties? Does it aggressively tax and regulate or nurture free enterprise? The field of public health law presents complex trade-offs and poses enticing intellectual challenges that are both theoretical and essential to the body politic.

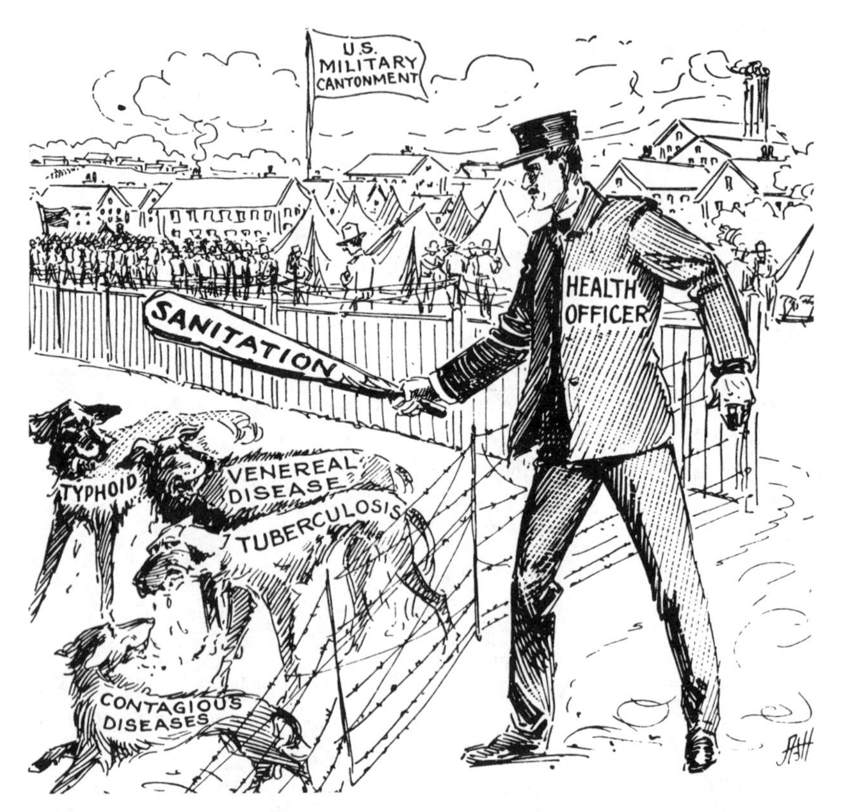

Photo 4. Containment of infectious disease around military training camps. During the First World War, the U.S. Public Health Service cooperated with local health departments to contain infectious diseases, which were assumed to be the principal threats to public health in the areas around the military training camps. Sanitation and public health regulation were health officers' principal weapons against these diseases.

CHAPTER 2

Public Health Regulation

A Systematic Evaluation

There are deep and fundamental and intuitively understood grounds for rejecting the view that confines itself merely to checking the parity of outcomes, the view that matches death for death, happiness for happiness, fulfillment for fulfillment, irrespective of how all this death, happiness and fulfillment comes about.

Amartya Sen (1994)

Public health regulation entails potential trade-offs between public goods and private interests. When public health officials act, they face troubling conflicts between the collective benefits of population health on the one hand, and personal and business interests on the other. Public health regulation is designed to monitor health threats and intervene to reduce risk or ameliorate harm within the population. At the same time, public health powers encroach on fundamental civil liberties such as privacy, bodily integrity, and freedom of movement, association, or religion. Sanitary regulations similarly intrude on basic economic liberties such as freedom of contract, pursuit of professional status, use of property, and competitive markets. Table 2 summarizes the major trade-offs in public health regulation. For each public health activity, one side of the table explains the probable public benefits and the other side explains the probable burdens on private interests.

These trade-offs between the collective benefits of population health and personal interests in liberty and property are much discussed within public health literature. But how do we know when the public good to be achieved is worth infringing upon individual rights? In this chapter, I propose a systematic evaluation of public health regulation that analyzes

TABLE 2. Public health regulation: Trade-offs between public benefit and private interests and rights

Public Benefits	←—— Public Health Activity ——→	Public Interests/Rights
	Surveillance	
· Identify injuries and diseases · Understand prevalence and incidence in the population · Understand causes of disease	· Reporting · Outbreak investigations · Case control studies	· Physician-patient confidentiality · Health information privacy
	Case Finding	
· Counseling · Education · Treatment · Support services	· Testing · Screening · Partner notification	· Personal autonomy · Bodily integrity · Health information privacy
	Medical Interventions	
· Prevent and diagnose disease · Reduce infectiousness · Reduce drug-resistant strains of pathogens	· Physical examination · Compulsory treatment · Immunization · Directly observed therapy	· Personal autonomy · Bodily integrity · Religious freedom
	Personal Control Measures	
· Prevent or reduce spread of infectious diseases	· Cease-and-desist orders · Isolation · Quarantine · Compulsory hospitalization	· Personal autonomy · Liberty · Travel
	Prohibition of Behavior	
· Protect health and safety of person or others by restricting risk behaviors	· Illicit drug use · Driving while intoxicated · Smoking in public places	· Personal autonomy and freedom of action
	Required Behavior	
· Prevent personal injury and health care costs by requiring safer behaviors	· Seat-belt use · Motorcycle helmet use	· Personal autonomy · Freedom of action

TABLE 2. *(continued)*

	Product Design	
· Prevent injuries by regulation or incentives for safer product design · Compensate injured persons	· Passive restraints in cars · Locks on firearms · Negligence under tort law · Product liability under tort law	· Freedom of contract (manufacturer-consumer) · Business interests · Property uses · Consumer costs
	Informational Constraints and Required Disclosures	
· Restrict content of commercial messages that encourage harmful behavior · Provide consumer information to avoid hazards	· Advertising restrictions · Labeling requirements · Mandated warnings	· Freedom of speech · Freedom of press · Business and property interests
	Youth and Access Restrictions	
· Reduce health and safety risks among children and adolescents	· Cigarettes · Alcoholic beverages · Firearms · Automobiles	· Autonomy of youth · Spillover effects in denying access to adults
	Nuisance Abatement	
· Reduce health/safety risks in: Businesses Recreational facilities Homes Other places	· Closure/regulation of: Bathhouses Adult theaters Food establishments Unsafe premises	· Property and business interests · Consumer costs · Free association
	Regulation of Businesses, Professionals, Food, Drugs, and Medical Devices	
· Reduce health/safety risks in: The conduct of business The provision of health care services The sale of drugs and medical devices	· Inspection of premises · Business permits · Professional licenses · Approval of pharmaceuticals	· Property and business interests · Freedom of contract · Consumer costs · Freedom to engage in occupations

TABLE 2. *(continued)*

Environmental Regulation		
· Prevent acute and long-term risks to health · Beautify the environment · Preserve habitat and animal life	· Emission controls of pollutants · Toxic waste cleanup · Drinking water standards	· Business and property interests · Consumer costs
Occupational Health and Safety		
· Reduce health and safety hazards in the workplace, such as: Exposure to toxic materials Dangerous workplace environments Stressful conditions	· Infection control · Health and safety standards · Maximum work hours	· Freedom of contract (employer-employee) · Business and property interests · Consumer costs
Taxation		
· Reduce demand for hazardous products · Create incentives for healthier behavior	· Taxes on cigarettes · Taxes on alcoholic beverages	· Consumer costs · Business and property interests · Possible fairness problem with regressive taxation

regulatory justifications, risks to health, the effectiveness, economic costs, and personal burdens of the intervention, and the policy's fairness. The chapter concludes with two principles of governance—transparency and precaution—that help inform decision-making processes in public health.

This chapter, unlike the previous one, is more prescriptive than descriptive. I suggest criteria for courts and policymakers to adopt in reviewing public health regulation. I do not mean to suggest, however, that these standards are already part of existing legal doctrine; nor do I mean to argue that these standards, if conscientiously applied, will lead to the "correct" public health policy. Public health problems and interventions are too diverse and complicated to meet a single ordered test of any kind. My claim, therefore, is that the following standards are important but not determinative in analyzing complex problems at the intersection of law and population health.

GENERAL JUSTIFICATIONS FOR PUBLIC HEALTH REGULATION

Convention holds that government intervention designed to promote population health and well-being is an unmitigated good. Why wouldn't society want to organize itself in ways that maximize the health of populations? To fulfill many of the aspirations of human life requires a healthy mind and body.[1] Because health is so highly valued, sometimes public health officials assume they need not justify their beneficent interventions. But government should justify interventions, because, almost invariably, they intrude on individual rights and interests and incur economic costs. Before proposing a systematic evaluation of public health regulation, it will be helpful to think about three general justifications for intervention: risk to others, protection of incompetent persons, and risk to self. The first justification is the standard, well-accepted idea that government may intervene to prevent harm to others or punish individuals for inflicting harm. The second justification supports government action to protect the health and safety of those who are incapable of safeguarding their own interests. The third justification, and by far the most controversial, is paternalism—the protection of the health or safety of competent individuals irrespective of their own expressed wants and desires.

The "Harm Principle": Risk to Others

> One very simple principle [justifies state coercion]. That principle is, that the sole end for which mankind are warranted, individually or collectively, in interfering with the liberty of action of any of their number, is self-protection. That the only purpose for which power can be rightfully exercised over any member of a civilized community, against his will, is to prevent harm to others. . . . His own good, either physical or moral is not a sufficient warrant. He cannot be rightfully compelled to do or forbear because it will be better for him to do so, because it will make him happier, because, in the opinion of others, to do so would be wise, or even right.
>
> John Stuart Mill (1856)

The risk of serious harm to other persons or property is the most commonly asserted and accepted justification for public health regulation.

The so-called harm principle holds that competent adults should have freedom of action unless they pose a risk to others.[2] Harm to self or immoral conduct is insufficient to justify state action: "Over himself, over his own body and mind, the individual is sovereign."[3] Liberal conceptions of autonomy and pluralism support granting individuals such a wide sphere of freedom.

Autonomy, literally "self-governance," has acquired meanings as diverse as liberty, privacy, individual choice, and even economic freedom.[4] The legal community uses autonomy to support rules such as informed consent and confidentiality. At its core, autonomy is personal governance of the self free from controlling interferences.[5] Autonomous persons are free to hold views, make choices, and take actions based on personal values and beliefs.[6] Respect for autonomy, according to Immanuel Kant, demands respect for a person's unconditional worth and freedom of will; persons should be treated as an end and never simply as a means.[7] Thus, an individual should not be exclusively used for furtherance of others' objectives without regard to her own goals.

The liberal principle of pluralism also supports a strong sphere of personal sovereignty. Pluralism recognizes that individuals have different conceptions of a satisfying life and that each conception deserves equal respect. According to liberal theory, government should remain neutral about the meaning of a good life, allowing individuals a private sphere to choose among their different conceptions.[8] Freedom to implement these choices by engaging in personal and economic activities is the hallmark of pluralism.

Theories of autonomy and pluralism maintain that government, or others, should not restrain competent adults in the absence of some overriding justification. Liberals have traditionally viewed a significant risk of harm to others as adequate justification for constraining liberty. Philosophers from John Stuart Mill[9] to Joel Feinberg[10] argue that persons should be free to think, speak, and behave as they wish, provided they do not interfere with a like expression of freedom by others. This is a classic argument that personal freedoms extend only so far as they do not intrude on the health, safety, and other legitimate interests of other individuals. Under this view, public health regulation is justified by the competing and overriding obligation not to harm or interfere with the rights of the community. If autonomy extended so far as to permit the invasion of others' spheres of liberty, there would be an overall diminution of freedom in the population. Seen in this way, genuine freedom requires a certain amount of security so that persons are free to live without risk of serious injury or disease.

The regulation of infectious disease provides a classic illustration of the harm principle. If a person behaves in a way that carries real risk of transmission of a serious infection, the harm to others is palpable. It does not matter whether the behavior is innocent or deliberate; the state may use force to avert the threat to the public's health. Consequently, even those who adhere to a minimalist view of the state's powers endorse liberty-limiting infectious-disease-control measures (e.g., vaccination, physical examination, treatment, and quarantine), at least in high-risk circumstances.[11]

"Best Interests": Protection of Incompetent Persons

The second justification for public health regulation (also well accepted) is protection of the health and safety of incompetent persons. Individuals, according to this theory, should be free not only from controlling interferences by others but also from internal limitations that impede meaningful choice. Persons who have insufficient understanding to make informed choices, to deliberate, and to act according to their desires or plans have diminished autonomy. Thus, two conditions are essential for autonomy: freedom from external control and internal capacity for deliberative action. Children and persons with mental or intellectual disabilities may, to a greater or lesser degree, have diminished capacity. In these circumstances, government may step in to ensure their health or safety, for instance by civilly committing a person with mental illness, controlling the financial affairs of a person with an intellectual disability, or granting parents or guardians a measure of control over the lives of their children.[12]

A justification for personal regulation based on incapacity does not give the state license to restrict freedoms without purpose. Rather, the state has a fiduciary duty to act for the welfare of the individual. Traditionally, two standards are used to make decisions on behalf of incompetent persons: substituted judgment and best interests. Under the first standard, the state makes decisions the individual would have made if she were competent. The substituted judgment standard makes most sense if the decision is consistent with the person's known wishes. Under the second standard, the state makes decisions that are in the person's best interests. This standard makes most sense if the person was never competent or if her wishes were unclear when she was competent. Under either standard, since the rationale for interference with autonomy is to ensure the person's well-being, the government should act beneficently. (For a constitutional explanation, see the discussion of *parens patriae* powers in the next chapter.)

A decision to find individuals incompetent can have far-reaching consequences because it justifies fundamental control over their lives. It is for this reason that decisions about incompetence need to be made, whenever possible, using a formal legal process characterized by impartiality and fundamental fairness. Moreover, a finding of incompetence should be as narrow as possible. Individuals are seldom wholly incompetent but may have difficulty making certain decisions at certain times. Fair and narrow incompetence determinations are most likely to show respect for the dignity of the individual.

Paternalism: Risk to Self

> This way of thinking and speaking [the "right" to take risks] ignores the fact that it is a rare driver, passenger, or biker, [or smoker] who does not have a child, or a spouse, or a parent. It glosses over the likelihood that if the rights-bearer comes to grief, the cost of his medical treatment, or rehabilitation, or long-term care will be spread among many others. The independent individualist, helmetless and free on the open road, becomes the most dependent of individuals in the spinal injury ward.
>
> Mary Ann Glendon (1991)

Of the three traditional justifications for public health regulation, risk to self is by far the most controversial. Risk to self is highly contentious because the behavior is "self-regarding"—that is, the conduct appears to affect only or at least primarily the person concerned and not others. Classical regulation of self-regarding behavior includes mandatory motorcycle helmet[13] and seat-belt laws,[14] gambling prohibitions,[15] criminalization of recreational drugs,[16] and fluoridation of drinking water.[17] Taxes on unhealthy products such as cigarettes, alcoholic beverages, or high-calorie foods also have a paternalistic quality, because they create marked disincentives for self-regarding behavior.[18] Paternalism is also used as a justification for protecting persons other than the class subject to the regulation. For example, health professional licensing requirements and FDA approval of pharmaceuticals are intended to protect consumers. Consumers cannot purchase unapproved drugs or the services of unlicensed practitioners even if they are informed about the risks and willingly assume them.[19]

Paternalism is the intentional interference with a person's freedom of action exclusively, or primarily, to protect the health, safety, welfare, and happiness or other interests or values of the person subject to coercion.[20] The state overrides a competent person's known preferences in order to confer a benefit or prevent harm to the subject herself.[21] (Paternalism, of course, also presents a hard problem in the private sector, such as when an employee is fired to protect that employee's health or safety. Should the courts allow an employer to discriminate on grounds of paternalism?)[22] The case against paternalism rests on the assumption that individuals are self-interested and most informed about their own needs and value systems.[23] After all, a person declines to wear a motorcycle helmet not because he is oblivious to the risk but presumably because he places one value (freedom) above another (physical security). Antipaternalists are not simply saying that individuals make wiser decisions by taking into account their own value systems. Rather, they find intrinsic value in permitting an individual to decide for himself even if, objectively, he makes the "unhealthy" choice. In short, allowing individuals to make decisions respects the person as an autonomous agent whereas coercion undermines dignity. For this reason liberal scholars maintain that "as long as individuals understand the hazards involved, they should be free to engage in [any] risky activity that provides them with personal satisfaction."[24]

A defense of paternalism usually relies on the fact that people face constraints (both internal and external) on the capacity to pursue their own interests.[25] Because personal behavior is heavily influenced and not simply a matter of free will, state regulation is sometimes necessary to protect the individual's health or safety. Individuals have to make decisions despite cognitive limitations. Most people cannot process complex scientific information to arrive at an informed choice. They also face informational deficits—decision making without full and accurate information about the risks. Not everyone knows that children are at risk of severe injury from front-seat air bags or that radon is prevalent and dangerous in homes. Even when information is available, consumers may misapprehend the risks. Media discussions of a "good diet" or the health effects of vigorous exercise are at best contradictory and confusing. Some information is provided precisely to persuade consumers to make unhealthy decisions, including advertisements for tobacco, alcoholic beverages, and fast food.

In addition to cognitive and informational constraints, individuals have limited willpower. They may objectively know what is in their best interests but find it difficult to behave accordingly. This point is obvious in the case of physical and psychological dependencies on illicit drugs, alcoholic beverages, tranquilizers, or nicotine. But individuals may also have difficulty controlling many behaviors that are not conventionally regarded as addictive. A person understands that high-fat foods or a sedentary lifestyle will cause adverse health effects or that excessive spending or gambling will cause financial hardship, but it is not always easy to refrain. The activities themselves may be so enjoyable in the short term that long-term consequences are insufficiently considered.

Finally, individuals face social and cultural constraints on their behavior. Human behavior is influenced by many external factors, including parents and family, peers and community, media and advertising. An adolescent's decision about whether to use a condom is affected not only by what he knows about sexually transmissible infections (STIs), but also by the social meaning associated with condoms among his peers and particularly his sexual partners.[26] Similarly, a person's decision about what to eat and whether to smoke cigarettes or drink alcoholic beverages (and what brand) is, at least in part, culturally determined. State paternalism has the potential to alter the culture in a positive direction, making it easier for individuals to make healthier or safer choices. Bans on smoking in public places, for example, have contributed to a shift in social norms about tobacco.

Although regulation of self-regarding behavior is pervasive in law and widely judicially sanctioned, few people are willing to concede that their beliefs or actions are paternalistic; seldom does one see a frank defense of paternalism. Instead, scholars, practitioners, and judges usually justify regulation of self-regarding behavior as if the real reason were protection against harm to others. After all, harm to others, or in economic terms, "negative externalities,"[27] can be found in almost any activity.[28] Commentators support the regulation of classically self-regarding behaviors by emphasizing the aggregate consequences for society's health and economic resources. Common sense tells us that bans on smoking in public places are intended to discourage tobacco use, but they are usually justified by the risks of sidestream smoke.[29] The same can be said of helmet or seat-belt laws where the unprotected motorist is said to present a traffic hazard[30] or pose an economic burden (e.g., urgent care costs and government expenditures under Medicaid).[31] Consider one court's view of motorcycle helmet laws:

> From the moment of the [motorcycle] injury, society picks the person up off the highway; delivers him to a municipal hospital and municipal doctors; provides him with unemployment compensation if, after recovery, he cannot replace his lost job, and, if the injury causes permanent disability, may assume the responsibility for his and his family's continued subsistence. We do not understand a state of mind that permits plaintiff to think that only he himself is concerned.[32]

These kinds of explanations for regulation of self-regarding behavior fail to confront the real issue of paternalism.[33] They reduce the justification to a strained conception of social harms rather than recognizing certain public health interventions as justified paternalism. Too often, paternalism is not candidly evaluated in scholarly and judicial discourse. Rather, it is masked by a legal fiction that the real reason is control of "other-regarding" behavior. Yet the principal reason that society requires conformance with an array of health and safety standards is to protect the person himself.

Perhaps it is not even accurate to think of public health paternalism as directed to the individual at all; perhaps it is instead directed toward overall societal welfare. Dan Beauchamp notes that public health practices are "communal in nature, and concerned with the well-being of the community as a whole and not just the well-being of any particular person. Policy, and here public health paternalism, operates at the level of practices and not at the level of individual behavior."[34] Public health aims its policies toward the community, and it counts its results in improved health and longevity in the population. Even if conduct is primarily self-regarding, the aggregate effects of persons choosing not to wear seat belts or helmets can be thousands of preventable injuries and deaths (see box 2).[35] Thus, while risk-to-self is often the least politically acceptable reason for regulation, it is nonetheless clear that paternalistic policies can be highly effective in preventing injury and death in the population.

The three principal justifications for public health regulation, then, are to prevent harm to others, protect the incompetent, and prevent risk to self. Having considered these general justifications for public health regulation,[36] it is important to systematically evaluate whether particular interventions are warranted. I propose that policymakers evaluate public

BOX 2

THE AGGREGATE HEALTH IMPACT OF REPEALING MOTORCYCLE HELMET LAWS

Paternalistic policies such as seat-belt or motorcycle laws save many lives, and repeal of these laws can have a significant adverse impact on the public's health.[1] More than 4,500 Americans died on motorcycles in 2005—nearly double the number in 1997. Almost half the people who died were not wearing helmets.[2] Yet, bowing to concerns about paternalism, state legislatures have repealed or weakened helmet laws: In 1975, forty-seven states mandated helmets for all riders, but now only twenty states require helmet use for all operators and passengers, three states have no requirements whatsoever,[3] and the remaining states have laws that apply only to certain classes of motorcyclists—usually those under eighteen years of age.[4] National Highway Transportation Safety Administration (NHTSA) data reveal that nine of the ten states with the highest numbers of fatalities do not require adults to wear helmets, while seven of the ten states with the fewest deaths do require helmets. For example, as a result of the repeal of the all-rider helmet law in Florida, NHTSA reported that of the 551 motorcyclist deaths in the three years preceding repeal of the law, 9 percent of the victims did not wear helmets; after the law was repealed, 61 percent of the fatally injured riders were not wearing helmets.[5] The agency concludes: "The states have been repealing the universal helmet laws. Whenever a state does that, the observed rate of helmet use drops in half almost immediately and motorcycle fatalities and injuries skyrocket."[6] Pittsburgh Steelers quarterback Ben Roethlisberger's motorcycle crash in 2006 rekindled debate about the need for tougher laws, but even Pennsylvania, where the crash occurred, did not enact a mandatory helmet law.[7]

1 Marion Moser Jones and Ronald Bayer, "Paternalism and Its Discontents: Motorcycle Helmet Laws, Libertarian Values, and Public Health," *American Journal of Public Health* 97 (2007): 208–17.

2 Micheline Maynard, "Death Rate on Highways Rises, and Motorcycles Are Blamed," *New York Times*, August 8, 2006.

3 Colorado, Illinois, and Iowa do not have a motorcycle helmet use law.

4 National Highway Traffic Safety Administration, Motorcycle Helmet Use Laws, January 1, 2006, http://www.nhtsa.dot.gov/staticfiles/DOT/NHTSA/Rulemaking/Articles/Associated%20Files/03%20Motorcycle%20Helmet%20Use.pdf.

5 National Highway Traffic Safety Administration, *Evaluation of the Repeal of the All-Rider Motorcycle Helmet Law in Florida*, DOT HS 809 849 (Washington, DC: Department of Transportation, 2005); National Highway Traffic Safety Administration, Motorcycle Helmet Use Laws; University of California, Berkeley, "Easy, Rider," *Wellness Letter* 21 (2005): 8.

6 Thomas Hargrove, "A Fatal Freedom: Deaths in Motorcycle Crashes on Rise," Scripps Howard News Service, May 25, 2006, http://www.shns.com/shns/g_index2.cfm?action = detail&pk = FATAL-FREEDOM-05-25-06.

7 Tracie Mauriello, "Lawmakers Divided on Revisiting Helmet Law," *Pittsburgh Post-Gazette*, June 14, 2006, http://www.post-gazette.com/pg/06165/698022-85.stm.

health regulation under the following criteria: significant risk, effectiveness, economic cost, burden on individuals, and fairness (see figure 9).

STEP 1: IS THE RISK SIGNIFICANT? RISK ASSESSMENTS

Risk. A concept used to give meaning to things, forces,
or circumstances that pose danger to people or to what

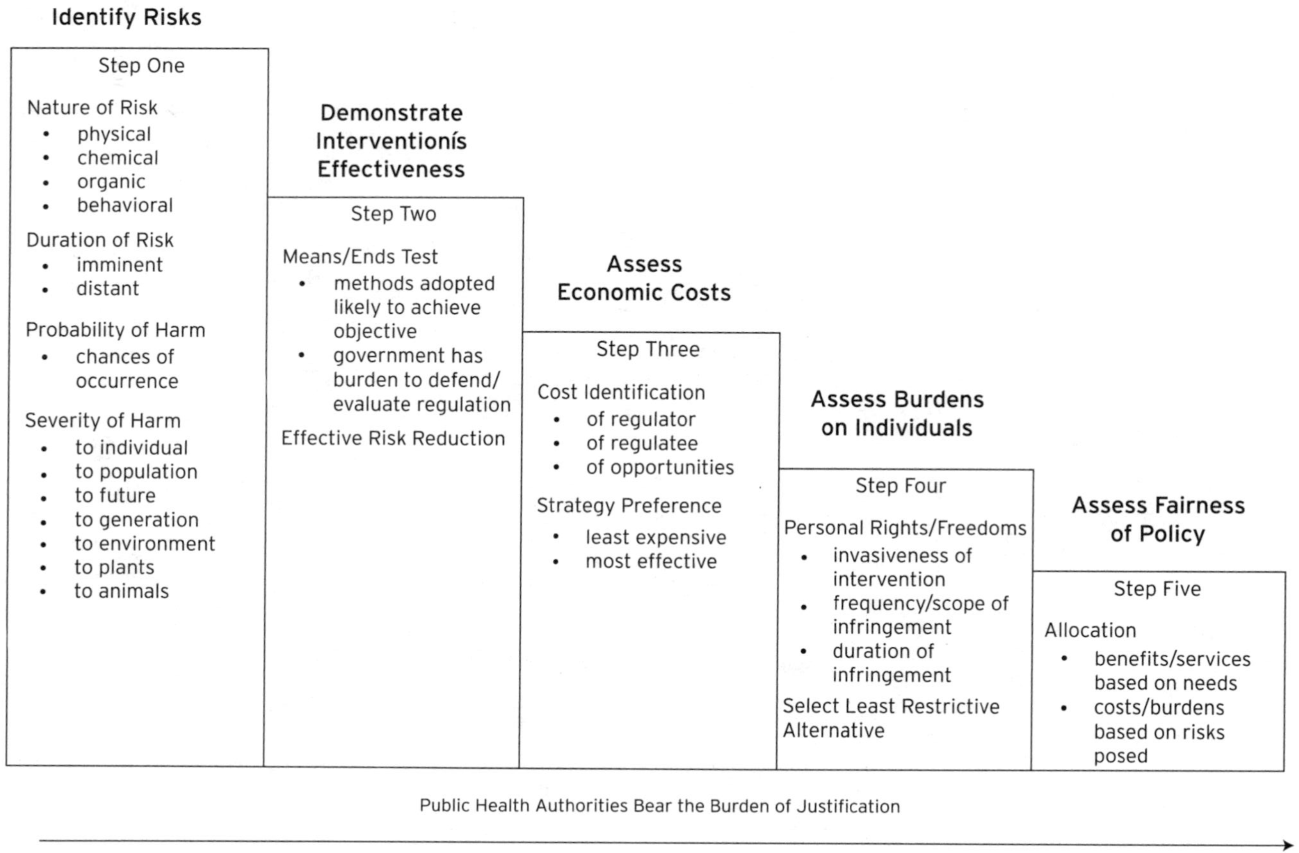

Identify Risks

Step One

Nature of Risk
- physical
- chemical
- organic
- behavioral

Duration of Risk
- imminent
- distant

Probability of Harm
- chances of occurrence

Severity of Harm
- to individual
- to population
- to future
- to generation
- to environment
- to plants
- to animals

Demonstrate Interventionís Effectiveness

Step Two

Means/Ends Test
- methods adopted likely to achieve objective
- government has burden to defend/ evaluate regulation

Effective Risk Reduction

Assess Economic Costs

Step Three

Cost Identification
- of regulator
- of regulatee
- of opportunities

Strategy Preference
- least expensive
- most effective

Assess Burdens on Individuals

Step Four

Personal Rights/Freedoms
- invasiveness of intervention
- frequency/scope of infringement
- duration of infringement

Select Least Restrictive Alternative

Assess Fairness of Policy

Step Five

Allocation
- benefits/services based on needs
- costs/burdens based on risks posed

Public Health Authorities Bear the Burden of Justification

Figure 9. Public health regulation: A stepwise evaluation.

> they value. Descriptions of risk are typically stated in terms of the likelihood of harm or loss from a hazard and usually include: an identification of what is "at risk" and may be harmed or lost (e.g., health of human beings or an ecosystem, personal property, quality of life, ability to carry on an economic activity); the hazard that may occasion this loss; and a judgment about the likelihood that harm will occur.
>
> National Research Council (1996)

The mission of public health is to identify risks and prevent or ameliorate harms or other undesirable consequences to humans and what they value. Populations face hazards from many different sources: from physical forces (e.g., radioactivity, sound waves, and magnetic fields), chemicals (e.g., ozone, mercury, dioxins, and drugs), organisms (e.g., viruses, bacteria, and prions),[37] and human behavior (e.g., sex, smoking, drunk driving, and firearm use).[38] Hazards may be incurred accidentally (e.g., a chemical spill), naturally (e.g., an infectious disease outbreak, earthquake, or hurricane), or intentionally (e.g., bioterrorism).[39]

Risk is a highly complex concept, and a vast literature exists about the analysis,[40] perception,[41] characterization,[42] communication,[43] and management[44] of risk. I will not attempt to systematically synthesize the extant literature regarding risk. However, I will propose a framework for risk analysis, discuss value choices in risk regulation, and explain the difficult trade-offs among competing risks to health.

Risk Analysis in Public Health Regulation

Public health regulation is an attempt to understand and control risk. However, we need to know more about the evidence needed to assess the risk and the level, or seriousness, of the risk that warrants regulation. Risk assessments are often made under circumstances of scientific uncertainty, so an accurate calculation can be difficult (see the discussion of the "precautionary principle" below). Nevertheless, to the extent possible, risk assessments should be based on objective and reliable scientific evidence provided by the multiple disciplines of public health, including medicine, virology, bacteriology, and epidemiology.[45] Science-based risk assessments provide a surer grounding for decision making and avoid reflexive actions based upon irrational fears, speculation, stereotypes, or pernicious mythologies.[46]

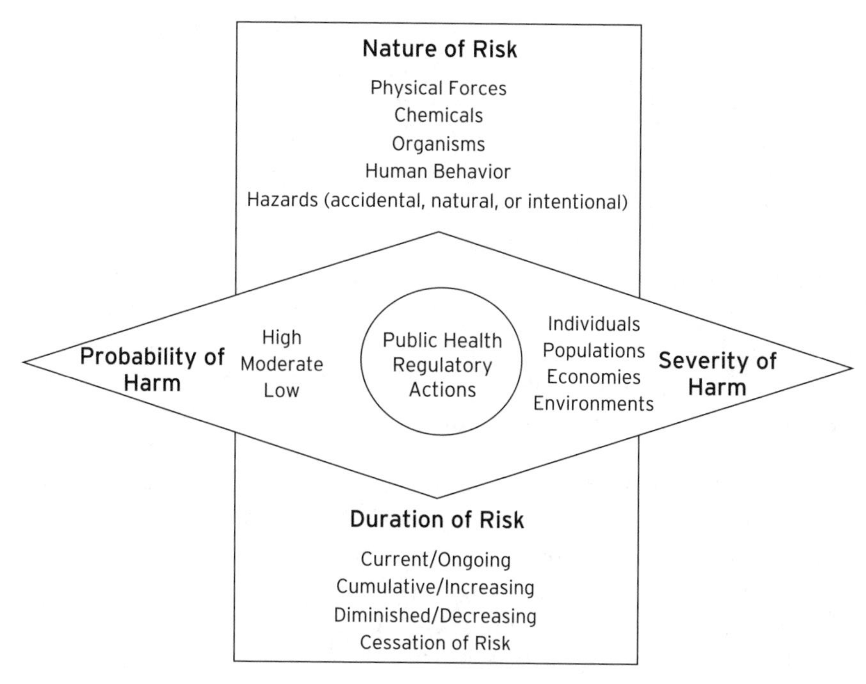

Figure 10. Public health risk assessment.

Risk assessments should also be made on a case-by-case basis. Individualized risk assessments avoid decisions made under a blanket rule or generalization about a class of persons. A fact-specific, individualized inquiry is more likely to result in a well-informed judgment grounded in a careful and open-minded weighing of risks and alternatives.

Finally, public health regulation should be based on risks that are "significant," not speculative, theoretical, or remote.[47] The level of risk needed to justify a regulatory response varies depending on the policy's economic costs and human burdens. If the costs and burdens are small, public health officials need to demonstrate lower levels of risk to justify the intervention. As the policy's costs and burdens increase, public health officials need to demonstrate ever-greater levels of risk. For example, where individual liberty is at stake, the risk justifying regulation should be substantial. Four factors are helpful in risk assessments: the nature of the risk, the duration of the risk, the probability that harm will occur, and the severity of the harm if the risk were to materialize (see figure 10).

The Nature of the Risk. As suggested above, populations face hazards from varying sources, each presenting a different kind of risk. It matters whether the danger is from exposure to an environmental carcinogen, ingestion of genetically modified plants or animals, or infection with an organism. Assessing the risk of an environmental carcinogen requires understanding the toxicity of the particular substance, the dose, and the length of exposure. The harm to any individual may be impossible to quantify; disease may not occur at all or it may take decades to develop, and even if the person does become ill, other causes cannot be eliminated. The risk, therefore, may be realized only in the aggregate based upon epidemiological investigations of various populations. Risk assessments for genetically modified plants and animals may be concerned not so much with the harm to those who ingest the food but with difficult-to-measure effects on the ecosystem.[48] Potential harms, such as global warming, may even affect future generations. Risk assessments for infectious diseases depend on the mode of transmission of the organism. Risks vary depending on whether the mechanism of transmission is sexual, airborne, bloodborne, waterborne, or foodborne. A significant risk can only be established in cases involving a primary mode of transmission, rather than a theoretical or inefficient mode.

The Duration of the Risk. Risks are rarely all-or-nothing events. Rather, risks change over time: A risk may remain constant, it may diminish or end, or it may increase. Assessments should take account of the risk as it exists at the moment and how it is predicted to change over time. Risks of radiation, radon, and tobacco smoke, for example, are cumulative and would be expected to increase the longer the person or population is exposed. Risks of infectious disease, however, exist only so long as the person remains contagious. A person should be subject to compulsory public health powers only if he or she has been exposed to infection or is infectious, and only for the period of time that the risk persists.[49]

The Probability of Harm. The probability of harm is an important aspect of risk assessment. Risk assessors seek to determine the chance that a particular harm will occur and, if so, when. For example, we know that measles and influenza are readily transmissible by airborne droplets and pose a significant risk to others in close proximity to the infected person. We also know that airborne transmission of HIV, or even bloodborne transmission in a health care setting, is highly unlikely. The "probability of harm" standard involves a prediction of the future and therefore requires rigorous scientific evaluation. As the probability of a harmful event increases, so does the justification for a regulatory response.

The Severity of Harm. The seriousness of harm represents an important calculation in assessing public health regulation. The probability of a harmful event does not tell us a great deal about its severity if the harm were to materialize. Severity of harm may be measured by its effects on an individual: It matters when the disease or injury occurs (young or old age), whether the effects are debilitating (physically or mentally), how long the effects persist, and whether it will result in death. Severity of harm may also be measured by its effects on populations. The harm to any single individual may be relatively small, but if the harm occurs to large populations, the severity is greater. Harm to populations includes not only adverse health effects but also socioeconomic effects on trade, travel, and tourism (e.g., the economic upheaval caused by SARS or avian influenza). Finally, severity of harm may be measured by its detrimental effects on the things human beings value. Degradation of the environment, the ecosystem, or animal life may or may not have measurable effects on human health. Yet, to the extent that people value intangible aspects of life like natural beauty, wilderness, or continuation and diversity of species, we count these harms in our risk calculations.

In assessing whether a particular risk justifies the exercise of a public health power, it is important to examine both the severity of the harm and the probability of its occurrence. A rough inverse correlation exists between probability and harm. As the seriousness of potential harm to the community rises, the level of probability needed to justify the public health intervention decreases. Bioterrorism, for example, presents a relatively small probability of occurring, but the consequences of an attack can be extraordinarily high, not only in human life but in social and economic disruption, as was illustrated during the anthrax attacks in October 2001. Central to understanding the "significant risk" standard is the fact that even the most serious potential for harm does not necessarily justify public health regulation in the absence of reasonable probability that it will occur.[50] Early in the HIV epidemic, for example, parents had difficulty comprehending why children who are infested with lice are excluded from school, but not those infected with HIV. The reason is that a very high probability exists that other children will become infested with lice, but the risk of contracting HIV in that setting is remote.

Risk assessments can be deeply complex, and it is not always clear whether the level of risk justifies an intervention. Modern controversy has swirled as to whether risk assessments are materially different when a health hazard presents the potential for catastrophic harm to the population, such as the risk of bioterrorism.

Social Values in Risk Assessment

> Should the government concern itself with public opinion when addressing public health risks such as cancer? What if the public opinion is at odds with all the best scientific evidence? Suppose the public demands extensive government regulation or even prohibition of a valuable substance or activity, when scientific studies indicate that the substance or activity presents little or no risk. The result is a conflict between the goals of a democratically responsive government and an effective public heath protection program. Because it is impossible to reduce all human health risks, as publicly perceived or as scientifically identified, a trade-off is unavoidable. This problem is complicated because the general populace and scientists do not even agree on the meaning of the term "risk."
>
> Frank B. Cross (1994)

The risk analysis offered so far is closely aligned to science. Science understands risk according to probabilistic assessments of the chance a dangerous event will occur, and if it does, the severity of its effects.[51] The scientific risk assessor generally considers risk in an objective and narrow context. The lay public's understanding of risk, however, accounts for more than statistical likelihood; it includes personal, social, and cultural values.[52] The differences between lay and expert perceptions of risk lead to interesting questions about which perspective should prevail and, more importantly, the implications for democratic values: Should science trump popular judgment? How much weight should elected leaders give to public opinion when it is at odds with scientific assessments?[53]

Scholars argue that lay judgments are prone to inaccuracy, leading to exaggerated perceptions of small risks and underestimations of larger risks.[54] Laypersons use heuristics, or rules of thumb, to make judgments about risk. They make simplifying assumptions: Toxic waste is harmful to health, so all toxic material must be removed; or, nuclear disasters occur, so all nuclear power must be dangerous.[55]

The public's perception of risk is influenced by its salience. The more the media draws attention to statistically low risks, the more the public becomes concerned. One can recount numerous examples of the media focusing on small risks: streptococcus A infection ("flesh-eating" disease),[56] the pesticide alar (in apples),[57] bovine spongiform encephalopathy (BSE),[58] infectious disease outbreaks (e.g., Ebola, SARS, or avian influenza), or bioterrorism (e.g., anthrax or smallpox).[59] The public understandably becomes alarmed when a dramatic event is reported, such as the disasters at Love Canal, Three Mile Island, and Chernobyl. In each of these cases, government reacted to heightened public concern with additional resources and other policy shifts.

Heuristics, salience, and other "unscientific" lay perceptions may skew the regulatory agenda, resulting in selective attention to relatively remote risks.[60] Though lay judgments are often "unscientific," they are not necessarily irrational. The public tolerates certain hazards because they voluntarily assume the risk, feel they can control the risk, or derive benefit from the activity. Laypersons, for example, may reject extensive regulation of grave risks that are voluntarily incurred, controllable, and enjoyable (e.g., smoking and automobile travel) but insist on extensive regulation of relatively low risks they feel are inescapable, unmanageable, or not tangibly valuable (e.g., hazardous waste sites, electromagnetic power lines, or air travel).[61]

The public also adopts other values in risk assessments: Do the risks occur "naturally" or are they introduced by novel technologies (e.g., nuclear power, cloning, transgenic foods)? Does the behavior conform to community standards of morality (e.g., sexuality, drug use, abortion)? Are the risks fairly distributed among the population (e.g., disproportionate burdens on women or racial minorities)? If, as Amartya Sen suggests in the epigraph at the beginning of this chapter, the scientific method of comparing "death for death" is deeply unintuitive, it may be because, on occasion, the public has a richer, more contextual understanding of risk that deserves attention in a democratic society.[62] The public, therefore, need not routinely cede moral judgments to public health's claims of value-free science. Nor is it wrong for democratically responsive government to weigh benefits to the public's health against harm to traditional values.

I am not suggesting that lay perceptions should supplant risk assessments derived from scientific methodologies. Public health officials gain their legitimacy by making sound scientific assessments. I am suggesting that, in a democratic society, public health has a political dimension that reasonably takes into account community values such as voluntariness, personal benefit, and fair distribution in risk assessments.

Risk-Risk Trade-Offs

Public health regulation entails trade-offs between competing risks to health. Frequently, when government intervenes to diminish one risk, it simultaneously increases another risk.[63] Thus, drinking water standards requiring chemical disinfection decrease risks of waterborne disease (*Guardia* and *Cryptosporidium*) but increase risks of cancer.[64] Universal precautions in medical settings decrease risks of bloodborne infection but increase costs, and thus make health care less widely available.[65] Nuclear power regulation reduces radiation risks but drives the market toward coal- or oil-based energy, thus increasing other hazards to humans and the environment.[66] A long-running lawsuit brought by environmental groups over New York's insecticide-spraying for West Nile virus illustrates the political nature of health trade-offs: Public health groups emphasize the risk of mosquito-borne diseases, while environmental groups focus on the risks of respiratory diseases and cancer.[67]

Risk-risk trade-offs occur in several contexts, making the problem difficult to resolve. Most often, regulators are aware of the trade-offs but have insufficient scientific data to choose the most serious risk among several hazards. It is not always possible, for example, to compare the immediate risk of a waterborne disease outbreak and the latent risk of introducing a carcinogen into the drinking water supply. Sometimes regulators are simply unaware of competing risks. Since civil servants usually are responsible for one set of health problems, they may have "tunnel vision" and fail to notice other risks. Similarly, agencies may have narrow regulatory authority that does not permit them to consider risks outside their jurisdiction. Environmental agencies, for example, may have jurisdiction to reduce exposure to lead or radon in homes but lack authority to prevent an overall decrease in housing stock resulting from environmental regulation. Ideally, public health officials should undertake a coordinating function among health and social services agencies so that they could consider aggregate rather than isolated risks.

STEP 2: IS THE REGULATION EFFECTIVE? THE "MEANS/ENDS" TEST

As we have just seen, the objective of public health regulation is to avert or diminish significant risks to health. Though courts and the public readily understand the need for a substantial health objective, they pay less attention to the methods used to achieve the goal. Instead, the intervention's effectiveness simply is assumed; or, more likely, the courts and the public trust the experts to develop, implement, and evaluate the intervention. It is unwise to assume that public health interventions are always effective. In fact, since proposed regulation entails personal burdens and economic costs, government should affirmatively demonstrate through scientific data that the methods adopted are reasonably likely to achieve the public health objective.[68] This is called the "means/ends test": It is the government's burden to defend and rigorously evaluate the effectiveness of regulation. The fact that government regulates in a particular area does not necessarily mean it is "doing something" about the problem. The better questions are whether public health officials accurately measure the health hazard, effectively reduce the risk or ameliorate the harm, and rigorously evaluate the intervention.

Public health officials should accurately measure relevant health risks as a prerequisite to meaningful action. If a regulatory response to radioactivity, magnetic fields, or lead paint is considered, public health officials should understand the health risks posed. How much is known about the hazard? How much exposure, and of what duration, is safe? How much reduction in exposure is necessary to reduce the risk to acceptable levels? If the hazard is not well understood, risk reduction strategies are less likely to be successful.

Public health officials should not simply measure the health risk but in fact reduce that risk or ameliorate the ensuing harm. Regulatory activities are frequently justified by historical convention. The need to demonstrate an intervention's effectiveness therefore requires ongoing evaluation. The Institute of Medicine proposes the adoption of performance monitoring, a process of selecting and analyzing indicators to measure the outcomes of an intervention strategy for health improvement.[69] Admittedly, scientific evaluation is complex, because many behavioral, social, and environmental variables confound objective measurement of the causal connection between an intervention and a health outcome. Nevertheless, asking public health officials to demonstrate an intervention's effectiveness is necessary to ensure that the community health benefits outweigh the personal burdens and economic costs.

STEP 3: IS THE REGULATION COST-EFFECTIVE?

> *Cecil Graham:* What is a cynic? [Sitting on the back of the sofa.]
>
> *Lord Darlington:* A man who knows the price of everything and the value of nothing.
>
> Oscar Wilde (1892)

Public health regulations impose economic costs: agency resources to devise and implement the regulation, costs to individuals and businesses subject to the regulation, and lost opportunities to intervene with a different, potentially more effective, technique (opportunity costs). A major issue, much debated in the literature, is the relevance of cost in regulatory decisions designed to safeguard the public's health.[70] Under standard accounts, government should prefer regulatory responses that provide the most health benefits[71] at the least cost.[72] Cost-effectiveness analysis (CEA) is an analytic tool that can be used to evaluate the outcomes and costs of interventions designed to improve health:[73]

> CEA provides ratios that show the cost (in monetary terms) of achieving one unit of health outcome. The measures of health outcomes most commonly employed are the number of lives, life-years (LYs), disability-adjusted life-years (DALYs), and quality-adjusted life-years (QALYs) gained. . . . Interventions can be ranked according to their cost-effectiveness ratios and a fixed budget can then be allocated to achieve maximum effectiveness.[74]

Society cannot escape the role that cost plays. Few people question the premise that society has finite and relatively scarce resources available for public health regulation.[75] Given the reality of scarcity, hard choices must be made between regulatory alternatives. Do we spend large sums to avert relatively trivial risks or do we devote resources to more serious risks that can be ameliorated at significantly lower cost? Although society cannot tally up costs and benefits into a tidy number, it can make sensible choices in prioritizing regulatory expenditures. Despite the importance of cost as a relevant factor, the Supreme Court has held that absent explicit permission in its enabling statute, an agency may not consider cost in setting health and safety standards.[76] Many statutes, however, do authorize agencies to consider the economic effects of regulations.[77]

The Standard Economic Account

Under the standard economic account, three serious problems exist with the regulatory state: inordinate costs for small health benefits (low cost-effectiveness), regulation carried to illogical extremes ("going the last mile"), and arbitrary selection of regulatory topics ("random agenda selection").[78] The principal critique of the regulatory process is that government often requires enormous expenditures to achieve relatively small health benefits. Focusing mostly on environmental regulations designed to reduce cancer risks, economists estimate that government spends, in some cases, millions of dollars to save a single human life.[79]

Regulators exacerbate the costs of intervention by "going the last mile"—insisting on near-zero risk from a particular hazard. Sometimes an agency is so single-minded in its pursuit of safety that it imposes high costs without achieving significant additional benefits. Trying to remove the last vestiges of risk often involves extraordinary technological measures, high cost, and legal fees. For example, in one federal case, the EPA required an expenditure of $9.3 million to eliminate the last remnants of toxic material at a swamp site so that children could safely eat dirt for 245 days a year, rather than only 70 days per year.[80]

Finally, extreme disparities in regulatory decisions make the process appear arbitrary. Humans face innumerable hazards, and only a small fraction are regulated. Even among those hazards that are regulated, little consistency exists in the costs incurred and the benefits achieved. When economists compare the resources that the government commits to eliminate different kinds of risks, the results are striking: Small risks, such as the carcinogenic effects of toxic substances, entail enormous regulatory cost, whereas large risks, such as injuries from unsafe product design, entail modest regulatory cost.[81] From a strict cost-benefit perspective, agencies devote dramatically different attention to different kinds of death.

Can Human Health and Life Be Reduced to a Numerical Ratio of Costs and Benefits?

Though these economic critiques of public health regulation are powerful, CEA is deeply controversial. First, market exchanges are not the principal measure of the value of a human life. Lives are not commensurate with dollars, and precise monetary valuation of human life cannot account for the hopes, fears, and fragilities of people, their families, and the things that humans value.[82] Second, public health regulation cannot be compressed, through ever more complex economic methods, into one aggregate number such as costs per quality-adjusted life saved.[83] Estimates of cost per life saved are not objective scientific facts susceptible to precise quantification.[84] Technical CEA is imbued with social values, such as the worth of human lives, the appropriate policy response to scientific uncertainty, and the importance of intangible regulatory benefits (e.g., ecological improvements).[85] Finally, scholars sharply question the underlying assumptions and data supporting CEA. The standard economic account often ignores risks and benefits other than human deaths (e.g., nonfatal harms to human health or harms to ecosystems); deeply discounts the benefits of regulations that save lives in the future (e.g., cancer risks from exposure to toxins); and most remarkably, decries exorbitantly costly regulations that were never adopted, including those that were never even proposed by the agency.[86]

Ackerman and Heinzerling provide particularly egregious illustrations of cost-effectiveness analysis gone awry.[87] They have concluded that government:

- actually *saves* money when citizens smoke, because the premature deaths reduce health care and social security costs (concluding that "cigarette smoking should be subsidized rather than taxed");
- devotes *too much* effort to controlling lead exposure among children, because their parents do not spend a great deal of money on treatment to excrete lead from their bodies (concluding that "agencies should consider *relaxing* lead standards");
- values children's lives *too highly,* because mothers do not take sufficient time to properly fasten car seats (concluding that mothers implicitly place a finite monetary value on the life-threatening risks to their children posed by car crashes).[88]

Despite the deeply divisive and troublesome implications of some CEA, regulatory costs do need to be considered. Maximization of health benefits within a relatively fixed budget remains an important social and political value, as the following discussion of opportunity costs suggests.

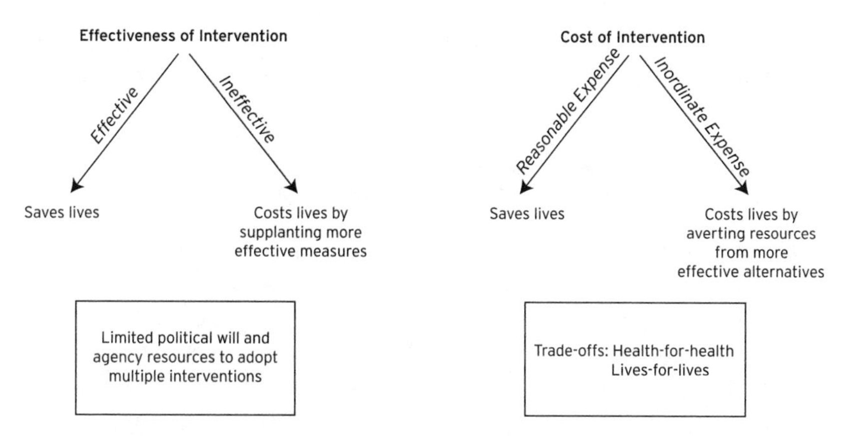

Figure 11. Opportunity costs in risk regulation.

Opportunity Costs

Why is it a problem if public health regulations impose inordinate expense with relatively modest benefits? At least part of the answer is that whenever government regulates, it forgoes opportunities for other interventions that improve community health. It is helpful to look at both sides of the effectiveness-expense equation to understand opportunity costs (see figure 11). If government adopts an ineffective strategy, it loses opportunities to intervene with a different, potentially more beneficial technique. Political will and agency resources are usually too limited to adopt multiple methods of intervention simultaneously. Consequently, government adoption of ineffective methods means it must forgo or delay more beneficial strategies, thus adversely affecting community health.

Now consider the expense side of the effectiveness-expense equation. A decision to devote extensive resources to avert trivial risks means government is forgoing opportunities to regulate far more serious risks. Legislatures allocate limited resources to public health regulation. Decisions to spend in one area mean that the money may not be available to spend in another more problematic area. Government can reduce morbidity and premature mortality by concentrating on serious hazards that are amenable to reduction at a reasonable cost. For example, irradiation of meat to prevent foodborne infection (a common health hazard) is much more cost-effective than measures to prevent BSE (a rare event).[89] When expensive regulations are seen as lost opportunities, it becomes clearer that the operable trade-off is not "money-for-lives," a choice that understandably generates public concern. Rather, the trade-off is "health-for-health" or "lives-for-lives," because a choice to spend excessively wastes not only dollars but also opportunities to promote health and longevity.

STEP 4: IS THE REGULATION THE LEAST RESTRICTIVE ALTERNATIVE? PERSONAL BURDENS

Public health regulations impose not only economic costs but also human rights burdens. A public health policy may be well designed, cost-effective, and likely to promote the health and well-being of the population, but still be unacceptable from an individual rights perspective. Table 2 (p. 44) lists many of the ways in which public health interventions invade personal rights, such as autonomy, privacy, expression, association, and religion. It also lists many of the ways in which public health regulations interfere with proprietary interests, such as the pursuit of trade and professional opportunities, the value of land or personal property, and commercial interests.

The following chapters offer a more detailed account of these personal rights and freedoms. For now, it is necessary to emphasize the importance of personal burdens in evaluating public health regulations. In each case, public health officials should consider the (1) invasiveness—to what degree does the public health intervention intrude on the right in question? (2) frequency and scope—does the infringement of rights apply to one person, a group, or an entire population? and (3) duration—how long is the person or group subject to the infringement?

Public health agencies should adopt the policy that is most likely to promote health and prevent disease while incurring the fewest possible personal burdens. The least restrictive alternative does not require public health agencies to adopt policies that are less likely to protect the population's health. Rather, health officials should prefer the least intrusive and burdensome policy that achieves their goals as well as, or better than, possible alternatives. For example, if public health officials could control a TB outbreak either with isolation or directly observed therapy (DOT), it should choose DOT because it is less intrusive.

STEP 5: IS THE REGULATION FAIR? JUST DISTRIBUTION OF BENEFITS, BURDENS, AND COSTS

Public health policy allocates benefits, burdens, and costs. Everyone realizes that to achieve the common good, it is sometimes necessary to confer benefits and impose regulatory costs and burdens. The mark of a desirable public health policy is its equitable distribution of benefits, burdens, and costs. But how are we to judge whether these distributions among populations are inherently just? The final step in a systematic evaluation of public health policy is an examination of fairness (see further, the discussion of social justice in chapter 1).

Public health policy conforms to the principle of social justice when, to the extent possible, it provides services to those in need and imposes burdens and costs on those who endanger the public's health.[90] Services provided to those without need are wasteful and, given scarce resources, may deny benefits to those with genuine need. Regulation aimed at persons or businesses where there is no danger imposes costs and burdens without a corresponding public benefit. Ideally, services should be allocated on the basis of need, and burdens imposed only where necessary to prevent a serious health risk.

Another way to think about equitable allocation is to consider the policy's target population. Most policies target a particular population by creating a class of people to which the policy applies. Well-conceived policies should avoid both under- and overinclusiveness (see chapter 4 for the constitutional implications). A policy is underinclusive when it reaches some but not all persons it ought to reach. Thus, a policy is underinclusive if government provides services to only a subgroup of those in need or if it regulates only a subgroup of those who are dangerous. By itself, underinclusion is not necessarily a problem because government may tackle a public health problem gradually or in stages. For example, STI counseling and education targeted to high-prevalence urban areas but not rural communities simply reflects reasonable government priorities. However, certain kinds of underinclusiveness mask discrimination, such as when government exercises coercive powers against politically powerless groups (e.g., the homeless, prisoners, or sex workers) but not others who engage in similar behavior.

A policy is overinclusive if it extends to more people than necessary to achieve its purposes. The policy unnecessarily benefits or penalizes a group of people. Overinclusiveness with regard to services is not cost-effective, because some people receiving services are not in need. Overinclusiveness with regard to coercive regulation unnecessarily imposes economic costs and human rights burdens by penalizing persons who pose no health risk. Consider a policy that prohibits all physicians with a bloodborne infection from practicing medicine. The policy penalizes an entire class, even though most physicians in the class pose virtually no risk to patients.

In summary, public health officials should justify regulation by demonstrating a significant risk, the intervention's effectiveness, reasonableness of economic costs and human rights burdens, and fundamental fairness. This proposed evaluation will not invariably lead to the best policy, because any analysis is fraught with judgments about politics and values and is confounded by scientific uncertainty. Nevertheless, the proposed criteria at least require systematic thought and consistent standards. I conclude this examination of regulation by examining two governance principles for public health policymakers: transparency and precaution.

"TRANSPARENCY": A PRINCIPLE OF GOOD PUBLIC HEALTH GOVERNANCE

> Transparency is a value? Five years ago, that idea would have been incomprehensible, like saying, "one of our values is suede." The transparency metaphor is inexact. It is not that people should be able to see right through you. It is that they should be able to see through to the real you.
>
> Michael Kinsley (2005)

> The right to search for truth . . . implies also a duty: one must not conceal any part of what one has recognized to be true.
>
> Albert Einstein (1954)

It is often said that when government operates in all of its spheres, it should do so transparently, and this is certainly true in the case of public health.[91] What do scholars mean when they urge transparency, and why is the principle important in public health? Transparency, literally truthfulness and openness to view, has no fixed meaning, but most definitions include the following overlapping features: open governance, free flow of information, civic participation, and public accountability.[92]

Open Governance. Open forms of deliberation and decision making are central characteristics of transparent government.[93] The relevant publics (e.g., those with a stake in the decision as well as the more generally interested public) should understand the factors that go into making a decision or rule: (1) the facts and evidence that support the judgment (e.g., the strength of the science); (2) the goals of the intervention (the specific public goods expected to emerge); (3) the steps taken to safeguard individual rights (e.g., methods to safeguard privacy); (4) the reasons for the decision (honest disclosure of relevant justifications); and (5) the procedures for appealing or revising decisions (fair processes to hear challenges by stakeholders).[94] Open governance may be accomplished in many ways, including open forums with advance notification to the public, publication of regulatory proposals in a public register, and the right of citizens to make verbal and written comments.

Free Flow of Information. Public health officials should fairly and honestly disclose relevant information to the public, including written documents, oral communications, and data. Citizens should have access to public health officials, the right to request and receive information, and input into decision-making and rule-making processes. Public health officials should also have affirmative and ongoing obligations to keep the community informed about data and actions that affect their lives. For example, agencies have a responsibility to fully and honestly disclose aggregate health data relevant to the causes, incidence, and prevalence of injuries and diseases in a community. Rarely, it may be ethically justifiable to limit disclosure of some information for a period of time—to safeguard personal privacy (e.g., medical record disclosure), protect vulnerable communities (e.g., negative effects of data about sensitive topics, such as STIs, substance abuse, or suicide), and defend national security (e.g., a credible threat of bioterrorism).

Civic Participation. Open deliberation and free flows of information are necessary to support public participation in public health governance. Public health officials should encourage the input of interested parties in the formulation of policy. Listening to citizens' concerns is an expression of an agency's commitment to fairness and justice. Civic participation also gives citizens a stake in their own health so that they can take responsibility for their behavior and provide support to members of their community.[95]

Public Accountability. Transparent government is accountable to the electorate. This certainly occurs through a democratic process as the public considers public health policies at the ballot box. However, public accountability goes beyond elections. It comes from checks and balances among the three branches of government. Thus, public health officials are politically accountable to the chief executive, must act within the scope of legislative authority, and are subject to judicial oversight. Public accountability also comes from having to justify governmental decisions to the public generally and affected communities in particular. Finally, public accountability comes from protection of "whistle-blowers"—people within agencies who speak out about illegal, improper, or secretive conduct.[96] Since the public cannot know when public officials are concealing important information, it is imperative to encourage insiders to reveal matters of public concern.

Transparency is important to public health governance because of its intrinsic value and its capacity to improve decision making. Citizens gain a sense of satisfaction by participating in policymaking and having their voices heard. Even if government decides that personal interests must yield to common needs, the individual feels acknowledged if she is listened to and her values are taken into account. Transparency also has instrumental value because it provides a feedback mechanism—a way of informing public policy and arriving at more considered judgments. Open forms of governance engender and sustain public trust, which benefits the public health enterprise more generally.[97]

Despite its undoubted value, transparency may be hard to achieve in the real world of politics. How do we know when public officials are simply feigning transparency—making it look as if they were open and fair? The reasons given for their decisions may simply be "spin," which is becoming ubiquitous in our democracy. "The whole point of spin is opacity: a no-see-through skin of your own design between the real you and the outside world."[98] And though officials may hold open meetings, how do we know they are not unduly influenced by economically powerful special interests acting behind the scenes—for example, large industries making profits from selling oil, tobacco, firearms, or even pharmaceuticals? It is for these reasons that citizens should not become complacent about transparency but should insist that public health officials adhere to the literal meaning of the term—truth and openness.

THE "PRECAUTIONARY PRINCIPLE": ACTING UNDER CONDITIONS OF SCIENTIFIC UNCERTAINTY

> Where there are threats of serious or irreversible damage, lack of full scientific certainty shall not be used as a reason for postponing cost-effective measures to prevent environmental degradation.
>
> Rio Declaration (1992)

> A clear distinction should be made between what is not found by science and what is found to be non-existent

> by science. What science finds to be non-existent, we must accept as non-existent; but what science merely does not find is a completely different matter. . . . It is quite clear that there are many, many mysterious things.
>
> His Holiness the Dalai Lama (1999)

If there is one article of faith in public health, it is that policy should be based on objective and rigorous scientific methodologies. If public health is not grounded in science, its utility is diminished and its legitimacy tarnished. But what if society faces hazards that are not fully understood but require that action be taken? That is, what principle should guide public health decision making under conditions of scientific uncertainty? Many of public health's most pressing judgments have to be made with incomplete knowledge.

The SARS outbreaks in 2003, for example, brought public health professionals back to a "pretherapeutic" era. There was no definitive test for the SARS corona virus, no vaccine, and no treatment. Even the modes and efficiency of transmission of infection were poorly understood. The widespread use of ancient methods, such as border screenings, travel advisories, and quarantine, were assumed but not known to be effective.[99] Indeed, although it was widely believed that these measures brought the outbreaks under control, researchers have subsequently questioned whether some were effective at all.[100]

What is the appropriate course of action in the face of scientific uncertainty?[101] The public health community sometimes advocates use of the "precautionary principle" for risk management.[102] The precautionary principle stipulates an obligation to protect populations against reasonably foreseeable threats, even under conditions of uncertainty.[103] The idea is intended to convey not passivity but rather active social "foresight," stimulating planning, innovation, and sustainability.[104] The four components of the precautionary principle are these: Apply preventive action in the face of uncertainty, shift the burden of proof to the proponent of an activity, explore a wide range of alternatives to possibly harmful actions, and increase public participation in decision making.[105]

First articulated in environmental policy, the precautionary principle seeks to forestall disasters and guide decision making in the context of insufficient data. Given the potential costs of inaction, the failure to implement preventive measures requires justification. Proponents of the precautionary principle explicitly defend their position by noting that entities which threaten the environment are best able to bear the burdens of regulation.[106] Opponents warn that the imposition of regulatory burdens may stifle economic progress and scientific innovation, perhaps even perverting risk assessments.[107]

Arguably, the precautionary principle should apply to environmental hazards to human health (e.g., toxic exposures and unsanitary conditions) and to ecosystems (e.g., burning fossil fuels leading to global warming). In such cases, the rationale is that businesses should not place their economic interests above the community's interests in health and the environment. The precautionary principle has not been explicitly invoked in the context of epidemic threats, however, where preemptive actions may burden individuals and impose limits on their freedom (e.g., mandatory testing, reporting, and quarantine). It is one thing to restrict economic freedom in the environmental context and quite another to restrict personal freedom in the infectious disease context. This still leaves a hard problem when public health officials are charged with limiting or forestalling serious health hazards such as epidemic outbreaks.[108]

There is no way to avoid the dilemmas posed by acting without full scientific knowledge. Failure to move aggressively can have catastrophic consequences. Actions that prove to have been unnecessary will be viewed as draconian and based on hysteria. The only safeguard is transparency. Public health agencies must be willing to make clear the bases for restrictive measures and openly acknowledge when new evidence warrants reconsideration of policies. Public health decisions will reflect in a profound way the manner in which societies both implicitly and explicitly balance values that are intimately related and inherently in tension.

Having considered the meaning, values, and scope of public health law, as well as the criteria for evaluating public health interventions, I now turn to the legal foundations of the field. In Part 2, I examine the constitutional design, constitutional limits on public health powers, administrative law, indirect regulation through the tort system, and the increasing importance of international law in safeguarding global health.

PART TWO

Law and the Public's Health

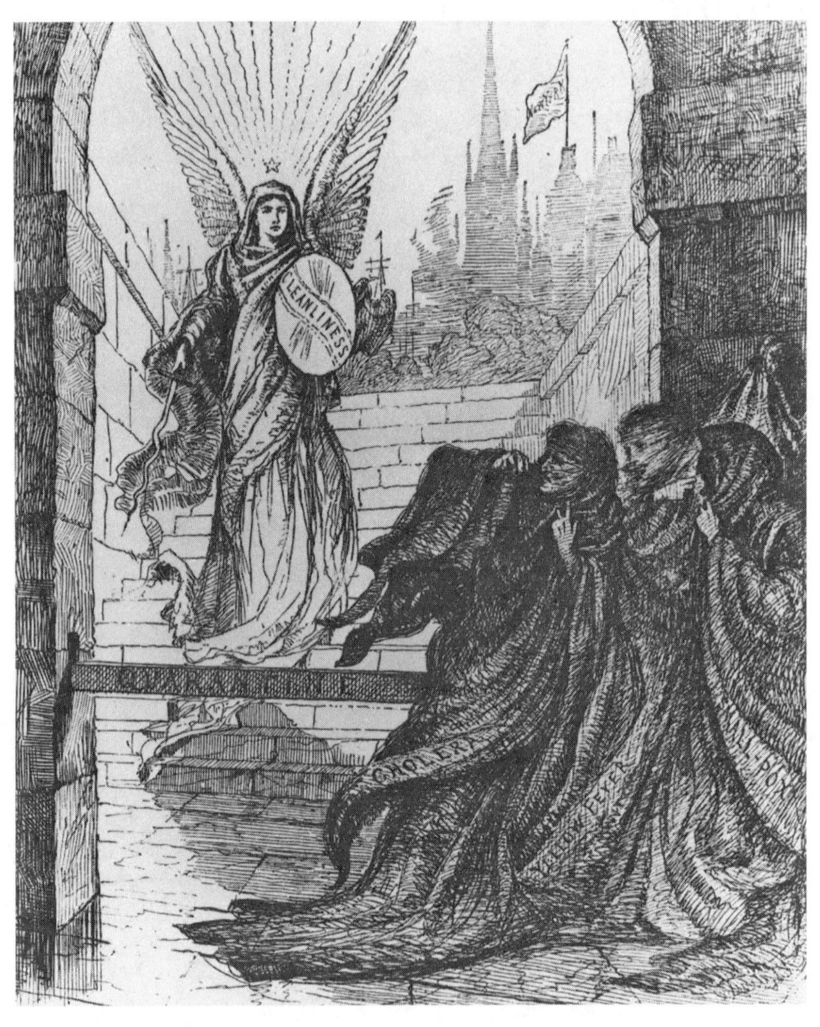

Photo 5. Print showing an angel defending New York City against the cholera epidemic. This print, entitled "At the gates—our safety depends on official vigilance," comes from an 1885 issue of *Harper's Weekly*. The angel holds a shield at the port of New York, defending the city against cholera, yellow fever, and smallpox. Courtesy of the National Library of Medicine.

CHAPTER 3

Public Health Law in the Constitutional Design

Public Health Powers and Duties

No inquiry is more important to public health law than understanding the role of government in the constitutional design. If, as I argue in chapter 1, public health law principally addresses government's assurance of the conditions for the population's health, then what activities must government undertake? The question is complex, requiring an assessment of duty (what government must do), authority (what government is empowered but not obligated to do), and limits (what government is prohibited from doing). In addition, this query raises a corollary question: Which government is to act? Some of the most divisive disputes in public health take place among the federal government, tribal governments, the states, and the localities regarding which government has the power to intervene.[1]

Legal reasoning in public health embraces constitutional doctrine, legislation, regulation, and common law. This chapter and the next view public health through the lens of constitutional law by exploring government duty and power, the division of powers under our federal system, and the limits on government power. I begin with a general discussion of constitutional functions and their application to public health.

CONSTITUTIONAL FUNCTIONS AND THEIR APPLICATION TO PUBLIC HEALTH

The Constitution serves three primary functions: to allocate power between the federal government and the states (federalism), to divide power among the three branches of government (separation of powers), and to limit government power (protection of individual liberties).[2] These functions are critical to the public's health. The Constitution enables government to act to prevent violence, injury, and disease, and to take measures to promote health. At the same time, the Constitution limits government's power to interfere with a personal sphere of liberty and autonomy. In the realm of public health, then, the Constitution acts as both a fountain and a levee: It originates the flow of power (to preserve the public's health) and curbs that power (to protect individual freedoms).[3]

American Federalism: Reserved Powers and Preemption

> Federal environmental and health rules have historically provided a floor of minimum protection. States, for their part, have led the way on countless matters, from requiring health insurers to cover mammograms to stringently regulating mercury emissions from power plants. So why is the federal government suddenly trying to block state efforts to protect public health—through bureaucratic actions largely outside the public view? The unfortunate result is that big businesses' revenues are being shielded, while protections for consumers and the environment are being stripped away.
>
> Nina Mendelson (2006)

If the Constitution is a fountain from which governmental powers flow, federalism is its foundation or structure.[4] Federalism separates the pool of legislative authority into two tiers of government: federal and state.[5] American federalism, as a precept of constitutional design, preserves the balance of power among national and state authorities (see figure 12).[6]

Theoretically, American federalism grants the national government only limited powers, while the states possess plenary powers. Under the doctrine of enumerated powers, the U.S. Congress is granted certain specific powers. For public health purposes, the chief powers are the power to tax and spend and to regulate interstate commerce. These powers provide Congress with independent authority to raise revenue for public health services and to regulate, both directly and indirectly, private activities that endanger the public's health. The Necessary and Proper Clause in Article I, §8 of the Constitution permits Congress to employ all means reasonably appropriate to achieve the objectives of the enumerated national

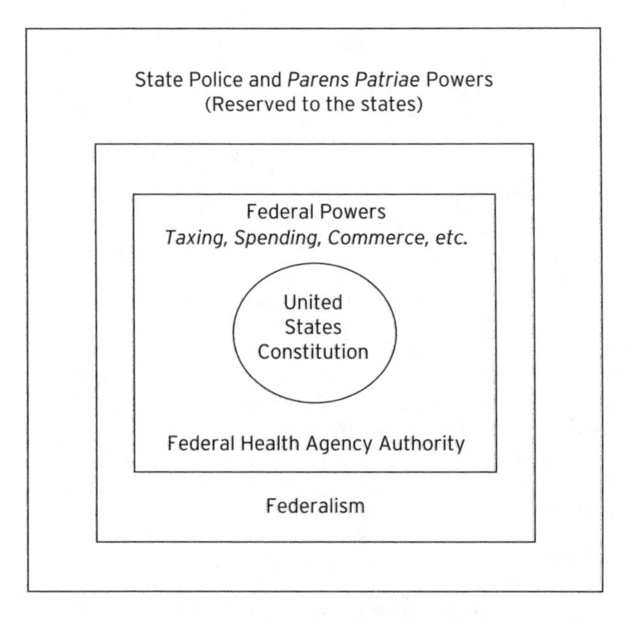

Note: This document represents an overhead view of the principle of federalism. Federal public health powers flow from the U.S. Constitution. Limited federal powers are circumscribed by the source of the constitutional power (e.g., taxing and spending powers and interstate commerce). State governmental powers exist outside the federal sphere (i.e., state police and *parens patriae* powers). Federalism is represented by the solid boundary dividing the pool of governmental powers. This line represents a permeable boundary between federal and state governmental powers. In theory, neither federal nor state powers may impede on one another, but the federal judiciary has often permitted federal public health activities to invade traditional state territory.

Figure 12. Public health and federalism in the constitutional design.

powers.[7] This "implied powers" doctrine has enabled the federal government to expand greatly the network of public health regulation.

The federal government is a government of limited power whose acts must be authorized in the Constitution to be valid. The states, in contrast, retain the power they possessed as sovereign governments before the Constitution was ratified.[8] The Tenth Amendment enunciates the plenary power retained by the states: "The powers not delegated to the United States by the Constitution, nor prohibited by it to the States, are reserved to the States respectively, or to the people."

The "reserved powers" doctrine holds that states may exercise all the powers inherent in government—that is, all the authority necessary to govern that is neither granted to the federal government nor prohibited to the states. Two specific powers—the police power (protecting the

BOX 3

FEDERAL PREEMPTION

Preemption is a rule of law stating that if Congress has enacted legislation on a subject matter, it takes precedence over state or local laws. Federal preemption effectively expands the jurisdiction of Congress to the detriment of states and local governments. Congress's power to preempt state and local laws stems from the Supremacy Clause in the Constitution.

In an *express preemption*, the federal statute explicitly declares that it supersedes state or local law. In an *implied preemption*, the language of the statute and the legislative history make clear Congress's intent to supersede state or local law. Two forms of implied preemption exist: field preemption and conflict preemption. In *field preemption*, the scheme of federal regulation is so pervasive as to make reasonable the inference that Congress left no room for the states to supplement it. As a result, the states may not regulate in that sphere. In *conflict preemption*, compliance with both federal and state regulations is a physical impossibility, or state law stands as an obstacle to the accomplishment and execution of the full congressional objectives.

Congress's purpose in preempting federal law may be to set a minimal standard of protection, leaving states to create stronger protection. Alternatively, the congressional purpose may be to assure national uniformity, severely restricting the ability of states to regulate at all. In most consumer and civil rights legislation (e.g., the Americans with Disabilities Act or the HIPAA Privacy Rule [see chapter 8]), federal law serves as a floor of protections. This "federal floor preemption" only supersedes weaker state laws, and it allows states and local governments to pass stronger laws. Conversely, "federal ceiling preemption" prevents states and other political entities from passing stronger laws. It can act as an effective bar to state and local legislation or enforcement.

health, safety, and morals of the community) and the *parens patriae* power (protecting the interests of minors and incompetent persons)—express the state's inherent sovereignty to safeguard the community's welfare.

Federalism functions as a sorting device for determining which government, federal or state, may legitimately respond to a public health threat. Often, the national and state governments exercise public health powers concurrently. A national, state, and local presence exists in most spheres of public health (e.g., injury prevention, clean air and water, and infectious disease control). Pursuant to the Supremacy Clause, however, conflicts between national and state regulation are resolved in favor of the federal government. The Supremacy Clause, found in Article VI, declares that the "Constitution, and the Laws of the United States . . . and all Treaties made . . . shall be the supreme law of the Land."

By authority of the Supremacy Clause, Congress may preempt, or supersede, state public health regulation, even if the state is acting squarely within its police powers.[9] Federal preemption may seem like an arcane doctrine, but it has powerful consequences for the public's health and

BOX 4

FEDERALISM: NATIONAL, STATE, AND LOCAL PUBLIC HEALTH FUNCTIONS

The arguments for and against the centralization of political power have remained largely the same over the course of American history, and are part of entrenched political ideologies.[1] Amelioration of ill health arises at every level of governmental intervention. Rigid ideological preferences for particular units can undermine just and effective public health policy. The government best situated for dealing with public health threats depends on the evidence identifying the nature and origin of the specific threat, the resources available to each unit for addressing the problem, and the probability of strategic success.

National Obligations

The national government has a duty to create the capacity to undertake essential public health services. A national commitment to capacity-building is important because public needs for health and well-being are universal and compelling. Certain problems demand national attention. The health threat may span many states, regions, or the whole country, as in the case of epidemic disease or environmental pollution. Further, the solution may be beyond the jurisdiction of individual states, as in problems related to foreign or interstate commerce. Finally, states simply may not have the expertise or resources to mount an effective response in a public health emergency such as a natural disaster, bioterrorism, or an emerging disease. For example, constructing levees to stem floodwaters or rebuilding cities devastated by a category 4 or 5 hurricane is beyond the capacity of any single city or state.

State and Local Obligations

Armed with sufficient resources and tools, states and localities have an obligation to fulfill core public health functions. States and localities are closer to the people and to the problems causing ill health. Delivering public health services requires local knowledge, civic engagement, and direct political accountability. States and localities are also often the preferable unit of government when dealing with complex, poorly understood problems. In such cases, the idea of a "laboratory of the states" enables local officials to seek innovative solutions.

Filling Public Health Policy Vacuums

Government at all levels has a duty to fill conspicuous vacuums in public health policy. If a particular unit of government fails to act in a sphere of high health importance, other units must fill the void. Federal intervention in civil rights was necessary precisely because states neglected this responsibility. Today, states are acting in the areas of the environment, food safety, occupational safety, and minimum wage because the federal government has pulled back.[2] California's vehicle emissions standard for greenhouse gases (which several other states are adopting) is a prime illustration. The automobile industry, supported by the Bush administration, litigated to bar implementation of these state regulations, claiming the need for national uniformity. However, these pending cases were undermined by a recent Supreme Court decision in *Massachusetts v. EPA*, which held that the Environmental Protection Agency has the authority to issue automobile emission standards based on policy considerations not

[1] Deborah Stone, *Policy Paradox: The Art of Political Decision Making* (New York: W.W. Norton, 1997): 351-72 (arguing that federalism debates are about empowering some people at the expense of others rather than about the effectiveness of the resulting policies).

[2] Lawrence O. Gostin, "The Supreme Court's Impact on Medicine and Health: The Rehnquist Court, 1986-2005," *JAMA*, 294 (2005): 1685-87.

enumerated in the Clean Air Act.[3] In this landmark decision, the Court did not force the EPA to regulate auto emissions, but did strongly suggest that a failure to act could only be justified by the agency's scientific determination that "greenhouse gases do not contribute to climate change."[4] The decision was viewed as a strong rebuke of the Bush administration's unwillingness to issue stringent automobile emission regulations. In an opinion by Justice Stevens, the Court explained that "EPA has offered no reasoned explanation for its refusal to decide whether greenhouse gases cause or contribute to climate change. Its action was therefore 'arbitrary, capricious . . . or otherwise not in accordance with the law.'"[5]

Harmonized Engagement

A system of overlapping and shared responsibility among federal, state, and local governments will most often be required. The root causes of ill health arise as a consequence of policy choices at all levels. Poor health is a function of many things, including education, income policy, environmental exposure, public sanitation, and access to health care. Government at all levels has responsibility to differing degrees. This insight was illustrated poignantly during the response to the Gulf Coast hurricanes in 2005. It is not that a particular political unit (federal, state, or local) should have had primacy. Rather, each should have played a unique role in a well-coordinated effort.

3 *Massachusetts v. EPA*, 127 S. Ct. 1438 (2007). Also see *Environmental Defense v. Duke Energy*, 127 S. Ct. 1423 (2007), a companion case that held a similarly broad view of the EPA's authority to regulate factories and power plants that produce air pollutants.

4 *Id.* at 1463.

5 *Id.*

safety. The Supreme Court's preemption decisions can effectively foreclose meaningful state regulation and bar persons from suing for their injuries.[10] Preemption has had antiregulatory effects in fields ranging from tobacco control,[11] occupational health and safety,[12] and motor vehicle safety[13] to employer health care plans[14] and pharmaceutical regulation.[15] Indeed, from 2001 to 2006, Congress enacted twenty-seven statutes that preempt state health, safety, and environmental regulations or other social policy.[16] This demonstrates the potentially broad sweep of federal supremacy that enables Congress to override state public health safeguards (see box 3).[17]

American federalism, then, ensures limited powers to national authorities and plenary powers to the states. However, federal constitutional authority is far-reaching, and where it has the power, congressional action trumps state public health regulation. (For a discussion of the various strengths of each level of government in matters of public health, see box 4.)

Separation of Powers

In addition to establishing a federalist system, the Constitution creates a national government, dividing power among three branches. Article I vests all legislative powers in the Congress of the United States; Article II vests executive power in the president of the United States; and Article III vests judicial power in one supreme court and in such inferior courts as the Congress may establish. The states, pursuant to their own constitutions, have adopted similar schemes of governance. This separation of powers provides a system of checks and balances, where no single branch of government can act without some degree of oversight and control by another, thereby reducing the possibility of government oppression (see figure 13).

The separation of powers doctrine is essential to public health, for each branch of government possesses a unique constitutional authority to create, enforce, or interpret health policy. The legislature creates health policy and allocates the resources necessary to effect it. Some commentators contend that legislators are ill equipped to make complex public health decisions: Legislators often fail to dwell sufficiently or carefully enough on any single issue to gather the facts and consider the implications; they characteristically lack expertise in the health sciences; and they are influenced by popular beliefs that may be uninformed, prejudicial, or both. Yet the legislature, as the only "purely" elected branch of government, is politically accountable to the people. If the legislature enacts an ineffective or overly intrusive policy, the electorate has a remedy at the ballot box. In addition, legislatures are responsible for balancing public health services with competing claims—say, for tax relief, national defense, transportation, and education.

The executive branch enforces health policy but has come to occupy a far greater role in modern America. Most of the influential public health agencies reside in the executive branch—for example, the Department of Health and Human Services at the federal level and public health departments at the state and local levels (see chapter 5). Executive agencies have far-reaching responsibilities on matters of health. Although the legislature establishes general policy goals, agencies frequently devise a network of rules and conduct detailed oversight and enforcement. The executive branch possesses many attributes for effectively governing public health: Agencies are created for the very purpose of advancing the public's health within their jurisdiction; agencies focus on the same set of problems for extended periods of time; and agency officials possess specific expertise and have the resources to gather facts, develop theories, and generate policy alternatives. Agency officials are not elected, however, and the long tenure in office of nonpolitical civil servants can result in stale thinking and complicity with the subjects of regulation. In

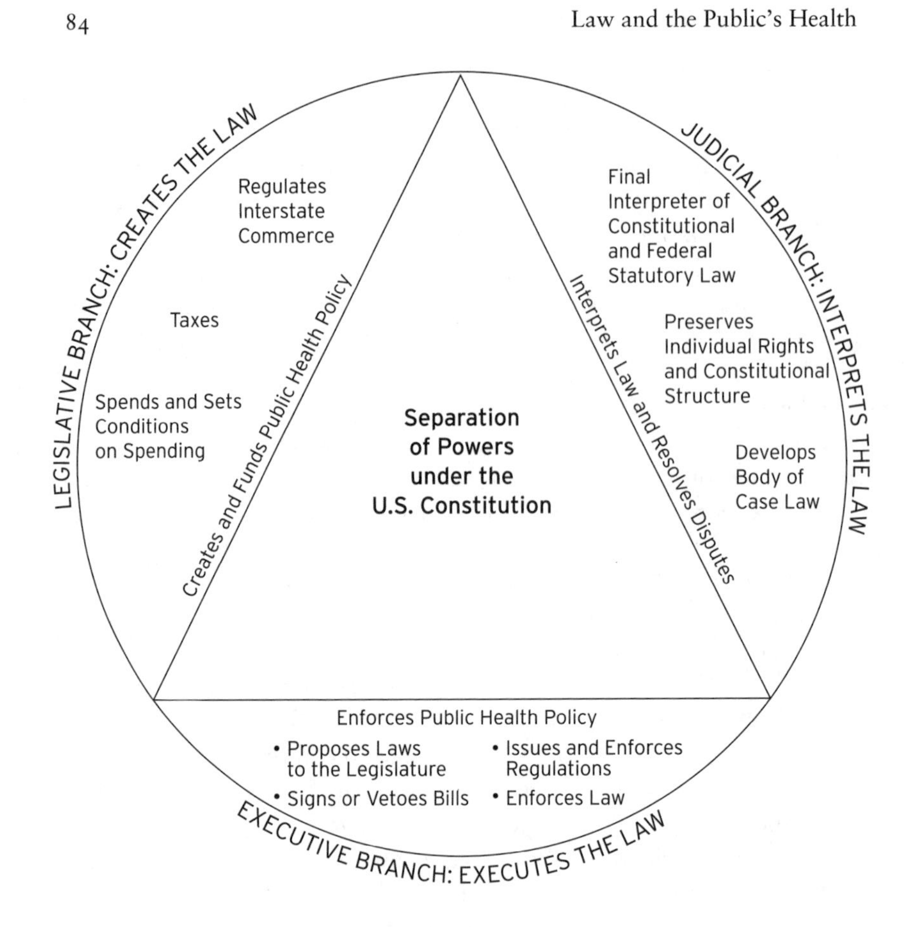

Figure 13. Separation of powers under the U.S. Constitution.

addition, they are not positioned politically to balance competing values and claims for resources.

The judiciary's task is to interpret laws and resolve legal disputes. These may appear to be sterile pursuits, devoid of much policy influence, but the courts' role in public health is actually quite broad. Increasingly, the courts have exerted substantial control over public health policy by determining the boundaries of government power. The judiciary erects a zone of autonomy, privacy, and liberty to be afforded to individuals, and economic freedoms to be afforded to businesses. The courts decide whether a public health statute is constitutional, whether agency action is authorized by legislation, whether agency officials have marshaled sufficient evidence to support their actions, and whether government officials and private parties have acted negligently. The judicial branch has the independence and legal training to make thoughtful decisions about constitutional claims regarding, for example, federalism or individual rights. Courts, however, may be less equipped to review critically the substance of health policy choices: Judges may be less politically accountable,[18] are bound by the facts of a particular case, may be influenced by expert opinion that is unrepresentative of mainstream public health thought, and may focus too intently on individual rights at the expense of communal claims to public health protection (or vice versa).[19]

Is it possible to conclude from this brief discussion which branch of government, if any, is best suited for formulating and executing public health policy?[20] Public health practitioners from time to time lament the influence wielded by legislators and judges in matters of public health. They claim that legislation and adjudication are time-consuming and costly endeavors, legislators and judges are not trained or experienced in the sciences of public health, and legislatures devote insufficient resources to the public health infrastructure.[21] Yet the separation of powers doctrine does not aspire to achieve maximum efficiency or even the best result in public health governance. Rather, the constitutional design appears to value restraint in policymaking: Elected officials reconcile demands for public health funding with competing claims for societal resources, the executive branch straddles the line between congressional authorization and judicial restrictions on that authority, and the judiciary tempers public health measures with its focus on individual rights. As a society, we forgo the possibility of bold public health governance by any given branch in exchange for constitutional checks and balances that prevent overreaching and ensure political accountability.

Limited Powers

A third constitutional function is to limit government power for the purpose of protecting individual liberties. When government acts to promote the communal good, it frequently infringes upon the rights and freedoms of individuals and businesses. For example, isolation and quarantine restrict liberty; cigarette advertising restrictions limit free expression; bathhouse closures constrain free association; and product regulation impedes economic freedom. Consequently, public health and individual rights conflict, at least to some extent; efforts to promote the common welfare may compel a trade-off with personal and proprietary interests.

Protection of "rights" is commonly regarded as the Constitution's most important function. The Constitution grants extensive government power but curtails it as well. The Bill of Rights (the first ten amendments to the Constitution), together with other constitutional provisions, creates a zone of individual liberty, autonomy, privacy, and economic freedom that exists beyond the reach of the government. The Framers believed, moreover, that people retain rights not specified in the Constitution. The Ninth Amendment states, "The enumeration in the Constitution, of certain rights, shall not be construed to deny or disparage others retained by the people." Although the Supreme Court has rarely interpreted the Ninth Amendment as granting an independent source of rights, some scholars argue that the Framers intended to protect "natural rights."[22]

The constitutional design, then, is one where government is afforded ample power to safeguard the common weal but is prohibited from exercising it to trample individual rights. The constant quest of students of public health law is to determine the point at which government authority to promote the population's health should yield to individual rights claims. Put another way, to what degree should individuals forgo freedom to achieve improved health, a higher quality of life, and enhanced safety for the community? Much of the remainder of this book strives to answer that question.

THE NEGATIVE CONSTITUTION: THE ABSENCE OF GOVERNMENT'S DUTY TO PROTECT HEALTH AND SAFETY

> Poor Joshua! Victim of repeated attacks by an irresponsible, bullying, cowardly, and intemperate father, and abandoned by respondents who placed him in a dangerous predicament and who knew or learned what was going on, and yet did essentially nothing except, as the Court revealingly observes, "dutifully recorded these incidents in [their] files." It is a sad commentary upon American life, and constitutional principles—so full of late of patriotic fervor and proud proclamations about "liberty and justice for all"—that this child, Joshua DeShaney, now is assigned to live out the remainder of his life profoundly retarded.
>
> Justice Blackmun (1989)

Individuals rely on government to organize social and economic life to promote healthy and safe populations. Given the importance of government in maintaining the public's health and safety (and many other communal benefits), one might expect the Constitution to create affirmative obligations to act. Although the Constitution does require government to take action in narrow circumstances, such as a right to an attorney in a criminal trial,[23] the Constitution is cast in largely negative terms.[24] Most of the Bill of Rights places restraints on state action; for example, the First Amendment declares that government may not abridge the freedom of speech. The Constitution does not provide a general affirmative state obligation to provide services or to protect people from harm.

There are two exceptions to the "no duty to protect" rule.[25] First, the government has a duty to a person placed in a custodial setting such as a prison[26] or mental institution[27] who, by reason of the deprivation of liberty, is unable to care for himself.[28] The state must provide humane conditions of confinement, including adequate food, clothing, shelter, medical care, and protection from violence.[29] Second, the government has an obligation to protect a person if the state increased the threat of harm so that it is responsible for creating the danger.[30] Many such cases have tragic facts involving government officials acting with deliberate indifference to the health and safety of vulnerable people.[31]

The Supreme Court remains faithful to a negative conception of the Constitution, even in the face of dire personal consequences.[32] In *DeShaney v. Winnebago County Department of Social Services* (1989), a state court granted a divorce and awarded custody of a one-year-old child, Joshua DeShaney, to his father. Two years later, county social workers in Wisconsin began receiving reports that Joshua's father was physically abusing him. The suspicious injuries were carefully noted, but the Department of Social Services took no action. Eventually, at four years of age, Joshua was beaten so badly that he suffered permanent brain injuries. He was left profoundly retarded and institutionalized. The *DeShaney* Court found no government obligation to protect children from harm of which the state is acutely aware. The Court held that, since no affirmative government duty to protect exists, citizens have no constitutional remedy.[33]

The Supreme Court has applied this line of reasoning in cases that bitterly divided the Court and the nation. In *Webster v. Reproductive Health Services* (1989),[34] the majority saw no government obligation to provide services—in this case, medical services—for the poor[35] when a Missouri statute barred state employees from performing abortions and banned the use of public facilities for such procedures. Referring to *DeShaney,* the Court rejected a positive claim for basic government services: "Our cases have recognized that the Due Process Clause generally confers no affirmative right to governmental aid, even where such aid may be necessary to secure life, liberty, or property interests of which the government itself may not deprive the individual."[36] According to the Court, if "no state subsidy, direct or indirect, is available, it is difficult to see how any procreational choice is burdened by the State's ban on the use of its facilities or employees for performing abortions."[37] The majority found irrelevant the fact that, if a woman is poor, her only realistic access to medical services may be through government assistance.

Procedural Due Process: Domestic Abuse Orders

> NOTICE TO LAW ENFORCEMENT OFFICIALS: You shall use every reasonable means to enforce this restraining order. You shall arrest, or, if an arrest would be impractical under the circumstances, seek a warrant for the arrest of the restrained person when you have information amounting to probable cause that the restrained person has violated or attempted to violate any provision of this order and the restrained person has been properly served with a copy of this order or has received actual notice of the existence of this order.
>
> Colorado Judicial Protective Order
> (quoted in *Castle Rock*, 2005)

The Supreme Court based its decisions in *DeShaney* and *Webster* on the Fourteenth Amendment Substantive Due Process Clause. The Court declined to address the claim that victims may have a *procedural* due process right of protection against private violence. In *Castle Rock v. Gonzales*, the Supreme Court held that state law requiring the police to enforce domestic abuse restraining orders does not confer the type of entitlement required to establish a property interest protected by the Procedural Due Process Clause. The case is based on a set of heart-wrenching facts, and bears important public health and constitutional implications.

Simon Gonzales, who had a history of erratic and suicidal behavior, violated a restraining order by abducting his three young daughters. His estranged wife, Jessica Gonzales, made repeated pleas to the police to enforce the restraining order, but to no avail. Nearly eight hours after she first contacted police, her husband opened fire on the police station with a semiautomatic handgun he had purchased after abducting his daughters. He was fatally shot, and police found the bodies of the three young girls, who had been murdered by their father, in the cab of his truck.

By framing her case as one of process rather than substance, Ms. Gonzales sought to circumvent the holding in *DeShaney.* But the Court saw little difference between the two cases. Under Supreme Court precedent, Ms. Gonzales was "deprived of property" warranting due process protection only if she had an "entitlement" to police enforcement of the restraining order.[38] Justice Scalia, writing for the majority, said that the arrest of a person who violates a protective order is discretionary, so there was no entitlement.[39]

The idea that police enforcement of restraining orders was discretionary in Colorado is a strained interpretation of state law. The Colorado statute declares that a peace officer "shall" arrest a person who violates a restraining order. The protective order itself had "NOTICE TO LAW ENFORCEMENT OFFICIALS" in large block letters, as shown in the epigraph, requiring them to arrest the restrained person should they have probable cause. The Court of Appeals in *Castle Rock* stressed that the restraining order "specifically dictated that its terms must be enforced" and a state statute commanded enforcement.[40] If the state had promised its eligible citizens a service (e.g., education) or a benefit (e.g., Medicaid), there clearly would be an "entitlement."[41] Police protection against violence is just as valuable as any other government service or benefit. Property rights should extend beyond ownership of real estate, chattels, or money.[42]

The state, through its statutes and enforcement procedures, in effect made an unambiguous promise to protect women and children subject to domestic violence. That was a promise that Ms. Gonzales relied on, yet the Court held there was no deprivation of life, liberty, or property under the Due Process Clause of the Fourteenth Amendment. The Supreme Court made it clear that the Constitution does not offer vulnerable people a remedy, even in the face of the direst need.

The Duty to Protect from a Public Health Perspective

In *DeShaney, Webster,* and *Castle Rock,* the judiciary has disavowed the idea of positive social rights by finding that the Constitution rarely affords affirmative obligations but principally negative liberties; government inaction is constitutionally immaterial, and government's failure to act brings no constitutional remedy. This negative theory of constitutional design is oversimplified and, in the words of Justice Blackmun, represents "a sad commentary upon American life and constitutional principles."[43] The U.S. Supreme Court has taken a position at odds with international human rights. The European Court of Human Rights, in cases strikingly similar to *DeShaney* and *Castle Rock,* has emphasized that the state's obligation to protect its citizens from harm is a fundamentally important governmental activity.[44]

A weakness of the negative theory of constitutional law is that its distinctions, as between action and inaction, are difficult to sustain.[45] The Supreme Court has repeatedly held that a government act that causes harm is actionable, while government passivity in an existing state of affairs is not. Although the Court appears to know instinctively what constitutes a governmental act, the difference between an act and an omission is often difficult to determine. Any government failure to act is usually embedded in a series of affirmative policy choices (e.g., which agency will be established; what the agency's objectives are and how its staff will be trained; what resources, if any, will be devoted to certain problems). When government deliberately chooses to intervene (or to allocate scarce resources) in one sphere and conspicuously fails to perform in another, can that fairly be characterized as "inaction"?

Another problem with the negative constitution is that citizens rely on the protective umbrella of the state. When the state establishes an agency to detect and prevent spousal or child abuse (or to prevent any other cause of injury or disease), it promises, at least implicitly, that it will respond in case of obvious threats to health. If an agency represents itself to the public as a defender of health and safety, and citizens justifiably rely on that protection, is government "responsible" when it knows that a substantial risk exists, fails to inform citizens so they might initiate action, and passively avoids a state response to that risk?

Finally, judicial refusal to examine government's failure to act, irrespective of the circumstances, leaves the state free to abuse its power and cause harm to citizens. Government more often exerts its power, and its potential to harm, by withholding services in the face of obvious threats to health.[46] The state's neglect of the poor and vulnerable, its calculated failure to respond to obvious risk, or its arbitrary or discriminatory enforcement of public health law is a certain, and direct, cause of harm. Professors Seidman and Tushnet suggest that the Fourteenth Amendment's historical purpose is consistent with the view that "the state is inflicting . . . deprivation [of life, liberty, or property] when officials organize their activities so that people fall prey to private violence."[47] A constitutional rule, moreover, that punishes government misfeasance (when the state intentionally or negligently causes harm) but not nonfeasance (when the state simply does not act) provides an incentive to withhold services and interventions. The rule requiring an affirmative state act as a prior condition for judicial review offers an uninspired vision of the Constitution.

STATE AND LOCAL POWER TO ENSURE THE CONDITIONS FOR THE PUBLIC'S HEALTH: *SALUS POPULI EST SUPREMA LEX*

The states and localities have had the predominant public responsibility for population-based health services since the founding of the republic. Early public health law employed a legal maxim that embodied the intrinsic purposes of a sovereign government: *Salus populi est suprema lex*, the welfare of the people is the supreme law.[48] *Salus populi* demonstrates the close connection between state power and historic understandings of the public's well-being. From a constitutional perspective, there exist historic wellsprings of state authority to protect the common good: the police power to protect the public's health, safety, and morals, and the *parens patriae* power to defend the interests of persons unable to secure their own interests.

Police Powers: Regulation for Health, Safety, and Morals: Sic Utere Tuo ut Alienum non Laedas

> Of OFFENCES against the PUBLIC HEALTH, and the PUBLIC POLICE or ŒCONOMY. [A] species of offences, more especially affecting the commonwealth, are such as are against the public health of the nation; a concern of the highest importance. . . . By public police and œconomy I mean the due regulation and domestic order of the kingdom: whereby individuals of the state, like members of a well-governed family, are bound to conform their general behaviour to the rules of propriety, good neighbourhood, and good manners; and to be decent, industrious, and inoffensive in their respective stations.
>
> William Blackstone (1769)

The "police power" is the most famous expression of the natural authority of sovereign governments to regulate private interests for the public good (see figure 14). I define police power as:

> The inherent authority of the state (and, through delegation, local government) to enact laws and promulgate regulations to protect, preserve, and promote the health, safety, morals, and general welfare of the people. To achieve these communal benefits, the state retains the power to restrict, within federal and state constitutional limits, private interests—including personal interests in autonomy, privacy, association, and liberty, as well as economic interests in freedom to contract and uses of property.

The linguistic and historical origins of the concept of *police* demonstrate a close association between government and civilization: *politia* (the state), *polis* (the city), and *politeia* (citizenship).[49] *Police* traditionally connoted social organization, civil authority, or formation of a political community—the control and regulation of affairs affecting the general order and welfare of society.[50] Such was the context in which Hamilton used the term in the Federalist Papers, to suggest civil peace and public law.[51] *Police* was meant to describe those powers that permitted sovereign government to control its citizens, particularly for the purpose of promoting the general comfort, health, morals, safety, or prosperity of the public.[52] The word had a secondary usage as well: "cleansing" or "keeping clean." This use resonates with early twentieth-century public health connotations of hygiene and sanitation.

The police power represents the state's authority to further the goal of government: to promote the general welfare of society.[53] States possess the police power as an innate attribute of sovereignty. As sovereign governments before the formation of the United States, the states still retain sovereignty except as surrendered under the Constitution.[54] Part of the constitutional compact of our Union was that states would remain free to govern within the traditional sphere of health, safety, and morals. All states, to a greater or lesser degree, delegate police powers to local government: counties, parishes, cities, towns, or villages.[55]

The definition of *police power* encompasses three principles: The governmental purpose is to promote the public good; the state authority to act permits the restriction of private interests; and the scope of state powers is pervasive.[56] States exercise police powers to ensure that communities live in safety and security, in conditions conducive to good health and with moral standards, and generally speaking, to promote human well-being. Police powers legitimize state action to protect and promote broadly defined social goods.

Government, in order to achieve common goods, is empowered to enact

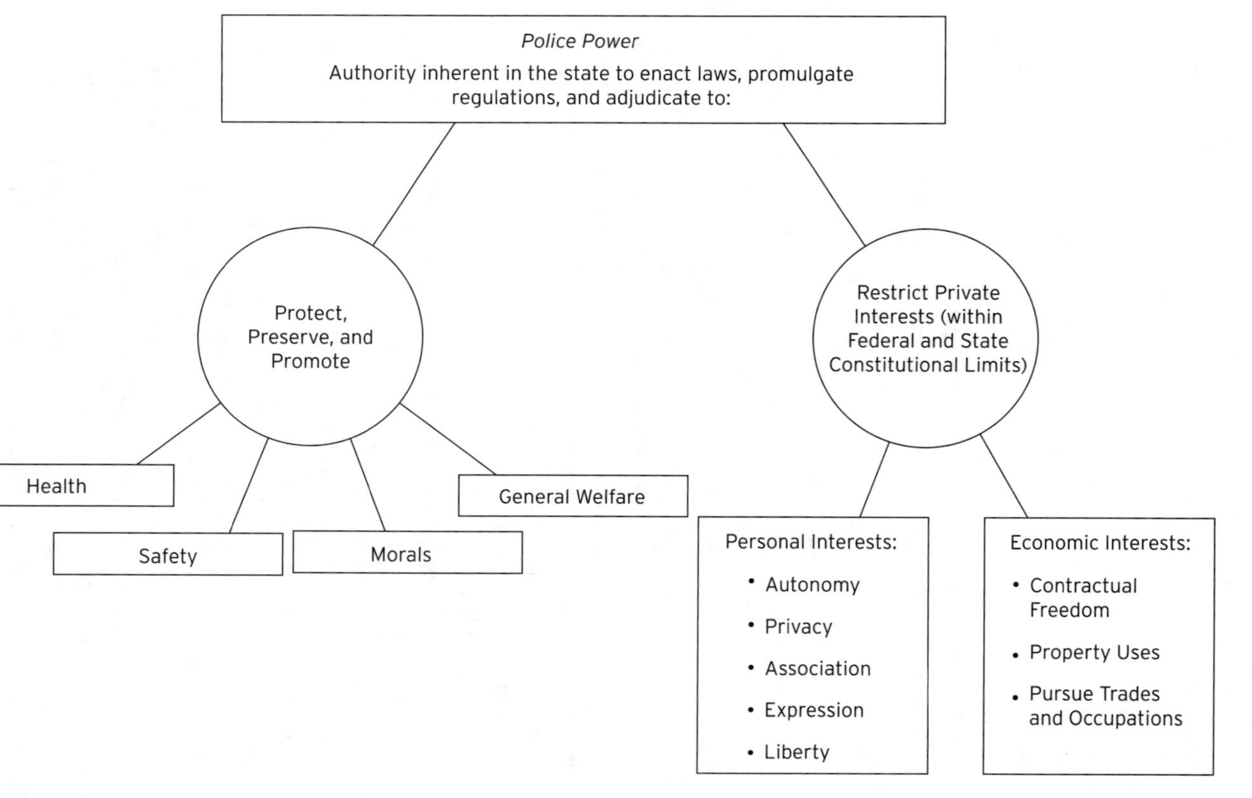

Figure 14. Police power.

legislation, regulate, and adjudicate in ways that necessarily limit private interests. Thus, government has inherent power to interfere with personal interests in autonomy, privacy, association, and liberty, and with economic interests in ownership, use of private property, and freedom to contract. State power to restrict private rights is embodied in the common law maxim *Sic utere tuo ut alienum non laedas*—use your own property in such a manner as not to injure that of another. The maxim supports the police power, giving government authority to determine safe uses of private property to diminish risks to others of injury and ill health.[57] More generally, the police power affords government the authority to keep society free from noxious exercise of private rights. The state retains discretion to determine what is considered injurious or unhealthful and the manner in which to regulate, consistent with constitutional protections of personal interests.

Police powers are so pervasive that they defy orderly or systematic description. The police power evokes images of an organized civil force for maintaining order, preventing and detecting crime, and enforcing criminal laws. But the origins of "police" are deeper and far more textured than notions of basic law enforcement and crime prevention. The police power in early American life, according to Novak, was part of a well-regulated society, a "science and mode of governance where the polity assumed control over, and became implicated in, the basic conduct of social life. . . . No aspect of human intercourse remained outside the purview of police science."[58]

Countless judicial opinions and treatises articulate police powers as a deep well of public authority granted to the body politic.[59] In *Gibbons v. Ogden* (1824), Chief Justice Marshall conceived of police powers as an "immense mass of legislation, which embraces every thing within the territory of a state, not surrendered to the general government. . . . Inspection laws, quarantine laws, health laws of every description . . . are components of this mass."[60] In the *Slaughter-House Cases* (1873), Justice Miller asserted that the police power was preeminent because "upon it depends the security of social order, the life and health of the citizen, the comfort of an existence in a thickly populated community, the enjoyment of private and social life, and the beneficial use of property."[61]

Police powers in the context of public health include all law and regulation directly or indirectly intended to improve morbidity and mortality in the population. Police powers have enabled states and their subsidiary municipal corporations to promote and preserve the public's health in areas ranging from injury and disease prevention[62] to sanitation, waste disposal, and clean water and air.[63] Police powers exercised by the states include vaccination,[64] isolation and quarantine,[65] inspection of commercial and residential premises,[66] abatement of unsanitary conditions or other health nuisances,[67] regulation of air and surface water contaminants and restriction of public access to polluted areas,[68] standards for pure food and drinking water,[69] extermination of vermin,[70] fluoridation of municipal water supplies,[71] and licensure of physicians and other health care professionals.[72]

The courts have often used the police power as a rough sorting device to separate authority rightfully retained by the states from that appropriately exercised by the federal government. If the authority exercised was traditionally part of the corpus of police powers, states, at least presumptively, were thought to have a valid claim of jurisdiction. Although the extent of permissible state public health regulation has not been easy to measure, a state's power is "never greater than in matters traditionally of local concern" to the health and safety of its population.[73] Courts in many contexts, such as the quality of meat,[74] fruits, and vegetables,[75] have emphasized the legitimacy of state authority. Even in assessing express federal preemption, courts acknowledge that police powers are "primarily, and historically, . . . matters of local concern."[76] Thus, the judiciary adopts a presumption that "the historic police powers of the States [are] not to be superseded by the Federal Act unless that is the clear and manifest purpose of Congress."[77]

Parens Patriae *Powers: State Power to Protect Children and Incompetent Persons*

> This prerogative of *parens patriae* is inherent in the Supreme power of every state, whether that power is lodged in a royal person, or in the legislature . . . [and] is a most beneficent function . . . often necessary to be exercised in the interests of humanity, and for the prevention of injury to those who cannot protect themselves.
>
> Joseph P. Bradley (1890)

Parens patriae—literally, parent of the country—refers to the state's role as sovereign and guardian of persons under legal disability (principally minors and incompetent persons).[78] *Parens patriae* powers derive from the Royal Prerogative in England, which arose in the early years of Edward I (1275–1306).[79] The Statute de Prerogativa Regis[80] recognized the existence of the Prerogative and imposed limits on its operation: "The King shall have the custody of the lands of natural fools, taking the profits of them without waste or destruction, and shall find them their necessaries." It was the job of the crown "to take care of people legally unable, on account of mental incapacity, whether it proceed[ed] from 1. nonage 2. idiocy or 3. lunacy: to take proper care of themselves and their property."[81]

In America, the *parens patriae* function belongs to the states, which have the power to protect and care for those who cannot care for themselves. The *parens patriae* power is traditionally invoked in two contexts: to make decisions on behalf of individuals who are incapable of doing so for themselves,[82] and to assert the state's general interest and standing in communal health, comfort, and welfare (see figure 15).[83]

The state, as *parens patriae,* has the authority to protect the welfare of persons who are unable to understand the nature and consequences of their decisions and who require protection in their own interests. The *parens patriae* power is used in diverse contexts, including custody and other decisions relating to children;[84] guardianship over money, property, and personal affairs for incompetent persons;[85] treatment decisions for incompetent or comatose patients;[86] and civil commitment of persons with mental illness.[87]

The exercise of *parens patriae* powers in this individualized context can deprive individuals of autonomy, privacy, and liberty: "An inevitable consequence of exercising the *parens patriae* power is that the ward's personal freedom will be substantially restrained, whether a guardian is appointed to control his property, he is placed in the custody of a private third party, or committed to an institution."[88] Consequently, courts adopt legal standards and processes for decision making to safeguard individuals' interests,[89] and they require fair treatment.[90] Depending upon the circumstance, the legal standards adopted may be either the person's best interests (the decision that would best secure the individual's welfare) or substituted judgment (the decision the person would have made were she competent to decide for herself).[91] Courts also require procedural due process, depending upon the context and the potential burden on individual interests.[92] Because of the potential for diminution of individual rights, then, courts adopt standards and procedures to ensure that the state's *parens patriae* powers, intended to be wielded beneficently, do not inflict harm.

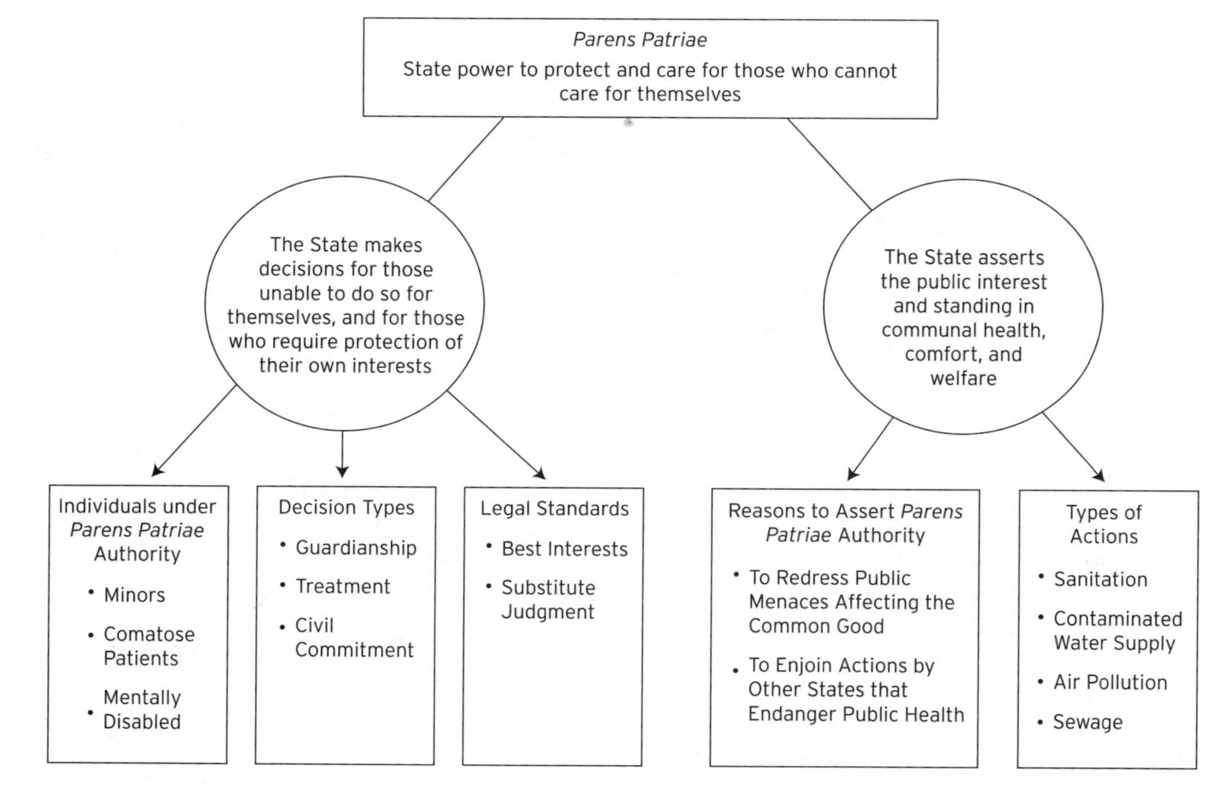

Figure 15. *Parens patriae* power.

Parens Patriae: *A State's Standing to Sue for the Communal Interest*

The *parens patriae* function is asserted not only to protect incompetent individuals but also to safeguard the general community interest in health, welfare, and economic benefit.[93] This meaning of *parens patriae* is quite different from the first; it is a concept used to describe a state's standing or right to sue in court to promote the communal interest. The legal theory is that the state litigates to defend the well-being of its citizens, not to defend the economic interests of the state.[94] Likewise, in situations where a state cannot legislate or institute a regulatory scheme to protect its citizens, it can sue in federal court under the *parens patriae* doctrine to enjoin another state from actions that pose a threat to health or welfare (e.g., where polluted water from another state threatens the health of its citizens).[95] At the turn of the century, the Supreme Court accepted this understanding of the *parens patriae* power in a quarantine case,[96] setting in motion a chain of litigation dealing with matters of public health: sanitation,[97] water supply,[98] air pollution,[99] and sewage.[100]

The state's ultimate goal in utilizing *parens patriae* is to protect individuals who are unable to protect themselves. For example, the state of New York sued to redress the denial of a zoning approval for a residence for homeless persons living with HIV/AIDS.[101] The "quasi-sovereign" interest alleged by the state was the damage to its population's health and welfare by the denial of benefits that a residential care facility would provide.

FEDERAL POWER TO SAFEGUARD THE PUBLIC'S HEALTH

Article I, §1 of the Constitution endows Congress with the "legislative Powers herein granted"—not with plenary legislative authority, as with the exercise of state police powers. The federal government must draw its authority to act from specific, enumerated powers. Thus, before an act of Congress is deemed constitutional, two questions must be asked: Does the Constitution affirmatively authorize Congress to act, and does the exercise of that power improperly interfere with any constitutionally protected interest?

In theory, the United States is a government of limited powers, but the reality is quite different. The federal government possesses considerable authority to act and exerts extensive control in the realm of public health and safety. The Supreme Court, through an expansive interpretation of Congress's enumerated powers, has enabled the federal government to maintain a vast public health presence in matters ranging from biomedical research and health care to infectious diseases, occupational health and safety, and environmental protection (see box 9, p. 174).

Congress derives its sweeping powers, in part, from Article I, §8 of the Constitution: Congress may "make all Laws which shall be necessary and proper for carrying into Execution" all powers vested by the Constitution in the government of the United States. The Necessary and Proper Clause, the subject of many great debates in American history, incorporates the doctrine of implied powers. Thus, the federal government may employ all means reasonably appropriate to achieve the objectives of constitutionally enumerated national powers. Chief Justice Marshall's authoritative construction of the Necessary and Proper Clause in *McCulloch v. Maryland* (1819) suggests that Congress may use any reasonable means not prohibited by the Constitution to carry out its express powers: "Let the end be legitimate, let it be within the scope of the constitution, and all means which are appropriate, which are plainly adapted to that end, which are not prohibited, but consistent with the letter and spirit of the constitution, are constitutional."[102]

The Constitution delegates diverse authority to the United States (see table 3). The foremost federal powers for public health purposes are the authority to tax and spend and to regulate interstate commerce. Additionally, Congress has authority "to promote the progress of Science and useful Arts."[103] Intellectual property protection provides incentives for scientific innovation, such as vaccines, pharmaceuticals, and medical devices.[104] The presidential authority "to make Treaties" with the Senate's advice and consent also has public health significance in such areas as tobacco, infectious disease, and global warming (see chapter 7).[105]

The Power to Tax Is the Power to Raise Revenue, Regulate Risk Behavior, and Induce Health-Promoting Behaviors

> No attribute of sovereignty is more pervading [than taxation], and at no point does the power of government affect more constantly and intimately the relations of life than through the exactions made under it.
>
> Thomas M. Cooley (1890)

Article I, §8 of the Constitution states that "Congress shall have Power To lay and collect Taxes, Duties, Imposts and Excises, to pay the Debts and provide for the common Defence and general Welfare of the United States." Congress has broad authority to tax and spend, and wide discretion

TABLE 3. Federal constitutional powers to protect the public's health

Federal Power	Constitutional Authority	Public Health Application
Regulate Interstate Commerce	Congress has the authority "to regulate Commerce with foreign Nations, and among the several States, and with the Indian Tribes." Art. I, § 8	The commerce power has been used in the fields of environmental protection, food and drug safety, occupational health, and other public health matters.
Tax and Spend	Congress "shall have Power To lay and collect Taxes, Duties, Imposts and Excises, to pay the Debts and provide for the common Defence and general Welfare of the United States." Art. I, § 8	To raise revenue to provide for the good of the community. Affords financial resources to provide health services; also affords power to regulate risk behavior and influence health-promoting activities.
Protect Intellectual Property	Congress has authority "to promote the Progress of Science and useful Arts." Art. I, § 8	Patents for vaccines, pharmaceuticals, and medical devices
Ratify Treaties	The president "shall have Power, by and with the Advice and Consent of the Senate, to make Treaties, provided two thirds of the Senators present concur." Art. II, §2	Framework Convention on Tobacco Control (U.S. signed but not ratified) Framework Convention on Climate Change (Kyoto Protocol) (U.S. signed but not ratified)
Enforce Reconstruction Era Amendments (Slavery, Equal Protection, Voting)	"Congress shall have power to enforce, by appropriate legislation, the provisions of this article." Amends. 13, 14, 15.	Civil rights and disability rights legislation

NOTE: The enumerated powers of Congress include the power to tax, borrow money, regulate interstate commerce, establish rules for naturalization and bankruptcies, coin money, punish counterfeiting, establish post offices, promote the progress of science and art by securing rights in intellectual property, constitute the judiciary, punish piracy and felony on the high seas, declare war, provide for and maintain (in various ways) the military of the United States, and exclusively legislate in the District of Columbia. Congress, moreover, may enact all laws that are "necessary and proper" to carry out its enumerated powers. U.S. Const. art. I, § 8. Apart from Article I, § 8, the provisions of the Constitution delegating power to Congress include Article IV (the manner in which full faith and credit shall be given to the acts of every state); Article V (ratification of constitutional amendments); the Sixteenth Amendment (national income tax); and various amendments that recognize individual rights that authorize Congress to enforce their provisions by "appropriate legislation."

to determine what contributes to the nation's general welfare.[106] The taxing power provides an independent source of federal legislative authority. Congress may regulate through the tax system for purposes that may not be authorized under its other enumerated powers.[107]

The power to tax is closely aligned with the power to spend.[108] Economists regard congressional decisions to provide tax relief for certain activities as indirect expenditures because government is, in fact, subsidizing the activity from the national treasury. Economists project, for example, that favorable tax treatment afforded to employer-sponsored health care plans will cost the federal government $760 billion between the years 2006 and 2010.[109]

On its face, the power to tax has a single overriding purpose—to raise revenue to provide for the good of the community. Absent the ability to generate sufficient revenue, the legislature could not provide services such as transportation, education, medical services to the poor, sanitation, and environmental protection. Historically, constitutional constraints have been imposed on Congress's revenue-raising capacity. Drawing a distinction between direct taxes (imposed upon property) and indirect taxes (imposed on the performance of an act),[110] the Supreme Court, at the turn of the twentieth century, declared a federal income tax unconstitutional.[111] The Sixteenth Amendment, ratified in 1913, restored the federal income tax and made possible an almost limitless revenue-raising potential within the federal government.

The taxing power, while affording government the financial resources to provide health services, has another, equally important purpose. The power to tax is also the power to regulate risk behavior and influence health-promoting activities. The Supreme Court, in its early jurisprudence, was concerned about federal taxes that were designed to punish or regulate rather than to raise revenue. Thus, the Court distinguished between revenue-raising taxes, which it upheld, and purely regulatory taxes, which it found constitutionally troubling.[112] This distinction, however, has all but disappeared. For example, the Court has upheld federal taxes on firearms capable of being concealed and on persons who "deal in" or prescribe marijuana, stating that a "tax does not cease to be valid because it regulates, discourages, or even definitely deters the activities taxed."[113] Today, a federal tax is likely to be constitutional unless it requires behavior conformance extraneous to any tax need.[114]

Virtually all taxes achieve ancillary regulatory effects by imposing an economic burden on the taxed activity or providing economic relief for certain kinds of private spending. Consequently, the tax code provides incentives and disincentives to perform, or to refrain from performing, certain acts. The more onerous the tax (in terms of the economic and administrative costs) or the more generous the tax relief, the more powerful the ancillary regulatory effects. Broadly speaking, the tax code influences health-related behavior through tax relief and tax burdens: Tax relief encourages private health-promoting activity and tax burdens discourage risk behavior.

Through various forms of tax relief (e.g., excluding benefits from taxable income, deducting spending from gross income, and providing credits against tax owed), government provides incentives for private activities that it views as advantageous to the public's health. The generous tax incentive for employer-sponsored health plans, for example, "deeply affects how health care is provided in the United States, to whom it is provided, and who provides it."[115] The tax code influences private health-related spending in many other ways: child care,[116] low-income housing,[117] pharmaceuticals for rare diseases,[118] and charitable spending for research and care.[119]

Public health taxation also regulates private behavior by economically penalizing risk-taking activities. Tax policy discourages a number of activities that government regards as unhealthy or dangerous.[120] Consider excise or manufacturing taxes on tobacco,[121] alcoholic beverages,[122] firearms,[123] or gambling.[124] Tax policy also influences individual and business decisions that adversely affect health or the environment; examples are taxes on gasoline[125] or on ozone-depleting chemicals[126] that contribute to environmental degradation. It is difficult to imagine a public health threat caused by human behavior or business activity that cannot be influenced, for good or bad, by the taxing power.

The power to tax, then, is the power to govern. Taxes amass the resources necessary for public health services and provide an effective regulatory mechanism for controlling individual and corporate behavior. Tax incentives and disincentives are powerful tools for promoting or discouraging anything legislators deem important for the health and well-being of the population.

The Power to Spend Is the Power to Allocate Resources and Induce Conformance with Public Health Standards

The powers to tax and spend both are found in the same constitutional phrase of Article I, §8: "Congress shall have Power To lay and collect Taxes . . . and provide for the common Defence and general Welfare of the United States." The spending power provides Congress with independent authority to allocate resources for the public good; Congress need not justify its spending by reference to a specific enumerated power.[127] Closely connected to the power to tax, the spending power has two purposes. First, it authorizes expenditures expressly for the public's health, safety, and well-being. Second, it effectively induces state conformance with federal regulatory standards.

The power to spend is expressly to promote the "general welfare," which would include all reasonable public health purposes. Theoretically, the spending power may be exercised only to pursue a common benefit, as distinguished from a local purpose, but Congress determines whether expenditures are for the common benefit, and the Supreme Court has historically concurred: "Nor is the concept of the general welfare static. Needs that were narrow or parochial a century ago may be interwoven in our day with the well-being of the Nation."[128]

The spending power does not simply grant Congress the authority to allocate resources; it is also an indirect regulatory device. Congress may prescribe the terms upon which it disburses federal money to the states. The conditional spending power is akin to a contract: In return for federal funds, the states agree to comply with federally imposed conditions.[129] The Supreme Court permits conditional appropriations, provided the conditions are clearly expressed in the statute and a reasonable relationship exists between the condition imposed and the program's purposes.[130] However, government may not condition a grant or a tax on the requirement that the person give up a constitutional right. Known as the "unconstitutional conditions" doctrine, the Court has declared that the state may not act indirectly to "produce a result which [it] could not command directly."[131]

If Congress wants states to conform to federally imposed standards to receive federal funds, it must say so clearly enough to permit the states to make an informed choice.[132] The "clear intent" rule means that Congress must convey its purpose in unambiguous terms to confer enforceable, individual rights under federal law. In recent years, the judiciary has refused to permit private enforcement of a variety of important rights because Congress was insufficiently clear—e.g., disability discrimination,[133] student privacy,[134] and Medicaid benefits.[135]

The strings attached to federal resources must also bear some reasonable relationship to the purposes of the grant. The conditional spending cannot be so coercive as to pass the point at which "pressure turns into compulsion."[136] Despite these theoretical limits, the Supreme Court grants Congress substantial leeway and appears to search for permissible relationships between the appropriation and the conditions.[137] For example, the Court saw a direct relationship between the appropriation of highway funds and the states' acceptance of a drinking age of twenty-one. Since a major purpose of highway funds is traffic safety, the drinking age limits were deemed constitutionally acceptable.[138]

Congress's power to set the terms upon which state appropriations shall be distributed is an effective regulatory device. States and localities can seldom afford to decline federal public health grants.[139] Congress and the federal agencies use conditional appropriations to induce states to conform to federal standards in numerous public health contexts, including HIV/AIDS,[140] Medicare and Medicaid,[141] abortion counseling and referral,[142] and land use and solid waste management.[143]

It is obvious from this discussion that the power to tax and spend is not value-neutral, but rather is laden with political overtones. Collection of revenues and allocation of resources go to the very heart of the political process. Legislators, as influenced by the public and interest groups, purport to promote the public's health, safety, and security. Many of their economic decisions, such as taxes on cigarettes and expenditures for antismoking campaigns, do promote the common good. But their vision is also influenced by moral, cultural, and social values, so that government's economic power may be used to *discourage* activities that many public health advocates support: safe abortion, fetal stem cell research, sex education, needle exchange, and so on. At the same time, government may create incentives for unhealthy or risky behavior. The tax code, for example, grants tax preferences to heavy-duty SUVs, which are detrimental to the environment, highway safety, and traffic congestion.[144]

The Power to Control Commerce Is the Power to Broadly Regulate

The Commerce Clause, more than any other enumerated power, affords Congress potent regulatory authority. Article I, §8 states that "the Congress shall have the power . . . to regulate Commerce with foreign Nations, and among the several States, and with the Indian Tribes." On its face, the Commerce Clause is limited to controlling the flow of goods and services across federal or state borders. Yet, as interstate commerce has become ubiquitous, activities once considered purely local have come to have national effects and have, accordingly, come within Congress's commerce power.[145]

Since Franklin Delano Roosevelt's New Deal era, the Supreme Court has interpreted the commerce power broadly, giving Congress the ability to regulate in almost any sphere. The Court's post-1937 jurisprudence has described "commerce among the states" as "plenary," or all-embracing,[146] applying it to virtually every aspect of social life.[147] Indeed, from 1937 to 1995, the Supreme Court did not find a single piece of social or economic legislation unconstitutional on the basis that Congress had exceeded its commerce power.

This expansive constitutional construction has enabled national authorities to reach deeply into traditional realms of state public health power and has significantly diminished the force of the Tenth Amendment. The courts have upheld exercises of the commerce power in the fields of environmental protection,[148] food and drug safety,[149] occupational health,[150] and infectious disease.[151]

The Supreme Court's 1995 decision in *United States v. Lopez* signaled a change in the Court's view about the balance of federal and state powers in the constitutional design.[152] In *Lopez,* the Court held that Congress exceeded its commerce authority by making gun possession within a school zone a federal offense. Concluding that possessing a gun within a school zone did not "substantially affect" interstate commerce, the Court declared the statute unconstitutional.

The Court continued to narrow the scope of the commerce power in *United States v. Morrison* (2000) when it struck down the private civil remedy in the Violence against Women Act.[153] The act created a civil rights remedy, permitting survivors to bring federal lawsuits against perpetrators of sexually motivated crimes of violence. Congress proclaimed that violence impairs the ability of women to work, harms businesses, and increases national health care costs. But the Court, reiterating its arguments in *Lopez,* found no national effects.

In *Lopez* and *Morrison,* the nation's highest court invalidated politically popular measures thought to be important to the public's safety. The Court did not invalidate these statutes on grounds that regulating guns in school zones or violence against women were unimportant aims of government, but only that they were outside the reach of the federal government. States would still be free to legislate in traditional realms of public health, but *Lopez* and *Morrison* left little doubt that the Court would henceforth examine the exercise of federal police power authority.[154]

Lopez and *Morrison* probably do not indicate a wholesale retreat from the liberal interpretation of the commerce power. The Supreme Court in the post-*Lopez* era has upheld social and public health activities ranging from the privacy of drivers' licenses[155] and protection of traffic safety data[156] to federal regulation of marijuana for medical purposes.[157] The medical marijuana case, *Gonzales v. Raich* (2005), was particularly telling because Justice Stevens explicitly said that *Lopez* and *Morrison* had been read "far too broadly."[158] The Court upheld Congress's commerce power to prohibit purely local cultivation and use of marijuana approved by a physician and in compliance with California law.[159]

Justice Sandra Day O'Connor, the Rehnquist Court's most ardent federalist, retired in 2005 right after her strident dissent in *Raich*, lamenting that the Court had extinguished an innovative state experiment on a difficult social issue. Whether the Roberts Court continues the federalism revolution or allows it to fade will depend in large part on its conception of the commerce power.[160]

The Dormant Commerce Clause

The Commerce Clause, in addition to affording Congress police power authority, implicitly narrows the states' public health power. The "Dormant" or "Negative" Commerce Clause limits state authority to regulate in ways that place an undue burden on interstate commerce. Thus, even if Congress has not entered a field of public health, states may not regulate if doing so obstructs commerce among the states.[161] The Supreme Court has a history of invalidating state public health legislation on Dormant Commerce Clause grounds. Thus, the Court has struck down state or local police power regulation involving milk sales;[162] liquor taxes;[163] shipping restrictions on wine;[164] groundwater use;[165] and solid,[166] liquid,[167] or hazardous waste[168] disposal and processing. The Constitution, therefore, does not simply empower Congress to control "commerce among the states" but implicitly limits state public health authority that unduly burdens interstate commerce.

Cooperative Federalism

Where Congress is acting under the commerce power, it may offer states the choice of either regulating according to federal standards or having federal regulation preempt state law. This model, known as "cooperative federalism," is found in federal public health statutes concerning water quality,[169] occupational health and safety,[170] and conservation.[171] It is the predominant approach to federal-state relations in environmental law. Under this model, federal agencies (e.g., the EPA) establish minimum national standards, and states retain the choice to administer the federal standards themselves or have federal authorities implement national standards.[172]

The Power to Abrogate State Sovereign Immunity: The Eleventh Amendment

The Eleventh Amendment grants states immunity from certain lawsuits in federal court without the state's consent.[173] Known as "sovereign immunity," this doctrine is important to states' autonomy because it limits Congress's power to authorize private lawsuits against states.[174] The modern Court perceives the states' immunity from suit to be a fundamental precept of sovereignty: "Federalism requires that Congress accord States the respect and dignity due them as residuary sovereigns and joint participants in the Nation's governance."[175] Congress's power to abrogate sovereign immunity depends on the constitutional power upon which it is acting:

Spending Power. Congress may require a waiver of state sovereign immunity as a condition of receiving federal funds, even though it may not order the waiver directly.[176] As with all conditional spending, Congress's waiver will be effective only if the statutory language is unequivocal.[177]

Commerce Power. In *Seminole Tribe of Florida v. Florida* (a case of great significance in American federalism that was decided in 1996),[178] the Supreme Court held that Congress lacks the power, when acting under the Commerce Clause, to abrogate the states' sovereign immunity in federal court.[179] Three years later, the Court extended *Seminole* by declaring that states cannot be sued, without their consent, by private parties in the states' own courts for violations of federal law.[180] These cases effectively preclude Congress from authorizing private individuals to sue states for infringing important federal rights, such as patent protection,[181] consumer protection,[182] or civil rights.[183]

Reconstruction Amendments. Although Congress may not abrogate state immunity based on its commerce powers, it may subject nonconsenting states to suit in federal court when it does so pursuant to its power to remedy and deter violations of the Reconstruction Amendments through "appropriate legislation"[184] regarding slavery,[185] equal protection,[186] and voting.[187] The Supreme Court, however, has interpreted these amendments narrowly, invigorating the doctrine of state sovereign immunity.[188] In *Board of Trustees of the University of Alabama v. Garrett*

(2001), the Court held that Congress exceeded its Fourteenth Amendment power by authorizing state workers to sue for discrimination under Title I (employment discrimination) of the Americans with Disabilities Act (ADA).[189] The Court, however, has been more willing to allow abrogation of sovereign immunity in cases involving race or sex discrimination[190] or the exercise of fundamental rights such as access to the courts.[191]

Injunctive Relief. The Eleventh Amendment creates a major hurdle for persons seeking to enforce federal public health or antidiscrimination laws against state governments. The issue of sovereign immunity, however, would not be so grave if plaintiffs were permitted to sue state officials rather than the state itself. The doctrine of *Ex parte Young* (1908) permits injunctive relief against state officials in certain circumstances, even when the state itself is immune from suit.[192] It is therefore feasible that "indirect" suits may be permitted against state officers, even if suits against the state itself are barred.[193]

The Reserved Powers Doctrine

Even if the federal government is acting under a valid grant of constitutional authority, such as the commerce power, there is another way in which the Court can strike down public health regulation: the reserved powers doctrine. In *New York v. United States* (1992), the Supreme Court, for only the second time in more than half a century,[194] invalidated a federal statute on Tenth Amendment grounds.[195] Congress had enacted monetary and other incentives to induce states to provide for disposal of radioactive waste generated within their borders. To ensure effective action, if a state was unable to dispose of its own waste, it was required under the statute to "take title" and possession of the waste. The Court invalidated the "take title" provision because the Constitution does not confer upon Congress the ability to "commandeer the legislative processes of the States by directly compelling them to enact and enforce a federal regulatory program." According to the Court, although Congress may exercise its legislative authority directly over private persons or businesses, it lacks the power to compel states to regulate according to the federal standards.[196] The Court's theory is that state officials "bear the brunt of public disapproval, while the federal officials who devised the regulatory program may remain insulated from the electoral ramifications of their decision."[197]

In *Printz v. United States* (1997), the Supreme Court used its reasoning in *New York* to overturn provisions in the Brady Handgun Violence Prevention Act, which directed state and local law enforcement officers to conduct background checks on prospective handgun purchasers.[198] The *New York* Court held that state legislatures are not subject to federal direction. In *Printz,* the Court held that federal authorities may not supplant the state executive branch. In this instance, Congress did not require the state to make policy, but only to assist in implementing the federal law. The Court rejected the distinction between "making" law or policy on the one hand and merely enforcing or implementing it on the other hand.

As a result of *New York* and *Printz,* the Tenth Amendment has become a vehicle for challenging federal statutes that compel state legislative or administrative action. In an era of "new federalism," a body of public health law may be vulnerable to challenges on Tenth Amendment grounds.[199]

NEW FEDERALISM AND THE PUBLIC'S HEALTH

This nation has long struggled with the problem of attaining the proper balance of powers between the federal government and the states.[200] This problem is particularly acute in matters of public health, because both levels of government want to be seen as responding to the electorate's concerns about health and safety. States and localities are closer to the people and better understand threats to their health. Because they are closer to the community, they can adapt prevention strategies to meet the needs of localities. States also are better placed to experiment with solutions to complex health problems. Federalism has the advantage of permitting states to act as laboratories for innovative health policies.

The federal government, on the other hand, has greater resources and scientific expertise with which to tackle complicated health policy problems. Many public health problems, moreover, transcend state borders, including pollution, infectious disease, and traffic hazards. Other public health problems are so worrying or pervasive that they demand a national response—e.g., the Virginia Tech tragedy in 2006, or the terrorist attacks in 2001.

It would be comforting to think that the struggles between federal and state public health authorities have been resolved by force of logic—that is, by systematically determining which level of government is likely to be more effective in reducing health threats. The reality, however, is that this struggle has been fought more on political than on policy grounds. The Supreme Court, moreover, has dramatically shifted its stance as the ideological composition of the Court has changed, and will continue to change with the appointments of Chief Justice Roberts and Associate Justice Alito in 2006.

Beyond the political and legal debates about federalism lies an important question about the population's health and safety. If the states do not act effectively or uniformly to reduce health threats such as firearms, cigarettes, or pollution, will the judiciary permit national authorities to exercise a police function? The current political thrust evident in the judiciary may impede the federal government's power to act for the health of the population. At the same time, an activist court is invalidating social legislation enacted through the democratic process, not to safeguard individual liberty but to pursue an ideal of governance that is much disputed within the nation.

The constitutional design is complex, seeking a balance between federal and state power (federalism); legislative, executive, and judicial power (separation of powers); and government authority and individual liberties (limited government). In this chapter, I have explored federalism and the separation of powers, both of which pose intriguing problems in the context of public health. Much of the history of public health, however, involves earnest debate over the relationship between the power of government and the freedom of individuals. That debate has only intensified with the contemporary concerns over emerging infectious diseases and bioterrorism. How much power should we afford government to act for the collective good? How important are individual values of liberty, privacy, association, and expression, or economic values of control of property and freedom of contract? How shall we balance personal liberty and business interests against communal goods of health, safety, and well-being? These are the questions that I turn to in the next chapter.

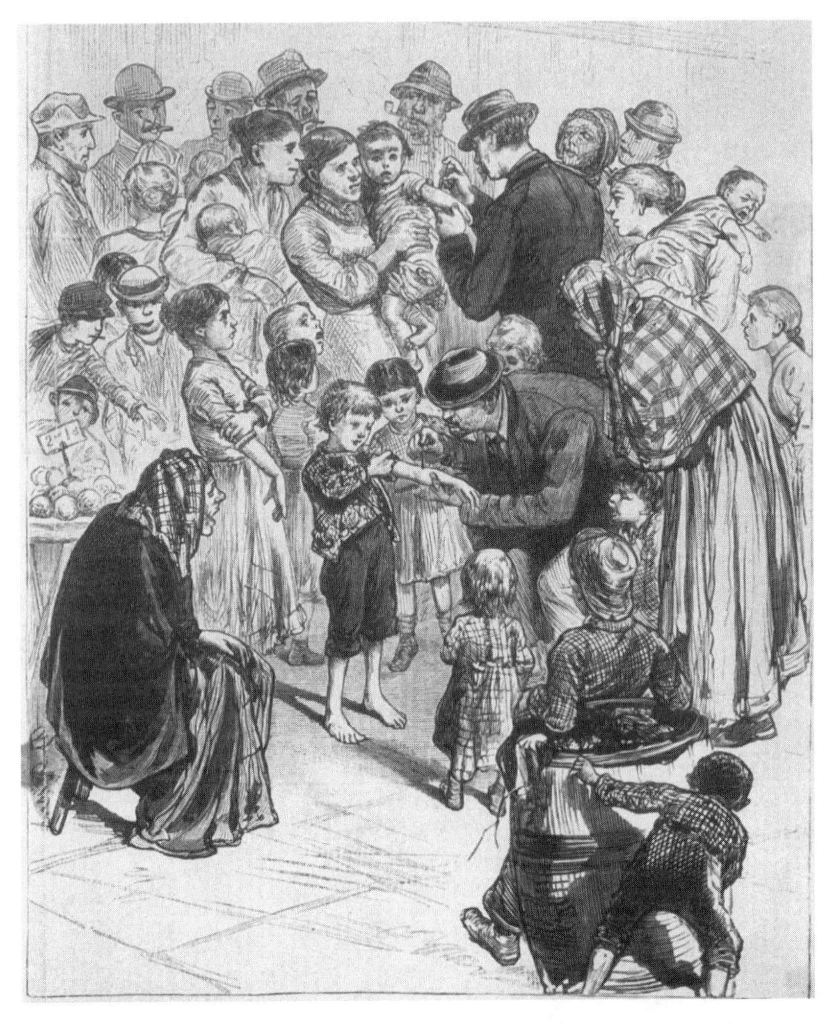

Photo 6. Public smallpox vaccinations in Jersey City. An 1800s engraving depicting smallpox vaccination in Jersey City, New Jersey: a street scene during the smallpox scare. By 1905, in *Jacobson v. Massachusetts*, the Supreme Court would find compulsory smallpox vaccination constitutional. Courtesy of the National Library of Medicine.

CHAPTER 4

Constitutional Limits on the Exercise of Public Health Powers

Safeguarding Individual Rights and Freedoms

The very existence of government presupposes the right of the sovereign power to prescribe regulations demanded by the general welfare for the common protection of all. This principle inheres in the very nature of the social compact. . . . This power of government, the power, as expressed by Taney, C.J., "inherent in every sovereignty, the power to govern men and things," is not, however, uncontrollable or despotic authority, subject to no limitation, exercisable with or without reason in the discretion or at the whim or caprice of the legislative body. . . . [The constitutional guaranty] was designed for the protection of personal and private rights against encroachments by the legislative body . . . as held and understood when the Constitution was adopted.

John A. Andrews (1889)

Regulation of persons and businesses historically has been a staple of public health practice.[1] Public health officials, in response to epidemics, exercise powers to test, vaccinate, physically examine, treat, isolate, and quarantine. Government agencies license health care providers, inspect food establishments, approve pharmaceuticals, monitor occupational health and safety, control pollutants, and abate nuisances. Public health regulation may not be the preferred strategy for ameliorating health threats; education and incentives often are more effective. Nevertheless, the legal basis of regulatory power and the trade-offs between personal freedom and the common good are core concerns of public health law.

The last chapter examined the broad powers of the federal and state governments to act for the public good. But there are also limits on government power to protect the public's health. This chapter, and much of the remainder of this book, examines those limits—that is, under what circumstances may the government interfere with a person's autonomy, privacy, liberty, or property to achieve a healthier and safer population?

PUBLIC HEALTH AND THE BILL OF RIGHTS: THE INCORPORATION DOCTRINE

The Bill of Rights, the first ten amendments to the Constitution, was ratified by the states in 1791. The first eight amendments guarantee certain fundamental rights and freedoms.[2] Table 4 describes the Bill of Rights, presents selected public health issues, and summarizes relevant case law.[3] The Bill of Rights is directed to the federal government, not the states.[4] However, the Fourteenth Amendment, ratified after the conclusion of the Civil War, has been interpreted as applying the Bill of Rights to the states. Under "incorporation," the Supreme Court applies most of the Bill of Rights to the states.[5] However, some constitutional rights, such as the Second Amendment's right to bear arms (see box 5), have not yet been incorporated and therefore apply only to the federal government and not to the states.[6]

The Constitution prohibits government, at every level, from invading certain fundamental rights and freedoms. But the Constitution does not constrain mere private conduct, however discriminatory or wrongful.[7] The public/private distinction in constitutional law may at first appear straightforward. However, the activities of government, private ("for profit" and charitable), and community actors are frequently intertwined in public health; it can be difficult to separate public from private activities.

Any affirmative measure taken by government constitutes "state action"—including public health statutes enacted by the legislature, regulations issued by the health department, and nuisance abatements adjudicated through the courts. The Constitution affords full protection to individuals adversely affected by governmental acts.[8] Additionally, if the state mandates a private breach of constitutional norms—for instance, an environmental agency that requires a private contractor to discriminate in access to public lands—there is state action.[9] Beyond these obvious forms of governmental activity, there exist numerous ambiguities (see box 6).[10]

TABLE 4. Public health and the Bill of Rights

Selected Public Health Issues	Selected Public Health Cases
First Amendment: Freedom of Religion, Speech, Press, Assembly, Petition	
Religious exemption to vaccination	*Mason:*[a] religious exemption to vaccination requirement constitutional
Advertising restrictions (e.g., cigarettes, alcoholic beverages)	*44 Liquormart:*[b] ban on advertising price of alcoholic beverages unconstitutional
Closure of bathhouses	*St. Mark's:*[c] closure of private bathhouses as a public health nuisance constitutional
Second Amendment: Right to Keep and Bear Arms	
Gun control legislation	*Fresno Rifle & Pistol Club:*[d] regulation of gun manufacture and sale constitutional
	Parker v. District of Columbia:[e] gun control held unconstitutional
Third Amendment: Right to Refuse to Quarter Soldiers in Home	
Not directly applicable to public health	
Fourth Amendment: Freedom from Unreasonable Search and Seizure	
Compulsory testing and screening (e.g., drug, alcohol, HIV testing)	*Skinner:*[f] upholding drug tests following train accidents
Inspection of premises / Administrative searches	*Camara:*[g] routine housing and building code inspections require search warrants
Fifth Amendment: Due Process, Equal Protection of the Law, and "Just Compensation" for Private Property Taken for Public Use	
Public health regulation that deprives a person of liberty or property must provide procedural due process	*Greene:*[h] fair procedures for quarantine *Addington:*[i] fair procedures for civil commitment of the mentally ill *Goldberg:*[j] fair procedures for denial of welfare benefits
Public health regulation must not be arbitrary or discriminatory	*Jacobson:*[k] compulsory vaccination is a legitimate use of state's police power
Just compensation for land-use restrictions for environmental and other public health purposes	*Lucas:*[l] landowner entitled to "just compensation" for environmental land-use restrictions that deprived land of all value

TABLE 4. *(continued)*

Sixth Amendment: Right to Speedy and Public Trial by an Impartial Jury in Criminal Prosecution
Not directly applicable to public health
Seventh Amendment: Trial by Jury in Civil Cases
Not directly applicable to public health
Eighth Amendment: Prohibition against Excessive Bail or Fines, or Cruel and Unusual Punishment
Not directly applicable to public health

[a] *Mason v. General Brown Cent. Sch. Dist.*, 851 F.2d 47 (2d Cir. 1988). See chapter 10.
[b] *44 Liquormart, Inc. v. Rhode Island*, 517 U.S. 484, 513–514 (1996). See chapter 9.
[c] *City of New York v. New St. Mark's Baths*, 562 N.Y.S.2d 642 (N.Y.A.D. 1 Dept., 1990). See chapter 12.
[d] *Fresno Rifle & Pistol Club, Inc. v. Van de Kamp*, 965 F.2d 723 (9th Cir. 1992). See box 5.
[e] *Parker v. District of Columbia*, 478 F.3d 370 (D.C. Cir. 2007). See box 5.
[f] *Skinner v. Railway Labor Executives' Assn.*, 489 U.S. 602, 613–14 (1989). See chapter 10.
[g] *Camara v. Municipal Court of the City & County of San Francisco*, 387 U.S. 523 (1967). See chapter 5.
[h] *Greene v. Edwards*, 265 S.E. 2d 662 (W. Va. 1980). See chapter 11.
[i] *Addington v. Texas*, 441 U.S. 418, 425 (1979). See chapter 11.
[j] *Goldberg v. Kelly*, 397 U.S. 254 (1970). See chapter 4.
[k] *Jacobson v. Massachusetts*, 197 U.S. 11 (1905). See chapter 4.
[l] *Lucas v. South Carolina Coastal Council*, 505 U.S. 1003 (1992). See chapter 5, table 5.

Private entities that exercise "public functions" are bound by the Constitution, but the definition of "public functions" is so narrow that it is unlikely to include the private exercise of many public health services. Public functions are "traditionally exclusively reserved to the State,"[11] but private actors undertake many public health services, such as vaccination, testing, and treatment. The Supreme Court finds state action only where there is such a "close nexus" between the state and private action that it "may be fairly treated as that of the State itself."[12] The Supreme Court, for example, has held that education[13] and other important public services[14] are not public functions.

JACOBSON V. MASSACHUSETTS: POLICE POWER AND CIVIL LIBERTIES IN TENSION

Jacobson v. Massachusetts (1905)[15] is thought to be the most important judicial decision in public health.[16] Why? Is it because of the Supreme Court's deference to public health decision making? Is it because the Court enunciated a framework for the protection of individual liberties

BOX 5

THE "RIGHT TO BEAR ARMS"

The Second Amendment

Firearms control and injury prevention are major public health objectives, so the application and scope of the Second Amendment is a salient concern.[1] The Second Amendment states: "A well regulated Militia, being necessary to the security of a free State, the right of the people to keep and bear Arms, shall not be infringed."[2] A nineteenth-century Supreme Court decision expressly declined to incorporate the Second Amendment to the states.[3] Consequently, states and localities possess broad powers to limit access to and possession of firearms.[4]

Even as applied to the federal government, the Court narrowly construes the Second Amendment to prohibit federal gun regulation that would interfere with effective state militias and police forces.[5] Considerable political tension exists over the scope of the Second Amendment.[6] The opposing theories concern whether the clause confers an individual or collective right.[7] "Individual rights" theorists believe the Second Amendment protects ownership, possession, and transportation of firearms. "Collective rights" theorists believe the clause only protects the states in their authority to maintain formal, organized militia units—a purely civic purpose.[8] The Supreme Court has given effect to the dependent clause of the amendment, suggesting that individual protection is afforded only in the context of the maintenance of a militia or other public force.[9]

The majority of federal circuits favor the collective rights approach.[10] However, the Fifth and D.C. Circuits recently declared that the Second Amendment protects an individual's right to own firearms, and the Supreme Court has heard an appeal from the D.C. Circuit case.[11] At what point federal regulation or prohibition of what kinds of firearms would conflict with the Second Amendment, if at all, remains a live question, particularly with the more conservative composition of the Supreme Court. Even if the Roberts Court were to find that the Second Amendment confers an individual right, it should still defer to legislatures seeking reasonable regulation of firearms in America.[12]

[1] Jon S. Vernick, Stephen P. Teret, "Firearms and Health: The Right to Be Armed with Accurate Information about the Second Amendment," *American Journal of Public Health,* 83 (1993): 1773-77; Jon S. Vernick and Julie Samia Mair, "How the Law Affects Gun Policy in the United States: Law as Intervention or Obstacle to Prevention," *Journal of Law, Medicine and Ethics,* 30 (2002): 692-704; Stephen P. Teret, Daniel W. Webster, Jon S. Vernick, et al., "Support for New Policies to Regulate Firearms: Results of Two National Surveys," *New Eng. J. Med.,* 339 (1998): 813-18; David Hemenway, "Regulation of Firearms," *New Eng. J. Med.,* 339 (1998): 543-45; Michael C. Dorf, "What Does the Second Amendment Mean Today?" *Chicago-Kent Law Review,* 76 (2000): 291-348.

[2] See generally H. Richard Uviller and William G. Merkel, *The Militia and the Right to Arms, or How the Second Amendment Fell Silent* (London: Duke University Press, 2002).

[3] *United States v. Cruikshank,* 92 U.S. 542 (1875), held that the Second Amendment operates as a limitation on the powers of the federal government only, and does not affect those of the states.

[4] See, e.g., *Presser v. Illinois,* 116 U.S. 252 (1886) (upholding a state law prohibiting all bodies of men except those comprising the regular organized militia of the state and U.S. troops from associating, drilling, or parading with arms in any state without license from the governor); *Quilici v. Village of Morton Grove,* 695 F.2d 261 (7th Cir. 1982), *cert. denied,* 464 U.S. 863 (1983) (upholding the constitutionality of a control ordinance prohibiting citizen ownership of handguns); *Miller v. Texas,* 153 U.S. 535 (1894) (upholding a state law forbidding the carrying of dangerous weapons on the person); *Robertson v. Baldwin,* 165 U.S. 275, 281-82 (1897) (stating, "The right of people to keep and bear arms [article 2] is not infringed by laws prohibiting the carrying of concealed weapons").

[5] See, e.g., *United States v. Romera-Pina,* 166 Fed. Appx. 34 (4th Cir. 2006) (holding that federal law which prohibited firearm possession by certain aliens did not violate the Second Amendment); *United States v Jackubowski,* 63 Fed. Appx. 959 (7th Cir. 2003), *cert. denied,* 540 U.S. 993 (2003) (finding that a federal statute prohibiting possession of a firearm after a felony conviction does not violate the Second Amendment); *Hickman v. Block,* 81 F.3d 98 (9th Cir. 1996), *cert. denied,* 519 U.S. 912 (1996) (stating that the plaintiff lacked standing to challenge denial of a permit to carry a concealed weapon because Second Amendment is a right held by states, not by private citizens); *Love v. Pepersack,* 47 F.3d 120 (4th Cir. 1995), *cert. denied,* 516 U.S. 813 (1995) (upholding officers' denial of an application for a

handgun on grounds of prior arrests); *Fresno Rifle & Pistol Club, Inc. v. Van de Kamp,* 965 F.2d 723 (9th Cir. 1992) (stating that a law proscribing sale and possession of guns does not violate the Second Amendment because it is limited to federal action).

[6] Dan Eggen, "Ashcroft–Gun Ownership an Individual Right: Letter to NRA Sparks Debate over Second Amendment, Long Interpreted as Applying Collectively," *Washington Post,* May 24, 2001; "Symposium on the Second Amendment: Fresh Looks," *Chicago-Kent Law Review,* 76 (2000); "Symposium on the Second Amendment and the Future of Gun Regulation: Historical, Legal, Policy, and Cultural Perspectives," *Fordham Law Review,* 73 (2004): 475-840.

[7] Adam Liptak, "A Liberal Case for Gun Rights Sways Judiciary," *New York Times,* May 6, 2007.

[8] The debate is heated, with commentators drawing strikingly different conclusions from the same language and history. See, e.g., Staff of Subcommittee on the Constitution, Senate Committee on the Judiciary, 97th Congress, 2d Sess., *The Right to Keep and Bear Arms* (Comm. Print 1982); Don B. Kates, Jr., "Handgun Prohibition and the Original Meaning of the Second Amendment," *Michigan Law Review,* 82 (1984): 204-73; Robert J. Cottrol, ed., *Gun Control and the Constitution: Sources and Explorations on the Second Amendment* (New York: Garland Pub., 1994); Stephen P. Halbrook, *That Every Man Be Armed: The Evolution of a Constitutional Right,* 2d ed. (California: Independent Institute, 1994); "Symposium, Gun Control," *Law and Contemporary Problems,* 49 (1986): 1-268; Sanford Levinson, "The Embarrassing Second Amendment," *Yale Law Journal,* 99 (1989): 637-60; Paul Finkelman, "Well Regulated Militia: The Second Amendment in Historical Perspective," *Chicago-Kent Law Review,* 76 (2000): 195-236.

[9] *United States v. Miller,* 307 U.S. 174, 178 (1939) (upholding a statute requiring registration under the National Firearms Act of sawed-off shotguns and stating that the Second Amendment must be interpreted "with that end [an efficient militia] in view"); *Cases v. United States,* 131 F.2d 916, 922 (1st Cir. 1942), *cert. denied,* 319 U.S. 770 (1943) (upholding a similar provision of the Federal Firearms Act and stating, "[Under the Second Amendment] the federal government can limit the keeping and bearing of arms by a single individual as well as by a group of individuals, but it cannot prohibit the possession or use of any weapon which has any reasonable relationship to the preservation or efficiency of a well-regulated militia"); *Lewis v. United States,* 445 U.S. 55, 65 n. 8 (1980) (stating in dictum that *Miller* holds that the "Second Amendment guarantees no right to keep and bear a firearm that does not have 'some reasonable relationship to the preservation or efficiency of a well regulated militia'"); *United States v. Parker,* 362 F.3d 1279 (10th Cir. 2004), *cert. denied,* 125 S.Ct. 88 (2004) (federal prosecution for violating a state gun-control statute by carrying a loaded firearm on a military base in that state does not violate the Second Amendment because neither the defendant nor his weapon was shown to have any connection with a state militia).

[10] See, e.g., *Silveira v. Lockyer,* 312 F.3d 1052 (9th Cir. 2002), *cert. denied,* 540 U.S. 1046 (2003) (rejecting the view that the Second Amendment provides any type of individual right to own or possess weapons and reaffirming earlier decisions holding that the Second Amendment confers a collective right only).

[11] *United States v. Emerson,* 270 F.3d 203 (5th Cir. 2001), *cert. denied,* 536 U.S. 907 (2002) (holding that the Second Amendment protects the individual's right to keep and bear arms, but the right is subject to reasonable restrictions); *Parker v. District of Columbia,* 478 F.3d 370 (D.C. Cir. 2007) (invalidating a D.C. law barring all handguns unless they were registered before 1976, on grounds that the Second Amendment conveys an individual right to bear arms), *cert. granted, District of Columbia V. Heller,* 128 S. Ct. 645 (2007).

[12] Erwin Chemerinsky, "A Well-Regulated Right to Bear Arms," *Washington Post,* May 14, 2007 (arguing that the courts should give deference to the legislature and uphold firearm control laws that are reasonably related to the legitimate government purpose of safeguarding public safety).

that persists today? Perhaps it is because *Jacobson* was decided during the same term as *Lochner v. New York* (1905)—the most infamous Supreme Court case of its era.[17] If *Lochner* exemplified judicial activism at its extreme for striking down reasonable economic regulation, then *Jacobson* showed judicial recognition of the police power, the most important aspect of state sovereignty. There is a further question that deserves attention: Would *Jacobson* be decided the same way today? What is the enduring meaning of the most famous decision in the realm of public health law? In 2005, the hundredth anniversary of *Jacobson,* scholars took a close look at this foundational case.[18]

BOX 6

THE PUBLIC/PRIVATE DISTINCTION

Five public health law problems

Official State Acts by Health Care Professionals

Health care professionals who are employed by the government and act in an official capacity are "state actors."[1] Consequently, professionals who work in prisons, state mental hospitals, or municipal STI clinics and who act in an official capacity are bound by the Constitution.

Licensed, Inspected, or Regulated Private Entities

Private individuals and businesses that are subject to government licensing, inspection, or regulation are not "state actors."[2] A regulatory scheme, "however detailed it may be in some particulars," does not, by itself, invoke the state action doctrine.[3] There may be no state action, for example, if a licensed, inspected, or regulated entity discriminates on grounds of race or sex,[4] censors certain sexually explicit or politically sensitive material,[5] or fails to provide fair procedures.[6] The government, through its regulatory network, must be "entangled" with the private entity to establish state action; a "close nexus" must exist between the state and the regulatory entity.[7]

Organizations in Receipt of Government Funding

The Supreme Court rarely finds state action based solely on government funding, even if subsidies are substantial: "Acts of . . . private contractors do not become acts of the government by reason of their significant or even total engagement in performing public contracts."[8] Thus, private health care providers, businesses, researchers, and community organizations that are funded by public health agencies are not bound to conform with constitutional norms.

Private Conduct Authorized by Law

To what extent is there state action if the government authorizes or empowers a

[1] *Home Telephone and Telegraph Co. v. City of Los Angeles*, 227 U.S. 278 (1913) (holding that even if a state officer misuses his power, state action still exists).

[2] See, e.g., *Reichley v. Pa. Dep't of Agric.*, 427 F.3d 236 (2005) (holding that there was no state action when a poultry producers' trade association purchased and destroyed a population of chickens that was suspected of being infected with avian influenza); *American Mfrs. Mut. Ins. Co. v. Sullivan*, 526 U.S. 40 (1999) (finding no state action in an insurance company decision to deny payment for medical treatment pending utilization review); *Blum v. Yaretsky*, 457 U.S. 991 (1982) (holding that a private nursing home decision to transfer patients to other facilities, thereby terminating their Medicaid benefits, did not constitute state action); *Jackson v. Metropolitan Edison Co.*, 419 U.S. 345 (1974) (finding no state action when a privately owned utility company terminated an individual's electric service); *Leshko v. Servis*, 423 F.3d 337 (3d Cir. 2005) (holding that comprehensive state regulation of foster care did not constitute a sufficient nexus to make foster parents state actors).

[3] *Moose Lodge No. 107 v. Irvis*, 407 U.S. 163, 176 (1972) (holding that a private club that discriminated on the basis of race did not implicate the state by simply adhering to state liquor laws).

[4] *Moose Lodge*, 407 U.S. 163.

[5] *Columbia Broadcasting System, Inc. v. Democratic National Committee*, 412 U.S. 94 (1973) (finding no state action in the FCC's refusal to require broadcast licensees to accept editorial advertising).

[6] *Jackson*, 419 U.S. at 345.

[7] *Blum*, 457 U.S. at 1004; *Burton v. Wilmington Parking Authority*, 365 U.S. 715, 725 (1961) (finding that the city was so "entangled" with a restaurant to which it leased space that there was a "symbiotic relationship" sufficient to constitute state action).

[8] *Rendell-Baker v. Kohn*, 457 U.S. 830 (1982).

private entity to cause harm? The test used by the Supreme Court is "whether the State provided a mantle of authority that enhanced the power of the harm-causing individual actor."[9] Additionally, a state is responsible for a private party's violation of constitutional rights when it enacts and enforces a law "requiring" violation of those rights, "compelling" a discriminatory act, or "commanding" a particular result.[10] The U.S. Court of Appeals for the Third Circuit, for example, held that the federal privacy rule that authorizes "routine uses" of medical records for "treatment, payment, and health care operations"[11] does not involve state action. The privacy rule does not compel or enhance the power of private entities to disclose private health information without the patient's consent.[12]

Privatization of Public Health Functions

Government may not privatize the exercise of powers traditionally associated with sovereignty.[13] Consequently, delegation of legislative, regulatory, or judicial powers to the private sector is impermissible (e.g., granting private entities police power authority to quarantine, compel medical treatment, or regulate businesses).[14] Although government may not delegate police powers, there is ample scope for delegation of a broad range of public health services to the private sector.[15]

[9] *Nat'l Collegiate Athletic Ass'n v. Tarkanian,* 488 U.S. 179, 192 (1970) (holding that the university's imposition of disciplinary sanctions against a basketball coach in compliance with National Collegiate Athletic Association rules and recommendations did not turn the association's otherwise private conduct into state action, and thus the association could not be held liable for violation of the coach's civil rights).

[10] *Adickes v. S.H. Kress & Co.,* 398 U.S. 144 (1970) (holding that the plaintiff could make a civil rights claim for deprivation of rights by showing existence of a state-enforced custom of segregating races in public eating places in the city at the time of the incident and that the defendant's refusal to serve the plaintiff was motivated by that state-enforced custom).

[11] *Health Insurance Portability and Accountability Act Privacy Rule,* 45 C.F.R. §164.506.

[12] *Citizens for Health v. Leavitt,* 428 F.3rd 167 (3rd Cir. 2005) (finding that the state actor requirement was not satisfied because the Secretary of Health and Human Services did not provide authority to enhance the power of private parties, and the fact that a private party changes behavior in response to the law does not itself provide state action).

[13] *Jackson,* 419 U.S. at 345.

[14] *Carter v. Carter Coal Co.,* 298 U.S. 238 (1936) (invalidating a congressional delegation of regulatory power to private parties); Leroy Parker and Robert H. Worthington, *The Law of Public Health and Safety and the Powers and Duties of Boards of Health* (New York: M. Bender, 1892): 12-13 ("The police power is so clearly essential to the well-being of the State, that the legislature cannot, by any act or contract whatever, divest itself of the power").

[15] René Bowser and Lawrence O. Gostin, "Managed Care and the Health of a Nation," *Southern California Law Review,* 72 (1999): 1209-96.

Jacobson: *Separation of Powers and Federalism*

Massachusetts enacted a law at the turn of the twentieth century empowering municipal boards of health to require the vaccination of inhabitants, if necessary for the public's health or safety. The Cambridge Board of Health, under authority of this statute, adopted the following regulation: "Whereas, smallpox has been prevalent . . . in the city of Cambridge and still continues to increase; and whereas, it is necessary for the speedy extermination of the disease . . . ; be it ordered, that all inhabitants of the city be vaccinated." Reverend Henning Jacobson, who refused the vaccination, was convicted by the trial court and sentenced to pay a fine of five dollars. The Massachusetts Supreme Judicial Court upheld the conviction, and the U.S. Supreme Court decided the case in 1905. Jacobson's legal brief asserted that "a compulsory vaccination law is unreasonable, arbitrary and oppressive, and, therefore, hostile to the inherent right of every freeman to care for his own body and health in such way as to him seems best."[19] His was a classic claim in favor of a laissez-faire society and the natural rights of persons to bodily integrity and decisional privacy.

Jacobson is a quintessential case about separation of powers and federalism, and these doctrines were used to support deference to the legislative branch and to the states. The Court's political theory about separation of powers led to an almost unquestioning acceptance of legislative findings of scientific fact. Quoting the New York Court of Appeals (which had recently upheld compulsory vaccination as a condition of school entry),[20] Justice Harlan suggested that

> the legislature has the right to pass laws which, according to the common belief of the people, are adapted to prevent the spread of contagious diseases. In a free country, where the government is by the people, through their chosen representatives, practical legislation admits of no other standard of action; for what the people believe is for the common welfare must be accepted as tending to promote the common welfare, whether it does in fact or not. Any other basis would conflict with the spirit of the Constitution, and would sanction measures opposed to a republican form of government.[21]

Under a theory of democracy, Justice Harlan would grant considerable leeway to the elected branch of government to formulate public health policy. The Supreme Court, relying on principles of federalism, also asserted the primacy of state over federal authority in the realm of public health. "It is of last importance," wrote Justice Harlan, that the judiciary "should not invade the domain of local authority except when it is plainly necessary. . . . The safety and the health of the people of Massachusetts are, in the first instance, for that Commonwealth to guard and protect. They are matters that do not ordinarily concern the National Government."[22]

Jacobson *in Historical Context: The Immunization Debates*

> The contention that compulsory vaccination is an infraction of personal liberty and an unconstitutional interference with the right of the individual to have

> the smallpox if he wants it, and to communicate it to others, has been ended [by the U.S. Supreme Court]. . . . [This] should end the useful life of the societies of cranks formed to resist the operation of laws relative to vaccination. Their occupation is gone.
>
> Editorial, *New York Times* (1905)

Jacobson v. Massachusetts was decided just a few years after a major outbreak of smallpox in Boston that, from 1901 to 1903, resulted in 1,596 cases and 270 deaths.[23] The outbreak reignited the smallpox immunization debate, and there was plenty of hyperbole on both sides. Antivaccinationists launched a "scathing attack":[24] Compulsory vaccination is "the greatest crime of the age"; it "slaughter[s] tens of thousands of innocent children," and "is more important than the slavery question, because it is debilitating the whole human race."[25] The antivaccinationists gave notice that compulsory powers "will cause a riot."[26] Their influence was noticeable, resulting in a "conscience clause" in the British Parliament, exempting any parent who can "satisfy Justices in petty sessions that he conscientiously believes that vaccination would be prejudicial to the health of the child."[27]

The response of the mainstream press was equally shrill, characterizing the debate as "a conflict between intelligence and ignorance, civilization and barbarism."[28] The *New York Times* remarked that "no enemy of vaccination could ask better than to have England's compulsory vaccination law nullified by that [conscience] clause"; the paper referred to antivaccinationists as a "familiar species of crank," whose arguments are "absurdly fallacious."[29] The mainstream media continued its campaign against the "jabberings" of "hopeless cranks" for years,[30] continuing to depict them as "ignorant" and "deficient in the power to judge [science]."[31]

The state courts, prior to *Jacobson,* were heavily engaged in the vaccination controversy, and their judgments were markedly deferential to public health agencies: "Whether vaccination is or is not efficacious in the prevention of smallpox is a question with which the courts declare they have no concern."[32] The courts routinely found school vaccination requirements constitutional.[33] To be sure, some courts invoked a standard of "necessity," but without strong safeguards of individual liberty.[34] The courts decided vaccination cases based more on administrative than constitutional law. They recognized the state's police power to delegate authority to public health agencies or boards of health.[35] In the rare instances where limits on a state's power were imposed, it was because a board exceeded its statutory authority or because the courts construed that authority as requiring a state of emergency.[36] A person's bona fide belief against vaccination was not a sufficient excuse for noncompliance; however, a person could be exempted due to a physical condition posing a particular risk of adverse effects.[37] The states compelled vaccination only indirectly—by imposing penalties, denying school admission, or quarantining. The courts, therefore, could avoid ruling on the constitutionality of physically requiring vaccination, as this would directly affect a person's control over his or her body.[38]

It was within this historical context that the U.S. Supreme Court decided *Jacobson v. Massachusetts.* Justice Harlan's opinion had many faces and was, at some points, in tension. Relying on social compact theory, Harlan displayed strong deference to public health agencies. Relying on a theory of limited government, Harlan set standards to safeguard individual freedoms. This was a classic case of reconciling individual interests in bodily integrity with collective interests in health and safety. In the hundred years following *Jacobson,* the case has been cited in sixty-nine Supreme Court cases—most in support of the police power and a minority in support of individual freedom (see table 5). (A more comprehensive table of Supreme Court cases citing *Jacobson* appears on the *Reader* Web site.)

Social Compact Theory: The Police Power and Public Health Deference

In early American jurisprudence, before *Jacobson,* the judiciary staunchly defended the police power. The judiciary even periodically suggested that public health regulation was immune from constitutional review,[39] expressing the notion that "where the police power is set in motion in its proper sphere, the courts have no jurisdiction to stay the arm of the legislative branch."[40] The core issue, of course, was to understand what was meant by the "proper legislative sphere," for it was not supposed, at least since the enactment of the Fourteenth Amendment in 1868, that government could act in an arbitrary manner free from judicial control.[41]

The *Jacobson* Court's use of social compact theory to support this expansive understanding of police power was unmistakable. Justice Harlan preferred a community-oriented philosophy, where citizens have duties to one another and to society as a whole:

> The liberty secured by the Constitution . . . does not import an absolute right in each person to be . . . wholly freed from restraint. . . . On any other basis

TABLE 5. U.S. Supreme Court decisions citing *Jacobson v. Massachusetts*, 1905–2006

Context of Citation to *Jacobson*	Assertion Cited to *Jacobson*	Majority Opinions	Concurring Opinions	Dissenting Opinions	Total Cases
Public Health Deference: Social Compact Theory	State can regulate individuals and businesses to protect public health and safety[a]	8	1	—	8
	Liberty interests can be limited by the state[b]	22	7	9	34
	Questions of policy and science are for the legislature, not the courts[c]	12	—	1	13
	State can delegate police powers to agencies[d]	5	—	—	5
Individual Rights: Theory of Governmental Restraint	Liberty interests safeguarded by the Constitution[e]	4	2	—	6
	Police power regulation must have real and substantial relationship to state interest[f]	5	1	—	6
	State must demonstrate compelling state interest in exercise of police power[g]	1	—	—	1
	Evaluate exercise of police power by balancing state interest against implicated individual interest[h]	4	—	—	4
	Police power cannot be exercised in an unreasonable or arbitrary manner[i]	6	—	1	7
	Federal government lacks the police power[j]	1	—	—	1
Statutory Construction	Courts should avoid absurd results in interpreting statutes[k]	2	—	—	2
Total[l]		58	7	8	69

[a] *German Alliance Insurance. Co. v. Hale* cites *Jacobson* when asserting that "all corporations, associations, and individuals . . . are subject to such regulations, in respect of their relative rights and duties, as the state may, in the exercise of its police power, . . . prescribe for the public convenience and the general good." 219 U.S. 307, 317 (1911).

[b] *Williams v. Arkansas* quotes *Jacobson* as saying, "The liberty secured by the Constitution . . . does not import an absolute right in each person to be at all times, and in all circumstances, wholly freed from restraint." 217 U.S. 79, 88 (1910).

[c] *South Carolina State Highway Department v. Barnwell Bros.* cites *Jacobson* when saying that where legislative action is "within the scope of [the police] power, fairly debatable questions as to its reasonableness, wisdom, and propriety are not for the determination of courts, but for the legislative body." 303 U.S. 177, 191 (1938).

[d] *Plymouth Coal Co. v. Pennsylvania* cites *Jacobson* when saying, "It has become entirely settled that [police powers] may be delegated to administrative bodies." 232 U.S. 531 (1914).

[e] *Roe v. Wade* notes, "As stated in *Jacobson* . . . 'There is, of course, a sphere within which the individual may assert the supremacy of his own will.'" 410 U.S. 179, 213 (1973) (Douglas, J., concurring).

[f] *California Reduction Co. v. Sanitary Reduction Works* cites *Jacobson* when saying courts will not strike down a regulation for the protection of the public health that "has a real, substantial relation to that object." 199 U.S. 306, 318 (1905).

[g] *Bates v. City of Little Rock* cites *Jacobson* when asserting that the state interest must be "compelling" for a "significant encroachment on personal liberty" to stand. 361 U.S. 516, 524 (1960).

[h] *Cruzan v. Director, Missouri Department of Health* notes that in *Jacobson* "the Court balanced an individual's liberty interest in declining an unwanted smallpox vaccine against the State's interest in preventing disease." 497 U.S. 261, 278 (1990).

[i] *Price v. Illinois* cites *Jacobson* when saying that unless a prohibition "is palpably unreasonable and arbitrary we are not at liberty to say that it passes beyond the limits of the state's protective authority." 238 U.S. 446, 452 (1915).

[j] *Carter v. Carter Coal Co.* notes that the federal government lacks the broad police power of the states that was recognized in *Jacobson*. 298 U.S. 238, 292 (1936).

[k] *Sorrells v. United States* cites *Jacobson* to support the assertion that courts should read statutes so as to avoid unreasonable or absurd results. 287 U.S. 435, 447 (1932).

[l] *Jacobson* was cited in a total of seventy-seven Supreme Court cases, but citations in Supreme Court memoranda (eight) were excluded from this analysis. *Jacobson* was sometimes cited for more than one assertion in a case or was cited in the majority opinion as well as concurring or dissenting opinions. Where *Jacobson* was cited for more than one assertion in a case or was cited in a concurring or dissenting opinion as well as the majority opinion, each reference was indicated separately on the table, but the case was only counted once in the total cases and total opinions.

> organized society could not exist with safety to its members. . . . [The Massachusetts Constitution] laid down as a fundamental principle of the social compact that the whole people covenants with each citizen, and each citizen with the whole people, that all shall be governed by certain laws for the "common good," and that government is instituted "for the protection, safety, prosperity and happiness of the people, and not for the profit, honor or private interests of any one man."[42]

The Court's opinion is filled with examples ranging from sanitary laws and animal control to quarantine, demonstrating the breadth of police powers. Justice Harlan granted considerable leeway to the elected branches of government. The distinct tenor of the opinion was deferential to agency action.

A primary legacy of *Jacobson,* then, surely is its defense of social welfare philosophy and police power regulation. The Supreme Court during the *Jacobson* era upheld numerous public health activities, including regulation of food,[43] milk,[44] and garbage disposal.[45] Although the Progressive Era appeal to collective interests no longer has currency, most of the sixty-nine cases citing *Jacobson* do so in defense of the police power and public health deference (see table 5). Post-*Jacobson* courts have affirmed the state's authority to regulate individuals and businesses for the public's health and safety (eight); limit liberty to achieve common goods (thirty-four); permit legislatures to delegate broad powers to public health agencies (five); and defer to the judgment of legislatures and agencies in the exercise of their powers (thirteen).

Theory of Limited Government: Safeguarding Individual Liberty

Jacobson's social compact theory was in tension with its theory of limited government. Beyond its passive acceptance of state legislative discretion in matters of public health, however, was the Court's first systematic statement of the constitutional limitations imposed on government. *Jacobson* established a floor of constitutional protection. Public health powers are constitutionally permissible only if they are exercised in conformity with five standards, which I call public health necessity, reasonable means, proportionality, harm avoidance, and fairness. These standards, though permissive of public health intervention, nevertheless require a deliberative governmental process to safeguard liberty.

Public Health Necessity. Public health powers are exercised under the theory that they are necessary to prevent an avoidable harm. Justice Harlan, in *Jacobson,* insisted that police powers must be based on the "necessity of the case" and could not be exercised in "an arbitrary, unreasonable manner" or go "beyond what was reasonably required for the safety of the public."[46] Early meanings of the term *necessity* are consistent with the exercise of police powers: To necessitate was to "force" or "compel" a person to do that which he would prefer not to do, and the "necessaries" were those things without which life could not be maintained.[47] Government, in order to justify the use of compulsion, therefore, must act only in the face of a demonstrable health threat.[48] The standard of public health necessity requires, at a minimum, that the subject of the compulsory intervention actually pose a threat to the community.

Reasonable Means. Under the public health necessity standard, government may act only in response to a demonstrable threat to the community. The methods used, moreover, must be designed to prevent or ameliorate that threat. The *Jacobson* Court adopted a means/ends test that required a reasonable relationship between the public health intervention and the achievement of a legitimate public health objective. Even though the objective of the legislature may be valid and beneficent, the methods adopted must have a "real or substantial relation" to protection of the public health, and cannot be "a plain, palpable invasion of rights."[49]

Proportionality. The public health objective may be valid in the sense that a risk to the public exists, and the means may be reasonably likely to achieve that goal. Still, a public health regulation is unconstitutional if the human burden imposed is wholly disproportionate to the expected benefit. "The police power of a State," said Justice Harlan, "may be exerted in such circumstances, or by regulations so arbitrary and oppressive in particular cases, as to justify the interference of the courts to prevent wrong, and oppression."[50] Public health authorities have a constitutional responsibility not to overreach in ways that unnecessarily invade personal spheres of autonomy. This suggests a requirement that a reasonable balance be achieved between the public good and the degree of personal invasion. If the intervention is gratuitously onerous or unfair, it may overstep constitutional boundaries.

Harm Avoidance. Those who pose a risk to the community can be required to submit to compulsory measures for the common good. The control measure itself, however, should not pose a health risk to its subject.

Justice Harlan emphasized that Henning Jacobson was a "fit subject" for smallpox vaccination; he asserted that it would be "cruel and inhuman in the last degree" to require a person who would be harmed to be immunized.[51] If there had been evidence that the vaccination would seriously impair Jacobson's health, he might have prevailed in this historic case.[52] *Jacobson*-era cases reiterate the theme that public health actions must not harm subjects. For example, a quarantine of a district in San Francisco was held unconstitutional, in part because it created conditions likely to spread bubonic plague.[53] Similarly, courts required safe and habitable environments for persons subject to isolation on the theory that public health powers are designed to promote well-being, and not to punish the individual.[54]

Fairness. The facts in *Jacobson* did not require the Supreme Court to enunciate a standard of fairness under the Equal Protection Clause of the Fourteenth Amendment because the vaccination requirement was generally applicable to all inhabitants of Cambridge. Nevertheless, the federal courts had already created such a standard in *Jew Ho v. Williamson* in 1900. A quarantine for bubonic plague in San Francisco was made to operate exclusively against Chinese Americans. In striking down the quarantine, the federal district court said that health authorities had acted with an "evil eye and an unequal hand."[55]

Several of these standards for protecting liberty have been discernible in cases citing *Jacobson* from 1905 through 2004 (see table 5). Some cases cite *Jacobson* for the simple, albeit important, proposition that bodily integrity is a constitutionally protected liberty interest (six); others do so to require the state to have an important interest (real and substantial [six], compelling [one], or fairly balanced with individual interests [four]); and still others cite *Jacobson* to prevent the state from acting arbitrarily or unreasonably (seven). Federalism is also used as a tool to rein in the national government, with one court arguing that the federal government lacks the police power.

Lochner v. New York: *The Antithesis of Good Judicial Governance*

Jacobson v. Massachusetts was decided in the same term as *Lochner v. New York*[56]—the beginning of the so-called *Lochner* era in constitutional law (1905–37).[57] In *Lochner,* the Supreme Court held that a limitation on the hours that bakers could work violated the Due Process Clause of the Fourteenth Amendment. The Court perceived a limitation on bakers' hours as an interference with the freedom of contract rather than as a legitimate police power regulation.[58] Yet Justice Harlan, in a powerful dissent, professed that the New York statute was expressly for the public's health: "Labor in excess of sixty hours during a week . . . may endanger the health of those who thus labor."[59] Quoting standard public health treatises, Harlan observed that "during periods of epidemic diseases the bakers are generally the first to succumb to disease, and the number swept away during such periods far exceeds the number of other crafts."[60]

The *Lochner* era posed deep concerns for those who realized that much of what public health does interferes with economic freedoms involving contracts, business relationships, the use of property, and the practice of trades and professions. *Lochner,* in the words of Justice Harlan's dissent, "would seriously cripple the inherent power of the states to care for the lives, health, and well-being of their citizens."[61] So it did. For in the next three decades, the Supreme Court struck down important health and social legislation protecting trades unions,[62] setting minimum wages for women,[63] protecting consumers from products that posed health risks,[64] and licensing or regulating businesses.[65]

At the time of the New Deal, however, those who believed that people did not have unfettered contractual freedom and that economic transactions were naturally constrained by unequal wealth and power relationships challenged the laissez-faire philosophy that undergirded Lochnerism. This was also a time when people looked toward government to pursue actively the values of welfare, health, and greater social and economic equity. It was within this political context that the Supreme Court repudiated the principles of *Lochner:* "What is this freedom? The Constitution does not speak of freedom of contract. It speaks of liberty and prohibits the deprivation of liberty without due process of law."[66] The post–New Deal period led to the resurgence of a permissive judicial approach to public health regulation, irrespective of its effects on commercial and business affairs.[67]

Why have legal historians viewed *Jacobson* so favorably and *Lochner* so unfavorably? *Lochner* represented an unwarranted judicial interference with democratic control over the economy to safeguard the public's health. *Lochner* was a form of judicial activism that was unreceptive to protective and redistributive regulation. The *Lochner* court mistakenly saw market ordering as a state of nature rather than a legal construct.[68] *Jacobson* was the antithesis of *Lochner,* granting democratically elected officials discretion to pursue innovative solutions to hard social problems.

THE ENDURING MEANING OF *JACOBSON*

Supreme Court jurisprudence has progressed markedly from the deferential tone of *Jacobson* and its Progressive Era embrace of the social compact. The Warren Court, within the context of the civil rights movement, transformed constitutional law. The Court developed its "tiered" approach to due process and equal protection, which placed a constitutional premium on the protection of liberty interests. The question arises, would *Jacobson* be decided the same way if it were presented to the Court today? The answer is indisputably "yes," even if the style and reasoning would differ.

The validity of *Jacobson* as a sound modern precedent seems, at first sight, almost too obvious. The federal and state courts, including the U.S. Supreme Court,[69] have repeatedly affirmed its holding and reasoning, describing them as "settled" doctrine.[70] The courts have upheld compulsory vaccination in particular on numerous occasions.[71] Even the rare judicial reservations about compulsory vaccination focus on religious exemptions and do not query the state's authority to create a generally applicable immunization requirement.[72]

During the last several decades, the Supreme Court has recognized a constitutionally protected "liberty interest" in refusing unwanted medical treatment. The Court accepted the principle of bodily integrity in cases involving the rights of persons with terminal illness[73] and mental disability.[74] Outside the context of reproductive freedoms,[75] however, the Court has not viewed liberty interests in bodily integrity as "fundamental."[76] Instead of heightened scrutiny, the Supreme Court balances a person's liberty against state interests.[77] In fact, when it adopts a balancing test, the Court usually sides with the state.[78] The Court has held that health authorities may impose serious forms of treatment, such as antipsychotic medication, if the person poses a danger to himself or others.[79] The treatment must also be medically appropriate.[80] The lower courts, using a similar harm prevention theory, have upheld compulsory physical examination[81] and treatment[82] of persons with infectious diseases.

Jacobson began a debate about the appropriate boundaries of the police power that is still evolving today. Americans strongly support civil liberties, but they equally demand state protection of public health and safety. The compulsory immunization controversy still swirls, with flare-ups ranging from childhood[83] and school[84] vaccinations to counter-bioterror vaccinations for anthrax[85] and smallpox.[86] Despite the discordance in public opinion, *Jacobson* endures as a reasoned formulation of the boundaries between individual and collective interests in public health.

PUBLIC HEALTH POWERS IN THE MODERN CONSTITUTIONAL ERA

Jacobson, as explained earlier, established a floor of constitutional protection for individual rights, including five standards of judicial review: necessity, reasonable methods, proportionality, harm avoidance, and fairness. Arguably, these standards remain in the modern constitutional era, but the Supreme Court has developed a far more elaborate system of constitutional adjudication. Modern constitutional law is complicated, and the analysis of public health measures affecting personal autonomy, liberty, privacy, and property will unfold in subsequent chapters. For now, I will review "first principles": due process of law (both substantive and procedural), equal protection of the laws, and levels of scrutiny used by the Court to balance public goods and individual rights.

It will be obvious from the discussion of federalism in the last chapter and of the *Jacobson* and *Lochner* era in this chapter that the march toward more rigorous constitutional scrutiny of governmental action has been slow, cyclical, and politically charged. During the two decades beginning in the 1960s, constitutional doctrine changed markedly. It is important to remember that constitutional law reflects culture, society, and politics. Many cultural developments brought about this revolutionary shift: the civil rights movement for African Americans, protests against the Vietnam War, and the reemergence of feminism.[87] Responding to these and other social movements, the Supreme Court, principally under Chief Justice Earl Warren, revitalized and strengthened the Court's position on issues of equality and civil liberties. The Warren Court set a liberal agenda that prized personal freedom and nondiscrimination, and exhibited a healthy suspicion of government. The Burger and Rehnquist Courts, however, were less sympathetic to liberal constitutional construction, and the Roberts Court could go farther in reversing late twentieth-century jurisprudence.[88]

Procedural Due Process

The Fifth and Fourteenth Amendments prohibit government from depriving individuals of "life, liberty, or property, without due process of law." The Due Process Clause imposes two separate obligations: a "substantive" element that requires government to provide a sound justification for invading personal freedoms, and a procedural element that requires government to provide a fair process for individuals subject to state regulation or coercion.[89] Consider a state requirement for the licensing of physicians or the inspection of food establishments: These governmentally imposed conditions on the ability to practice a profession or to run a business meet the substantive part of the test if the state has a legitimate public health rationale (e.g., to assure the competent practice of medicine or the safe preparation of food). Actual decisions to deny or withdraw the license meet the procedural part of the test if the state affords professionals or businesses a reasonable opportunity to be heard.[90]

The procedural element of due process requires government to provide a fair process before depriving a person of life, liberty, or property—principally notice, a hearing, and an impartial decision maker. Affording individuals an opportunity to present their case is so essential to basic fairness that Europeans refer to procedural due process as "natural justice." Procedural due process is important in many different public health contexts, ranging from licenses and inspections of businesses to isolation of persons with infectious disease. This section explains "property" and "liberty" interests in the context of public health, and briefly discusses the kinds of procedures that are required in particular cases.

Property Interests. Government must provide a fair process before depriving individuals of property. Health departments possess the statutory authority to take, destroy, or restrict property uses to prevent risks to the health or safety of the community.[91] Except in urgent cases,[92] due process generally requires notice and an opportunity to be heard before the deprivation of a property interest.[93] Deprivations of property interests, which trigger procedural due process safeguards, occur in a variety of public health contexts: inspections of goods and buildings;[94] licenses of health care professionals,[95] hospitals and clinics,[96] nursing homes,[97] or restaurants;[98] and staff privileges in public hospitals.[99]

The Supreme Court defines a "property interest" as more than an abstract need, desire, or unilateral expectation. The person must "have a legitimate claim of entitlement."[100] Certainly, an individual has an "entitlement" to the legitimate ownership of real or personal property. However, does a person have an entitlement to a benefit, a job, a professional license, a business permit, or even government protection against private violence?

The Supreme Court, until the 1970s, limited "property interests" to cases where the person had a legal right and not a simple privilege. However, in *Goldberg v. Kelly* (1970), the Supreme Court abandoned the "rights/privilege" distinction, holding that individuals have a property interest in the continued receipt of welfare benefits.[101] Though the Court has officially rejected the distinction between rights and privileges, demonstrating an "entitlement" can be difficult. Under the reasoning of *Goldberg*, an entitlement is measured by the importance of the interest to the person's life; without welfare, for example, a person may not obtain the necessities of life. The modern Court's preferred approach is to examine whether the person has a legitimate claim of entitlement to the property interest based on an independent source, such as state law.[102]

The Supreme Court has held that a benefit is not a protected entitlement if government officials may grant or deny it at their discretion.[103] In *Castle Rock v. Gonzales* (2005), discussed in the last chapter, the Court found that police had "discretion" not to enforce a domestic violence restraining order, even though the order specifically declared and a state statute commanded that it must be enforced.[104] The Court said that even if enforcement was "mandatory," "it is by no means clear" that the individual has "property interest" for the purposes of due process: "Such a right would not, of course, resemble any traditional conception of property," wrote Justice Scalia.[105]

Liberty Interests. Government must provide procedural due process before depriving individuals of liberty.[106] A person who is imprisoned, of course, is deprived of liberty—even, for example, U.S. citizens detained as "enemy combatants" in the "war on terror."[107] However, the Supreme Court broadly defines a "liberty interest" as "not merely freedom from bodily restraint but also the right to contract, to engage in any of the common occupations of life, to acquire useful knowledge, to marry, establish a home and bring up children, to worship God . . . , and generally to enjoy those privileges long recognized . . . as essential to the orderly pursuit of happiness by free men."[108]

Procedural due process classically is required in any case where public health authorities interfere with freedom of movement (e.g., isolation and quarantine) or bodily integrity (e.g., compulsory physical examination and medical treatment).

The Elements of Procedural Due Process. Fair procedures are constitutionally required if an individual or business suffers a deprivation of property or liberty.[109] However, this does not decide the question of exactly what kinds of procedures the government must provide. Due process is a flexible concept that varies with the particular situation. The Supreme Court has said that, in deciding which procedures are required, courts should balance several factors.[110] First, the courts consider the nature of the private interests affected. The more intrusive or coercive the state intervention, the more rigorous the procedural safeguards. In cases of plenary deprivation of liberty,[111] such as civil commitment of a person with mental illness[112] or tuberculosis,[113] the state must provide the full panoply of procedures—notice, counsel, impartial hearing, cross-examination, written decision, and appeal. The justification for rigorous procedural protections is found in the fundamental invasion of liberty occasioned by long-term detention.[114]

Second, the courts consider the risk of an erroneous deprivation and the probable value, if any, of additional or substitute procedural safeguards. Here, the courts are concerned with the value of procedures as a method of protecting against erroneous decision making. If the court feels that an informal process is likely to lead to a "correct" result, it will not require procedural formalities that it regards as unnecessary. In *Parham v. J. R.* (1979), "mature minors" were "voluntarily" admitted to a mental hospital by their parents, although the minors opposed the admission. The Supreme Court ruled that the hearing did not have to be formal or conducted by a court. Since juvenile admission was "essentially medical in character," an independent review by hospital physicians was sufficient for due process purposes.[115]

Third, the courts consider the fiscal and administrative burdens in providing additional procedures and the extent to which the government's interests would be undermined. Most mental health or public health statutes permit an expedited form of due process in cases of emergency. Reduced due process is justified by the fact that the state's interests in rapid confinement of immediately dangerous persons would be undermined by elaborate, time-consuming procedures.

In sum, in ascertaining what procedures are constitutionally required, the courts weigh three factors—the extent of the deprivation of liberty or property, the risk of an erroneous decision, and the burdens that additional procedures will entail. Thus, the procedures in any given circumstance depend on the public health context and vary from case to case. The process required can range from a full-blown hearing to an informal, nonadversarial review.[116]

Substantive Due Process

Substantive due process is a legal theory that requires government to justify any deprivation of life, liberty, or property. Under this theory, government must have adequate reasons for its interventions.[117] The police power represents a classically adequate justification under substantive due process. Thus, government may act for the purposes of protecting the health, safety, or morals of the community. Depending on the level of judicial scrutiny applied, government action must be justified by a legitimate, a substantial, or even a compelling public interest.[118]

Another way of thinking about substantive due process is its proscription of arbitrary and capricious government activity.[119] Because government must produce adequate reasons, it cannot intervene in ways that are indiscriminate, haphazard, or purposeless. If public health officials coerce without a comprehensible rationale, they violate substantive due process. Similarly, the state must avoid regulation influenced by animosity toward a politically unpopular constituency. In cases where the government's principal purpose is to disadvantage a person or population, the Court might conclude that "enactment [is] divorced from any factual context from which [the Court] could discern a relationship to legitimate state interests."[120]

Substantive due process is controversial because it permits the judiciary to find constitutional rights where none are expressed in the Constitution. The modern Court has repeatedly declared its reluctance to expand substantive due process "because guideposts for responsible decision-making in this unchartered area are scarce and open-ended."[121] The Court sees substantive due process as being in conflict with democratic values because the doctrine places policy questions outside the "arena of public debate and legislative action."[122] The Court's concern is that, absent objective criteria, substantive due process would permit members of the Court to inject their policy preferences. The Supreme Court's substantive due process analysis has two features designed to facilitate objective reasoning. The Court requires, first, a "careful description" of the asserted liberty interest and, second, that the interest be "deeply rooted in the Nation's history and traditions."[123]

The ongoing debate between those with an expansive view of due process and those who favor a more restrictive application is highly important in public health. Few public health measures directly infringe on a right or freedom declared in the Bill of Rights. The Constitution, for example, does not explicitly mention bodily integrity, which is implicated in mandatory testing and treatment, or privacy, which is implicated in mandatory reporting and partner notification. Moreover, since groups at risk of certain diseases have never gained protection within our constitutional history (e.g., gays and prostitutes), the Court might not see their freedoms as "deeply rooted in the Nation's history."

In a deeply divisive case, *Lawrence v. Texas* (2003), the Supreme Court acknowledged that history and tradition are the starting point but not necessarily the ending point of substantive due process inquiry.[124] The Court, in overturning *Bowers v. Hardwick* (1986),[125] held that a Texas statute which made it a crime for two persons of the same sex to engage in intimate sexual conduct violated the Due Process Clause.[126] In a departure from its narrow reading of substantive due process, the Court said that criminal penalties against same-sex sodomy touched upon "the most private human conduct, sexual behavior, and in the most private of places, the home." Adults, wrote Justice Kennedy, have the "liberty" and "dignity as free persons" to enter into personal relationships that injure no other person.[127] The Court cited with approval a ruling by the European Court of Human Rights that homosexual adults have a right to engage in intimate, consensual conduct.[128] This *dicta* is controversial because it raises the question of when, and to what extent, the Supreme Court should pay attention to settled international law. *Lawrence* makes clear, however, that a law will not satisfy due process simply because a governing majority has traditionally viewed a personal behavior as immoral, particularly when the law implicates basic human rights.

Equal Protection of the Laws

The Fourteenth Amendment commands that no state shall "deny to any person within its jurisdiction the equal protection of the laws." The Supreme Court, in a 1954 school segregation case, held that the federal government must also afford persons equal protection of the laws.[129]

The law usually classifies for one purpose or another, with resulting disadvantage to various persons or groups.[130] The law can discriminate among people in two ways. First, the law can expressly make distinctions among persons or groups. This kind of discrimination is called a facial classification because the distinction among people is "on the face" of the statute. A statute that requires searches of persons of Middle Eastern descent facially discriminates on the basis of national origin. Second, the law can be "facially neutral" in that it applies one standard to all people. Statutes of general applicability nonetheless often disproportionately affect particular persons or groups. For instance, a law that requires prenatal screening in all communities with a high prevalence of HIV infection will have a disparate impact on women of color and low-income women. The Supreme Court may not find that a law of general applicability violates equal protection even if it would have a demonstrably inequitable effect on vulnerable groups. If a law is facially neutral, the disproportionately burdened class must demonstrate that the government's actual purpose was to discriminate against that group, which can be exceedingly difficult to prove.[131]

If a law expressly discriminates or if a facially neutral law adversely affects persons or groups against whom the government intended to discriminate, an equal protection problem exists. Contrary to popular belief, however, government is not obliged to treat all people identically. Instead, the Equal Protection Clause requires that government treat like cases alike, but permits government to treat unlike cases dissimilarly.[132] Virtually any public health policy establishes a class of people that receives a benefit or burden and a class that does not. The critical question is whether sufficient justification exists for the distinction among classes. Put another way, do public health authorities have a valid reason for distinguishing among people, and if so, how substantial is that reason? Medicare eligibility, for example, is based on a person's age, but the government has a plausible reason for offering the benefit to the elderly and excluding others. On the other hand, quarantining Asian Americans but not Caucasians in an area where disease is endemic has no justification.[133]

If the government engages in particularly pernicious forms of discrimination or infringes on particularly important rights, it must provide a more cogent justification for the unequal treatment. Equal protection analysis therefore requires an examination of the class created by the statute and the right denied to that class. The Court strictly scrutinizes laws that create "suspect classifications" (e.g., race, national origin, or alienage) or burden "fundamental rights" (e.g., procreation, marriage, interstate travel, and voting) (see "Levels of Constitutional Review of Public Health Activities" below). For example, the courts would closely examine a policy that required all African Americans to be tested for sickle cell disease. Similarly, the courts would carefully examine a quarantine placed at the border of New York and New Jersey that inhibited movement across state lines.

Levels of Constitutional Review of Public Health Activities

As this brief discussion of substantive due process and equal protection suggests, the Supreme Court adopts different levels of constitutional review, depending on the form of discrimination and the nature of the civil liberty in question. The level of review signals how the courts will balance the various interests in a particular case—the government's interest in preventing injury or disease and the individual's interest in avoiding infringement of autonomy, privacy, or liberty. The level of review also signals how carefully the Court will examine the public health policy, or to put it another way, how much deference the courts will give to public health regulation. The lower the level of scrutiny, the greater the Court's presumption of constitutionality. The three formal levels of constitutional review, ranging from the most to the least deferential, are rational basis (minimum rationality), intermediate, and strict scrutiny.

Rational Basis Review. The Court's lowest, and most commonly used, standard of constitutional review is the rational basis test. All public health regulation must at least comply with this minimum rationality standard. Rational basis review requires both a legitimate government objective and means that are reasonably related to attaining that objective. Police power regulation is a classically valid objective: "Public safety, public health, morality, peace, law and order—these are some of the more conspicuous examples of [legitimate governmental interests]."[134] The Court has expressly upheld numerous public health objectives, including traffic safety,[135] detection of underdiagnosed disease,[136] and disease prevention.[137] Not only must the government's purpose be valid, but the means adopted must be reasonably directed toward achieving the public health objective.[138] For example, an ordinance requiring owners of vacant lots to clear-cut all vegetation was invalidated because the town's claim that noxious vines could grow was implausible.[139]

Rationality review is highly permissive of public health regulation, with the Court granting a strong presumption of constitutionality.[140] Constitutional review "is not a license for courts to judge the wisdom, fairness, or logic of legislative choices."[141] The judiciary leaves the desirability of public health regulation to the legislature. Further, the legislature need not "actually articulate at any time the purpose or rationale" for its public health policy.[142] Rather, public health regulation is upheld if there is "any reasonably conceivable state of facts that could provide a rational basis for the classification."[143]

Scientific evidence of risk is the raison d'être of public health action. Yet, in a rational basis review, the state is not obliged to produce scientific evidence.[144] "A legislative choice is not subject to courtroom fact finding and may be based on rational speculation unsupported by evidence or empirical data."[145] Indeed, the courts often defer to expert agencies on matters of public health policy because agencies are faced with complex practical problems that require "rough accommodations—illogical, it may be, and unscientific."[146] The courts, under rationality review, have upheld a wide spectrum of public health regulations, ranging from infectious disease screening,[147] mandatory treatment,[148] and vaccine compensation[149] to regulation of landfills[150] and licensing of fishermen.[151]

Rationality review almost always results in a finding that police power regulation is constitutional. However, several Supreme Court decisions suggest that rational basis review may be more rigorous when the government engages in invidious discrimination. In 1938, in a famous footnote in the *Carolene Products* case, the Court hinted that it might engage in a more searching judicial inquiry when legislation discriminates against "discrete and insular minorities" who could not easily redress their injuries through democratic processes.[152] Though the modern Court seldom, if ever, applies the *Carolene Products* standard, it has on several occasions engaged in more exacting scrutiny of discriminatory government action, while purporting to apply the rational basis test—so-called rational basis with a bite.[153]

In *City of Cleburne v. Cleburne Living Center, Inc.* (1985),[154] the Supreme Court, using rational basis review, declared unconstitutional a zoning ordinance that effectively prevented the operation of a group home for persons with mental retardation. Under conventional rationality review, the judiciary would be deferential, but the Court believed that the legislature was motivated by animosity toward a traditionally disenfranchised group. Similarly, in *Romer v. Evans* (1996),[155] the Supreme Court saw prejudice against homosexuals, another group that is disadvantaged in the political process. Colorado had amended its state constitution to prohibit all legislative, executive, or judicial action designed to protect lesbians or gay men from discrimination. The Court held that the state constitutional amendment "fails, even defies," the rational basis test.[156] The state's reason, said the Court, "seems inexplicable by anything but animus toward the class that it affects; it lacks a rational relationship to legitimate state interests."[157] The Supreme Court in *Lawrence v. Texas,* which cites *Romer,* similarly found no rational basis for singling out gay men under a criminal sodomy statute. *Cleburne, Romer,* and *Lawrence* suggest that there may be areas where legislatures act against politically disfavored groups with such hostility that the Court is prepared to examine legislative motives more carefully than in conventional applications of rationality review. In the Court's words, "A bare congressional desire to harm a politically unpopular group cannot constitute a legitimate government purpose."[158]

Rationality review is extraordinarily important in public health because most prevention strategies are measured against this standard. Because risk assessment and scientific evidence are so important in evaluating public health measures, rationality review hardly seems sufficient.[159] This lowest standard of review does not force public health authorities to justify their actions by demonstrating a significant risk and showing the intervention is likely to ameliorate that risk; nor does it usually require authorities to justify targeting particularly vulnerable or unpopular groups, such as gays, prostitutes, homeless persons, or drug users. Discrimination on the basis of sexual orientation, disability, and socioeconomic class has played an important role in the history of public health. In the wake of cases such as *Cleburne, Romer,* and *Lawrence,* the future will show whether the Court is prepared to look more carefully at disfavored treatment of politically unpopular groups.

Intermediate Review. The Supreme Court adopts an intermediate level of review where government discriminates on the basis of sex[160] or against "illegitimate" children.[161] Gender discrimination triggers this intermediate scrutiny, whether the discrimination is against women or men.[162] Under this middle level of constitutional review, the state must establish that its classification serves important governmental objectives and that the classification is substantially related to those objectives.[163] Thus, the government's interest must be "important," not simply legitimate, and the relationship between means and ends must be "substantial," not merely reasonable. The Court exercises great care in examining government policy under this middle tier of review. In invalidating gender discrimination at the Virginia Military Institute, Justice Ginsberg emphasized that the state must demonstrate "an exceedingly persuasive justification. . . . The burden of justification is demanding and rests entirely on the State."[164]

Public health actions that classify on the basis of sex, therefore, are subject to a rigorous form of judicial review. Consider, for example, mandatory syphilis testing of female, but not male, applicants for a marriage license. This sexual classification probably would be unconstitutional because it does not serve a substantial public health purpose.[165] Prenatal HIV testing of women, however, might withstand constitutional scrutiny, because the state could demonstrate a substantial reason for focusing the intervention on women.[166]

Strict Scrutiny. As explained earlier, the Supreme Court strictly reviews laws that create "suspect" classifications or burden "fundamental" rights and liberty interests. The Court has given several reasons why it might find a classification suspect: (1) immutable characteristics—personal statuses acquired at birth that individuals do not choose and cannot change; (2) political powerlessness—discrete minorities who have ineffective access to the political process to safeguard their own rights; (3) history of discrimination—groups that have suffered from long periods of prejudice and unfavorable treatment; and (4) stereotypes—classifications that are rarely justified by rational public policy choices. The Court has decided that race,[167] national origin,[168] and with some exceptions, alienage[169] are suspect classes.[170]

The Court also strictly reviews government actions that burden fundamental rights and liberty interests, including procreation,[171] marriage,[172] interstate travel,[173] and child rearing.[174] (The Court has used an "undue burden" standard to review state regulation of abortions,[175] but the Roberts Court has begun eviscerating this standard.[176]) The Court has found a constitutionally protected liberty interest in bodily integrity, but it has yet to hold that such an interest is "fundamental."[177] Fundamental rights and interests receive heightened protection because of their value in our constitutional system. The Supreme Court, during its modern history, has used different forms of reasoning to determine if a right is "fundamental." Liberties that are explicitly protected within the text of the Constitution, such as the freedoms of expression and religion, or the right to vote, are always regarded as fundamental. Other liberties, such as the right to procreate, are deemed fundamental because they involve "the most intimate and personal choices a person may make in a lifetime, choices central to personal dignity and autonomy."[178] Finally, as explained earlier, rights are deemed fundamental if they "are deeply rooted in this Nation's history and tradition."[179]

Under strict scrutiny, the government must demonstrate a "compelling interest" and a tight relationship between means and ends, and show that its objectives could not be achieved by less restrictive or discriminatory purposes. First, the government must demonstrate an interest that is "compelling" or truly vital to community well-being. Public health and safety are quintessentially regarded as compelling interests. Second, the government must demonstrate that the methods chosen are strictly necessary to achieve its objectives. Thus, legislation must avoid underinclusiveness and, particularly, overinclusiveness. Policies that are underinclusive apply to certain individuals or groups but not to others who are in a similar position; for example, the policy may use compulsion against one group but not against another group that poses the same risk to the public. By itself, underinclusiveness is not necessarily fatal from a constitutional position. Government may use its limited resources "one step at a time" to address part of a public health problem without having to address the entire problem. Overinclusiveness, or overbreadth, occurs when a policy extends to more people than it needs to in order to achieve the public health objective. An overinclusive exercise of a compulsory power is frequently unacceptable because it subjects individuals who pose no health risk to loss of liberty. For example, isolation of all persons with tuberculosis infection who are not contagious could be fatally overinclusive because most people in this population do not pose a risk.[180]

Finally, strict scrutiny requires the adoption of the "least restrictive alternative." Thus, the government must demonstrate that its public purpose could not be achieved as well through less restrictive or less discriminatory policies. The principle of the least restrictive alternative does not require public health authorities to adopt policies that are less effective than the proposed policy. It simply requires government to utilize the policy that achieves the public health objective with the least intrusion on personal rights and freedoms.

When the Court adopts strict scrutiny, it almost invariably strikes down the statute. A deeply controversial exception, however, is affirmative action based on race. In its 2004–5 term, a bitterly divided Court rejected a university admissions policy that automatically granted twenty points to minority applicants because the policy made race a decisive factor.[181] In a second case, the Court upheld a narrowly tailored use of race without quotas in university admissions to further the compelling interest of diversity in higher education.[182] The Roberts Court will struggle with affirmative action, recalling Justice O'Connor's premonition that "twenty-five years from now, the use of racial preferences will no longer be necessary."[183] In the 2007–8 term, the Court again broached this issue and decided by a five–four vote that local school districts unlawfully made student assignment decisions based in part on race.[184]

Beyond Levels of Constitutional Scrutiny

Constitutional scholars, and members of the Court itself, often criticize the levels of review because they are inflexible and outcome-determinative.[185] Where the Court sees certain touchstones of constitutional concern, such as a suspect classification or the violation of a fundamental right, the government almost invariably loses; strict scrutiny is "strict in theory, but fatal in fact."[186] In the absence of these specific gauges of constitutional concern, the Court uses the rational basis test and the government almost invariably wins. Certainly, different standards ought to apply depending on the class affected or the right infringed, yet it is far from clear why such sharply different constitutional standards and outcomes should result. Strict scrutiny is invoked for classifications based on race, national origin, and alienage, but not sexual orientation,[187] disability,[188] socioeconomic status,[189] or geographical location.[190] Yet each of these groups has experienced discrimination based on irrational fears and prejudices. Similarly, strict scrutiny is invoked for invasions of fundamental interests like contraception, abortion, interstate travel, and access to medicine, but not for breaches of confidentiality[191] or interference with the doctor-patient relationship.[192] Yet each of these liberty interests has importance to human dignity and individual freedom. Whatever differences exist between various status classifications and liberty interests, they are differences of degree, not of kind.

At the same time, when the Court applies rationality review, it fails to ask public health authorities to justify their actions in the most elemental ways: What are the specific public health goods sought by the intervention? What scientific evidence demonstrates a significant health risk? Are the interventions proposed likely to be effective?

Two problems, then, are evident in constitutional analysis. First, the standards provide a rigid "all-or-nothing" assessment rather than a graduated examination based on the burdens posed by discriminatory classifications or infringements on autonomy, privacy, and liberty. Second, rationality review, by far the most common form of scrutiny, places few demands on public health authorities to justify their actions based on scientific evidence of risk reduction.

For a different way of thinking about levels of constitutional review, think of a sliding scale that subjects public health policies to increasingly demanding levels of constitutional review. As the intrusiveness and unfairness of the public health policy grows, so would the level of scrutiny. As

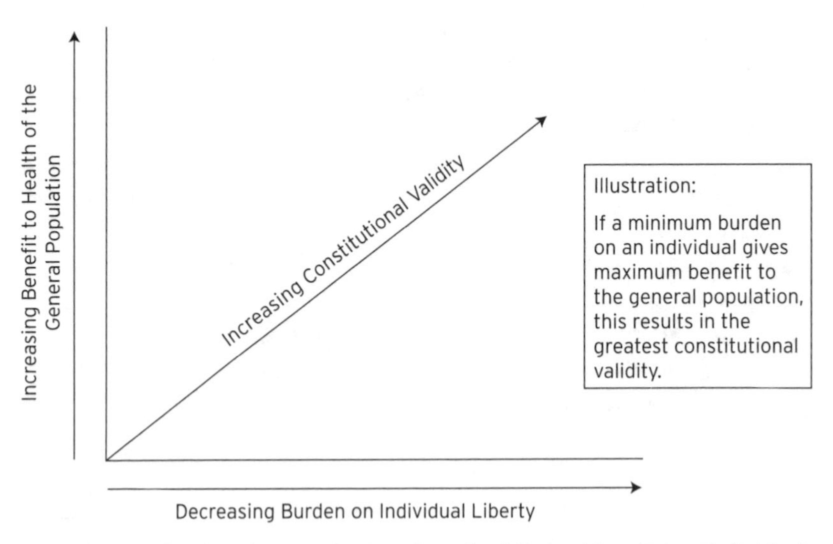

Figure 16. Evaluating the constitutionality of public health policies: Individual liberties versus public benefit.

a policy moves across the continuum because of its restrictive or discriminatory quality, public health would gradually give way to individual liberty (see figure 16).

Constitutional powers, duties, and limitations are critical for understanding public health law. However, constitutional law is not the only field of domestic law with high relevance to public health. In the following two chapters, I examine the fields of administrative law and tort law, both of which are important to the study of public health.

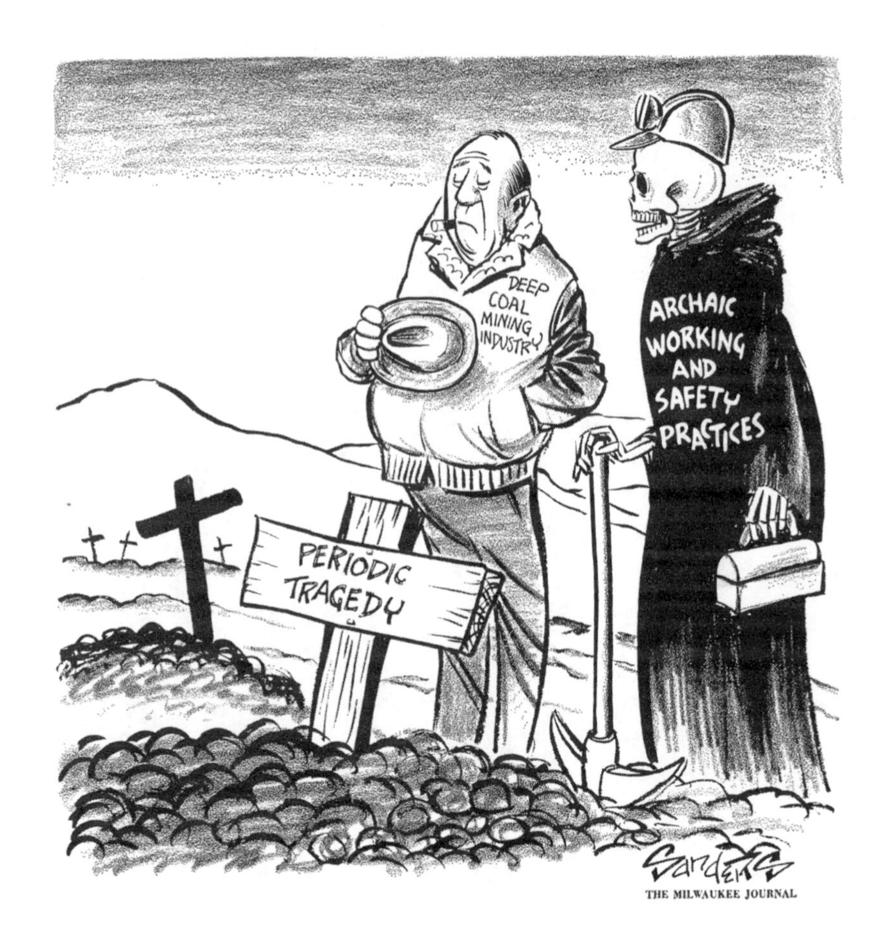

'We'd best get back to business, pardner'

Photo 7. Cartoon deriding the dangerous state of mine safety practices. In the wake of the Sago Creek Mine disaster of 2006, this cartoon derides the mine's safety violations that may have been responsible for seriously injuring one miner and killing twelve others. Weeks later, West Virginia enacted new mine safety laws, including requirements for better communication, underground oxygen supplies, and faster emergency responses. A few months thereafter, President Bush signed the Mine Improvement and New Emergency Response Act of 2006 (the MINER Act), which required mines to have emergency response plans, improved communication, and increased supplies of oxygen. The Act also increased fines for mine safety violations. Courtesy of the *Milwaukee Journal Sentinel*. Artist: Sanders. © 2007 Journal Sentinel, Inc. Reproduced with permission.

CHAPTER 5

Public Health Governance

Direct Regulation for the Public's Health and Safety

The protection and promotion of the public health has long been recognized as the responsibility of the sovereign power. Government is, in fact, organized for the express purpose, among others, of conserving the public health and cannot divest itself of this important duty.

James Tobey (1927)

Constitutional law and democratic theory support the basic power or obligation of organized society (principally through government) to protect and preserve the health and safety of populations. Governmental health activities form part of the fabric and experience of public health. Over the history of public health, the line between public and private action has never been hard and fast. Moreover, private, charitable, and religious influences have been manifest.[1] Still, from the colonial and framing eras to the Progressive Era and New Deal—and continuing in modern times—government in all its various forms has assumed responsibility for the public's health. This chapter on direct regulation by public health agencies and the next, on indirect regulation through the tort system, examine further the political and legal structures and mechanisms of regulation.

Traditional public health governance relies on direct government regulation of industry and professions. State regulation has value because market forces do not always ensure the health and safety of workers, consumers, and the general public—as evidenced by the death of fourteen West Virginia miners in 2006.[2] Theories of modern regulation are changing, however. Scholars are proposing an array of "new governance" mechanisms—including market-based incentives, disclosure requirements, negotiated or self-regulation, and public/private partnerships.[3] The

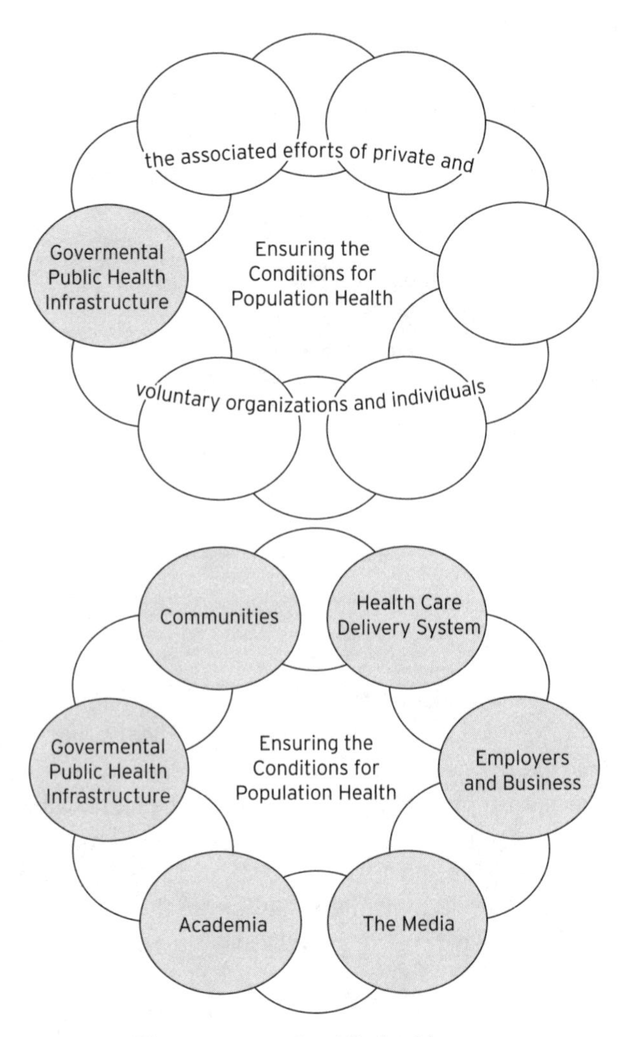

Figure 17. The intersectoral public health system.

Institute of Medicine, recognizing broader influences on governance, thinks of public health as a "system" with government at its center but also comprising health care institutions, the community, businesses, the media, and academia (see Figure 17).[4]

This chapter explores both traditional forms of direct regulation and new governance theory and practice. Government should not be wedded to any particular form of regulation. Rather, the state has an abiding interest in effective, efficient, and economical interventions to improve the public's health. "Smart regulation" may entail a combination of approaches and stakeholders with the one objective of ensuring the public's health and safety.[5]

The deep-seated problems of safety and health pose complex, highly technical challenges that require expertise, flexibility, and deliberative study over the long term. Solutions cannot be found within traditional government structures, such as representative assemblies or governors' offices. As a result, governments have formed specialized entities, usually within the executive branch, to pursue the goals of population health and safety.[6] These administrative agencies form the bulwark for public health activities in the United States. It is for this reason that administrative law (the body of law formed by administrative agencies established by the legislature, and subject to review by the courts) lies at the heart of public health.[7]

This chapter first presents a brief history of public health regulation of commercial activities, showing the long-standing and pervasive interest of public health agencies in regulating trades and professions, health institutions, and businesses. Second, it examines the structure and powers of modern public health agencies at the federal, state, and local levels. Third, the chapter explains administrative law as it relates to public health: legislative delegation of authority, restraints on power, and the processes of rulemaking, adjudication, and enforcement. Finally, the chapter examines new governance theory and practice—the effort to find innovative ways of improving health and safety through involvement of stakeholders and public/private collaborations. (Chapter 12 reviews the law relating to three of the most common forms of commercial regulation—licenses, inspections, and nuisance abatements—and assesses the value of economic freedom.)

A BRIEF HISTORY OF PUBLIC HEALTH REGULATION

A distinctive and powerful governmental tradition devoted in theory and practice to the vision of a well-regulated society dominated United States social and economic policymaking from 1787 to 1877. . . . At the heart of the well-regulated society was a plethora of bylaws, ordinances, statutes, and common law restrictions regulating nearly every aspect of early American economy and society. . . . Taken together they explode tenacious myths about nineteenth-century government (or its absence) and demonstrate the

> pervasiveness of regulation in early American versions of the good society: regulations for public safety and security . . . and the open-ended regulatory powers granted to public officials to guarantee public health (securing the population's well-being, longevity, and productivity). Public regulation—the power of the state to restrict individual liberty and property for the common welfare—colored all facets of early American development. It was the central component of a reigning theory and practice of governance committed to the pursuit of the people's welfare and happiness in a well-ordered society and polity.
>
> William J. Novak (1996)

Much public health regulation takes place at the local level and involves the status of cities. Cities in colonial America had the primary governmental responsibility for public health. Early legislative activities were organized around reducing filth and regulating dangerous trades.[8] Perhaps the oldest sanitary law, enacted in 1634, prohibited residents of Boston from depositing fish or garbage near the common landing.[9] Beginning in 1652, a series of ordinances were enacted to control the sanitary condition and location of privies, prohibit the dumping of rubbish onto public thoroughfares and waterways, and impound stray animals from the streets and remove dead animals and offal.[10]

Regulation of hazardous trades and businesses limited the location and methods of operation of butchers, blubber-boilers, slaughterhouses, tanners, and other enterprises. For example, the first Massachusetts General Assembly, in 1692, empowered selectmen in market towns to prohibit slaughterhouses, the drying out of tallow, and the currying of leather, except in assigned locations.[11] At the same time, legislatures were also overseeing the production of food (principally bread and meat) by requiring inspections and enforcing standards.[12]

By the mid-nineteenth century, the Industrial Revolution was transforming societies in Western Europe and North America, making possible substantial advances in prosperity. Laissez-faire politics reinforced belief in free markets, and led to the expansion of industry and a consequent migration of workers to the city to secure jobs and livelihood.[13] The United States was becoming one of the most successful industrial economies in the world.

The sheer success of industrialization and urbanization posed such momentous hazards to community health and well-being that it made possible a political shift in favor of extensive commercial regulation. Public health advocates, a progressive coalition of sanitary engineers, physicians, and public-spirited citizens known as "Sanitarians,"[14] observed and documented the profound health and safety risks that arose from the new industrial civilization (see box 7).[15] The engine of industrial growth, the factory, was causing injury to workers and harm to communities. Migration to the cities for work resulted in overcrowding, slum conditions, homelessness, squalor, and violence. There existed a growing realization that disease caused by garbage, sewage, pollution, and contaminated food and drinking water affected the entire community and was within the proper sphere of government control. By the end of the century, the Sanitarians were pressing for an ambitious regulatory agenda to control noxious substances and unsanitary conditions, as well as to promote town planning.[16] The most important public health report of the time, written by Lemuel Shattuck in 1850, commenced with a call for sanitary legislation:

> The condition of perfect public health requires such laws and regulations as will secure to man associated in society the same sanitary enjoyments that he would have as an isolated individual; and as will protect him from injury from any influences connected with his locality, his dwelling house, his occupation, . . . or from any other social causes. It is under the control of public authority, and public administration; and life and health may be saved or lost, as this authority is wisely or unwisely exercised.[17]

A pervasive regulatory system evolved in state and local governments to ameliorate the health effects of industrialization and urbanization. Even the most casual perusal of treatises on city government in the late nineteenth century reveals the extensive regulatory system that controlled every aspect of civil society.[18] Public health regulations extended to dangerous buildings, public conveyances, corporations, use of travel ways (e.g., streets, highways, and navigable waters), objectionable trades, disorderly houses, storage of gunpowder, sale of food, sale and prescription of dangerous drugs, health and safety of workers, and many other commercial activities.[19]

During the latter half of the nineteenth century, criminal law was the preferred method of sanctioning violations of health and safety regulations. Violation of these laws was usually a misdemeanor, but conviction

BOX 7

THE GREAT NINETEENTH-CENTURY PUBLIC HEALTH CAMPAIGNERS

In the nineteenth century, great figures in public health devoted their lives to sanitary reform, including Villermé in France, Shattuck in the United States, Chadwick in England, and Virchow in Germany. Each of these campaigners stressed the devastating effects of urbanization, industrialization, and poverty on the morbidity and mortality of populations.

Louis-René Villermé (1782-1863) argued that life and death are not primarily biological phenomena but are closely linked to social circumstances. He showed that "arrondissements" in Paris with lower socioeconomic status (SES) had systematically higher mortality rates than higher SES neighborhoods. Villermé's famous study on the link between cotton production and pneumonia and his campaign against excessive child labor in manufacturing resulted in the enactment of the Child Labour Act of 1841.[1]

Lemuel Shattuck's (1793-1859) greatest work was his 1850 "Report of the Sanitary Commission of Massachusetts," in which he linked environmental and social conditions to health, and recommended the establishment of a state board of health. Although the report has since been hailed as a milestone in American public health, Shattuck's failure to implement the reforms led some to conclude that he was "good at diagnosis, but weak on therapy."[2] After his death, in 1869, the first state board of health in the United States was established in Massachusetts.

Edwin Chadwick (1800-1890) published his famous "Report into the Sanitary Conditions of the Labouring Population of Great Britain" in 1842.[3] The Chadwick Report demonstrated that life expectancy was much lower in towns than in the countryside and challenged the laissez-faire attitude of the time: "The various forms of epidemic, endemic, and other disease caused, or aggravated, or propagated chiefly amongst the labouring classes by atmospheric impurities produced by decomposing animal and vegetable substances, by damp and filth, and close and overcrowded dwellings prevail amongst the population in every part of the kingdom." In 1848, in response to the report and partly through fear of cholera, Parliament passed the first British Public Health Act, which is still largely in effect.[4] Chadwick had a bold, abrupt personality, lecturing the masses about health. Some said that they would rather take their chances with cholera than be told what to do by Chadwick!

Rudolf Ludwig Karl Virchow (1821-1902), perhaps best known for championing cell theory, also campaigned for public health measures, such as sewage disposal, hospital architecture, improvement of meat inspection techniques, and school hygiene. He argued that high infant mortality was due to poor housing, declining milk supply, and sepsis. He famously stated that "medicine is a social science, and politics nothing but medicine at a larger scale."[5]

[1] Louis-René Villermé, *Tableau de l'état physique et moral des ouvriers employés dans les manufactures de coton, de laine et de soie* (Paris: J. Renouard, 1840).

[2] Marie E. Daly, "Disease and Our Ancestors: Mortality in the Eighteenth and Nineteenth Centuries," *New England Historical Genealogical Society*, June 13, 2006, http://www.newenglandancestors.org/publications/NEA//disease_and_our_ancestors_mortality_in_the_eighte_607_1807.asp.

[3] Edwin Chadwick, *Report into the Sanitary Conditions of the Labouring Population of Great Britain* (1842; rpt. Edinburgh: University Press, 1965).

[4] A proposal for a new Health of the People Act in the United Kingdom has not been successful. Stephen Monaghan, Dyfed Hughes and Marie Navarro, *The Case of a New UK Health of the People Act* (London: Nuffield Trust, 2003).

[5] Russel Viner, "Abraham Jacobi and German Medical Radicalism in Antebellum New York," *Bulletin of the History of Medicine*, 72 (1998): 434-63; Theodore Brown and Elizabeth Fee, "Rudolf Carl Virchow: Medical Scientist, Social Reformer, Role Model," *American Journal of Public Health*, 96 (2006): 2104-5.

Historians have debated whether it was increasing income or public health reforms that produced the dramatic changes in mortality after the nineteenth century. However, there is consensus that public health reforms, such as clean water, food standards and inspections, underground sewage systems, and other hygiene measures, significantly improved the health of populations in the industrialized world.

was facilitated by the imposition of strict liability, and convicted entrepreneurs faced short terms of imprisonment.[20] The criminal method of enforcing health and safety laws (which would substantially, but not completely, give way to civil penalties in the twentieth century) was significant. Criminal penalties are more stigmatizing than civil remedies and undermine the prestige and status of businesspersons.[21] The transition from criminal to civil penalties also influenced social perceptions of harmful corporate behavior.

In summary, despite the prevalent contemporary belief that the nineteenth century was a time of free markets and undeterred entrepreneurs, in fact it was a well-regulated society. A range of sanitary legislation had been enacted to ensure that activity did not bring with it excessive risks to health and safety. Public health laws were often backed up with criminal penalties imposed on business executives. Finally, as the following discussion suggests, the infrastructure and powers of public health departments were extended to cope better with the growing regulatory system. Tighter control by well-organized government was grounded in the belief that commercial activities, while contributing to prosperity, created harms to the commons. Government's raison d'être was to protect the community's interests by curtailing individual freedoms.

PUBLIC HEALTH AGENCIES AND THE RISE OF THE ADMINISTRATIVE STATE

> The success or failure of any government in the final analysis must be measured by the well-being of its citizens. Nothing can be more important to a state than its public health; the state's paramount concern should be the health of its people.
>
> Franklin Delano Roosevelt (1932)

Sanitary regulation commenced even before cities and states had well-organized and effective public health infrastructures that could support regulation. During the early nineteenth century, public health administration was simple in organization and limited in scope. Only a few ma-

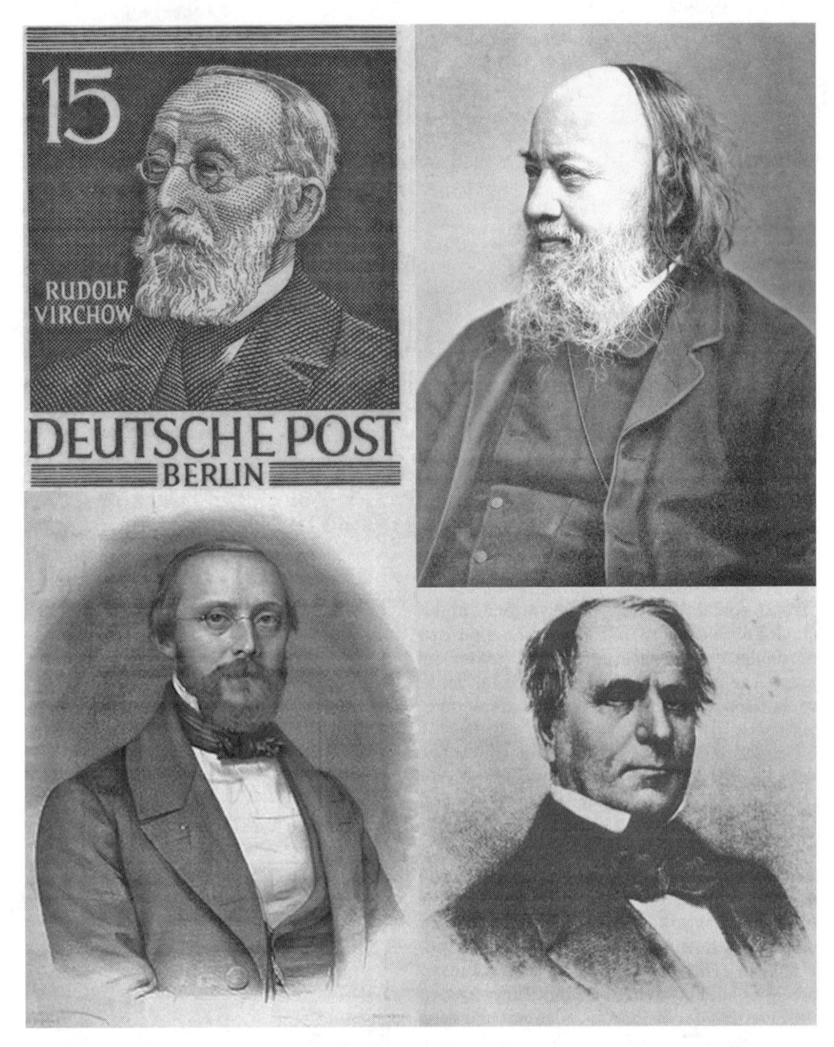

Photo 8. Portraits of the great nineteenth-century public health campaigners (top row, left to right): Virchow, Chadwick; (bottom row, left to right) Villermé, and Shattuck. Courtesy of the University of Tennessee Health Sciences Library and Biocommunications Center (Vichow) and the National Library of Medicine (Chadwick, Villermé, and Shattuck).

jor cities had established formal boards of health; the first local health departments were established in Baltimore in 1793, in Philadelphia in 1794, and in Massachusetts's municipalities in the late 1790s.[22] At this time, public health officials had no qualifications, no career advancement, and no job security.[23] Even in the latter part of the nineteenth century, many large urban areas had no health department, and expertise was only beginning to emerge among public health officials.[24]

The burgeoning social problems of the industrial cities convinced legislatures to form more elaborate and professional public health administrations within municipal government.[25] For example, a properly constituted health board was established in New York City in 1866 under An Act to Create a Metropolitan Sanitary District and Board of Health. The board comprised experts in medicine and public health and was granted extensive power both to create and to administer regulations relating to the preservation of the public's health.[26] This public health infrastructure was necessary to ensure careful regulatory scrutiny of the burgeoning industrial civilization. Therefore, boards of health were established to create an effective ministerial agency to supervise and direct the details of the execution of ordinances. To accomplish its tasks, state legislatures granted local boards of health the power to enact detailed administrative regulations, inspect businesses and property owners to ensure compliance, and adjudicate and sanction those who violated regulatory standards.[27]

Public health administrations within the states came even later than those in municipalities. It was not until after the Civil War that states formed boards of health. The first working state health board was formed in Massachusetts in 1869, followed by a number of other states in the 1870s, including California, Maryland, Minnesota, and Virginia.[28] County and rural health departments did not emerge until the early twentieth century.[29]

Despite the advances in public health administration, campaigners still observed patronage, inefficiency, and unprofessionalism in state and local health agencies into the twentieth century. Charles Chapin, the superintendent of health for Providence, Rhode Island, pressed for a corps of public health officials who were highly qualified and trained, with adequate compensation and opportunities for career advancement.[30] These challenges persist in public health professionalism to this day: the lack of leadership in public health, the failure to constructively engage with elected officials, and the short tenure of politically appointed public health officials.[31]

Federal Public Health Agencies

Many observers saw Franklin Delano Roosevelt's New Deal as an important juncture in developing an active federal role in public health.[32] During this period, the federal government asserted regulatory jurisdiction

BOX 8

THE FEDERAL PRESENCE IN PUBLIC HEALTH

On July 16, 1798, President John Adams signed "An Act for the Relief of Sick and Disabled Seamen," which established the U.S. Marine Hospital Service (USMHS) for merchant seamen. The USMHS—a forerunner of the present-day Public Health Service—became part of the Treasury Department.[1] Three-quarters of a century later, in 1862, a Bureau of Chemistry was founded, which eventually led to the creation of the Food and Drug Administration (FDA).[2]

The federal government's quarantine power can be traced to 1796, when the Fourth Congress authorized the president to assist states in enforcing their public health laws.[3] A Federal Quarantine Act "to prevent the introduction of contagious or infectious diseases into the United States" was passed on April 29, 1878.[4] A National Board of Health was created the following year principally for formulating a quarantine policy.[5] The board became embroiled in controversy about states' rights; it was disbanded in 1893 and its powers transferred to the USMHS.[6] In 1890, Congress gave the USMHS interstate quarantine authority,[7] and in 1893, following outbreaks of cholera in Europe, Congress granted the federal government the right of quarantine inspection.[8] (See the discussion of federal quarantine power in chapter 11.)

In 1887, a bacteriological laboratory known as the Laboratory of Hygiene was established at the Marine Hospital, Staten Island, N.Y., for research on cholera and other infectious diseases. This one-room laboratory would later become the National Institutes of Health (NIH).[9] In 1912 the USMHS was reorganized into the United States Public Health Service (USPHS).[10] Among its other responsibilities, the USPHS performed public health functions, such as imposing and enforcing quarantine regulations in immigration. The Public Health Service Act of 1944 defines the modern powers and duties of the USPHS.[11]

In the years following the New Deal, Congress greatly expanded the federal presence in public health. The Social Security Act of 1935 began to address problems of

[1] *An Act for the Relief of Sick and Disabled Seamen,* Pub.L. No. 77, 1 Stat. 605 (1798) (repealed). *The NIH Almanac—Historical Data,* March 16, 2006, http://www.nih.gov/about/almanac/historical/legislative_chronology.htm. See Elizabeth Fee, "Public Health and the State: The United States," in *The History of Public Health and the Modern State,* ed. Dorothy Porter (Amsterdam: Rodopi, 1994): 224, 233.

[2] C.C. Regier, "The Struggle for Federal Food and Drugs Legislation," *Law and Contemporary Problems,* 1 (1933): 3-15.

[3] 1 Stat. 474 (1796); see *Annals of Congress* 1349–59 (1796) (debating whether to authorize the president to impose quarantines at ports of entry, with opponents arguing that the authority belonged to the states).

[4] *Federal Quarantine Act,* 20 Stat. 37 (1878).

[5] *An Act to Prevent the Introduction of Infectious or Contagious Diseases into the United States, and to Establish a National Board of Health,* 20 Stat. 484 (1879).

[6] Fitzhugh Mullan, *Plagues and Politics: The Story of the United States Public Health Service* (New York: Basic Books, 1989).

[7] *An Act to Prevent the Introduction of Contagious Diseases from One State to Another and for the Punishment of Certain Offenses,* 26 Stat. 31 (1890).

[8] *Quarantine Act,* 27 Stat. 449 (1893), repealing the *Quarantine Act* of 1879, 20 Stat. 484 (1879).

[9] *Randell Act,* Pub. L. No. 71-25 (1930), 46 Stat. 379 (codified as amended at 42 U.S.C. §§21, 22, 23a-23g) (establishing NIH from the Hygienic Laboratory in 1930). See Ralph C. Williams, *The United States Public Health Service, 1798-1950* (Washington, DC: Commissioned Officers Association of the U.S. Public Health Service, 1951).

[10] *Public Law of 1912,* ch. 288, 37 Stat. 309, superseded by *Public Health Service Act,* 42 U.S.C.S § 202 (1944).

[11] *Public Health Service Act,* 42 U.S.C. § 201 (1944). See Williams, *The United States Public Health Service, 1798-1950;* Bess Furman, *A Profile of the United States Public Health Service, 1798-1948* (Bethesda, MD: National Institute of Health, Washington Printing Office, 1973); Fitzhugh Mullan, *Plagues and Politics.*

poverty and its harmful health effects, and the Federal Security Agency was established in 1939 to deal with health, education, social insurance, and human services. In 1946, the Communicable Disease Center was founded, which later became the Centers for Disease Control and Prevention (CDC).[12]

The Department of Health, Education, and Welfare (HEW), created in 1953, incorporated the USPHS. Since then, advancements in public health have continued. The 1960s saw the creation of Medicare and Medicaid, the Head Start program, and the Administration on Aging. In the 1970s, Congress established the National Health Service Corps, the Environmental Protection Agency (EPA), the Occupational Safety and Health Administration (OSHA), and the Health Care Financing Administration (now the Centers for Medicare and Medicaid Services [CMS]). In 1979, a reorganization split HEW into the Department of Education and the future Department of Health and Human Services (DHHS). In 2002, Congress established the Department of Homeland Security (DHS), which consolidated twenty-two agencies, unifying a variety of security functions in a single agency.[13] This reform reoriented the mission and functions of many health agencies to include a greater focus on public health preparedness. What began in the eighteenth century as a marine hospital has grown into a massive federal presence in the areas of health, safety, and security.

The modern role of the federal government in public health is broad and complex. Public health functions, which include public funding for emergency preparedness, health care, safe food, effective drugs, clean water, a beneficial environment, and prevention services, can be found in an array of agencies. Most public health functions are located under the umbrella of DHHS. Under the aegis of DHHS, various programs promote and protect health. The CMS administers the Medicare and Medicaid programs. The CDC provides technical and financial support to states for monitoring, controlling, and preventing disease. The CDC's efforts include population-based initiatives, such as childhood vaccination, prevention of chronic diseases and injuries, and emergency response to infectious diseases. The NIH conducts and supports research, trains investigators, and disseminates scientific information. The FDA ensures that food is pure and safe, and that drugs, biologicals, medical devices, cosmetics, and products that emit radiation are safe and effective. DHS's mission is risk assessment, prevention, protection, response, and recovery with respect to terrorism, natural disasters, and other health emergencies.[14]

As the United States has garnered more resources and the Supreme Court has permitted greater congressional authority, the federal presence in public health has grown. From modest beginnings, it is nearly impossible to find a field of public health that is not heavily influenced by the federal government.

[12] Elizabeth W. Etheridge, "History of the CDC," *Morbidity and Mortality Weekly Report,* 45 (1996): 526-28, 526.

[13] *Homeland Security Act of 2002,* 6 USC §§ 101-557 (2002). DHS's mission is "preventing terrorist attacks within the United States, reducing the vulnerability of the United States to terrorism at home, and minimizing the damage and assisting in the recovery from any attacks that may occur."

[14] U.S. Department of Homeland Security, *The DHS Strategic Plan: Securing Our Homeland,* February 24, 2004, http://www.dhs.gov/dhspublic/interapp/editorial/editorial_0413.xml.

over adulterated or otherwise harmful food, drugs, and cosmetics;[33] established national standards for drinking water;[34] enacted a venereal disease control program in response to a reemergent sexually transmitted disease epidemic;[35] and formed a federal grant-in-aid program requiring states to establish and maintain public health services and training for

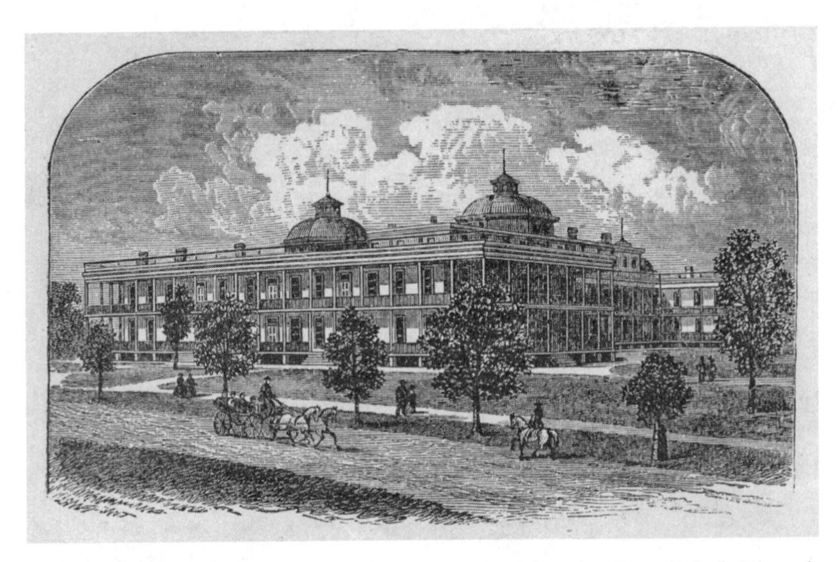

Photo 9. Marine hospital in New Orleans. A 1798 law for the relief of sick and disabled seamen created a major role for the federal government in the public health arena by establishing the Marine Hospital Service (forerunner of the Public Health Service). Marine hospitals such as this one in New Orleans were built in many American port cities. Used with permission of Documenting the American South, the University of North Carolina at Chapel Hill Libraries.

public health professionals.[36] The federal presence expanded during Lyndon Baines Johnson's "Great Society," with his antipoverty agenda of aid to education, urban renewal, and the establishment of Medicare and Medicaid.[37] President Nixon continued the trend of expansive federal regulation, forming new agencies to protect the environment and the safety of workers. By the time President Reagan took office, the nation was becoming disenchanted with the growth in federal bureaucracy. The Reagan administration ushered in increased oversight of executive agencies, particularly involving a mandate to conduct cost-benefit analysis—a requirement that remains robust to this day (see chapter 2).[38]

Federal agencies, part of the executive branch, are given the role of promoting the public's health and safety. Federal regulation now covers broad aspects of public health, such as air and water quality, environmental protection, food and drug safety, tobacco advertising, pesticide production and sales, consumer product protection, and occupational health and safety.[39] Federal health agencies, after the disaster of September 11, 2001, and the establishment of the Department of Homeland

MILESTONES IN FEDERAL REGULATION

1796 Following a debate on state's rights, the National Quarantine Act limits federal quarantine activities to cooperation requested by states to enforce their own quarantine laws.

1798 The Act for the Relief of Sick and Disabled Seaman lays down the groundwork for what will become the U.S. Public Health Service.

1813 The Act to Encourage Vaccination appoints an agent and provides for letters and packages containing vaccination materials, specifically smallpox, to be sent free of charge through the U.S. mail. Repealed in 1822 after inadvertent vaccinations with real smallpox scabs.

1878 The National Quarantine Act creates a "disease intelligence system" managed by the supervising surgeon general of the Marine Hospital Service (MHS) enabling the creation of rules and regulations at the federal level to detain ships with possible contagions on board. The reports of the surgeon general on these activities, "Bulletin of the Public Health," have transitioned into the *Morbidity and Mortality Weekly Report.*[1]

1879 A National Board of Health is created. The responsibilities of the board of health focus on preventing the introduction of contagious diseases to the United States, public health information gathering for states and the federal government, and quarantine procedures. Debate surrounding states' rights led to board disbandment in 1893 and its powers were transferred to the MHS.[2]

1891 An immigration act required MHS physicians to conduct immigrant health inspections and to exclude "all idiots, insane persons, paupers or persons likely to become public charges, *persons suffering from a loathsome or dangerous contagious disease,*" as well as criminals.

1892 The international cholera epidemic led to President Harrison signing a new national quarantine act, which included the requirement that all vessels from foreign ports have a bill of health signed by a U.S. consul and enabled the surgeon general to evaluate state and municipal quarantine procedures.

1902 MHS is renamed Public Health and Marine Hospital Service of the United States (PHMHS). The surgeon general is empowered to compile and collect data from states and territories on vital statistics.

1912 PHMHS is renamed the Public Health Service; it enables the study and investigation of the propagation of disease.

1918 July 1: Congress appropriates $1 million to promote cooperation of the federal government with states and municipalities to prevent the spread of disease through interstate traffic in order to safeguard "the health of military forces and Government employees."

1918 July 9: The Division of Venereal Disease is established, expanding joint efforts of states and the Public Health Service.

[1] Centers for Disease Control, "Notifiable Disease Surveillance and Notifiable Disease Statistics—United States, June 1946 and June 1996," *Morbidity and Mortality Weekly Report,* 45 (1996): 530-32.

[2] Fitzhugh Mullan, *Plagues and Politics: The Story of the United States Public Health Service* (New York: Basic Books, 1989).

1918 October 1: Congress appropriates $1 million to be managed by the Public Health Service's director of interstate quarantine, in response to the Spanish influenza pandemic.

1921 The Sheppard-Towner Act enables the establishment of state centers to educate mothers about prenatal and infant care through federal grants. A Federal Board of Maternity and Infant Hygiene is created to approve states' use of the funds.

1929 The Narcotics Division (the name is eventually changed to the Division of Mental Hygiene) of the Public Health Service is established. Two hospitals are created for the confinement and treatment of federal prisoners with drug addictions and those who voluntarily seek treatment for drug addiction.

1930 The Ransdell Act creates the National Institute of Health, to "establish and operate a National Institute of Health, to create a system of fellowships in said institute, and to authorize the Government to accept donations for use in ascertaining the cause, prevention, and cure of disease."

1935 Title VI of the Social Security Act, the Public Health Title, authorizes expenditures for investigating disease and sanitation, for the first time creating a national health program.

1939 The Reorganization Act transfers the Public Health Service from the Department of the Treasury to the Federal Security Agency (FSA). The FSA included the Children's Bureau and the Food and Drug Administration.

1943 In response to nursing shortages during World War II, Congress passes the United States Nurse Corps bill, which provides funding for nursing education to be administered through the PHS.

1944 The Public Health Service Act recodifies Public Health Service laws and creates the Division of Tuberculosis Control.

1946 The successful Malaria Control in War Areas program is converted into the Communicable Disease Center (CDC), which later becomes the Centers for Disease Control and Prevention.

1946 The National Mental Health Act supports research on mental illness and calls for the establishment of a National Institute for Mental Health.

1953 The Federal Security Agency is elevated to cabinet status as the Department of Health, Education, and Welfare.

1965 Medicare and Medicaid programs are created.

1970 The creation of the Environmental Protection Agency (EPA) leads to the loss of USPHS programs in such areas as air pollution and solid waste to the new agency.

1971 The Occupational Health and Safety Administration (OSHA) is established as part of the Department of Labor (DOL). Since its inception, OSHA has diminished workplace fatalities by 60 percent and injury and illness by 40 percent.[3]

1979 A major reorganization splits HEW into the Department of Education and the future Department of Health and Human Services (DHHS).

1988 Creation of the JOBS program and federal support for child care. Passage of the McKinney Act to provide health care for the homeless.

3 More facts on the Occupational Safety and Health Administration can be found on their Web site at http://www.osha.gov/as/opa/oshafacts.html.

1993 — The Vaccines for Children program is established, providing free immunizations to children in low-income families.

1996 — Enactment of the Health Insurance Portability and Accountability Act (HIPAA).

2002 — The establishment of the Department of Homeland Security (DHS) reorients the mission of many health agencies to a greater focus on terrorism.

2003 — Enactment of the Medicare Prescription Drug Improvement and Modernization Act, the most significant expansion of Medicare since its enactment.

SOURCE: Timeline adapted from Bess Furman, *A Profile of the United States Public Health Service, 1798-1948* (Bethesda, MD: National Institute of Health, Washington Printing Office, 1973), unless otherwise noted.

Security the following year, have increasingly focused on biosecurity—both intentional dispersal of pathogens and naturally occurring infectious diseases, such as highly pathogenic influenza. Federal funding to states and localities has similarly emphasized public health preparedness. (Box 8 and the accompanying timeline canvass milestones in federal regulation.)

State Public Health Agencies

The state's police powers to protect the health, safety, and welfare of its inhabitants are inherent aspects of sovereignty and not derived from another source. The state's plenary power to safeguard citizens' health, moreover, includes the authority to create administrative agencies devoted to that task.[40] State legislation determines the organization, mission, and functions of public health agencies.

Contemporary public health agencies take many different forms and defy simple classification.[41] Before 1960, state public health functions were primarily located in health departments, with policymaking functions residing in boards of health (e.g., issuance and enforcement of regulations).[42] As programs expanded through increased federal funding for categorical programs and block grants, certain public health functions relating to mental health, financing of medical care for the indigent, and environmental protection were assigned to other state agencies. Currently, fifty-five state-level health agencies exist (including the District of Columbia, American Samoa, Guam, Puerto Rico, and the U.S. Virgin Islands); these may be freestanding, independent departments or components of a larger state agency. The trend since the 1960s has been to merge state health departments with other departments—often social services, Medicaid, mental health, and substance abuse—to form superagencies.

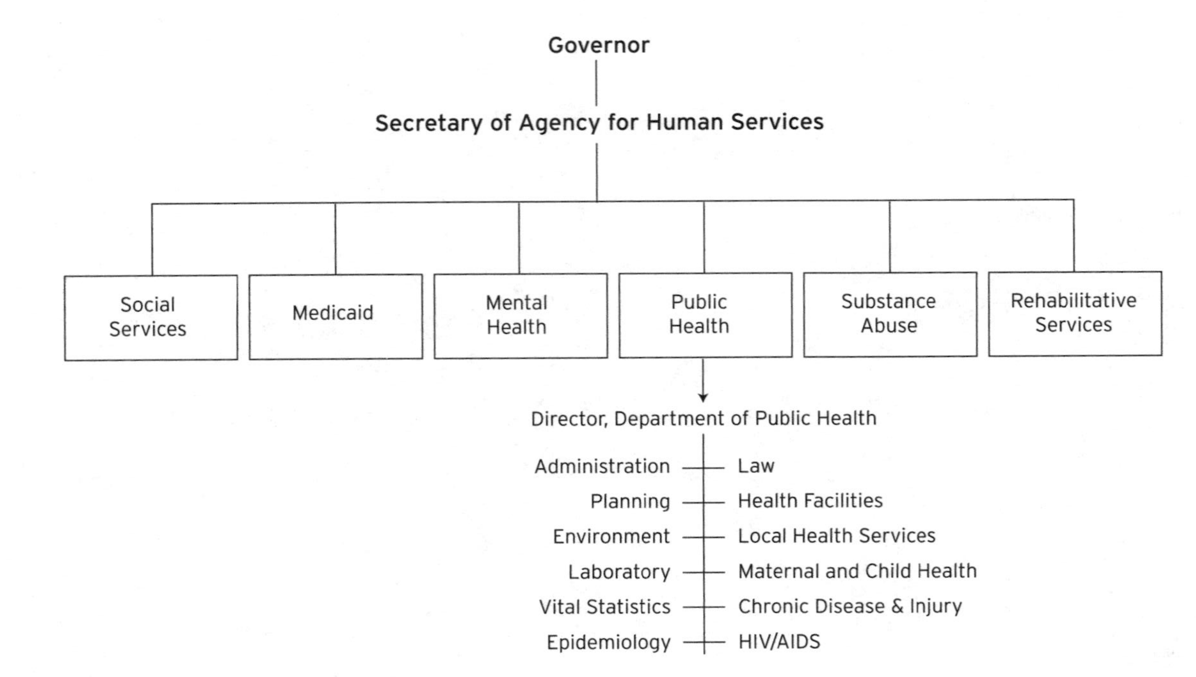

Figure 18. Public health as a division of a superagency.

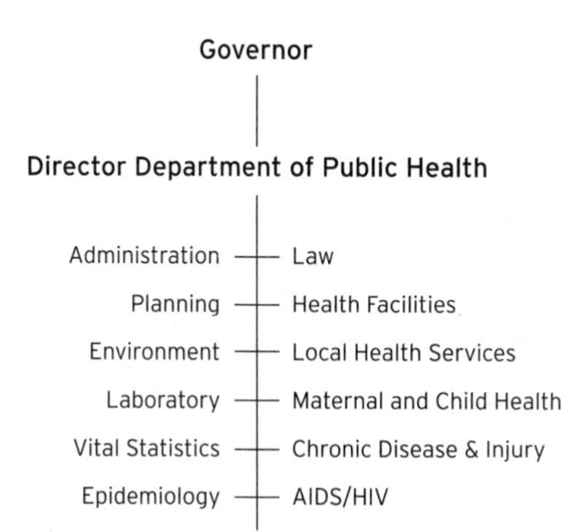

Figure 19. Public health as a cabinet agency.

Under this framework (Model 1), the public health unit is often called a Division of Health or Public Health (see figure 18). Another common framework is to assign public health functions to a cabinet-level agency (Model 2). Under this model, the public health unit is often called a Department of Health or Public Health (see figure 19).[43]

The trend has also been to eliminate or reduce the influence of boards of health. These boards, once ubiquitous and highly influential, are now often replaced or supplemented with specialized boards or committees established by state statute to oversee technically complex or politically controversial programs (e.g., genetics, rural health, and expansion of health care facilities).[44] The chief executive officer of the public health agency—the commissioner, director, or less often, the secretary—is usually appointed by the governor, but may be appointed by the head of a superagency or, rarely, the board of health. Qualification standards may include medical and public health expertise, but increasingly, chief executives with political or administrative experience are appointed.[45]

Local Public Health Agencies

To make everywhere available these minimum protections of the health and welfare of children, there should be a district, county or community organization for health, education and welfare, with full-time officials, coordinating with a statewide program. . . . This should include: trained, full-time public health officials, with public health nurses, sanitary inspection, and laboratory workers.

Herbert Hoover (1931)

The most pervasive and fundamental authority of local governments is the police power to protect the public's health, safety, morals, and general welfare (see chapter 3).[46] Local health departments provide a broad range of services to their communities, including data collection and analysis, disease control, epidemiology and surveillance, community and personal health, environmental health, and licensing.[47] They typically exercise numerous public health functions relating to air, water, and noise pollution; sanitation and sewage; smoking in public places; drinking-water fluoridation; firearm registration and prohibition; infectious diseases; rodents and infestations; housing codes; sanitary food and beverages; trash removal; and animal control.[48]

Municipalities and counties, like the states, have created public health agencies to carry out their functions.[49] Local public health agencies have varied forms and structures:[50] centralized (directly operated by the state), decentralized (formed and managed by local government), or mixed.[51] A minority of states have an intermediate administrative structure between the state-level agency and local health departments, often called district health departments.[52] Local boards of health or, less often, government councils still exist in most local public health agencies, with policymaking or advisory functions.[53] The courts usually permit local agencies to exercise broad discretion in matters of public health,[54] sometimes even beyond the geographic area if necessary to protect city or county inhabitants (e.g., during a waterborne disease outbreak).[55]

Local public health agencies serve a political subdivision of the state, such as a city (a municipality), town, township, county, or borough. Some local public health functions are undertaken by special districts, which are limited government structures that serve special purposes (e.g., drinking water, sewage, sanitation, or mosquito abatement).[56]

Local government entities are subsidiary and largely subordinate to the state.[57] They have delegated authority and may exercise only those police powers granted by the state. The sources of local government power are the state constitution (which delegates power directly from the people to municipalities), state legislation (which grants delegated power), and the municipal or county charter (which is usually approved by local voters and expresses the powers of the corporation).[58] Constitutional and statutory grants of generic authority to cities or counties can create autonomy, or home rule, over local affairs.[59] State constitutions sometimes grant considerable public health power to localities: "To exercise any power and perform any function pertaining to [local government and affairs] including . . . the power to regulate for the protection of the public health, safety, morals, and welfare."[60] This kind of constitutional authority can insulate cities and counties from state interference in purely local public health functions.

Courts construe state grants of police power to ensure that local governments act within the scope of the delegation. Judge Dillon formulated the conventional rule of interpretation of state-delegated powers.[61] Dillon's Rule holds that local governments can exercise only those powers expressly conferred, necessarily or fairly implied, or essential to the objects and purposes of the municipality. The strict construction of delegations to local governments during the nineteenth century was often used to block public health measures that judges regarded as unwarranted.[62] The modern judiciary appears split on whether to interpret strictly or liberally state delegation of powers to local government.[63] However, courts often find public health powers to be quintessentially within the local sphere.[64]

Relationships among states and localities are complex and highly political. Each level of government may fervently claim jurisdiction over public health matters such as smoking or infectious diseases. States may seek to deny cities or counties the power to exercise control by withholding grants of power or resources, or by preempting local regulation. Localities, on the other hand, may claim implied authority or assert home rule over public health matters of inherent local importance. Consider the political debate over firearm regulation, with the majority of states preempting local government regulation of gun sales.[65] In response, cities and counties have adopted innovative methods to regulate firearm violence through their traditional zoning and licensing authority (e.g., banning dealers in residential areas and creating strict licensing standards).[66]

In summary, states possess inherent, and localities delegated, police power to regulate for the common good. To achieve this goal, states and localities both have developed elaborate administrative agencies. Powers and duties of agencies are governed by law but are powerfully influenced by politics. One of the most fundamental issues in law and politics is the appropriate scope of agency power. Because agencies are not directly accountable to the voters, the amount of discretion they exercise is of enduring importance, as the following discussion illustrates.

ADMINISTRATIVE LAW: POWERS AND LIMITS OF EXECUTIVE AGENCIES

Administrative law is concerned primarily with the power and limits on power of executive agencies. The legislature delegates powers to administrative agencies; therefore, the most important tool of administrative law is statutory interpretation—ascertaining the authority that the legislature intended to grant to the agency.[67] The courts actively review the exercise of powers to ensure that legislatures appropriately delegate powers to the executive branch and that agencies act within the scope of their authority. For example, in *Food and Drug Administration v. Brown and Williamson Tobacco Corp.* (2000), the Supreme Court, with four justices in dissent, invalidated an FDA rule curtailing the promotion and accessibility of cigarettes to children and adolescents. The Court reasoned that, considering the Food, Drug, and Cosmetic Act as a whole, Congress intended to exclude tobacco products from the FDA's jurisdiction.[68] The courts, of course, can rule that an agency is obliged to regulate under a congressional grant of power.[69] The principal inquiry, therefore, is what powers the legislature intended to confer on the agency.[70]

The Powers of Administrative Agencies: Rulemaking, Enforcement, and Adjudication

Legislatures delegate broad powers to agencies. These delegations are remarkable because agencies possess powers that are characteristic of the three branches of government. Agencies may exercise *legislative power* to issue rules and regulations; *executive power* to investigate potential violations and sanction offenders; and *judicial power* to interpret legal norms and adjudicate disputes. Consequently, the lines between lawmaking, enforcement, and adjudication have become blurred with the rise of the administrative state (see figure 20). For example, the Occupational Safety and Health Act of 1970[71] authorizes the Secretary of Labor to promulgate mandatory workplace safety standards, enforce the law through inspections or monitoring, and adjudicate or arbitrate disputes.

Broad delegations raise important constitutional questions of separation of powers and the need for checks and balances. However, agencies have advantages over traditional forms of governance: specialization and expertise, ongoing commitment to a single set of health and safety issues, and flexibility in decision making. Agencies may need legislative,

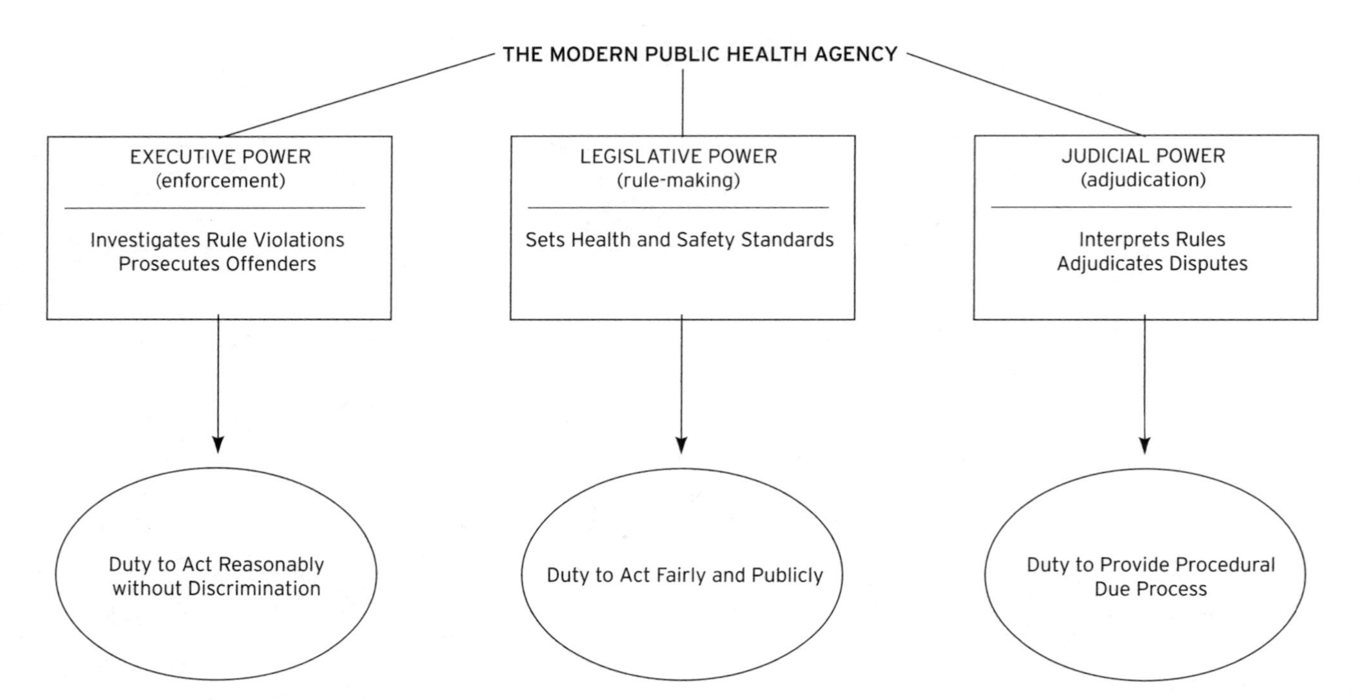

Figure 20. The modern public health agency.

executive, and judicial powers to deal comprehensively with complex health problems.

Rulemaking. Although agencies possess considerable power to issue detailed rules, they must do so fairly, publicly, and within the scope of the legislative delegation of authority. Federal and state administrative procedure acts (as well as agency-enabling acts) govern the deliberative processes that agencies must undertake in issuing rules.[72] As the Supreme Court ruled in *Vermont Yankee Nuclear Power Corp. v. NRDC* (1978), the federal Administrative Procedure Act (APA) "establishes the maximum procedural requirements that Congress was willing to have the courts impose upon federal agencies in conducting rulemaking proceedings."[73] (Procedural due process, under the federal or state constitution, does not apply to rulemaking as it does to adjudication—see the discussion of quasi-judicial functions below.)[74]

The federal APA requires two different procedural forms (and many state APAs follow similar paths): informal and formal. Some agency rulemaking is exempted from the act's notice and public procedure requirements.[75]

The APA's basic rulemaking procedure (called "informal" or "notice-and-comment" rulemaking) was intended to be a simple and flexible process, although in practice it is often unwieldy and cumbersome. It consists of three requirements:[76] prior notice (e.g., publication in the Federal Register), written comments by interested persons, and a statement of basis and purpose for the rule.[77] The formal rulemaking process ("rulemaking on the record") directs the agency to conduct a hearing and provide interested parties with an opportunity to testify and cross-examine adverse witnesses before issuing a rule.[78] Formal procedures can be costly and futile. For example, the FDA's proposed regulation of vitamin supplements involved eighteen months of hearings, and the agency lost on appeal because it had unduly restricted cross-examination of a government expert.[79]

Enforcement. Health departments possess not only legislative power to promulgate rules, but also executive power to enforce laws and regulations. Enforcement is squarely within the constitutional powers of executive agencies. Legislatures set the penalty for violation of health and safety standards; the executive branch monitors compliance and seeks redress against those who fail to conform. Pursuant to their enforcement power, health departments may inspect premises and businesses, investigate complaints, and generally monitor the activities of those who come within the orbit of health and safety statutes and administrative rules.

Quasi-Judicial. Modern administrative agencies do not simply issue and enforce health and safety standards; they also interpret statutes and rules as well as adjudicate disputes about whether standards are violated.[80] Federal and state administrative procedure acts and agency-enabling legislation often enumerate the procedures that agencies must follow in adjudicating disputes. Under the federal APA, formal adjudications ("evidentiary" or "on-the-record" hearings) apply only in the relatively rare cases where the agency's authorizing statute directs the agency to hold an evidentiary hearing.[81] Formal adjudications are typically conducted by an administrative law judge, followed by an appeal to the agency head.[82] Formal adjudications usually include notice, the right to present oral and written evidence, cross-examination of hostile witnesses, and agency findings of fact and law, as well as reasons for the decision. Even in the absence of statutory requirements, federal and state constitutions require fair hearings if the regulation deprives an individual of "property" or "liberty" (see chapter 4). Consequently, agencies are constitutionally obligated to provide due process for adjudicative hearings.[83]

In summary, modern administrative agencies exercise legislative power to issue rules that can carry heavy penalties, executive power to investigate potential violations of health and safety standards and to sanction offenders, and judicial power to interpret law and adjudicate disputes over violation of governing standards. Agency powers have developed for reasons of expediency (agency expertise) and politics ("specialists" presumed to act in accordance with disinterested scientific judgments).

Agency Decisions and Judicial Review

Although administrative agencies have considerable leeway in promulgating rules, enforcing norms, and adjudicating disputes, they are not entirely free from constraint. The language of the enabling statute that confers regulatory authority confines all agency action. Statutory language is often inherently broad or ambiguous (to varying degrees); hence there is a range of actions that an agency could take. As a result of ambiguities, agency regulations are often challenged, typically either by the industry being regulated (arguing that regulations are too stringent) or by public interest groups (arguing that regulations are too lax).

The Nondelegation Doctrine. Conventionally, representative assemblies may not delegate legislative or judicial functions to the executive branch. Known as "nondelegation," this doctrine holds that the legislative branch should make policy, and the judicial branch should adjudicate disputes,[84] because the legislature is deemed politically accountable and the judiciary independent. The nondelegation doctrine requires the legislature to provide reasonably clear standards for agency rulemaking—that is, the statutory criteria cannot be so vague as to give the agency unfettered discretion to set policy. However, federal courts rarely use the doctrine to limit agency powers.[85] In *Whitman v. American Trucking Associations* (2001), the Court held that the Clean Air Act's directive to the Environmental Protection Agency to devise air quality standards designed to protect the "public health" with "an adequate margin of safety" is not so "standardless" as to amount to an unconstitutional delegation of legislative power.[86] This ruling put the brakes on attempts by lower courts to invoke the nondelegation doctrine and overturn federal laws that grant agencies broad rulemaking authority.

The nondelegation doctrine has received varying interpretations at the state level:[87] Some jurisdictions liberally permit delegation,[88] while others are more restrictive.[89] New York state's highest court, for example, found a health department prohibition on smoking in public places unconstitutional because the legislature, not the health department, should make the "trade-offs" between health and freedom. "Manifestly," the court said, "it is the province of the people's elected representatives, rather than appointed administrators, to resolve difficult social problems by making choices among competing ends."[90]

Even if the courts do not rigidly apply the nondelegation doctrine, they may use it as an aid to statutory construction, interpreting agency authority narrowly if the grant of rulemaking power is vague. For example, the Supreme Court in the benzene case invalidated an OSHA rule that limited benzene in the workplace to no more than one part benzene per million parts of air. The Court reasoned that the broad congressional delegation of power did not permit OSHA to impose health standards for exceptionally low risks with inordinately high costs.[91]

Judicial Deference to Agencies. A key administrative law question is whether courts should grant "deference" to agency decisions; that is, should courts give special weight to an agency's interpretation of statutes or rules?[92] In *Chevron v. Natural Resources Defense Council* (1984), the Supreme Court created a two-step test.[93] Under *Chevron* Step 1, if Congress has "directly spoken to the precise question at issue," then the agency must give effect to that congressional intent and courts must enforce Congress's mandate.[94] Under *Chevron* Step 2, where there is statutory ambiguity, courts usually defer to agency action so long as the interpretation is not arbitrary or capricious, because Congress has delegated power to the agency to make a policy decision.[95] However, *Chevron* deference is granted only "when it appears that Congress delegated authority to the agency generally to make rules carrying the force of law, and that the agency interpretation claiming deference was promulgated in the exercise of that authority."[96] Otherwise, the interpretation is entitled to respect only to the extent it has the "power to persuade."[97]

Gonzales v. Oregon (2006) illustrates the complexity of judicial review of administrative action. In *Gonzales,* the Supreme Court held that the Controlled Substances Act does not allow the attorney general to prohibit physicians from prescribing controlled drugs for physician-assisted suicide under state law permitting their use for this purpose.[98] The Court refused to grant *Chevron* deference because Congress did not authorize the attorney general to make a rule declaring illegitimate a medical standard for patient care and treatment.

This framework governing judicial deference to agency action is important because it provides a system of "checks" on executive agencies. Administrative agencies wield considerable power over regulated entities. The nondelegation doctrine has not proven to be a check on agencies; thus, the Court has created a taxonomy of deference to ensure that agencies do not stray too far from the legislative directives that empower them to act.

NEW GOVERNANCE: THEORY AND PRACTICE

> Often, a logrolling process may end up as a redistributive scheme, where the winning coalition takes a bad initial proposal, and loads it with enough provisions that appeal to special-interest groups, until a solid majority has been obtained. . . . Before we race off to our federal, state, or local legislature, we should pause to recognize that there are *government failures as well as market failures.*
>
> Paul A. Samuelson and William D. Nordhaus (2004)

Is government regulation an effective response to complex social problems? Scholars and politicians routinely disparage the regulatory state, characterizing it as costly, inefficient, and intrusive. They point to extreme cases of government failure, such as policies that are highly cost-ineffective (inordinate sums to redress minute risks—see chapter 2); inefficient, such as the response of the Federal Emergency Management Agency (FEMA) to the Gulf Coast hurricanes; or intrusive, such as syndromic surveillance of personally identifiable medical records.

Even the labels used to describe agency action are pejorative: "big government," "centralized top-down," "bureaucratic," "command and control." These descriptions feed into deep-seated concerns about overbearing government, particularly at the national level. The standard critique, often framed as "public choice" theory,[99] is that legislators and administrators provide interest groups with favorable regulatory treatment rather than advance the public's health and safety. Interest groups (industry, lobbyists, and advocacy groups)—which are highly motivated, self-interested, and resourceful—"capture" regulatory agendas and decisions.

Although these characterizations are popular, most citizens rely on government in their everyday lives to ensure basic necessities, including clean air and water; hygienic restaurants; healthy workplaces; safe transport; control of infectious diseases; disaster preparedness; and efficacious pharmaceuticals, vaccines, and medical devices. Starved of resources and political support, administrative agencies could not offer the kind of comprehensive protection of health and safety that the citizenry expects. In short, sound regulation (setting standards and enforcing them) is still important in the lives of individuals and communities.

Despite the undeniable need for government to safeguard the public's health, the antigovernment narrative has had a political impact. The response to perceived government failure has been to call for *deregulation,* allowing the market to influence business and consumer behavior; *devolution,* so that residual regulation is focused at the local level; and *privatization,* so that traditional government functions are conducted by for-profit or voluntary entities.[100]

"New governance" theory positions itself between the two extreme characterizations of the regulatory state: traditional "command-and-control" rulemaking and enforcement on the one hand and deregulation, devolution, and privatization on the other.[101] This theory sees governance as more than state action, including a wide variety of stakeholders and actors that influence events and outcomes in society. It recognizes the powerful role of businesses, consumers, the community, nonprofit organizations, academia, and the media.[102] (At the international level, governance is multidimensional and complex. Sovereign states are important, but intergovernmental organizations, nongovernmental organizations, philanthropic foundations, and civil society also influence national and global health [see chapter 7].)[103]

New governance theorists pursue innovative ways to control individual and corporate behavior, with government playing a central, coordinating role but in collaboration with a variety of interested actors. A key feature of alternative forms of governance is to use the private market as a lever, but subject to the influence of government and its partners. These newer forms of governance are highly variable, and most have not been systematically studied for effectiveness. They include market- or incentive-based regulation, negotiated rulemaking, self-regulation, public disclosure, and other methods that prioritize the views and decisions of regulated entities instead of giving effect to the agency's own determination about what regulatory scheme works best (see box 9).

Emissions Trading. Economists often point to emissions trading permits as a prime illustration of market- or incentive-based regulation. A government agency caps emissions of a pollutant at a certain level and then issues permits to industries that grant the right to emit a stated amount of that pollutant over a time period. Firms may then trade these credits on the free market. Firms whose emissions exceed the amount of credits they possess are penalized. In some emissions trading systems, a portion of the traded credits are retired, thus achieving a net reduction in emissions. The Clean Air Act's Acid Rain Program, for example, uses a trading system designed to reduce sulfur dioxide (SO_2) emissions.[104] Similarly, the Kyoto Protocol to the U.N. Framework Convention on Climate Change allows States Parties to use carbon emissions trading as a way to meet their obligations under the treaty.[105]

In theory, by using the market, desired pollution reductions are met at the lowest cost to society. Some environmentalists, however, argue that emissions trading does not solve the problem of pollution. A reduction of permits available in the system is the only way to reduce overall pollution, which requires central regulation.

Negotiated Rulemaking. Negotiated rulemaking (sometimes known as "regulatory negotiation," or "reg-neg") is a voluntary process to promote interactive participation in drafting regulations, which is less adversarial. It brings interested parties together to negotiate the text of a proposed rule.[106] The negotiators seek consensus through a process of evaluating priorities and making trade-offs.[107] The agency publishes the

BOX 9

OSHA'S NEW GOVERNANCE STRATEGIES

The Occupational Safety and Health Administration exemplifies the transformation to new governance. In response to discontent with traditional regulation (universal standard-setting, random inspections, and prosecution of violators), OSHA radically changed its approach. In its Strategic Management Plan for 2003–8, the agency moved toward collaborative relationships with public and private institutions, flexible and noncoercive practices, and expanded outreach (e.g., fewer inspections, semivoluntary compliance, compliance assistance, and industry education).[1] The agency has similarly moved from formal adjudication of disputes to expanded use of voluntary Alternative Dispute Resolution (ADR) programs to resolve disputes.[2]

Bitter disagreement has ensued about the appropriateness and effectiveness of "soft" governance as opposed to conventional, well-enforced regulations. The agency reports that injuries and diseases have been cut nearly in half at work sites engaged in cooperative relationships.[3] Yet commentators point to an abysmal record of safety compliance, with virtual nonenforcement of violations, even in the face of worker injuries and deaths.[4]

[1] U.S. Department of Labor, Occupational Safety and Health Administration, *OSHA 2003–2008 Strategic Management Plan*, http://www.osha.gov/StratPlanPublic/strategicmanagementplan-final.html.

[2] *Expanded Use of Alternative Dispute Resolution in Programs Administered by the Department of Labor*, 62 Fed. Reg. 6690–95 (February 12, 1997).

[3] U.S. Department of Labor, Occupational Safety and Health Administration, *OSHA Enforcement: Effective, Focused, and Consistent*, January 31, 2006, http://www.osha.gov/dep/enforcement/enforcement_results_05.html.

[4] In 2003 the *New York Times* published "When Workers Die" by David Barstow, a three-part series exploring the failure of OSHA to prosecute employers for workers' work-related deaths: "The Plumber's Apprentice, a Trench Caves In; A Young Worker Is Dead, Is It a Crime?" *New York Times*, December 21, 2003; "Culture of Reluctance, U.S. Rarely Seeks Charges for Deaths in Workplace," *New York Times*, December 22, 2003; "The California Way, California Leads Prosecution of Employers in Job Deaths," *New York Times*, December 23, 2003. See David C. Vladeck and S. M. Wolfe, "The Politics of OSHA's Standard Setting," *American Journal of Industrial Medicine*, 19 (1991): 801–4; Stephen Labaton, "OSHA Leaves Worker Safety Largely in the Hands of Industry," *New York Times*, April 25, 2007.

proposed rule in the Federal Register and uses the normal procedure of soliciting and evaluating public comments. The Negotiated Rulemaking Act was enacted in 1990 to encourage federal agencies to use this process.[108] In 1996, Congress passed the Administrative Dispute Resolution Act, which authorizes agencies to employ ADR techniques, such as mediation, arbitration, and minitrials.[109]

The benefits of negotiated rulemaking include reduced time and resources to develop rules, earlier implementation, greater compliance, less litigation, and more cooperative relationships.[110] Critics, however, assert that it leads the agency to abandon its role as the guardian of the public interest by yielding to the interests of powerful stakeholders: "It sounds like an abdication of regulatory authority to the regulated, the full burgeoning of the interest-group state, and the final confirmation of the 'capture' theory of administrative regulation."[111] Does the "interest representation" model of administrative law view agency policymaking as more a political than a scientific process, and is that appropriate?[112] And do consensual mechanisms for developing regulations give sufficient weight to the public interest, which may be crowded out by the substantially greater expertise and resources of regulated industries?[113]

Self-Regulation. Industry itself may choose to adopt voluntary mechanisms for solving common problems. Forms of industry self-regulation include codes of conduct, product design, industry norms, collaborative agreements, accreditation, information disclosure, and ratings. These programs govern a wide array of domains, including worker and product safety, consumer protection, environmental management, fire prevention, and advertising. There are numerous illustrations of industry self-regulation in the fields of tobacco, firearms, motor vehicles, food and beverages, and other products and services. For example, trade associations representing sellers of beer, wine, and distilled spirits require member advertising to reach an audience composed of more than 50 percent adults.[114] And in 2006, the American Beverage Association issued highly publicized guidelines to sharply limit the sale of soft drinks in schools.[115] But even self-regulation can be controversial, as illustrated by this high school student's critique of school soda policy: "It is preposterous that I have the right to vote . . . but am unable to make lifestyle choices. Although some believe they are endowed with the wisdom to make daily choices for others, I would prefer personal freedom."[116]

Industry associations, through their power to repudiate and reward, can encourage compliance with their standards of competence, safety, or design. Companies often do not want to jeopardize their reputation with consumers by failing to abide by measures adopted by their peers. Government sanctions also can give self-regulation the force of law. For example, the Joint Commission for the Accreditation of Hospitals, a self-regulatory body, must accredit hospitals as a condition of their participating in Medicare and Medicaid.[117]

Well-constructed industry self-regulation offers possible advantages over government rulemaking, including speedy implementation, greater flexibility, less burden, and reduced political opposition. Self-regulation may be a particularly appropriate mechanism for curtailing advertising and promotion of hazardous products, because of First Amendment concerns inherent in government regulation of commercial speech (see chapter 9). Industry self-regulation also allows government to devote its scarce resources to policy matters for which government is best suited.[118]

Why would industry agree to constrain itself, potentially limiting its practices and profitability? Promarket advocates claim that industries self-regulate because consumers demand healthful and safe products, and full information to make informed choices. Market forces therefore spur self-regulation. Many in public health, however, argue that meaningful self-regulation often occurs in response to pressure by government or advocacy groups.[119] For example, the initiatives described above by the alcoholic beverage[120] and soft drink industries[121] both occurred directly after the publication of Federal Trade Commission reports highlighting product health hazards to children and young adults.[122] At the same time, advocates were threatening litigation for deceptive marketing practices.[123] Although technically not a form of self-regulation, the Master Tobacco Settlement Agreement is the quintessential illustration of industry capitulation to outside pressure for change (see chapter 6).

Public Disclosure. Government can influence behavior by requiring companies to disclose information. Public disclosure can take the form of product labeling, health warnings, conflict of interest statements, health outcomes data, adverse event reporting, and product safety information. Public information can be a powerful form of regulation. It can require companies to change product design to avoid having to disclose harmful ingredients (see box 10). It can promote honest dealings, such as the FDA requirement to disclose financial transactions between pharmaceutical companies and clinical investigators.[124] It can advise consumers about hazards and safe uses of products, such as warnings on drug packages or consumer goods. And it can create incentives for safer professional practices, such as public disclosure of the performance of physicians, hospitals, and managed health care plans.

Public disclosure is a politically palatable form of government regulation. It conforms to prevailing ideologies about consumer and patient rights to full information for autonomous decision making. It is also hard for industry to resist calls for providing accurate information. Since it does not require industry to alter its products and allows consumers to make informed choices, many consider disclosure preferable to command-and-control regulation. Finally, required disclosure is easier and less costly to administer because the government only has to take the minimal action of monitoring.

BOX 10

INFORMATION AS REGULATION: ZERO TRANS FAT OREO COOKIES

Recently, the food industry began producing and aggressively marketing foods without trans fatty acids (trans fat)—even the classic Oreo cookie: "At Kraft, we know the importance of good nutrition, and we are committed to helping people make healthy food choices . . . so we wanted to share some information about trans fat and Oreo cookies."[1] Was this in response to recent scientific evidence that trans fat causes the arteries to clog, increasing the risk of heart disease and stroke? No, actually the science had been well understood for years and health advocates had been urging reductions in trans fat, but the industry had taken no action. Perhaps it was because the government had compelled the food industry to reduce trans fat in its products? No, the FDA has never regulated trans fat in foods. But, on January 1, 2006, the FDA required food companies to list trans fat content separately on the Nutrition Facts panel of all packaged foods. Well before the rule's implementation, companies began to reduce trans fat. In fact, the FDA's disclosure rule permits companies to label a product "trans fat free" if it contains less than 0.5 grams per serving. The agency also does not require disclosure of a percentage daily value (%DV), which is required for other nutrients, such as saturated fat. The labeling requirement does not apply to foods served at restaurants. As a result, "trans fat free" packaged foods often contain just under 0.5 grams per serving of trans fat (which still has health risks); consumers are not informed of a safe recommended daily value for trans fat; and most restaurants have taken no action at all. Public information appears to be a powerful form of regulation, but only goes so far.[2]

[1] Kraft Foods, "Update: Trans Fat and Oreo Cookies," http://www.kraft.com/update/index.html.
[2] Dariush Mozaffarian, Martijn B. Katan, Alberto Ascherio, et al., "Trans Fatty Acids and Cardiovascular Disease," *New Eng. J. Med.*, 354 (2006): 1601–13 (elimination of trans fatty acids from partially hydrogenated oils would avert thousands of cardiovascular events each year in the United States).

From a public health perspective, public disclosure can be beneficial, but does it go far enough? Much depends on the meaning and content of the disclosure (what is "healthy," "lean," "natural," "organic," "low carb"?), the prominence of the disclosure (in bold letters or small print?), and the public's sophistication about the risk. For example, direct-to-consumer advertising of pharmaceuticals requires disclosure of risks in television ads. However, information about the drug's adverse effects is drowned out by positive images and sounds. As a result, physicians prescribe pharmaceuticals much more widely when the products are aggressively advertised to consumers.

While ample agency power is important for achieving public health goals, it is also troubling and perplexing in a constitutional democracy. The prevailing political narrative is that administrative regulation is costly, ineffective, intrusive, and stifling to innovation. There is an abiding concern that regulators too often accede to powerful private interests, failing to secure the higher public good. The very strengths of public health agencies (e.g., neutrality, expertise, and broad powers) can become liabilities if they appear politically unaccountable and aloof from the real concerns and needs of the governed. This is why governors' offices, representative assemblies, and courts struggle over the political and constitutional limits that should be placed on agency action.

As with most narratives, this negative picture of government is oversimplified. In truth, citizens' and politicians' historic reliance on administrative agencies to address important social problems, albeit in partial and imperfect ways, is telling.[125] New governance theory may provide a fresh perspective. Certainly, market incentives, stakeholder collaboration, self-regulation, and public information are valuable techniques for altering risky commercial behavior. However, it is unlikely that new governance can, or should, supplant traditional regulation when bright lines are needed to safeguard the public's health and safety.[126] Direct regulation will remain a staple of public health, as will indirect regulation through the tort system—the subject for discussion in the following chapter.

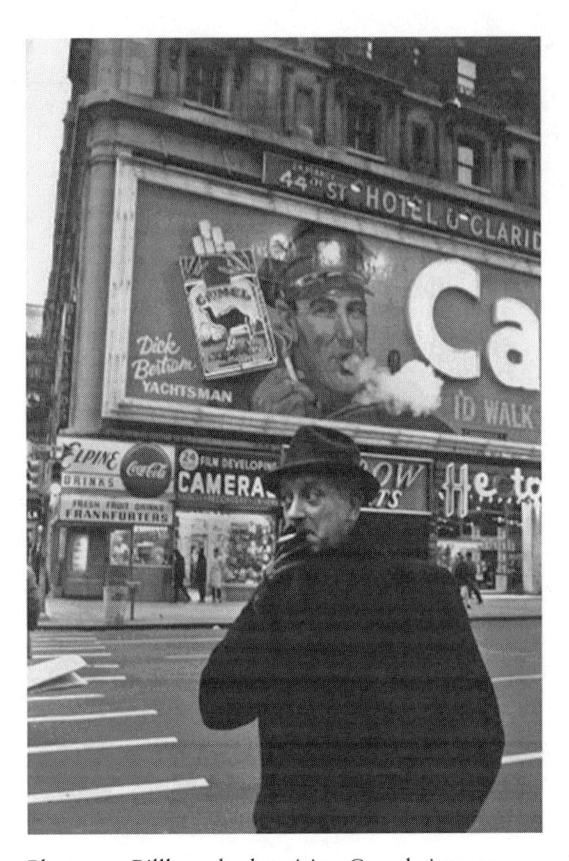

Photo 10. Billboard advertising Camel cigarettes in Times Square. This billboard advertisement for Camel cigarettes in Times Square is one of the images of tobacco products that pervaded the country's visual landscape during the twentieth century. However, on April 23, 1999, cigarette billboards were dismantled as part of a Medicaid cost reimbursement settlement reached in 1998 between tobacco producers and forty-six states. Eddie Hausner/New York Times Pictures.

CHAPTER 6

Tort Law and the Public's Health

Indirect Regulation

Both tort and statutory law have regulatory effects. Tort law can regulate behavior not only directly through providing injunctive relief, but indirectly—and more commonly—through the award of damages. Similarly, statutes can regulate behavior directly through standard setting and indirectly through fees [and] subsidies. . . . The line between common law tort actions and regulatory interventions has blurred in recent years as courts look for design defects, agencies propose incentive schemes, and statutes permit private rights of action.

Susan Rose-Ackerman (1991)

Thus far, I have considered regulation principally in terms of the actions taken by legislatures and administrative agencies to prevent injury or disease and to promote the public's health. The creation of private rights of action in the courts can also be an effective means of public health regulation.[1] This chapter concerns an important form of civil litigation: the role of tort law in redressing harms to people and the environment they inhabit.[2]

A tort, derived from the Latin *torquere,* "to twist," is a civil, non-contractual wrong for which an injured person or group of persons seeks a remedy, usually in the form of monetary damages.[3] Tort law, then, characteristically is a private rather than public right of action, and a civil rather than criminal proceeding. It remedies a wrong principally by awarding monetary damages. Tort law is composed of a series of related doctrines that impose civil liability upon persons or businesses whose (usually) substandard conduct causes injury or disease.

The functions, or goals, of tort law—although highly controversial and imperfectly achieved—are the (1) assignment of responsibility to individuals or businesses that impose unreasonable risks of causing injury or disease; (2) compensation of persons for loss caused by the conduct of individuals or businesses; (3) deterrence of unreasonably hazardous conduct; and (4) encouragement of innovation in product design, packaging, labeling, and advertising to reduce the risk of injury or disease.[4] In thinking about tort law as a tool of public health, it is important to emphasize the role of litigation in preventing risk behavior and providing incentives for safer product design.

Tort litigation can be an effective tool to reduce the burden of injury and disease.[5] Attorneys general, public health authorities, and private citizens resort to civil litigation to redress many kinds of public health harms: environmental damage (e.g., air pollution[6] or groundwater contamination[7]); exposure to toxic substances (e.g., pesticides,[8] radiation,[9] or chemicals[10]); unsafe pharmaceuticals, vaccines, or medical devices (e.g., diethylstilbestrol [DES],[11] live polio vaccines,[12] or contraceptive devices[13]); hazardous products (e.g., tobacco, firearms, or alcoholic beverages[14]); and defective consumer products (e.g., children's toys,[15] recreational equipment,[16] or household goods[17]).

While tort law can be an extremely effective method of advancing the public's health, like any form of regulation, it is not an unmitigated good. The tort system imposes economic costs and personal burdens on individuals and businesses that warrant careful consideration. The costs entailed in adjudication—transaction expenses (e.g., the court system and attorney fees) and liability—can discourage businesses from entering markets, render it economically burdensome to stay in markets, or increase consumer prices. Litigation as a form of regulation, then, holds enormous potential for improving the public's health but also entails economic costs and diminution of autonomy. Like any form of regulation, we trade off the public goods gained through civil litigation against the burdens.

The complexity of the tort system goes well beyond the scope of a text on public health law. Nevertheless, to understand tort actions designed to achieve a public good, I must first explain the major theories of liability. Next, I examine the complicated problems of scientific proof and uncertainty involved in bringing tort litigation. After examining the doctrine and scientific evidence, I demonstrate the value of tort law as a tool of public health. Two paradigmatic case studies are presented: one relating to chronic disease (tobacco lawsuits) and one relating to accidental and intentional injury (firearm lawsuits). Finally, I look at some of the limitations of traditional tort doctrine in addressing major public health problems, including the economic costs and burdens as well as the indirect regulatory effects. (See also box 12, p. 213, on obesity litigation.)

MAJOR THEORIES OF TORT LIABILITY

As explained above, the tort system is composed of a series of related doctrines that impose liability on persons, businesses, or governments whose conduct causes injury or disease. Tort law classifies cases according to the degree of culpability inherent in the risk-taking behavior—negligent, intentional, and no fault. Plaintiffs may adopt multiple theories of recovery but must prove each element in a cause of action by a preponderance of evidence.

Negligence

> The rule that you are to love your neighbor becomes in law, you must not injure your neighbor; and the lawyer's question, Who is my neighbor? receives a restricted reply. You must take reasonable care to avoid acts or omissions which you can reasonably foresee would be likely to injure your neighbor. Who, then, in law is my neighbor? The answer seems to be—persons who are so closely and directly affected by my act that I ought reasonably to have them in contemplation.
>
> James R. Atkin (1932)

The use of fault as a basis of civil liability is so much a part of the American experience with tort law that a New York judge was able to assert in 1873: "The rule is, at least in this century, a universal one, which, so far as I can discern, has no exceptions or limitations, that no one can be made liable for injuries to the person or property of another without some fault or negligence on his part."[18] It was not always this way. Though negligence has remained the dominant standard in tort law, prior to the nineteenth century persons were often held liable for harm caused by accidents irrespective of fault.[19] The transition from strict liability to fault is often attributed to private enterprise values designed to protect youthful industries from inordinate liability during the Industrial Revolution.[20]

TABLE 6. Negligence: The elements

Duty of Care	Legal obligation to protect others against unreasonable risks of harm
Breach of Duty	Defendant fails to conform to the legally recognized standard of safe behavior *Reasonable person standard:* Would a "reasonable person of ordinary prudence" have engaged in that risk behavior? *Rule of custom:* What is the usual and customary practice adopted in the industry or among fellow professionals? *Rule of law:* Did the person or business meet existing regulatory standards?
Causation	Reasonably close causal connection between unreasonably risky conduct and resulting injury *Causation "in fact"*: Would harm have occurred but for the defendant's conduct? *Proximate cause:* Was the injury a foreseeable consequence of the defendant's behavior?
Loss or Damage	Plaintiff must have suffered actual loss or damage and not mere insult to dignity

The modern elements of a cause of action based on negligence are duty of care, breach of duty, causation, and loss or damage (see table 6).[21]

Duty of Care. A duty of care is an obligation recognized in law to conform to a standard of conduct of protecting others against unreasonable risks of harm. Philosophically, the difference between an act ("misfeasance," or active misconduct) and an omission ("nonfeasance," or passive inaction) is far from clear, but the law traditionally draws a distinction. Generally, with respect to affirmative acts, we all owe a duty to every other person in the community to conduct our activities in reasonably safe ways to avoid foreseeable harm. A person usually is not liable for failing to take steps to protect others—that is, no general duty to rescue exists.[22] However, a person does have an affirmative duty to protect another from harm if—by custom, sentiment, or public policy—they share a special relationship, particularly where one person has expert knowledge and the other is vulnerable, such as in a physician-patient relationship.[23]

Breach of Duty. A breach of duty—that is, the person is "negligent"—occurs when a person fails to conform to the legally recognized standard of safe behavior. The standard of care is often characterized as the behavior that would be undertaken by a "reasonable person" or a person of "ordinary prudence."[24] The standard is intentionally vague, relying on the jury to make a normative judgment about the reasonableness of the activity—a legal fiction that randomly selected laypersons will act as the informed conscience of the community.

The notion of a "reasonable person" is informed by two concepts—objectivity and foreseeability.[25] Under the "objective" standard, the jury inquires whether a person of ordinary care and skill would have acted the same way under the circumstances. (Some professionals, such as physicians, are held to a higher standard derived from the skill that would be exercised by similarly situated professionals.) The law of negligence is not concerned with the particular actor's actual intent to do good or to cause harm, nor does the law take account of the actor's individual characteristics or capacity for safe behavior. Though allowance is made for physical disabilities (e.g., acts of the blind are compared with reasonable conduct of others who cannot see), no allowance is made for the actor's intelligence, character, or mental faculties. If a person exercises his judgment to the best of his ability, he will not necessarily avoid liability in negligence. The logic of reasonable care, however, does require that the harm be reasonably foreseeable. Thus, a person must know, or reasonably should know, that the behavior poses a risk of harm; failing to reduce a risk about which an individual does not and reasonably could not know is not negligence.[26]

Courts define negligence by reference to rules of custom and law. Since negligence is a community standard, evidence of the usual and customary conduct of others under similar circumstances is highly probative. Thus, courts examine the practices adopted in the industry or among fellow professionals. For example, medical malpractice law follows a strict rule of custom, so that physician behavior is measured against a national standard of how similar generalists or specialists practice in the country. In addition to custom, courts look to standards set by statutes, regulations, and guidelines. A breach of statutory or regulatory standards may be negligence per se or at least highly suggestive of negligence. If OSHA requires employers to reduce lead exposure to a specified level, failure to achieve that level may be conclusive evidence of negligence. Even the issuance of nonbinding guidelines by government agencies (e.g., the CDC) or professional organizations (e.g., the AMA) strongly influences legal standards of care in a negligence action.

Compliance with lax regulatory standards can, of course, also be used as a shield against liability. Tort litigation in areas ranging from environmental law[27] to automobile safety[28] and medical devices[29] sometimes founders because industry successfully argues that its conduct met low regulatory standards. For example, in 2006 the FDA announced that compliance with prescription drug labeling standards displaces, or preempts, state tort liability for failure to warn.[30] Artificially weak regulatory standards, therefore, can be doubly problematic for public health: Industry can cause unreasonable harm even while complying with the regulation, and individuals cannot effectively bring a tort action for their injuries.

Causation. Liability for negligence requires a reasonably close causal connection between the unreasonably risky conduct and the resulting injury. Causality is often examined in terms of "proximate" (or legal) cause, plus "causation in fact." Philosophically, causal relationships can be traced to innumerable antecedent events, but legal responsibility is limited to actions that actually cause harm and to sequences of events that are foreseeable. Courts often adopt a "but for" rule to explain causation in fact—that is, the harm would not have occurred but for the defendant's conduct; or, conversely, the harm would still have occurred without the defendant's conduct.[31] Proximate cause is difficult to define because the term is meant to convey the circumstances when, as a matter of law, it is fair to impose liability. Some courts hold that a defendant is liable if her conduct is the direct cause of the injury and not simply a remote one; others say that the harm must be a natural and probable consequence of the act. Most definitions of proximate cause, however, turn on whether the injury was a foreseeable consequence of the defendant's behavior—that is, whether the defendant reasonably could have anticipated the harm at the time she engaged in the risk behavior.

Loss or Damage. Finally, liability for negligence requires actual loss or damage and not a mere insult to dignity. (This separates negligence from "intentional torts," such as battery, where plaintiffs may recover nominal damages even if no tangible harm has occurred.) For example, a needlestick injury caused by a hospital's negligence will not result in liability unless the plaintiff actually contracted a bloodborne infection or at least was exposed and genuinely fears infection.[32]

In summary, negligence is a measure of legally acceptable risk; a person must exercise due care to avoid causing unreasonable risk of harm to others. The law of negligence does not require avoidance of all possibilities of harm; nearly all human activity carries risk, and only "unreasonable" risks are deemed negligent. There is much imprecision, of course, in separating "reasonable" from "unreasonable" risks. Some jurists and scholars propose a "negligence calculus" that assesses risk, benefit, and cost; this calculus takes into account the probability that the conduct may

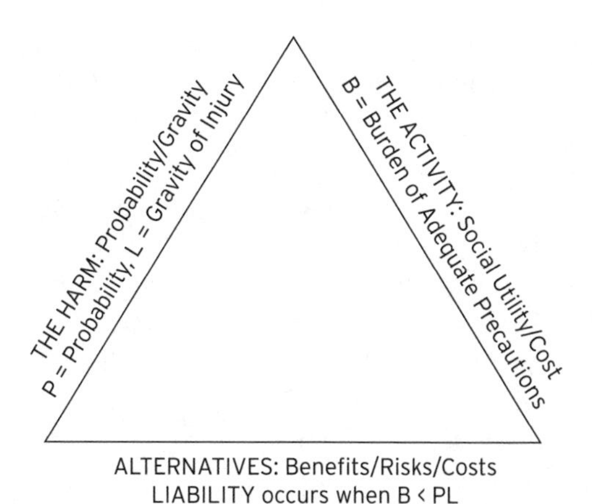

Figure 21. The "negligence calculus": Balancing risks, benefits, and costs.

cause harm; the severity of the harm should the risk materialize; the social utility and economic costs of the activity; and the benefits, risks, and costs of the alternatives available to the actor. Judge Learned Hand famously stated the negligence calculus as an algebraic formula: "If the probability [of harm] be called P; the [gravity of the resulting] injury, L; and the burden [of adequate precautions to avert the harm], B; liability depends upon whether B is less than L multiplied by P: i.e., whether B is less than PL" (see figure 21).[33]

Suppose a manufacturer foresees that an attenuated live vaccine will cause death in one in ten thousand cases. Should the manufacturer be liable to the person who contracts a vaccine-induced disease? The level of risk is mixed: Probability is very low, but severity of harm (death) is high. Balanced against the risk is the social utility, which, in the case of vaccines, is high. Perhaps the conclusive factors would be the costs and benefits of alternative vaccines. If a dead vaccine achieves the same protection and causes disease only in one case in a million, it may be unreasonable to use the live vaccine. However, if the live vaccine costs one dollar per dose and the dead vaccine twenty-five dollars per dose, should the manufacturer be liable? From a population-based perspective, the answer may be "no," but the parent of a child who contracts a vaccine-induced disease may think differently.

Private Nuisance

Private and public nuisances are distinct doctrines. Chapter 12 discusses public nuisances, which are principally legislative and are enforced by public health agencies. This chapter discusses private nuisances, which are principally part of the common law and are redressed through the tort system.

A private nuisance is an unreasonable interference with the possessor's use and enjoyment of land, such as contamination of adjoining property.[34] The components of a private nuisance are (1) the defendant intends to interfere with the use and enjoyment of land, and (2) the interference is substantial and unreasonable.[35] The intent requirement refers only to the defendant's knowledge of the nuisance—if he knows that his activity creates an interference with property use and he still continues, he has the requisite intent. For example, if a person continues the activity after he is notified that his emissions are polluting an adjoining stream, he is deemed to intend the result. It does not matter whether the person's motivation is to pollute or if it is the by-product of a socially desirable activity.

The interference must be substantial, not minor or ethereal. An invasion that affects the physical condition of land is almost always substantial, particularly if it results in measurable economic loss. For example, knowledge that pollution of soil or underground water affects natural resources has considerable weight in judicial thinking. It is more difficult to demonstrate that physical or psychological discomfort is a substantial interference. Modern society requires landowners to bear many annoyances due to noise, smells, and unsightly conditions. An annoyance of this kind must create an appreciable interference with property interests judged by the standard of an ordinary member of the community with normal sensitivity and temperament. Nuisances are measured in the context in which they occur, taking into account the neighborhood, property uses, and culture.

Closely associated with "substantiality" is the notion that interference with property uses must be unreasonable. The courts assess reasonableness by weighing the parties' interests, much as they would in a negligence action: the extent and duration of harm, the social value of the activity, the cost of avoiding or ameliorating the harm, and comparative economic effects (the relative capacity of the parties to bear the loss).[36]

Economists often reason that in a well-functioning market it is fairer and more efficient if companies "internalize" socially harmful activities as a cost of business.[37] Thus, an entrepreneur engaged in a socially useful activity, such as mining coal or refining petroleum, should pay for the harm caused to the surrounding community, even if modern scientific processes are used to reduce environmental harm.[38] Under this economic theory, monetary damages would be preferred over injunctive relief. A nuisance abatement stifles an enterprise rather than requiring it to bear the fair cost of the activity. Yet courts may grant injunctions in nuisance actions if an unreasonable activity is ongoing, particularly if a danger to humans or the environment persists. For example, in *United States v. Reserve Mining Company* (1974), a court enjoined a mining operation to prevent the discharge of carcinogenic fibers into the water supply. The court reasoned that "in matters of public health, by their very nature, monetary damages are usually incapable of compensating those who are or who will be injured by the nuisance."[39]

Courts, then, have three choices: Social equities may militate in favor of the plaintiff bearing the burden (no relief), the defendant internalizing the cost (monetary damages), or the defendant forbearing the harmful enterprise completely (injunction).

Strict Liability

> [My Lords], if the Defendants, not stopping at the natural use of their close, had desired to use it for any purpose which I may term a nonnatural use . . . [and the plaintiff was injured] . . . then for [that evil] the consequence . . . is that, in my opinion, the Defendants would be liable.
>
> Hugh McCalmont Cairns (1868)

Torts based on negligence can be difficult to prove due to lack of evidence of substandard care. For certain risk-taking behaviors, however, the judiciary affixes liability without regard to culpability (e.g., for unduly hazardous activities and for the sale of defective products). The law holds that even if the defendant exercises reasonable (or even extreme) care, she has to carry the cost of injuries. Strict, or no-fault, liability may be thought of as mandatory insurance against designated risks for reasons of social policy; it remains a highly controversial legal doctrine.

Strict liability does not impose absolute liability; it has the following limits: *intention*—the defendant must knowingly engage in the activity; *proximate cause*—liability is confined to the consequences caused by the activity and to persons foreseeably harmed; *public duty privilege*—liability is not imposed when the law expressly authorizes or imposes a duty to conduct the activity; and *sovereign immunity*—the Federal Tort Claims Act waives sovereign immunity, but not strict liability, for claims of government negligence.[40]

Abnormally Dangerous Activities. Strict liability in the modern era originated in the English case of *Rylands v. Fletcher* (1868), in which the House of Lords found that if "a person brings, or accumulates, on his land anything which, if it should escape, may cause damage to his neighbour, he does so at his peril."[41] Thus, if a nonnatural substance "does escape, and causes damage, he is responsible, however careful he may have been, and whatever precautions he may have taken."[42]

The rule of *Rylands v. Fletcher* found its way into American law through the doctrine of "abnormally dangerous activities," defined by reference to a number of factors:[43] high degree of risk, seriousness of resulting harm, inability to eliminate the risk by the exercise of due care, and the activity's danger compared with its value to the community. Lord Cairns's formulation of a "natural use" is reflected in the modern notion of "common usage." If an unsafe activity is prevalent (e.g., driving automobiles), it is not abnormally dangerous.[44] Common usage depends, in part, on whether the activity is inappropriate to the place where it is conducted. For example, storage of explosives may be abnormally dangerous in a densely populated area but not in a rural community.[45]

In summary, strict liability may be imposed where an activity, although lawful, is so dangerous, unusual, and inappropriate (within the context of its place and manner of use) as to justify allocating the risk of loss to the enterprise. Strict liability is particularly important in environmental law, where chemical production or disposal may be considered ultrahazardous.[46] Similarly, production of nuclear energy or transport of nuclear materials may be abnormally dangerous activities.[47]

Product Liability. The emerging market in consumer products at the turn of the twentieth century had enormous benefits for the population, but individuals injured by those products faced insuperable obstacles in gaining compensation. The extant law permitted actions for negligence only against a party with whom an injured person had a contractual relation, that is, "privity."[48] Contractual privity was abandoned in the famous 1916 decision *MacPherson v. Buick Motor Company,* which permitted consumers to sue automobile manufacturers.[49] Though *MacPherson* was a negligence action, no-fault product liability emerged later. Notably, consumers could sue under "implied warranty of merchantability," a contractual theory that did not require negligence.[50] Sellers, however, began to undermine implied warranty litigation by using safety disclaimers in consumer contracts. In response, strict liability for defective products emerged in the middle part of the century,[51] and by the 1970s, most states had adopted the theory.[52] The two most important concepts in product liability law are *products* and *defects*.

A product is broadly understood as tangible goods.[53] Product liability applies to virtually all goods capable of causing injury, ranging from motor vehicles,[54] household appliances,[55] and work[56] and recreational equipment[57] to pharmaceuticals,[58] vaccines,[59] and medical devices.[60] Activities (e.g., "abnormally dangerous" activities within the meaning of *Rylands v. Fletcher*) and services are not "products" and, therefore, are not covered under product liability law.[61] For example, blood is not a product: Statutes in every state stipulate that blood suppliers are deemed to provide services, so strict liability theory does not apply.[62]

The courts have adopted varied tests of a product "defect," and no single standard is universally accepted. A common standard is whether the product performed "as safely as an ordinary consumer would expect when used in an intended or reasonably foreseeable manner."[63] The "consumer expectation" test works well for manufacturing defects—for example, a consumer does not expect a food product to contain a foreign object such as animal feces. However, the consumer expectation test is less applicable to a design or informational defect, because most consumers lack the expertise to evaluate a product's design or safe use, particularly a complex or scientific product such as a medical device.

As a result, many courts use a "risk-utility" balancing test to determine if a defective product is "unreasonably dangerous to the consumer": Does the foreseeable risk of harm from the product outweigh the utility? The court might inquire, for example, whether the cost of making a product safer is greater than the danger from the product in its present condition.[64]

Product defects generally fall into three categories: manufacturing defects, design defects, and failures to warn.[65] Some courts also use a misrepresentation theory in finding products defective (see figure 22). The Restatement (Third) of Torts: Product Liability (hereafter Product Liability Restatement) creates a different standard of liability for each category of defectiveness.

A product contains a *manufacturing defect* when, as produced, it does not conform to the manufacturer's own design. This means that a flaw was not present in the product design, but despite due care, the defect

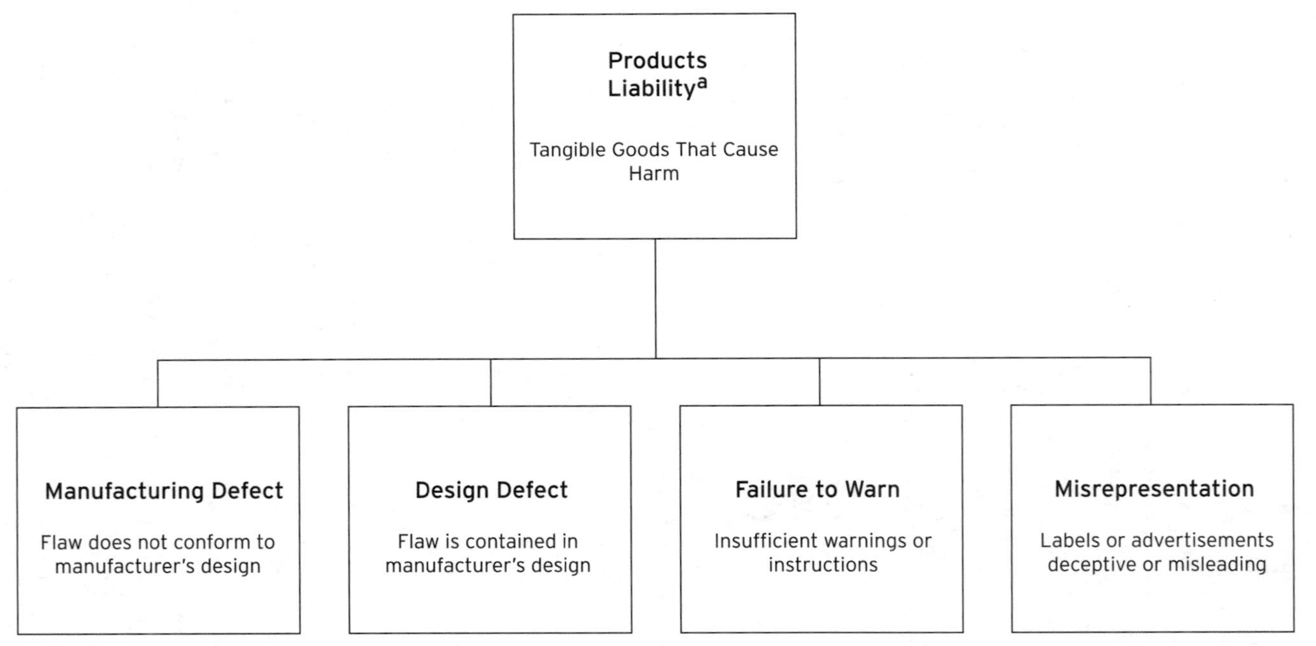

[a] Rules that shield manufacturers from strict liability: unavoidably unsafe products: products that are incapable of being made safe (e.g., pharmaceuticals and vaccines); products in common use: common and widely distributed products (e.g., alcoholic beverages and firearms).

Figure 22. Product liability theories.

resulted from the construction process. Manufacturing defects tend to be random and usually do not affect the entire product line.[66] Since it is usually difficult for consumers to detect a manufacturing flaw, courts impose liability on the seller. Thus, injured consumers do not have to demonstrate that the manufacturer used faulty materials, lacked due care in construction, or failed to inspect properly. The Product Liability Restatement imposes liability whenever a product "departs from its intended design even though all possible care was exercised."[67]

A product contains a *design defect* when it is defective although produced as planned by the manufacturer. Consequently, a design defect usually is apparent in an entire product line. Manufacturers are liable for design defects when "the foreseeable risks of harm posed by the product could have been reduced or avoided by the adoption of a reasonable alternative design . . . and the omission of the alternative design renders the product not reasonably safe."[68] "Reasonable design alternative" is a liability-limiting test (akin to negligence) because it requires the plaintiff to show that the product could have been made safer.[69] The design defect theory is controversial because the manufacturer often intentionally included the "defective" design feature after due consideration of price, attractiveness, and functionality. The defect, however, may be capable of causing great harm or injury, and it is important that the tort system effectively provide incentives for safer product design.

Strict liability for a design defect is not available for "unavoidably unsafe" products (e.g., pharmaceuticals, vaccines, and medical devices) or for inherently dangerous products in "common use" (e.g., alcoholic beverages or firearms). These exemptions from strict liability are very important to the public's health, and are explained in box 11.

A product has a *failure to warn* defect when the seller fails to inform consumers adequately about the risks or provide instructions for safe use.[70] The theory underlying this product defect is consumer sovereignty, the notion that customers deserve sufficient data to make informed purchasing choices.[71] Courts use a "reasonableness" test in evaluating failure to warn cases: Could the foreseeable risks have been reduced by reasonable instructions or warnings, and did the omission of instructions or warnings render the product unreasonably dangerous?[72] The fact that "failure to warn" cases often turn on the reasonableness of the action suggests a similarity to negligence theory. Some courts, however, unabashedly adopt strict liability for failure to warn even if the dangers were "undiscoverable at the time."[73]

Closely related to "failure to warn" theory is *misrepresentation,*

BOX 11

EXEMPTIONS FROM STRICT LIABILITY FOR A DESIGN DEFECT

"Unavoidably unsafe" or inherently dangerous products in "common use"

Strict liability for a design defect is not available for "unavoidably unsafe" products (e.g., pharmaceuticals, vaccines, and medical devices) and for inherently dangerous products in "common use" (e.g., alcoholic beverages or firearms). These exemptions from strict liability are important to the public's health because they make it extraordinarily difficult to successfully sue industries that affect the health and safety of the population.

"Unavoidably Unsafe" Products: Comment k

According to the Restatement (Second) of Torts § 402A, comment k, products that are highly beneficial to society but inherently risky escape strict liability if, "in the present state of human knowledge, they are quite incapable of being made safe for their intended and ordinary use." Pharmaceuticals, vaccines, and medical devices are classic illustrations of unavoidably unsafe products,[1] but courts have applied comment k also to dangerous products such as asbestos[2] and solvents.[3] Comment k "vindicates the public's interest in the availability and affordability" of a desirable consumer product.[4] The doctrine is intended to preserve incentives for socially useful products, but it also has the effect of shifting the risk of loss from manufacturers to injured consumers.

Courts in all jurisdictions that have ruled on the matter have adopted comment k, but they disagree on the scope of protection. Most courts apply comment k selectively, exempting from strict liability for defective design only prescription drugs, vaccines, and medical devices of high social utility.[5] However, a minority of courts exempt all such medical products from strict liability for defective design.[6] The majority view may be preferable because not every pharmaceutical is socially valuable—some are "me too" drugs that provide only small benefits over existing drugs at far greater cost, and others have principally cosmetic effects.

The Restatement (Third) of Torts: Products Liability proposes a standard by which prescription drugs may be considered to be defectively designed that is radically different from the majority view of comment k. Under the Third Restatement, a manufacturer will be exempted from strict liability on the basis of defective design if any reasonable health care provider would prescribe the pharmaceutical to any class of

[1] *Wilkinson v. Bay Shore Lumber Co.*, 227 Cal. Rptr. 327 (Cal. Ct. App. 1986) (stating that comment k cases overwhelmingly involve "prescription drugs, vaccines, blood, and medical devices such as intrauterine devices and breast implants"). The courts are divided, however, over whether comment k bars strict liability for all prescription drugs or whether the determination should be made on an individual basis by balancing utility and risk. Compare *Grundberg v. Upjohn Co.*, 813 P.2d 89 (Utah 1991) (favoring an across-the-board rule for all FDA-approved drugs) with *Hill v. Searle Lab.*, 884 F.2d 1064 (8th Cir. 1989) (adopting a case-by-case approach to deny comment k immunity for the CU-7 intrauterine device). In an attempt to narrow prescription drug and medical device liability, the revised restatement elaborates on comment k. Restatement (Third) of Torts: Prod. Liab. § 6, holds manufacturers of drugs and medical devices strictly liable only if a reasonable health care provider, informed of the risks and benefits of the therapy, would not prescribe it to any class of patient.

[2] *Borel v. Fibreboard Paper Products Corp.*, 493 F.2d 1076 (5th Cir. 1973).

[3] *Purvis v. PPG Industries, Inc.*, 502 So. 2d 714 (Ala. 1987).

[4] *Brown v. Superior Court*, 751 P.2d 470, 482 (Cal. 1988).

[5] See, e.g., *Feldman v. Lederle Labs.*, 479 A.2d 374, 382 (N.J. 1984) (rejecting the manufacturer's argument that all prescription drugs were unavoidably unsafe, and applying comment k only to drugs that were "more vital to the public health and human survival than others").

[6] See, e.g., *Brown*, 751 P.2d 470.

patient.[7] Scholars have criticized this standard as too lax and antithetical to the public's health.[8] It virtually forecloses the possibility of successful litigation relating to a drug that causes harm to a population, provided a reasonable physician could have prescribed it to a small class of patients. The Products Liability Restatement implicitly rejects a risk-utility analysis from a population perspective in favor of the prescribing physician's clinical judgment. To date, most states have not had the opportunity to consider the Third Restatement, and no state has yet formally adopted it.

Inherently Dangerous Products in "Common Use"

Strict liability is also unavailable for inherently dangerous products that are in common use and made according to the manufacturer's design (e.g., "good" whiskey and tobacco).[9] The Products Liability Restatement says that "common and widely distributed products such as alcoholic beverages, firearms, and above-ground swimming pools" may be held defective only if they are sold without reasonable warning or if reasonable alternative designs could have been adopted.[10] The rationale is that, since these hazardous products have received long-term market acceptance, the legislature is thought to be the appropriate regulatory agency. However, many would find it odd that tobacco and firearms are immunized from strict liability (along with vaccines and prescription drugs) while far safer and socially advantageous products, such as children's toys and food products, must meet rigorous strict-liability standards. If the functions of strict liability are to encourage safer product design and to spread the risk of injury and disease, then cigarettes, alcoholic beverages, and firearms would seem to be prime candidates for tort regulation. Yet tort law treats these hazardous products favorably, and the legislature has even shielded tobacco (through preemption—see box 3, p. 80) and firearm (see the case study later in this chapter) companies from liability. (Legislatures similarly have immunized the food industry against obesity lawsuits—see box 12, p. 213.)

[7] *Restatement (Third) of Torts: Prod. Liab.* §6(c) (1998).
[8] Mark D. Shifton, "The Restatement (Third) of Torts: Products Liability—The ALI's Cure for Prescription Drug Design Liability," *Fordham Urban Law Journal*, 29 (2001-2): 2343-86.
[9] *Restatement (Second) of Torts* § 402A, cmt. i (1965).
[10] *Restatement (Third) of Torts: Prod. Liab.* § 2, cmt. d (1998).

where the seller misinforms consumers orally, in writing, or through other conduct calculated to convey a false impression. Misrepresentation is established through labels, packet inserts, or advertisements that are inaccurate, deceptive, or misleading. Intentional concealment of the truth also can be considered misrepresentation, such as when a tobacco company fails to disclose internal research on the harmful effects of cigarettes on smokers.[74] Given the pervasive advertising of modern products, misrepresentation claims may become a significant theory of liability for advancing the public's health.[75]

Courts and scholars have criticized the reporters of the Product Liability Restatement for writing what amounts to "a wish list from manufacturing America."[76] The Restatement, critics suggest, does not faithfully record the state of the law as it existed at the time. More importantly, the Restatement retreats from strict liability in favor of negligence. It requires injured persons to demonstrate that manufacturers reasonably should have foreseen the dangers and failed to adopt a reasonable alternative design. The Restatement ignores the policy underlying strict liability: that manufacturers are in a better position than the consumer to evaluate their products, anticipate hazards, and make the necessary changes or improvements. As a result, several states have rejected the Third Restatement on the grounds that product liability should be strict, and that the danger need not be foreseeable.[77]

SCIENTIFIC CONUNDRUMS IN MASS TORT LITIGATION: EPIDEMIOLOGY IN THE COURTROOM

> Thus not only our reason fails us in the discovery of the ultimate connexion of causes and effects, but even after experience has inform'd us of their constant conjunction, 'tis impossible for us to satisfy ourselves by our reason, why we shou'd extend that experience beyond those particular instances, which have fallen under our observation. We suppose, but are never able to prove, that there must be a resemblance betwixt those objects, of which we have had experience, and those which lie beyond the reach of our discovery.
>
> David Hume (1739)

The cultures and purposes of law and science differ markedly, and these differences span centuries of interaction between the two fields.[78] Both fields seek the truth, but each gives truth a different meaning.[79] Whereas law seeks finality and closure, scientific inquiry is continuous; whereas law in civil litigation makes decisions based on the preponderance of evidence (greater than 50 percent), science uses statistical significance (greater than a 95 percent chance of a nonrandom finding); whereas law follows an adversarial method, science embraces the experimental design (the "scientific" method); whereas legal evidence is testimonial, scientific evidence is empirical. These different understandings do not mean that one field discovers truth and the other less than truth.[80] Rather, the two fields have different missions, but each operates, at least partly, in the other's environment. Science and law, therefore, must seek to understand the other, and each must accommodate the methods and cognitive processes of the other.

Interactions between law and science center on issues of causality: Did an act, event, or exposure produce a certain harm? The law's purpose is to assign responsibility for the harm. Problems of proof in traditional tort actions, such as motor vehicle accidents, are usually surmountable. If X hits Y, who sustains an immediate injury, causality can be readily established by an eyewitness who observed the event and a medical expert who testifies that the harm resulted from the impact. But what if a product (P) or activity (A) is associated only with an increased rate of harm (H) in the population, not an immediate injury? How difficult is it to marshal scientific proof that A or P caused H?

This is the kind of scientific conundrum that arises in so-called mass exposure ("toxic tort") litigation. Mass tort actions characteristically involve large populations that are exposed to one or more toxic substances. Toxic substances in mass exposure litigation are as diverse as commercial materials (e.g., lead paint), chemical compounds (e.g., dioxin), personal items (e.g., tampons or silicone breast implants), pharmaceuticals (e.g., Bendectin), vaccines (e.g., swine flu), and low-level radiation. Plaintiffs claim these substances cause a variety of health conditions ranging from carcinogenic (cancer), teratogenic (birth defects), and mutagenic (genetic mutations) effects to autoimmune and nervous system dysfunction. The health effects of exposure to toxic substances usually are not immediately apparent and may take a decade (e.g., asbestosis) or even a generation (e.g., birth defects) to emerge.

Problems of scientific proof in mass exposure litigation relate to the massive scope of the population, the exposure, the health conditions, and the latency period. First, a large number of people are exposed to the same toxic substance, but some of them have the alleged health effect and some do not (e.g., the massive exposure to methyl isocyanate from a Union Carbide plant in Bhopal, India).[81] Second, the population at risk probably has been exposed to many different toxic substances, and their levels (or doses) of exposure vary widely. Third, the health conditions from which the population claims to suffer also appear in background levels in groups who were not exposed.[82] Finally, because of the passage of time between the original exposure and the onset of symptoms, plaintiffs find it difficult to gather evidence and to discount the multiple intervening variables that might explain their present health condition. Consider a population that claims a higher prevalence of leukemia and other cancers due to exposure to radiation from a nuclear power plant. The same diseases occur in the general population and show complicated etiologies, including genetics, smoking, and exposure to radon. In such circumstances, it is extraordinarily difficult to prove that the exposure to atomic testing definitively caused the cancers.[83]

Plaintiffs in mass exposure litigation must establish two types of causation: general and specific.[84] General (or generic) causation assesses whether the substance (at the dosage to which the plaintiffs were exposed)[85] is capable of causing a harm found at increased levels in the population. Specific causation assesses whether exposure to the substance in fact caused the plaintiff's harm.[86] Professors Tom Christoffel and Stephen Teret explain that even if plaintiffs can show that factor X is responsible for a significant percentage of all cases of harm Y in a population (general causation), it can rarely be proven that the harm Y suffered by a particular individual was one of the cases caused by factor X (specific causation).[87]

Courts often favor single-cause explanations for injury and seek a traceable causal chain of events.[88] The preferred form of proof is the "eyewitness"—the treating physician who testifies that a specific event caused the patient's harm. Toxic tort plaintiffs, however, may use probabilistic evidence to establish a legally cognizable connection between the exposure and the harm (i.e., the likelihood that the exposure which caused the harm was sufficiently high to demonstrate cause and effect).[89] Certainly, as the epigraph by David Hume explains, positive correlations never establish causation; yet epidemiologists use statistical significance to explain positive correlations between two phenomena (the exposure and the harm) and to infer causality.[90]

The Admissibility of Scientific Evidence: "Junk Science" in the Courtroom

Issues of causation are often determined by scientific evidence, but the courts have struggled with the vexing question of when scientific testimony may be admitted in a trial.[91] In *Frye v. United States,* decided in 1923, the court set a standard for the admissibility of scientific evidence that lasted for more than seventy years. *Frye*'s "general acceptance" test permitted into evidence only "a well-recognized scientific principle or discovery . . . sufficiently established to have gained general acceptance in the particular field."[92] Thus, establishing a consensus within the scientific community was crucial to the admission of expert testimony. In 1975, Congress enacted the Federal Rules of Evidence, which reflected a more liberal attitude toward the admission of evidence: "If scientific, technical or other specialized knowledge will assist the trier of fact to understand the evidence . . . a witness qualified as an expert . . . may testify."[93] The Federal Rules favor the admission of relevant testimony, relying on the adversarial process to sort out strong and weak evidence.[94]

The Federal Rules' "let it all in" theory, however, makes it easier to introduce scientifically unfounded evidence (so-called junk science), with the effect that businesses are held liable for harms they did not create. Peter Huber argues that trial lawyers have an incentive to introduce scientific evidence irrespective of its rigor, medical experts are willing to testify for a fee, and juries are prone to decide against defendants with "deep pockets."[95] Marcia Angell chronicled the systematic use of pseudoscience in the silicone breast implant cases, where Dow Corning was held liable, even though independent scientific reviews showed that implants do not cause autoimmune or connective tissue diseases.[96] Unscientific evidence proffered by "hired guns" representing either industry or consumers remains a serious problem, although the Supreme Court, as the following discussion shows, is moving toward a more scientifically oriented approach to expert evidence (see figure 23).

After 1975, courts began to divide on whether the restrictive *Frye* test or the permissive Federal Rules test governed admissibility. The Supreme Court resolved the disagreement in *Daubert v. Merrell Dow Pharmaceuticals* (1993).[97] In this case, the Court held that the Federal Rules superseded the *Frye* "general acceptance" test,[98] but it shifted to a more scientific approach,[99] finding that the trial judge must assume a gatekeeping (or screening) role in assessing the admissibility of expert evidence: "The judge must ensure that . . . scientific testimony or evidence admitted is not only relevant, but reliable."[100]

Daubert—one of a long series of cases alleging that the antinausea drug Bendectin caused birth defects in children—established a two-part test to determine the admissibility of scientific evidence: reliability and relevancy (or "fit"). The Supreme Court suggested four factors, or "general observations," to assess the reliability of scientific evidence: (1) testing—whether the scientific theory or technique can be and has been tested; (2) peer review—whether the theory or technique has been subjected to the strictures of peer review and publication; (3) error rate—whether there is a high known or potential rate of error; and (4) general acceptance—whether the theory or technique enjoys general acceptance within a relevant scientific community.[101]

Daubert's four factors are illustrative and nonexclusive, and should be applied flexibly by the trial court; they "neither necessarily nor exclusively apply to all experts or in every case."[102] Federal courts, for example,

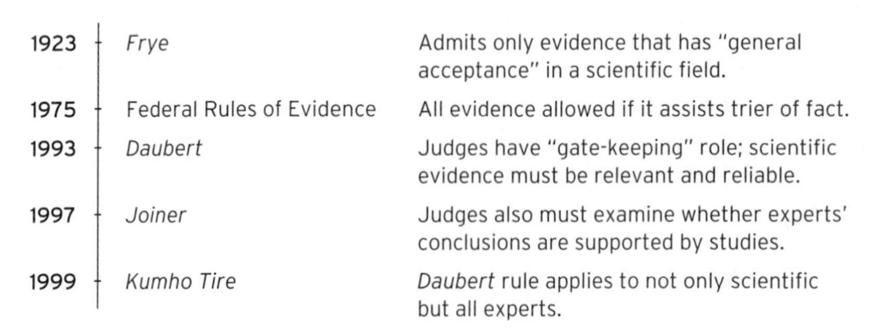

Figure 23. Admissibility of scientific evidence in the courtroom: A timeline.

have admitted expert testimony that does not meet all or even most of the *Daubert* factors.[103]

After considering the reliability of the scientific evidence, the trial court must consider the relevance, or "fit," of the evidence to the ultimate issue to be decided: The evidence must "assist the trier of fact to understand the evidence or to determine a fact in issue."[104] Thus, to be relevant, testimony must "logically advance a material aspect of the case."[105] In mass exposure cases, plaintiffs often rely on a complex chain of causation beginning with animal studies.[106] Plaintiffs must satisfy the *Daubert* test of reliability and relevance for each link in the causal chain; if they fail to do so, courts exclude the expert testimony.[107]

Appellate courts grant the trial judge considerable discretion in making decisions on whether to admit expert evidence.[108] All evidentiary decisions are reviewed under an "abuse of discretion" standard that is highly deferential.[109]

The Supreme Court in *Daubert* left unclear an important issue about inadmissibility: whether the standards of reliability and relevancy apply only to the expert's methodology or whether they apply to her conclusions as well. In other words, must the trial court accept anomalous conclusions from an expert who relies on valid studies?[110] The Supreme Court in *General Electric Company v. Joiner* (1997) held that the trial court could critically examine whether the expert's conclusions were supported by the studies cited: "Conclusions and methodology are not entirely distinct from one another. Trained experts commonly extrapolate from existing data. But . . . a district court [is not required] to admit opinion evidence which is connected to the existing data only by the ipse dixit of the expert. A court may conclude that there is simply too great an analytical gap between the data and the opinion proffered."[111]

The Supreme Court, in *Kumho Tire Company v. Carmichael* (1999),[112] held that the *Daubert* factors apply not only to scientific experts but to all experts, such as engineers. The Court reasoned that no clear line divides scientific knowledge from technical or other specialized knowledge, and no convincing need exists to make such distinctions.

In summary, the Supreme Court has progressively tightened the liberal admissibility standard in the Federal Rules, giving trial judges considerable discretion to exclude both scientific methodologies and expert opinions of all kinds that fail to meet tests of reliability and relevance. The Court itself said that the law must make certain that an expert "employs in the courtroom the same level of intellectual rigor that characterizes the practice of an expert in the relevant field."[113]

The major criticism of the "*Daubert* trilogy" (*Daubert, Joiner,* and *Kumho Tire*) is that judges do not possess adequate knowledge or scientific background to assess effectively the validity of theories and data offered by expert witnesses.[114] Courts, exhibiting a misunderstanding of scientific reasoning, have excluded evidence that appeared highly probative, such as animal studies,[115] epidemiological research that shows a relative risk of less than 2.0,[116] and even well-accepted studies with minor flaws.[117] To the dismay of environmental and public health advocates, courts have made it difficult to demonstrate causation between hazardous products or exposures and harms to the population.[118] Trial judges have also been inconsistent, with some including and others excluding substantially similar evidence—for example, whether PCBs or environmental tobacco smoke cause lung cancer.[119]

Although this critique of the *Daubert* trilogy is undoubtedly true, the courts should adopt some reasonable methodology for ensuring that judicial decision making is scientifically valid or at least does not fly in the face of science. The judge's role as gatekeeper—to ensure that experts base their opinions on scientifically rigorous data and draw reasonable inferences from those data—can be helpful. The judiciary has an even better method at its disposal for solving the problem of unscientific evidence, but judges would need to make greater use of it. Trial judges have the power to appoint independent experts to evaluate evidence for the jury. Independent experts could be chosen from a panel of scientists well regarded in their fields, without conflict of interest and independent from the parties to the case. The independent experts could then draw their conclusions from a wide breadth of peer-reviewed and other reliable data, applying scientifically sound principles to the facts of the case.

THE PUBLIC HEALTH VALUE OF TORT LITIGATION

Regulation can be as effectively exerted through an award of damages as through some form of preventive relief. The obligation to pay compensation can be, indeed is designed to be, a potent method of governing conduct and controlling policy.

Felix Frankfurter (1959)

Tort law can be an important tool for advancing the public's health.[120] Many public health issues are politically charged and powerfully affect businesses and consumers. As a result, it may be exceedingly difficult to regulate directly harmful products or activities through legislation or agency rules. Powerful interest groups, such as the tobacco, food, or firearms lobby, can thwart regulation through the political process. Consumers themselves may rise up in revolt against regulation and taxation of the products they desire. Consider the difficulty of imposing strict emission standards for automobiles and light trucks, higher taxes on cigarettes, restrictions on the fat content of fast foods, or safety locks on handguns. Where direct regulation through the political process fails, tort law can become an essential tool in the arsenal of public health advocates.

Tort law, used as a strategy complementary to direct regulation, serves several purposes: preventing dangerous products from being put in the market, increasing prices and thus decreasing consumers' willingness to purchase those products, limiting unsafe or misleading businesses practices, and forcing internalization of the social costs of high-risk activities.[121]

One major critique of tort law is that it is not a particularly effective deterrent. Some scholars assert that legal doctrine rarely controls human behavior: Laypersons are not usually aware of legal rules, and, even if they are, they are more likely to be influenced by normal human motivations—a sense of adventure, sexual desire, tolerance for risk, or desire for safety.[122] This critique has validity but misses the point. Tort law affects consumer behavior by altering the way businesses conduct their activities. Industry may react to tort law by making products safer, providing clearer warnings and instructions, or simply discontinuing product lines, all of which powerfully affect consumer choice and action. Alternatively, businesses may absorb the cost of liability, usually passing the cost on to consumers in the form of price increases. Price increases can reduce demand, particularly among young people, as the experience with cigarettes demonstrates.

Businesses are likely to adjust their behavior in response to legal norms, particularly if economic costs are associated with noncompliance. It matters to a business whether it must bear the cost of environmental damage or personal injury; an enterprise will weigh litigation and liability costs in deciding whether to emit a toxin or design a safer product. The tort system, then, can be a potent form of regulation because it imposes costs on individuals and businesses when they engage in risky behavior.

Perhaps the single greatest limitation of traditional tort law in advancing the public's health is the concept of fault under the negligence theory. It is not usually a problem to demonstrate that industry acts unreasonably when selling unsafe products or engaging in high-risk activities. The real difficulty arises from the notion that individuals contribute to their ill health through their own behavior—a persistent claim by industry in tobacco, firearms, and obesity litigation.[123] Two defenses in negligence actions can be fatal to public health: assumption of risk and contributory or comparative negligence.

The first defense, assumption of risk, holds that if individuals are aware of the risk but nonetheless engage in the activity, they cannot recover. In numerous situations, individuals understand the risks they face in smoking cigarettes, eating high-calorie foods, or purchasing and using a firearm. In these circumstances, it may be easy for industry to point the finger of blame at the consumer herself, suggesting she is responsible for her own condition. In thinking about assumption of risk, government-imposed labeling and disclosure requirements actually may be helpful to industry. For example, alcoholic beverage manufacturers can rely on government health warnings to resist liability. After all, they will argue, the dangers of the product were prominently displayed on the product package and advertising, so the consumer must accept responsibility for her own behavior.

The second defense, contributory or comparative negligence, holds that a damage award can be reduced or eliminated if the plaintiff's negligence contributed to a portion of the injury or disease she suffered. The contributory negligence defense allows industry to assert that the plaintiff's ill health was a product of her own lack of due care. A person who continues to smoke after she experiences extreme breathing difficulties, drinks excessively after experiencing liver damage, or eats unhealthy foods after being diagnosed with diabetes may easily be portrayed as acting unreasonably. Similarly, a person who stores her firearm without a lock and within reach of children will be seen as lacking common sense. In all these cases and many more, businesses seek to transfer responsibility from themselves to consumers in the minds of jurors. In this way, industry can argue that the harm results not from its own negligence in the design and marketing of a dangerous product but from the irresponsible behavior of the user of the product.

The skillful use of assumption of risk and comparative negligence by manufacturers may appear ruinous to public health strategies in tort law. However, upon more careful reflection, in a counterintuitive way, these limitations of tort doctrine may muster support for limiting health threats that appear to be self-imposed. [124] Because of these limitations, plaintiffs must frame their arguments in terms that make the threat seem to be inflicted from without rather than from within. This is one important reason tobacco, and now firearms and obesity, litigation has finally adopted the device of having governments, rather than injured consumers, sue for damages. Unfortunately, as we will see, even governments are finding it difficult to succeed in litigation involving personal risk behavior.

In any event, defenses in negligence actions, such as assumption of risk and comparative negligence, give a major incentive to plaintiffs and public health advocates to reframe the debate in a way that makes what once was a quintessentially voluntary risk, such as smoking or drinking alcoholic beverages, seem ambiguous at best, if not outright involuntary. Thus, public health threats that seem to be self-inflicted become more a matter of industry's efforts to mislead, cajole, and reassure the public;[125] sometimes consumers can point to the product's addictive qualities, as with alcoholic beverages or tobacco. This kind of thinking paves the way for public understanding of the true nature of risk and responsibility in tobacco, alcoholic beverages, firearms, and other major health threats. Similarly, it can be helpful in legislative and agency responses that, like tort doctrine itself, have also resisted regulation of perceived self-inflicted harms.

To illustrate the public health value of tort law, I present two case studies—one on tobacco and the other on firearm litigation. In these case studies, it is interesting to see how public health strategies have shifted over time to overcome, not always successfully, the nagging problem of personal blame and responsibility.

"THE TOBACCO WARS": A CASE STUDY

Who are these persons who knowingly and secretly decide to put the buying public at risk solely for the purpose of making profits and who believe that illness and death of consumers is an appropriate cost of their own prosperity? As the following facts disclose, despite some rising pretenders, the tobacco industry may be the king of concealment and disinformation.

Dolores K. Sloviter (1992)

In the early 1950s, before the first lawsuit against the tobacco industry was filed, the cigarette was a cultural icon—tobacco smoking was viewed as chic, promoted ubiquitously, and portrayed by sports and movie stars as an accoutrement of the good life. Epidemiologists, however, were already reporting an association between cigarettes and cancer,[126] and these data were soon published in the popular media.[127] The first tobacco lawsuit was filed in 1954,[128] initiating what torts scholar Robert Rabin called the first wave of tobacco litigation.[129] During this first wave, from 1954 to 1973, approximately 100–150 cases were filed; very few of these cases ever came to trial, and in no case did a plaintiff prevail over the tobacco industry (see figure 24).[130]

The first wave of cases was filed principally under theories of negligence, breach of warranty, and misrepresentation.[131] In retrospect, it is surprising that tobacco litigation was so unsuccessful. At that time, plaintiffs could not voluntarily assume the risks because they had begun smoking without knowledge of the harmful effects. The misrepresentation claims, moreover, appeared powerful because industry advertisements trumpeted product safety: "Play Safe, Smoke Chesterfield. Nose, throat, and accessory organs not adversely affected" (1952) and "More doctors smoke Camels than any other cigarette" (1955). Epidemiologists also were still working out the problem of causation, culminating in Luther Terry's landmark Surgeon General's report on smoking in 1964.[132] Ironically, around the same time the Surgeon General's report was dramatically changing the views of science and the public, the American Law Institute (ALI) all but absolved the tobacco industry from strict product liability. In the Restatement (Second) of Torts, the ALI stated, "Good tobacco is not unreasonably dangerous merely because the effects of smoking may be harmful."[133]

By the time of the second wave of litigation, from 1983 to 1992, cigarette smoking was becoming a hallmark not of elegance but of weak character and lower social class. The public had become far more health conscious, and cigarettes were thought to be a highly dangerous and addictive product. This new health consciousness was both a blessing and

1954	*Lowe v. R.J. Reynolds*	First suit filed by a smoker against cigarette companies for smoking-related injuries.
1963	*Lartigue v. R.J. Reynolds*	Court finds that "[cigarette] manufacturers are not insurers against unknowable risks." Tobacco industry found not liable.
1967	*Pritchard v. Liggett & Meyers*	Tobacco industry convinces jury that plaintiffs assume risks of smoking despite misleading advertisments.
1970	*Green v. American Tobacco*	Court finds that asserting "unwholesomeness of standardized product line" is legally insufficient for breach of warranty claim. Major ruling for tobacco industry.
1992	*Cipollone v. Liggett Group*	After eight years of litigation, jury awards the plaintiff's estate $400,000 for cigarette-related illness—the first damage award against the industry. On appeal, the U.S. Supreme Court holds that the federal cigarette labeling act preempts negligence, but not fraud, claims against the industry.
1994	Tobacco Papers	Disclosure of evidence that tobacco companies knew health risks and conspired to conceal information.
1997	Medicaid Settlements	Texas, Mississippi, and Florida attorneys general reach settlements for Medicaid medical cost reimbursement.
1998	Master Settlement Agreement	Forty-six states and tobacco companies reach $206 billion settlement.
1999	*Broin v. Philip Morris Co.*	Flight attendants sue for exposure to second-hand smoke. Tobacco companies settle.
	Individual suits	Several plaintiffs in Oregon, California, and Florida obtain large verdicts against cigarette manufacturers for tobacco-related illnesses.
	Federal government lawsuit	Department of Justice files civil action against tobacco companies for Medicare cost reimbursement.
	Engle v. R.J. Reynolds	All Florida smokers addicted to cigarettes and suffering from certain conditions are allowed to file claims.
2000	*Engle v. R.J. Reynolds*	First jury verdict for class action against tobacco companies.
2005	*United States v. Philip Morris*	The U.S. Department of Justice sought to force cigarette manufacturers to disgorge $280 billion in proceeds from their past unlawful activity. Instead of imposing billions of dollars in fines, the court ordered the tobacco companies to stop using deceptive terms such as "light."
2006	*Engle v. Liggett Group*	Florida Supreme Court throws out the largest punitive damage award in the history of cigarette litigation, $145 billion.

Figure 24. "The tobacco wars": A timeline.

a curse for litigants. While problems of causation were reduced, plaintiffs could no longer claim ignorance of the health risks. Instead, defense counsel portrayed plaintiffs as morally responsible for their own illness. Individuals, after all, made their own choice to smoke, fully apprised of the risks. Federal antitobacco regulation was used by the industry, moreover, as a shield against litigation. The Cigarette Labeling and Advertising Act, enacted in 1965, required warning labels on cigarette packages.[134] Defense counsel could point to those warnings as nearly definitive evidence that plaintiffs were informed of the risks.

During this second wave of litigation, nearly two hundred cases were filed, many under new theories of failure to warn and strict liability.[135] This was a time when litigants were making stunning advances in mass torts cases ranging from Agent Orange and DES to the Dalkon Shield and Bendectin. One would have thought that if any product would fare badly under the "risk-utility" analysis in this era of mass torts, it would be cigarettes: This product caused more illness and death than any other in American history, and its effects were disproportionately borne by young people, ethnic minorities, and the poor. Nevertheless, despite marked changes in science, tort theory, and social attitudes, the results were the same. It was not until 1990 that a New Jersey jury awarded damages of $400,000 to the estate of Rose Cipollone, a smoker who died of cancer at the age of fifty-eight. The jury verdict (which was overturned on appeal) was the first in the history of the extensive tobacco litigation in which a plaintiff was awarded damages.[136] To understand why the industry was so successful, it is important to examine its tactics.

"King of the Mountain": Industry Tactics in the Tobacco Wars

[The industry has prevailed] by resisting all discovery, thus requiring a court hearing before plaintiffs can obtain even the most rudimentary discovery . . . by getting confidentiality orders attached to the discovery materials they finally produce, thus preventing plaintiffs' counsel from sharing the fruits of discovery and forcing each plaintiff to reinvent the wheel . . . by taking exceedingly lengthy depositions and naming multiple experts of their own for each specialty, thereby putting plaintiffs' counsel [to inordinate expense] . . . [and] by taking dozens and dozens of

> oral depositions, all across the country, of trivial fact witnesses.
>
> William E. Townsley and Dale K. Hanks (1989)

> The aggressive posture we [the tobacco companies] have taken regarding depositions and discovery in general continues to make these cases extremely burdensome and expensive for plaintiffs' lawyers. . . . To paraphrase General Patton, the way we won these cases was not by spending all of [R. J. Reynolds's] money, but by making that other son of a bitch spend all his.
>
> J. Michael Jordan (1993)

The tobacco industry resorted to an unusual but highly effective strategy during the first two waves of tobacco litigation: aggressive and uncompromising litigation.[137] First, the industry was relentless in pretrial maneuvering, attempting to delay the trial endlessly and deplete plaintiffs' resources. Since plaintiffs' lawyers were characteristically situated in small firms and practiced on a contingency basis, they could not cope with large up-front expenses preceding a trial. The industry adopted a conscious policy of devoting inexhaustible resources, never settling a case, and always fighting to the bitter end. For example, the *Cipollone* case produced twelve federal opinions and cost the plaintiff's attorneys roughly $4 million; the attorneys withdrew from the case before it went to trial a second time.[138] Second, the industry adopted a no-holds-barred defense in which it probed the moral habits of the plaintiff, urging juries to find personal blameworthiness. Since risks of cancer and heart disease unfold over decades, it was easy for defense counsel to examine every possible behavioral risk factor. What was intended to be a sober adjudication of corporate responsibility became a searching examination of the plaintiff's morality. Finally, the industry consistently disputed the health risks. A 1972 memorandum outlined the industry's strategy of "creating doubt about the health charge without actually denying it; and advocating the public's right to smoke without actually urging them to take up the practice."[139]

The Preemption Battle: The Cigarette Labeling Act and Rose Cipollone

The Cigarette Labeling and Advertising Act of 1965,[140] subsequently amended as the Public Health Cigarette Smoking Act of 1969,[141] preempts state regulation based on "smoking and health." Following Rose Cipollone's jury verdict, the Supreme Court granted certiorari, setting the stage for the landmark decision in *Cipollone v. Liggett Group* (1992).[142] Justice John Paul Stevens, in a plurality decision, held that the 1969 act preempts tort claims based on "failure to warn and the neutralization of federally mandated warnings to the extent that those claims rely on omissions or inclusions in the [manufacturers'] advertising or promotions." However, the act does not preempt tort claims based on express warranty, intentional fraud and misrepresentation, or conspiracy.[143] The Supreme Court's decision left ample room for tobacco litigation based on theories of misinformation and deceit. During the third wave, plaintiffs succeeded in ways that scarcely could have been imagined.

The "Third Wave" of Tobacco Litigation

The third wave did not begin quietly. On May 12, 1994, a paralegal at the law firm representing Brown and Williamson Tobacco delivered over ten thousand pages of internal industry documents to Professor Stanton Glantz at the University of California, San Francisco. The "Tobacco Papers" contained damaging evidence about the tobacco industry's actual knowledge and intent.[144] Despite the industry's public claims, the Tobacco Papers demonstrated that executives understood the health effects of smoking, the addictive quality of nicotine, and the toxicity of pesticides contained in cigarettes. The industry, moreover, had manipulated the nicotine content of cigarettes and marketed their products to young persons. These documents, and others obtained through press reports[145] and discovery,[146] would be used with great effect in the ensuing litigation—notably medical cost reimbursement, class actions, and individual smoker lawsuits.

Medical Cost Reimbursement. Governments and other payers who sought reimbursement for paying the costs of tobacco-related illnesses became a dominant theme in the third wave. State attorneys general filed direct claims against the tobacco industry for reimbursement of public money that had been spent to pay for tobacco-related illness. Following the original Medicaid reimbursement suit, filed in Mississippi in 1994,[147] most states joined the litigation. On June 20, 1997, the tobacco industry and the attorneys general ended their negotiations and presented a settlement that required Congress to grant the industry immunity from certain forms of litigation. In exchange, the states would receive $368 billion over twenty-five years. However, federal attempts to codify the settlement ultimately failed. For example, a bill sponsored by Senator John McCain would have increased the tax on cigarettes, raised the settlement amount, and altered the civil immunity provisions.[148] As a result, RJR-Nabisco withdrew support for federal tobacco legislation, and the bill died in committee.

In the wake of federal failure, four states (Florida, Minnesota, Mississippi, and Texas) settled with the tobacco industry for a total of $40 billion.[149] As the cost of individual settlements mounted, the industry negotiated a Master Settlement Agreement (MSA) with forty-six states and six U.S. territories. The agreement, concluded on November 16, 1998, requires industry to compensate states in perpetuity, with payments totaling $206 billion through the year 2025; creates a charitable foundation to reduce adolescent smoking; disbands the Council for Tobacco Research; provides public access to documents through the Internet; and restricts outdoor advertising, the use of cartoon characters, tobacco merchandising, and sponsorship of sporting events. The industry received civil immunity for future state claims, but not for individual or class action lawsuits.[150]

Cigarette manufacturers and other stakeholders have challenged the lawfulness of the MSA on various theories: constitutional,[151] antitrust,[152] and unlawful exclusion of Indian tribes in the negotiations.[153] However, none of these suits was successful and the MSA has been consistently upheld.

The success of state attorneys general against the tobacco industry encouraged other groups to seek medical expense reimbursement. The most promising was a lawsuit by the federal government to recoup health care expenditures for past and future treatment of tobacco-related illnesses. The U.S. Department of Justice, in a RICO claim, sought to enjoin tobacco companies from engaging in fraudulent or other unlawful conduct, and to force companies to "disgorge" $280 billion in proceeds from their past unlawful activity. In a severe blow to the government's case, the U.S. Court of Appeals for the D.C. Circuit held in 2005 that disgorgement was not an available remedy because RICO provided jurisdiction only for forward-looking remedies aimed at future violations.[154] The Justice Department subsequently reduced its damages request from $130 billion to $10 billion, leading health advocates and Democratic lawmakers to accuse the White House of improper political interference.[155] In the end, the U.S. District Court ruled that companies had conspired to deceive the public, but that it was not permissible to impose billions of dollars in fines. However, in an attempt to prevent future harms, the court ordered the tobacco companies to stop using deceptive terms such as "low tar" or "light."[156]

The courts have been openly hostile to medical reimbursement suits by private parties. A court rejected a claim by individuals acting as private attorneys general to recoup Medicare costs.[157] And eight federal circuits have ruled against suits by labor unions and others to recoup health care costs for treatment of tobacco-related illnesses.[158] Even foreign countries have sought to obtain costs expended by their public health care systems, thus far without success.[159] Perhaps the most unusual plaintiffs were bankrupt asbestos companies, which had been found liable for causing lung cancer in workers. These companies sued the tobacco industry for contributions to the lung cancer burden that juries had attributed solely to asbestos, but they too have met with little success.[160]

Class Actions. Tobacco litigants have adopted a strategy of class action litigation. In 1994, nonsmoking flight attendants filed a class action against tobacco manufacturers alleging that they suffered injuries caused by inhalation of secondhand smoke in airplane cabins. The judiciary certified the class,[161] and the parties reached a settlement for a $300 million medical foundation; the settlement permits individual lawsuits.[162]

The judiciary, however, has thus far thwarted the most ambitious class actions. In *Castano v. American Tobacco Company* (1996),[163] the Fifth Circuit Court of Appeals decertified a class of all nicotine-dependent smokers in the United States because variations in state law would render the class impracticable. Similarly, in *Engle v. Liggett Group* (2006), the Florida Supreme Court affirmed the appellate court's decision to throw out the largest punitive damage award in the history of cigarette litigation, $145 billion. The court also affirmed decertification of the class because individualized issues, including proof of causation and apportionment of fault among the defendants, predominated over issues common to the class.[164] Courts in other jurisdictions have also rejected class action tobacco suits.[165]

Individual Smokers. The tobacco industry also faces litigation from individual smokers in the third wave. Plaintiffs in Oregon[166] and California[167] have won substantial verdicts, and numerous individual suits are pending.[168] Although the *Engle* decision has been cast as a victory for the tobacco industry, the court's ruling may also open the door for thousands of individual claims by Florida smokers.[169] Because the defendant cigarette manufacturers were found guilty of negligence, product liability, fraud, and breach of warranty, members of the decertified class need not prove these elements if they file individual claims in Florida within the year.[170] Individual nonsmokers have also successfully sued for exposure to environmental, or "secondhand," tobacco smoke.[171] Although these plaintiffs face difficult legal hurdles in proving a casual relationship between secondhand smoke and their ill health,[172] the 2006 Surgeon General's report decisively linking secondhand smoke to cancer and cardiovascular disease is likely to bolster these efforts.[173] With the formation of the Tobacco Trial Lawyers Association (a network that shares information, expert witnesses, and tactics), stricter judicial case management, and new rules regarding work-product discovery,[174] individual lawsuits may emerge as a force in the tobacco wars.[175]

Punitive Damages. The future of large punitive damage awards is uncertain in both class action and individual suits, however, as excessive awards may violate the constitutional guarantee of due process. The Supreme Court has suggested (without actually deciding) that punitive damages should not exceed compensatory damages by more than a single-digit ratio,[176] but state courts subsequently upheld jury awards far surpassing this limit.[177] The Supreme Court partially addressed this issue during the 2006–7 term, when it threw out a $79.5 million Oregon verdict against Philip Morris. The Court held that the Fourteenth Amendment's Due Process Clause bars state court juries from using punitive damages awards to punish defendants for harm done to nonparties.[178] Such awards deprive the defendant of a fair chance to defend against claims of absent victims whose circumstances are unknown. However, the Court sees no problem with allowing evidence of harm to nonparties as a means of showing reprehensibility, as long as the jury does not punish defendants for such harms. As the case is remanded to the Oregon Supreme Court, it is unclear whether the verdict will be reinstated or reduced, or whether a new trial will be ordered.[179]

The tobacco wars have been a stunning, and highly unexpected, public health success, but the success only goes so far. Considering that numerous tobacco suits over several decades failed to clear the obstacle of smoker responsibility, the Master Settlement Agreement is a remarkable achievement. The result of the cash settlement will certainly increase the price of cigarettes, thus decreasing consumer demand. Additionally, the voluntary ban on outdoor advertisements, cartoon characters, merchandising, and sports sponsorship will reduce the omnipresent images of tobacco in American culture.

BOX 12

OBESITY LITIGATION: PARALLELS TO "BIG TOBACCO"?

The National Restaurant Association is working closely with its state restaurant association partners to assist in introducing legislation around the country that will limit the civil liability of any manufacturer, distributor, seller, or retailer of food or nonalcoholic beverages in cases in which liability is based on an individual's weight gain, obesity, or obesity-related health condition that results from that individual's long-term consumption of a food or beverage.

National Restaurant Association (2006)

Tobacco litigation was perceived to be highly effective in increasing prices, deterring manufacturers from concealing risks, and changing the culture of smoking. Public health advocates would like to achieve similar results in combating obesity, and they see parallels between the tobacco and food industries. Before the risks were widely understood, the public objected to holding tobacco companies accountable for the consequences of what was seen as a purely personal choice. The tide of opinion changed, however, when people learned the extent to which the tobacco industry had deceived the public about known links between smoking and health. The executive and legislative branches failed to enact meaningful regulations, so the battle against "big tobacco" played out in the courts.

The consequences of obesity, like those of tobacco, similarly have become a public health concern—and ultimately a political concern.[1] Despite dire proclamations about the consequences of obesity in the United States[2] and globally,[3] and its economic effects,[4] the elected branches of government have not forcefully regulated food products. Although public opinion still is squarely against obesity litigation,[5] the tide may change if deception by the food and beverage industry is uncovered—such as manipulating sugar and fat content or portion size, targeting children, or misleading the public. Like tobacco claims, obesity claims lend themselves to judicial action because they produce an identifiable injured class and corporate targets.[6]

Litigation against McDonald's Corporation has given some hope to public health advocates. In *Pelman v. McDonald's* (2005), two teenagers brought suit alleging that

Epigraph source: National Restaurant Association, "State Frivolous-Lawsuit Legislation," Aug. 16, 2006, http://www.restaurant.org/government/state/nutrition/bills_lawsuits.cfm.

[1] Rogan Kersh and James A. Morone, "Obesity, Courts, and the New Politics of Public Health," *Journal of Health Politics, Policy and Law*, 30 (2005): 839–68 (regulating private behavior to reduce obesity alters the way society frames political issues and shifts important decisions from legislatures to courts).

[2] U.S. Department of Health and Human Services, "Overweight and Obesity: Health Consequences," June 2006, http://www.surgeongeneral.gov/topics/obesity/calltoaction/fact_consequences.htm; Institute of Medicine, *Preventing Childhood Obesity: Health in the Balance* (Washington, DC: National Academies Press, 2005).

[3] World Health Organization Regional Office for the Western Pacific, *Obesity*, September 20, 2005, http://www.wpro.who.int/health_topics/obesity.

[4] Kersh and Morone, "Obesity, Courts, and the New Politics" (estimating annual medical expenditures for obesity-related conditions at $92–$117 billion, and indirect costs—lost productivity, wages, and future earnings—at $56 billion).

[5] "Obesity Inc.," *New York Times*, seven-part series, April 3 to Sept. 22, 2005 (reporting 89 percent of respondents do not support obesity lawsuits); J. Eric Oliver and Taeku Lee, "Public Opinion and the Politics of Obesity in America," *Journal of Health Politics, Policy and Law*, 30 (2005): 923–54.

[6] Alyse Meislik, "Weighing in on the Scales of Justice," *Arizona Law Review*, 46 (2004): 781–815; Matthew Salzmann, "More Than a Fat Chance for Lard Litigation," *Rutgers Law Review*, 56 (2004); Michelle M. Mello, E. B. Rimm, and David M. Studdert, "The McLawsuit: The Fast-Food Industry and Legal Accountability for Obesity," *Health Affairs*, 22 (2003): 207–16; Caleb E. Mason, "Doctrinal Considerations for Fast-Food Obesity Suits," *Tort Trial and Insurance Practice Law Journal*, 40 (2004): 75–106.

McDonald's created the false impression that its food was part of a healthy lifestyle and nutritionally beneficial.[7] They charged that McDonald's failed to disclose adequately that its food additives and processing techniques were less healthy than represented. The complaint accused McDonald's of representing that it would provide nutritional information to customers but then failing to do so at a number of restaurants.[8] The U.S. Court of Appeals for the Second Circuit allowed the plaintiffs' claims alleging deceptive representation of the nutritional benefits of McDonald's food to go to trial. The court held that the plaintiffs must have the opportunity to prove in discovery the causal relationship between consumption of McDonald's food and their ill health.[9]

McDonald's also settled a lawsuit brought in 2005 by Ban Trans Fat for misleading consumers. Despite its public statement to the contrary, the company did not cut the level of trans fat in its french fries. The $8.5 million settlement will go toward health education about trans fat, a major contributor to heart disease.[10]

Public interest litigators have threatened lawsuits against other fast-food and beverage manufacturers under similar theories: beverages or foods dangerous beyond the extent ordinarily understood by consumers, negligent failure to warn consumers of the risks, and deceptive marketing and business practices under consumer protection laws.[11]

The food and beverage industry has struck back, waging an aggressive campaign to shield the industry from obesity lawsuits. Restaurant owners and food company executives personally lobbied states, donated millions of dollars, and even helped write legislation and conduct legwork in state capitols.[12] As of October 2006, twenty-one states had enacted "commonsense consumption" or "personal responsibility" laws that, with slight variations, prevent lawsuits seeking personal injury damages for obesity-related injuries.[13] In late 2005, the U.S. House of Representatives passed the Personal Responsibility in Food Consumption Act—nicknamed the "cheeseburger bill"—which would prevent lawsuits "relating to a person's weight gain, obesity, or any health condition associated with weight gain or obesity."[14]

Commonsense consumption laws may not foreclose some kinds of obesity litigation. Tort claims based on risk-utility assessments, for example, might be brought on the grounds that a product is unreasonably dangerous and a reasonable alternative design could have reduced foreseeable risks. Plaintiffs may be able to satisfy the first prong—that the product is unreasonably dangerous—by pointing to the nutritional information. A consumer who sits down to a McDonald's meal of a double quarter pounder with cheese, large fries, and a thirty-two-ounce shake ingests 2410 calories (120.5% Daily Value), 96 grams of fat (150% Daily Value), 41 grams of saturated fat (203% Daily Value), 2030 grams of sodium (85% Daily Value) and 260 milligrams of choles-

[7] *Pelman ex rel. v. McDonald's Corp.*, 237 F. Supp. 2d 512 (S.D.N.Y. 2003), *refiled as* 2003 WL 22052778 (S.D.N.Y. Sept. 3, 2003), *vacated in part,* 396 F.3d 508 (2d Cir. 2005), *remanded to* 396 F. Supp. 2d 439 (S.D.N.Y. 2005).

[8] *Pelman v. McDonald's Corp.*, 237 F. Supp. 2d 512 (S.D.N.Y. 2003) ("Pelman I"). Although the court dismissed the claims for lack of specificity, the court granted the plaintiffs leave to refile their case. However, the court dismissed the subsequent suit without leave to amend. *Pelman v. McDonalds,* 2003 WL 22052778 (S.D.N.Y. Sept. 3, 2003) ("Pelman II").

[9] *Pelman v. McDonald's,* 396 F.3d 508 (2005) (holding that allegations stated claim against the chain for violation of the deceptive trade practices provision of the New York Consumer Protection Act); *Pelman v. McDonald's,* 02 Civ. 7821 (RWS) (S.D.N.Y. 2006) (holding on remand that the plaintiff had stated a claim with sufficient specificity, thus allowing the suit to proceed).

[10] "McDonald's Settles Trans Fats Lawsuits," *New York Times,* February 12, 2005.

[11] Michelle M. Mello, David M. Studdert, and Troyen A. Brennan, "Obesity—the New Frontier of Public Health Law," *New Eng. J. Med.,* 354 (2006): 2601-10.

[12] Melanie Warner, "The Food Industry Empire Strikes Back: Lobbying Effort to Shield Companies from Court Action Is Gaining Ground," *New York Times,* July 7, 2005.

[13] National Restaurant Association, "State Frivolous-Lawsuit Legislation," August 16, 2006, http://www.restaurant.org/government/state/nutrition/bills_lawsuits.cfm.

[14] H.R. 554, 109th Cong. (2005).

terol (87% Daily Value).[15] A plaintiff may be able to demonstrate that a meal that contains more than the recommended allowance of calories, fat, and saturated fat, and most of the allowance of sodium and cholesterol for the entire day, without any warning, is unreasonably dangerous.

The second prong of the test—that a reasonable alternative design existed that could have reduced foreseeable risks of harm—is easier to satisfy. It would be easy, and arguably cheaper, for McDonald's to produce a meal that has less salt, less sugar, is smaller in size, and is made with healthier cooking oil. In fact, McDonald's has, on a number of occasions, changed its cooking oil and has said the change did not affect the taste. With the harm to be avoided (obesity and its attendant health risks) so well known, and the existence of alternative designs that are healthier and do not increase production costs, a successful lawsuit is not impossible.

Lawsuits could also be brought to prevent marketers of unhealthy food from targeting advertisements at children—one of the successful restrictions on big tobacco. Several studies have found a link between the number of commercials watched and the amount and type of food children consume.[16] It is estimated that the average child watches twenty-eight hours of television per week and sees ten thousand commercials per year for food, 95 percent of which are for fast food, sugary cereals, soft drinks, salty snacks, and candy. Selling food to children is a $13 billion dollar a year business.[17] Lawsuits could be brought against corporations marketing unhealthy food to youth—the population that is arguably least able to resist the commercial messages and has the least access to nutritional information in order to make healthy choices (see the case study on food marketing to children in chapter 9).

Although a number of policy choices could be made that would help fight obesity, partisan gridlock and interest group politics may prevent meaningful legislation from being enacted. Accordingly, the responsibility for dealing with the political, economic, and health consequences of obesity may, like tobacco before it, fall to the courts. This would infuriate conservatives, who see eating primarily as a matter of free will and personal responsibility.[18] And, of course, the analogy to tobacco only goes so far: Cigarettes are inherently dangerous, whereas food is essential for life.

[15] McDonald's USA, *McDonald's USA Nutrition Facts for Popular Menu Items,* June 20, 2006, http://www.mcdonalds.com/app_controller.nutrition.index1.html.

[16] Institute of Medicine, *Food Marketing to Children and Youth: Threat or Opportunity?* (Washington, DC: National Academies Press, 2005).

[17] W.P. Carey School of Business, Arizona State University, "Pediatric Studies Link TV Advertising with 'Global Fattening,'" August 11, 2006, http://knowledge.wpcarey.asu.edu/index.cfm?fa = viewArticle&id = 1213.

[18] Richard A. Epstein, "What (Not) to Do about Obesity: A Moderate Aristotelian Answer," *Georgetown Law Journal,* 93 (2005): 1361-86; Paul Campos, "The Legalization of Fat: Law, Science, and the Construction of a Moral Panic," Legal Studies Research Paper Series, Working Paper 06-16 (Boulder: University of Colorado Law School, 2006) (arguing that the obesity epidemic is "constructed" and not based on science); Radley Balko, "Does Obesity Justify Big Government?" *Cato Institute,* Dec. 9, 2005, http://www.cato.org/pub_display.php?pub_id = 5226 (arguing that Americans are getting healthier, not sicker, despite the rise in obesity); Katherine Mayer, "An Unjust War: The Case against the Government's War on Obesity," *Georgetown Law Journal,* 92 (2004): 999-1031.

Despite the undeniable benefits of the litigation, the victory is tarnished in several respects. First, the financial settlement offered a missed opportunity for investment in smoking prevention; experience with the fairness doctrine shows that counteradvertising is a highly effective technique.[180] Unfortunately, the states have used the discretionary funds primarily for general education, social programs, tax relief, and other political priorities.[181] In 2006, of the $21.3 billion in revenue they received from the tobacco settlement and tobacco taxes, the states spent only 2.6 percent on prevention and cessation programs.[182] Second, disbanding the Council for Tobacco Research actually may be advantageous to the industry. The council had become a vehicle for discovering harms from tobacco use and, eventually, industry concealment of those harms, which rebounded to the disadvantage of tobacco companies. Third, advertising restrictions still permit ample scope for creative industry promotion of its product in multiple forums accessible to young people. Cigarette advertisements are still pervasive in sporting activities, for example, which reach a wide television audience.[183] Finally, states argue that they are not receiving the full settlement amount due. States claim that they were shortchanged by $813 million in 2006, and that they would be underpaid by nearly $1 billion in 2007.[184]

Perhaps the most important effect of tobacco litigation was to transform public and political perceptions about risk and responsibility in smoking, making clear what manufacturers knew, how they concealed this knowledge, and how they manipulated consumers. Far-reaching tobacco legislation in the aftermath of the settlement seemed achievable but ultimately failed. Here we have a case where tort law reframed the debate from personal to corporate responsibility; yet the industry managed, at least in the political realm, to alter the discourse to one involving freedom of choice for the smoker, the evils of "big government," and unfair taxation. This case may be instructive for those who seek to use litigation to fight obesity (see box 12).

TORT LITIGATION TO PREVENT FIREARM INJURIES: A CASE STUDY

> A gun is an article that is typically and characteristically dangerous; the use for which it is manufactured and sold is a dangerous one, and the law reasonably may presume that such an article is always dangerous. . . . In addition, the display of a gun instills fear in the average citizen; as a consequence, it creates an immediate danger that a violent response will ensue.
>
> John Paul Stevens (1986)

Firearms are pervasive in the United States. The United States has more guns than any other developed nation. Private citizens own more than

Self-protection is more than your right... it's your responsibility.
You always have a right to protect yourself in your home. Even more important, you have a responsibility to be there for those who depend on you.
At Colt, we believe that the safe and responsible ownership of a firearm can play an important role in personal security. Like a home fire extinguisher, it may be better to have it and not need it, than to need it and not have it.
For protecting yourself and your loved ones, we recommend a dependable Colt semiautomatic pistol. Choose either the compact Colt 380 or the new Colt All American™ Model 2000, holding 15 rounds of 9mm ammunition, yet small enough to be easily handled.
Both Colt semiautomatics are dependable and easy to operate. Ask your Colt dealer to demonstrate the Colt 380 and All American Model 2000. Each is a responsible investment in protecting yourself and those for whom you care.
For free catalog write to: Colt's Manufacturing Company, Inc., Attn: Marketing Dept. LHJ, P.O. Box 1868, Hartford, CT 06144-1868.
COLT. The Legend Lives
Colt's Manufacturing Company, Inc. P.O. Box 1868. Hartford, CT 06144-1868

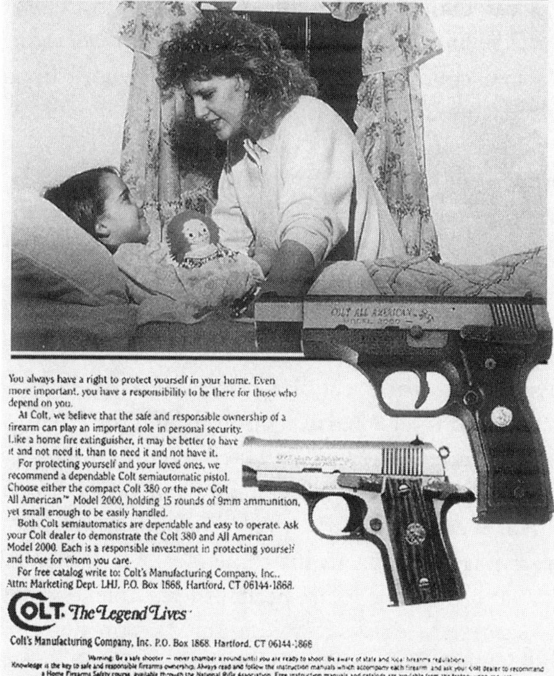

Photo 11. Advertisement for a Colt handgun. "Self-protection is more than your right . . . it's your responsibility." From *Ladies' Home Journal,* July 1992.

200 million firearms,[185] and this number is increasing by an estimated 4 million each year.[186] It is conceivable that within the next few decades, the number of guns could surpass the number of U.S. citizens.[187] Guns are owned by a large percentage of the population; 40 percent of all U.S. households own at least one firearm.[188]

Given the ubiquity of firearms in the United States, it is not surprising that they are a major cause of morbidity and mortality.[189] In 2003, over thirty thousand deaths were associated with firearms, which accounted for 18.4 percent of all injury deaths.[190] Twice as many nonfatal injuries required emergency care.[191] Firearm injuries particularly affect young persons (mainly homicides) and the elderly (mainly suicides),[192] with a disproportionate burden on males and African Americans.[193] The number of gun crime victims in the United States rose by 50 percent in 2005, to 477,040.[194] The public health burden of firearms is much greater in the United States than in comparable societies. For example, the firearm death rate for U.S. children is nearly twelve times higher than in twenty-five industrialized countries combined.[195] The overall firearm-related death rate in the United States is eight times higher than the average rate of other developed nations.[196]

Firearm injuries are increasingly being seen as a public health problem. In addition to regulation and educational programs, tort law provides a tool to help prevent many of the injuries and deaths due to firearms. Tort theorists might ask two related questions: From a public health perspective, which party could most effectively prevent these injuries and deaths? From a justice perspective, which party is best able to suffer the loss: manufacturer, retailer, owner, shooter, or victim?

The shooter could reduce harm by exercising greater care, but many shooters are children or suffer self-inflicted wounds. In any case, courts already impose liability in negligence on adults for the unintentional discharge of a firearm causing injury; a very high degree of care is required because a firearm is a dangerous instrument.[197] Victims usually are not in a position to avoid harm and are perhaps least able to absorb the loss.

Gun owners can reduce risks by taking care to store guns safely:[198] unloaded and in a locked area separate from ammunition so that they cannot be accessed by children or other unauthorized users.[199] Yet, many owners—even those with children[200]—store guns loaded or unlocked.[201] Several states have enacted child access prevention statutes that render gun owners criminally responsible for unsafe storage.[202] Other states, under the same theory of negligent entrustment applied to retailers,[203] impose liability if a child gains access to and uses a carelessly stored firearm.[204]

However, injury prevention programs often achieve the greatest success when they focus on safer product design and distribution rather than on safer operation. Though human behavior is difficult to control, manufacturers can create products that reduce injuries.[205] Manufacturers are the entity best able to abate harm and absorb loss, as they can limit distribution,[206] add safety devices, and control manufacturing quality. Public health advocates have argued that because the firearms industry is in the best position to prevent harm, it should be held accountable in civil litigation for gun-related morbidity and mortality.[207]

Early suits against gun manufacturers focused on dangerous aspects of the guns themselves, proceeding under product liability or design defect theories, but they were rarely successful. Since the late 1990s, however, the majority of suits against firearm manufacturers and sellers have focused on stopping marketing and distribution that facilitate access to illegal firearms by criminals, juveniles, and other prohibited purchasers. These more recent cases, based on negligent entrustment and public nuisance theories, have had an impact on the firearm industry's conduct. In 2000, Smith and Wesson, the largest gun manufacturer in the United States, agreed to a settlement in lawsuits brought by municipalities. The company agreed to include child safety locks, ensure background checks at retail stores and gun shows, and take so-called ballistic fingerprints of its guns.[208]

However, just as this litigation was beginning to succeed, politics intervened. Partially in response to this settlement and the limited success of other tort claims against the gun industry under negligent distribution and public nuisance theories, in October 2005, Congress passed and President Bush signed into law the Protection of Lawful Commerce in Arms Act (PLCAA).[209] The act gives the industry broad immunity from liability, dismissing all current civil actions against gun sellers and manufacturers in both federal and state court for damages resulting from unlawful use of a firearm by another, and preempting all future claims. Prior to the act, thirty states had similarly restricted the ability of individuals or municipalities to sue firearm dealers or manufacturers for crimes committed with firearms that were lawfully made and sold.[210] Yet, as discussed below, the PLCAA contains exceptions that may offer a ray of hope for public health advocates.

Even though the PLCAA preempted most tort suits against the firearms industry, it is useful to describe the four main legal theories that have been employed. The first two theories, product liability and defective design, relate to the safety issues associated with the design and manufacture of firearms. The second two theories, negligent entrustment and public nuisance, concern potentially unlawful marketing and distribution by gun manufacturers and distributors: oversupply, overpromotion, and failure to supervise retail dealers.

Dangerous by Design: Product Liability and Defective Design

Manufacturing Defects. Product liability claims seek damages for injuries caused by guns that malfunction (exploding barrels, etc.). These actions are fairly uncontroversial because they differ little from commonplace tort claims regarding ordinary products that do not perform in the manner intended. Although plaintiffs are reasonably successful in these claims,[211] they serve little public health value because firearms functioning as intended cause the vast majority of gun-related injuries.

Design Defects. Defective design suits argue that the intended design of firearms, rather than random or accidental malfunctions, contribute significantly to unintentional injuries and deaths.[212] Injury control experts regard at least three design features to be unsafe: (1) trigger devices sufficiently easy to pull so that young children can operate them, (2) no reliable indication of whether a round of ammunition is in the firing chamber, and (3) the universal ability of unauthorized users to operate the firearm.[213]

Some plaintiffs have pursued design defect suits under a risk-utility theory, arguing that the risks associated with aspects of firearms that make them attractive to criminals outweigh their useful purposes.[214] For example, many handguns are designed to be small and easily concealable (an asset for someone with criminal intent), and other weapons, such as those that permit fully automatic firing, appear to be designed to deliver mass injuries. However, courts have often rejected this argument, holding that liability for defective design applies only to products that malfunction in some way.[215] In other words, without something being functionally wrong with the product, the risk-utility balancing test should not even apply.[216] Other defective design suits argue that manufacturers are liable because they failed to equip their firearms with available safety devices, such as locks, loaded chamber indicators, or personalization technology.[217] These suits claim that failure to include such safety features constitutes a design defect because a reasonable alternative design existed that could prevent injuries. Overall, these suits have fared better than the risk-utility claims; two have reached juries, with one resulting in a verdict for the plaintiff.[218]

Generally, however, most firearm design defect cases fail.[219] Courts often find that consumers have a "reasonable expectation" that firearms will be dangerous.[220] Courts have concluded that firearm risks, for the most part, are open and obvious, and consumers do not require expert knowledge to assess the risks.[221] Firearms, moreover, are in "common use." If they are functioning properly, they may be exempt from strict liability based on the theory that they are "good" (well-made) guns.[222] Perhaps because of this judicial reluctance to hold the industry liable for the dangers inherent in guns themselves, the recent trend in tort suits against the firearms industry has been to argue that the industry's marketing, sales, and distribution behavior creates an unreasonable danger, as described in the next two sections.

Dangerous Distribution: Negligent Entrustment and Public Nuisance

Negligent Entrustment. The doctrine of negligent entrustment holds that a person in control of personal property owes a responsibility not to entrust that property to another that she knows, or should know, is apt to use it in a dangerous way. Once that duty of care is imposed, the negligent entrustment case is just like any other negligence case, with all the same elements (duty, breach, causation, damages).[223] For example, a person who lends his car to someone he knows is intoxicated would be liable to anyone injured by that driver. Gun retailers have been found liable for the sale of a weapon to a person who is known or reasonably should be known to be mentally ill, intoxicated, or underage.[224]

Recently, plaintiffs have tried to extend negligent entrustment or "negligent distribution" liability to encompass sales that foreseeably will result in mass distribution of handguns through the illegal secondary market.[225] In *Hamilton v. Beretta* (2001), the plaintiffs alleged that negligent marketing had bolstered an illegal underground market in handguns. The lower court found that manufacturers and distributors had the unique ability to guard against foreseeable risks, creating a special "protective relationship" with downstream distributors and retailers.[226] The New York Court of Appeals, however, reversed the decision, finding that manufacturers owe no duty of care to persons harmed by gun violence: "Judicial resistance to expansion of duty grows out of practical concerns both about potentially limitless liability and about the unfairness of imposing liability for the acts of another."[227]

Yet the court did not completely foreclose the use of negligent entrustment in future cases: "Negligent entrustment doctrine might well support the extension of a duty to manufacturers to avoid selling to certain distributors in circumstances where the manufacturer knows or has reason to know those distributors are engaging in substantial sales of guns into the gun-trafficking market on a consistent basis."[228] This situation was realized in *Ileto v. Glock* (2003), where plaintiffs alleged that manufacturers purposefully oversaturated the legal gun market to take advantage of resales to sellers that they knew or should have known would in turn sell to illegal buyers. The Ninth Circuit Court of Appeals reversed the lower court's dismissal of the lawsuit.[229]

Negligent entrustment cases, with the exception of *Ileto,* mostly have been unsuccessful. Plaintiffs' biggest challenge in pleading negligent entrustment or marketing is demonstrating the foreseeability of dangerous use—not by the initial purchaser of the firearm, but by some third party further down the distribution stream.[230] Plaintiffs can increase their chances of success by conducting a thorough investigation so that they will be able to plead in extensive detail the gun industry's knowledge of the dangers posed by the secondary market.[231]

Public Nuisance. Cities or states have brought public nuisance suits claiming that the industry's practices create an "unreasonable interference with a right common to the general public," including the right to health, safety, convenience, and public peace.[232] Public nuisance suits can be brought under criminal nuisance statutes or as civil actions, and usually seek an abatement of the nuisance. Cities often use this theory when seeking changes in marketing and distribution practices that contribute to gun-related violence, in some cases seeking damages for the increased costs of law enforcement and medical care. It is also possible for individual citizens to bring a public nuisance suit but only when they have suffered an injury that is distinct in kind from that experienced by the general public.[233]

Public nuisance suits are generally supported by three types of fact patterns. In oversupply cases, plaintiffs allege that a gun manufacturer or distributor knowingly oversupplies states with weak gun control laws, knowing that guns will be sold and resold into states with stricter laws, and ultimately used in crimes.[234] Overpromotion cases focus on a combination of design features and advertising that make firearms attractive to criminals. For example, the Tec-DC9 assault rifle was designed with fully automatic capabilities and can be easily outfitted with features such as silencers and flash suppressors. Other guns are advertised as being "resistant to fingerprints" or "tough as your toughest customers."[235] Under failure to supervise claims, manufacturers are allegedly at fault for not training or monitoring retail dealers to whom they distribute in order to prevent illegal sales. Most of these suits have been rejected, but a few are still pending.

The Protection of Lawful Commerce in Arms Act: The Loss of Tort Law as a Tool to Combat Firearm Injuries

The hopes in the public health community created by negligent entrustment and public nuisance lawsuits[236] were dashed by the passage of the

PLCAA. The act precludes lawsuits against firearm manufacturers or distributors "resulting from the criminal or unlawful use of . . . firearms, their parts, or ammunition."[237] However, the statute broadly defines "criminal or unlawful use." As a result, the PLCAA might even preclude suits where children have accidentally harmed themselves or others.

The act, however, does allow suits to proceed if they fall within one of six exceptions. The exceptions permit suits (1) when the transferor knew the firearm would be used in drug trafficking or a violent crime and the plaintiff's injury was a proximate result; (2) for negligent entrustment or negligence per se; (3) if the seller knowingly violated a federal or state statute applicable to firearm sale or marketing, and that violation was a proximate cause of the plaintiff's injury; (4) for breach of contract or warranty; (5) for design defects if the injury or property damage was not the result of intentional criminal conduct; and (6) under civil penalties already existing in the law, which the attorney general may still enforce.[238]

These exceptions are very narrow, and combined with the broad scope of the preclusions, the act has effectively halted suits against the firearms industry. [239] Since the act's passage, only one pending suit has survived the defendants' motion for summary judgment or dismissal: *City of New York v. Beretta* (2005).[240] In this case, the city sued the firearms industry, arguing that manufacturers improperly marketed and distributed their guns, creating an unnecessary hazard for the city's population.

Beretta is an interesting case because it demonstrates a potential loophole in the PLCAA, which may allow for the continued use of public nuisance as a tort litigation strategy. Under the law's third exception, suits are allowed "if the seller knowingly violates a federal or state statute applicable to firearm sale or marketing, and that violation is a proximate cause of the plaintiff's injury." New York state law makes the creation of a public nuisance a second-degree criminal offense.[241] Therefore, the court ruled that the suit is permitted under the PLCAA's third exception, since New York's nuisance law was capable of being applied to the alleged conduct of the defendant gun manufacturers and distributors.[242]

However, a district court in California reached the opposite conclusion in *Ileto v. Glock* on remand from the Ninth Circuit.[243] There, the court found that the examples given in the statute seemed strongly to suggest that the predicate exemption was intended to apply only to statutes specifically directed at the sale and marketing of firearms, not laws of general applicability. The court said that an expansive reading, such as that taken in *Beretta*, would undermine the express purpose of the act, which was to shield firearms manufacturers from liability for injuries caused by third parties using nondefective, legally obtained firearms.

This firearms case study demonstrates that tort law can be a useful, albeit contentious, tool for reducing injury and disease. To the public health community, the act is a prime illustration of the politicization of public health and the protection of a dangerous industry engaged in insidious practices. To conservative scholars, however, the act appropriately preempted frivolous lawsuits against the industry and was necessary to curtail judicial activism. Congress, in highly partisan fashion, decided that the social and economic costs of tort litigation outweigh the potential benefits. The following section discusses the costs of tort litigation in more detail.

THE LIMITATIONS OF TORT LAW: SOCIAL AND ECONOMIC COSTS

I have devoted this entire chapter to the idea that tort law is an important vehicle for advancing the public's health. However, I do not want to leave the impression that the tort system achieves only socially desirable results. Opponents argue that litigation usurps legislative authority to decide complex social questions in a democracy, and individual freedom to make self-regarding decisions in a free society. Additionally, tort litigation can divert resources from regulatory efforts, and it is often unsuccessful.[244] Tort costs (liability and litigation expenses) have potentially detrimental effects that warrant consideration.

Economic Burdens. Tort costs, as explained earlier, must be absorbed by the enterprise, which will often pass the costs on to its employees or consumers through loss of employment (or loss of benefits of employment, such as wages and health insurance) or higher prices.[245] Since socioeconomic status has important health effects (see chapter 1), lower employment or wages and higher consumer prices are important from a public health perspective. The advantages of deterrence, therefore, have to be weighed against the adverse effects on employment and prices. Imposing costs on a polluter or the supplier of an unsafe product may appear to be an unmitigated public good, but it does entail social cost. In 2005, Congress reacted to perceptions that class action lawsuits in state courts were unfairly burdening companies by passing the Class Action Fairness Act.[246] This legislation makes it much easier for defendants to remove claims to federal courts, which are seen as less favorable to plaintiffs.[247] The law has been criticized for making meritorious claims more difficult to file and for "reduc[ing] the accountability of corporations that violate laws protecting employees, consumers, and the environment."[248]

Penalizing Business Judgment. Suppose that the enterprise does not pass tort costs onto the consumer, but rather redesigns its products to avoid potential hazards. I have depicted this kind of redesign as clearly beneficial, but this is not inevitably the case. Businesses may forgo product features that are attractive, convenient, and offer better value for consumers in exchange for relatively small safety advantages. Certainly, safety is a fundamental public good, but it is not the only good.

Overdeterrence and Stifled Innovation. Tort costs may be, or may be perceived to be,[249] so high that businesses refrain from entering the market, leave the market, or curtail research and development.[250] Society, it may be argued, would not be any poorer if tort costs made it difficult for dangerous, socially unproductive enterprises (e.g., tobacco and firearms) to operate within the market. Tort costs appear to be just as high, however, for socially advantageous goods and services. While it is in society's interest to encourage safety in the production of health-related products and services, overdeterrence may result in less investment. It matters to society if industry cuts back on the research or marketing of childhood vaccines[251] or prescription drugs.[252] The same may be true of certain medical specialties, such as obstetrics, neurosurgery, and orthopedics, where malpractice insurance costs have potent deterrent effects.

Wrong Incentives. Sometimes the tort system sends the wrong deterrent signal, with the result that behaviors are changed in unintended ways. Consider the effects of medical malpractice litigation. Ideally, the tort system wants to send a signal that physicians should exercise due care to avoid medically induced injury. Physicians, however, sometimes understand the law to be encouraging the practice of defensive medicine (e.g., ordering intrusive diagnostic tests that are not clinically indicated). As a result, patients may have to undergo unnecessary procedures, and the health care system incurs unnecessary cost.[253]

These potential adverse consequences do not militate against using tort law to achieve important public health objectives. The judiciary, as an independent institution, can change social policy when the other branches are politically obstructed. Litigation can deter hazardous activities, penalize those who put the public at risk, and fund public health programs.

Just as important, lawsuits can be useful for focusing attention on health hazards, forcing the legislature to act, and changing public culture, as with tobacco. Discovery can also be used to gather information needed to inform the public and the political process.[254] However, I do want to make a point that recurs throughout this text and that applies with equal force to tort law: Regulation intended to promote the public interest has personal and economic consequences. Regulation may help solve a particular public health problem but create or exacerbate another problem for individuals or for society at large. The resulting dilemmas—legal, scientific, and ethical—are perplexing but exceedingly important to the study of public health law.[255]

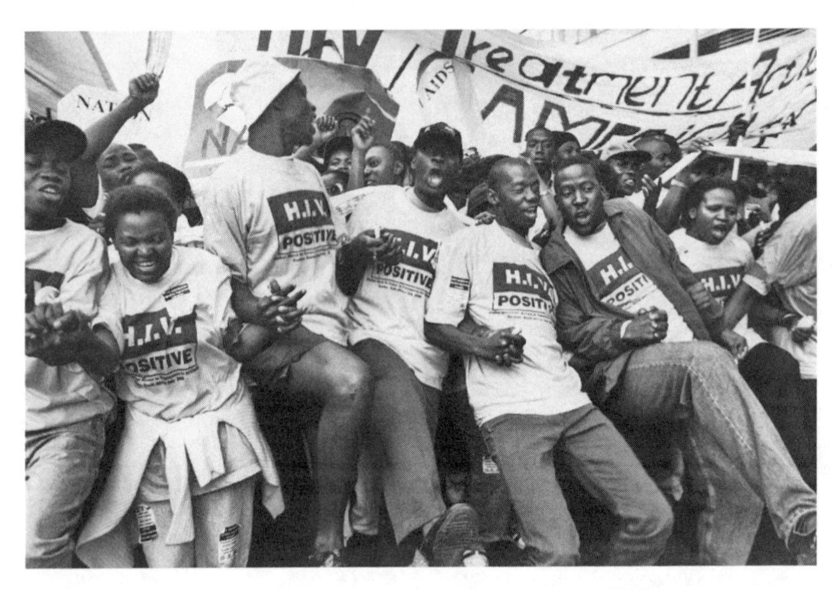

Photo 12. South African protest demanding free access to HIV drug therapy. Treatment Action Campaign March, Thirteenth International AIDS Conference, Durban, KwaZulu/Natal, South Africa, 2000. A protest march through the streets of Durban organized by Treatment Action Campaign (TAC) during the "Breaking the Silence" International AIDS Conference. The protesters were demanding free access to drug therapy for people with HIV or AIDS in Third World countries. Protesters wore HIV-positive T-shirts to challenge the stigma so often associated with the disease. © Gideon Mendel/CORBIS.

CHAPTER 7

Global Health Law

Health in a Global Community

If we believe that men have any personal rights at all as human beings, they have an absolute right to such a measure of good health as society, and society alone is able to give them.

Aristotle

The examination of public health law has thus far focused on constitutions, statutes, regulations, and common law at the national and subnational level, particularly in the United States. However, the determinants of health (e.g., pathogens, air, food, water, even lifestyle choices) do not originate solely within national borders. Health threats inexorably spread to neighboring countries, regions, and even continents. People's lives are profoundly affected by commerce, politics, science, and technology from all over the world. Global integration and interdependence occur "as capital, traded goods, persons, concepts, images, ideas, and values diffuse across state boundaries."[1] It is for this reason that law and policy need to be transnational—extending beyond sovereign nations.[2] There is no other way to truly ensure the public's health than through cooperation and global governance (see box 13).

This chapter searches for reasons as to why health hazards seem to change form and migrate everywhere on the earth; why extant global governance systems are frequently ineffective; and how international law can be used as a tool for improving the health of the world's population, especially the poorest and most vulnerable. This requires an understanding of the global dimensions of disease and of man's role in harming the planet; the meaning and sources of international law; and modern international regimes of high relevance to health, including infectious disease, tobacco, trade, and human rights.[3] Illuminating the complex and voluminous field of global health law is impossible in a single chapter,

BOX 13

GLOBAL GOVERNANCE FOR HEALTH

International law used to be defined as the law that governs relations between states, and undoubtedly, the rights and obligations of sovereign countries are still salient. However, global health governance is more broadly concerned with rules of conduct that influence or bind actors in activities, relations, and transactions that transcend national borders.[1] Thinking of global governance, however, only in terms of what governments do is unsatisfactory. Governance for health is complex and multifaceted. A broad range of stakeholders exert considerable power over events that influence health.[2] These stakeholders may act alone, in partnership, or in conflict; separately and together they influence the conditions in which people can be healthy or be placed at risk:[3]

- Intergovernmental organizations (IGOs)—see table 7
- Nongovernmental organizations (NGOs)—see table 8
- Multinational corporations—e.g., tobacco, food, energy, and technology
- Philanthropic organizations—e.g., Gates, Rockefeller, and Ford foundations and Clinton Global Initiative
- Public/private hybrids—e.g., Global Fund to Fight AIDS, TB and Malaria[4]
- Media outlets—e.g., CNN, BBC World, and al Jazeera

To demonstrate the power of nonstate actors, consider the influence of the Gates Foundation. With Warren Buffet's gift of $37 billion in 2006, the foundation has the capacity to donate $3 billion per year to improve global health equity. This single source of funding comprises nearly one-fourth of all financial assistance to developing countries, including funds provided by governments, IGOs, and private donors combined. Now consider that there are no international rules that require transparency, fairness, or accountability on the part of private foundations. International law does not usually reach private actors, even if they profoundly affect global health. Should global governance extend to nonstate entities, and if so, what innovative mechanisms could be established?

[1] Some scholars prefer the term *transnational law,* defined as "the law which regulates actions or events that transcend National frontiers . . . includ[ing] both . . . public and private international law." Philip C. Jessup, "Transnational Law 2," in *Storrs Lectures on Jurisprudence* (New Haven, CT: Yale University, 1956): 136. "The term 'transnational law' has been used to describe . . . the creation of law in the international context by governments, international organizations, and non-state actors." Matthias Lehmann, Comment, "A Plea for Transnational Approach to Arbitrability in Arbitral Practice," *Columbia Journal of Transnational Law,* 42 (2004): 753–81.

[2] For example, after Warren Buffet's gift, the Gates Foundation will donate $3 billion per year to improve global health equity. This single source of funding will comprise nearly a fourth of all health-related donations to developing countries. Susan Okie, "Global Health—the Gates-Buffet Effect," *NEJM,* 355 (2006): 1084–88.

[3] Scott Burris, "Governance, Microgovernance and Health," *Temple Law Review,* 77 (2004): 335–61; Nana K. Poku and Alan Whiteside, eds., *Global Health and Governance: HIV/AIDS* (London: Palgrave Macmillan, 2004).

[4] As a partnership between governments, civil society, the private sector, and affected communities, the Global Fund represents an innovative approach to international health financing. The fund was created to finance a dramatic turnaround in the fight against AIDS, tuberculosis, and malaria. These diseases kill over 6 million people each year. The Global Fund, "Investing in Our Future: The Global Fund to Fight AIDS, Tuberculosis and Malaria, 2002–2006," http://www.theglobalfund.org/en/; see also Allyn L. Taylor, "Public-Private Partnerships for Health: The United Nations Global Fund on AIDS and Health," *John Marshall Law Review,* 35 (2002): 400–407.

TABLE 7. Major intergovernmental organizations working on health

IGO	Mission	Major Health Initiatives
United Nations	Promote respect for human rights, protect the environment, fight disease, and reduce poverty	*Millennium Development Goals:* Eradicate extreme poverty and hunger Ensure universal primary education Promote gender equality Reduce child mortality Improve maternal health Combat HIV/AIDS and other diseases Ensure environmental sustainability Develop global partnership for development
UN Specialized Agencies		
World Health Organization (WHO)	Support attainment of the highest possible level of health for all people	Framework Convention on Tobacco Control International Health Regulations Global Strategy on Diet, Physical Activity and Health
Joint UN Programme on HIV/AIDS (UNAIDS)	Coordinate global response to HIV/AIDS	Declaration of Commitment on HIV/AIDS International Partnership against AIDS in Africa World AIDS Campaign
UN International Children's Emergency Fund (UNICEF)	Serve socioeconomic and health needs of women and children	Baby-Friendly Hospital Initiative Int'l Code of Marketing for Breast Milk Substitutes
UN Women's Fund (UNIFEM)	Reduce poverty, violence, HIV/AIDS, and gender inequality	Trust Fund to Eliminate Violence against Women

TABLE 7. *(continued)*

IGO	Mission	Major Health Initiatives
UN Development Programme (UNDP)	Reduce poverty, preserve the environment, and strengthen democratic governance	UN Capital Development Fund
UN High Commissioner for Refugees (UNHCR)	Provide legal protection and emergency relief for refugees	Research on mental and physical health of refugees, and policies on HIV/AIDS
UN High Commissioner for Human Rights (UNHCHR)	Monitor national efforts to meet obligations under human treaties	Special rapporteur monitors and recommends policies to advance the right to health
International Labor Organization (ILO)	Promote social justice and monitor compliance with human and labor rights treaties	Safety and Health at Work and in the Environment Program on HIV/AIDS and the World of Work
Food and Agriculture Organization (FAO)	Improve nutrition, agricultural productivity, and the lives of rural populations	Codex Alimentarius Commission develops safety standards and codes of practice under the Joint FAO/WHO Food Programme
World Organization for Animal Health	Promote animal welfare and prevent the transmission of disease between animals and humans	FAO Crisis Management Centre Global Early Warning System for Animal Diseases Transmissible to Humans
World Bank Group	Provide loans, grants, and advice to low- and middle-income countries	Int'l Bank for Reconstruction and Development Int'l Development Association
World Trade Organization (WTO)	Ensure smooth and predictable global trade flows	Trade Related Intellectual Property Agreement Doha Development Agenda

NOTE: Intergovernmental organizations (IGOs) are organizations of international scope whose members are sovereign nation-states. IGOs are established by treaties, which bring the organizations under the jurisdiction of international law and grant them powers to enter into agreements with states and other organizations. Membership in IGOs, such as UN specialized agencies and the WTO, is open to all nation-states.

TABLE 8. Major nongovernmental organizations (NGOs) working on health

NGO	Mission	Focus
Health Opportunities for People Everywhere (Project HOPE)	Health education, policy research, humanitarian relief, and socioeconomic development assistance	Infectious diseases (including HIV/AIDS), women's and children's health, humanitarian assistance, etc.
International Committee of the Red Cross (ICRC)	Assistance and protection for prisoners of war and civilians affected by war	State compliance with Geneva Conventions
Doctors without Borders/Médecins sans Frontières (MSF)	Medical care to communities affected by natural disasters, conflict, epidemics, and poverty	Campaign for Access to Essential Medicines: advocates for lower drug prices in developing countries and research on neglected diseases
Family Health International (FHI)	Prevention of HIV/AIDS and improvement of access to reproductive health care in developing countries	Reproductive health and HIV/AIDS
Global Health Council	Umbrella NGO whose members work to improve global health	Infectious diseases (including HIV/AIDS), women's and children's health
Population Council	Coordination of international public health and biomedical research, and strengthening of local health care	Reproductive health and HIV/AIDS
PATH International	Advancement of health care in developing countries	Health training and education, contraceptives, injection devices, and diagnostic tools

NOTE : Nongovernmental organizations (NGOs) are private organizations not affiliated with (though often in part funded by) governments; they typically pursue social justice, development, and humanitarian activities. More than 30,000 NGOs work internationally.

but this text will serve as an introduction to the impressive literature that is emerging.[4]

GLOBALIZATION AND THE SPREAD OF INFECTIOUS DISEASE, MAN-MADE AND CONTROLLABLE

Disease amplifiers are principally man-made and therefore controllable.[5] Human beings congregate and travel, live in close proximity to animals, pollute the environment, and rely on overtaxed health systems. This constant cycle of congregation, consumption, and movement allows infectious diseases to mutate and spread across populations and boundaries. The global population is also vulnerable to deliberate manipulation and dispersal of pathogens. Those engaged in bioterrorism have incentives to move pathogens to places where they will have the most destructive impact. These human activities and many more have profound health consequences for people in all parts of the world, and no country can insulate itself from the effects. The world's nations are interdependent and reliant on one another for health security (see figure 25).

Mass Congregation, Migration, and Travel. Infectious diseases spread among populations and geographic areas as human beings congregate, migrate, and travel. Mass movement of people occurs naturally as individuals travel to urban settings in search of livelihoods and social attachments.[6] People may also be compelled to travel in large numbers as they flee situations of famine, violence, civil unrest, or war.[7] The gross unsanitary conditions in refugee camps and other mass settings are deeply troublesome from public health and humanitarian perspectives.[8] Overpopulation, whether through voluntary or forced migrations, places a strain on drinking water, food supplies, and sewage systems, providing a breeding ground for infectious disease.

Human/Animal Interchange. People do not merely congregate together but do so in close proximity to animal populations through intensive farming, meat production (farming, slaughtering, and eating animals), and exotic animal markets.[9] Such interactions with animals entail serious risks as novel pathogens mutate and jump species.[10] For example, live bird markets, traveling poultry workers, fighting cocks, and migratory birds are vectors for spreading avian influenza A (H5N1).[11] Farmers contribute to microbial resistance through overuse or inappropriate use of pharmaceuticals.[12] Animal diseases have significant economic consequences, as illustrated by outbreaks of bovine spongiform encephal-

COMMONWEALTH Pharmaceutical ASSOCIATION
TB DRUG COMPLIANCE
Rx
A Pharmacist and Patient Alliance
WORLD STOP TB DAY 2006
"Actions for Life: towards a world free of tuberculosis"
Tobacco or Health:
Choose Health
World's 1st No Tobacco Day
7 April 1988
World Health Organization

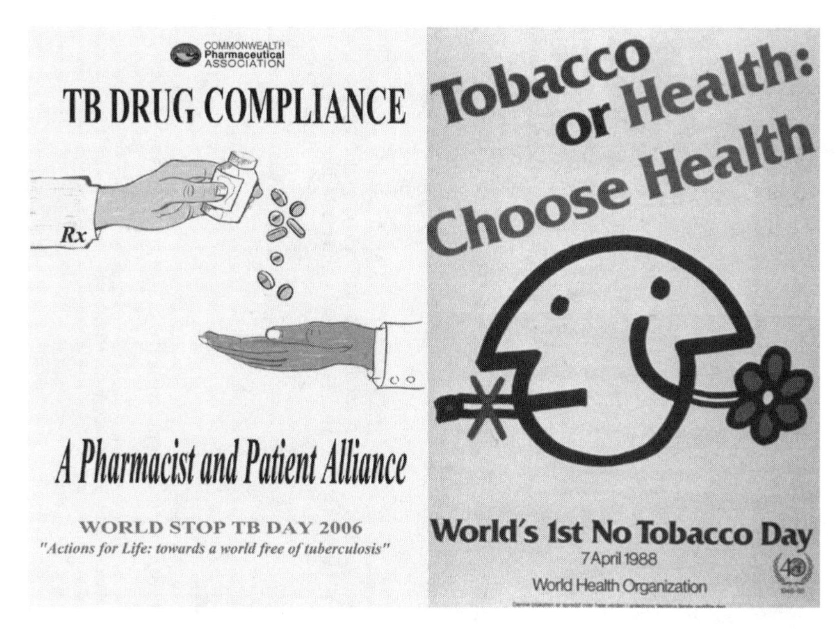

Photo 13. Health communication campaign posters: tuberculosis and tobacco. Posters encourage the public to take an active part in disease control. Courtesy of the Commonwealth Pharmaceutical Association and the World Health Organization.

opathy (BSE) and foot and mouth disease.[13] Animal diseases also affect human health; animals, particularly wild animals, are the source of 70 percent of all emerging infections.[14] These processes have transnational dimensions, as a result of thriving international markets in cattle, meat, and poultry.

Ecosystem Degradation. Human well-being is highly dependent on ecosystems, and ecosystems are sensitive to human activity. Ecosystem degradation in one geographic area affects other parts of the world; in this way, living systems (e.g., air, sea, forests, and soil) are interconnected, as are people and places in the world.[15] Ecosystem degradation has multiple adverse health effects. [16] For example, air and water pollution increases respiratory (e.g., asthma) and gastrointestinal (e.g., cholera and *E. coli*) diseases, as well as cancers. The emission of heat-trapping gases (e.g., carbon dioxide, methane, and nitrous oxides) contributes to global warming, which causes a number of health hazards: heat-related illnesses and deaths; infectious disease carried by insects and rodents (e.g., malaria and West Nile virus); droughts that result in famine and conflicts over

Mass Congregation

- The world's population grew from 1.6 billion at the beginning of the twentieth century to 6.1 billion by the century's end. Population is estimated to be 9.1 billion by 2050.
- The number of people living in urban centers has increased from 2.26 billion to 3.01 billion between 1990 and 2003. The rate of urbanization is highest in developing countries.

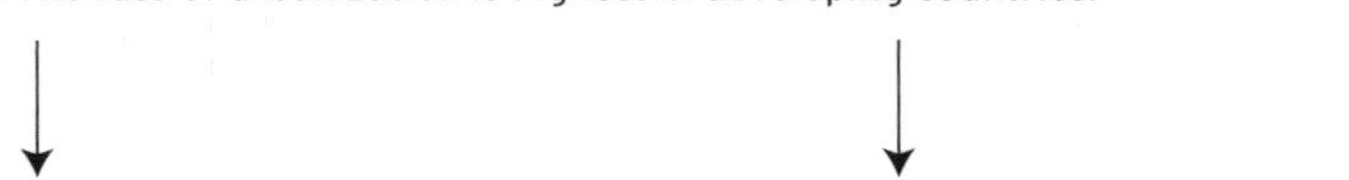

Environmental Degradation

- Water and air pollution increase respiratory and gastrointestinal diseases.
- Global warming results in extreme weather which creates breeding grounds for disease.

Human/Animal Interchange

- Many infectious diseases, including HIV/AIDS, Ebola, SARS, and avian influenza originated in animals but crossed over to humans.
- Cattle diseases endanger human health and stifle international trade.

Overtaxed Health Systems

- Overtaxed health centers lack equipment and training for sterilization and infection control.
- Health care providers improperly prescribe medicines, creating drug-resistant viruses and bacteria.

Spread of Infectious Diseases

- 75% of all deaths from infectious diseases occurred in Southeast Asia or sub-Saharan Africa.
- More than 90% of deaths from infectious disease are caused by lower respiratory diseases, HIV/AIDS, diarrhea, tuberculosis, and malaria.

Figure 25. The transnational spread of infectious diseases.

water resources; and natural disasters that produce floods and destruction (e.g., the Asian tsunami and Hurricane Katrina). Finally, excessive and unsustainable use of scarce resources (e.g., deforestation, strip-mining, and intensive farming or fishing) diminishes natural assets needed for healthy living.[17]

Health Systems. Health care systems themselves can contribute to poor health. The lack of sterilizing equipment, safe blood supplies, and basic infection controls in resource-poor hospitals puts both health care professionals and patients at risk for bloodborne diseases, such as HIV/AIDS and hepatitis B or C. Weak public health infrastructures can fail to detect and contain outbreaks of Ebola or SARS in their early stages, giving these diseases opportunities to spread. Lack of funding and infrastructure in turn creates human resource deficits, as trained health care professionals from poor countries leave for better-paying jobs in North America and Europe,[18] further deteriorating a country's capacity for surveillance, response, and treatment. Finally, health care systems, even in the developed world, often deliver antibiotic and antiviral medications indiscriminately, causing microbial adaptation. These practices can result in changes in the virulence of pathogens and development of resistance to frontline medications (e.g., multidrug-resistant TB, HIV, or streptococcal infections).

THE EPIDEMIOLOGIC TRANSITION FROM INFECTIOUS TO NONCOMMUNICABLE DISEASES: A DOUBLE BURDEN IN RESOURCE-POOR COUNTRIES

> Here [in Chennai, India], juxtaposed alongside
> the stick-thin poverty, the malaria and the AIDS, the
> number of diabetics now totals around 35 million
> and counting. . . . The conventional way to see India is
> to inspect the want—the want for food, the want for
> money, the want for life. . . . But there is another way
> to see it. In a changing India, it seems to go this way:
> make good money and get cars, get houses, get servants,
> get meals out, get diabetes.
>
> N. R. Kleinfield (2006)

The spread of infectious diseases in a changing and interdependent world is to be expected, given increased human migration and trade. Less obvious is how, and why, noncommunicable diseases (NCDs) seem to have global dimensions. Noncommunicable or chronic diseases include cardiovascular diseases, cancers, diabetes, respiratory diseases, and mental illness. Human behavior, such as high-fat/high-caloric diets, sedentary lifestyles, cigarette smoking, consumption of alcoholic beverages, and stressful lifestyles, is a primary cause of NCDs, which means that they are largely preventable.

The burden of NCDs was once felt disproportionately in highly industrialized countries. However, chronic diseases are now the major cause of death and disability worldwide and increasingly affect people from resource-poor countries.[19] The latest available data (from 2001) show that chronic diseases contributed to 59 percent of the 56.5 million total reported deaths in the world and 46 percent of the global burden of disease. If the trend continues, by 2020 NCDs will account for 80 percent of the global burden of disease, causing seven out of every ten deaths in developing countries.[20] The ability of resource-poor countries to prevent and treat NCDs is undermined by impoverished socioeconomic conditions and inadequate health systems.[21]

What is causing the epidemiologic transition from infectious to chronic diseases, and why have high-risk behaviors moved from richer to poorer countries? High-risk lifestyles were once thought to be associated with abundance and excessive consumption. The affluent were more likely to consume high-energy diets and work in white-collar jobs with less physical activity. Smoking cigarettes and drinking fine wine and spirits were glamorous pursuits. Cinema, television, and magazines displayed images of well-heeled men and women, with successful careers and vibrant lifestyles, smoking and drinking. The poor seemed to have a different set of problems: malnutrition rather than overeating, lives filled with hard work rather than leisure, and lives cut short from injuries and infections rather than chronic disease.

Yet, just as infectious diseases move and change, so do NCDs.[22] The global rise in NCDs reflects significant transformations in diet habits, physical activity levels, and tobacco use worldwide. The process of industrialization, urbanization, economic development, and increasing food market globalization has led to harmonization of behavior.[23] What was once culturally attractive primarily in industrialized countries has gained popularity all over the world. Visit any major city and witness the effects of a blended culture inspired by multinational corporations, media conglomerates, and the influence of tourists and immigrants as they travel

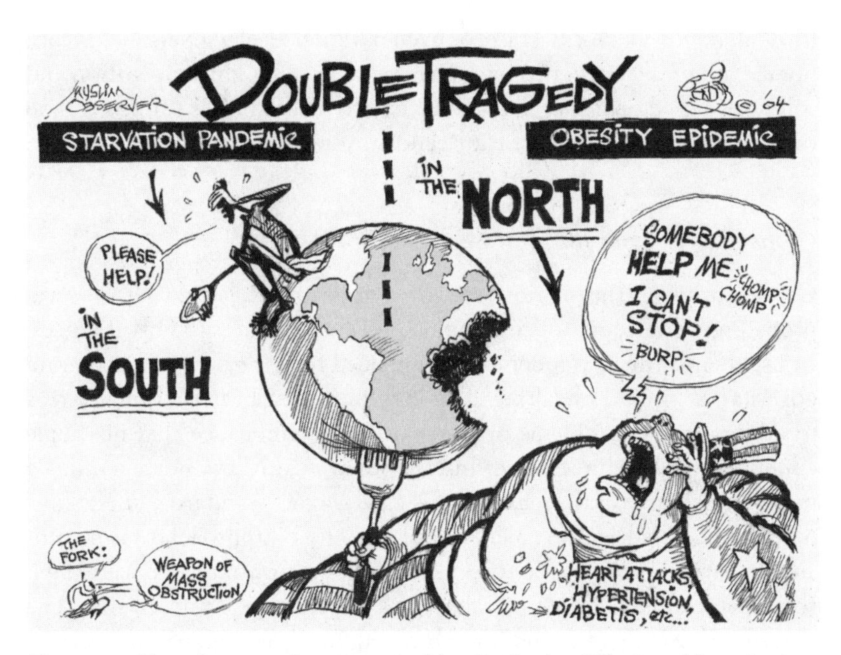

Photo 14. Chronic starvation versus epidemic obesity: Who's to blame? With the growing number of obese Americans and individuals suffering from heart attacks, hypertension, and diabetes, the U.S. government is criticized for its citizens' overconsumption and poor health.

globally. The High Streets are filled with food chains such as McDonald's, Burger King, KFC, and Dunkin' Donuts; the billboards display omnipresent images of Camel cigarettes, Hershey's chocolate, Coca-Cola, and Johnnie Walker whiskey; and movies and television continue to run attractive images of alluring people smoking cigarettes and drinking alcoholic beverages. This is how risk behavior migrates from place to place and permeates all people and cultures. Perversely, as developing countries begin to grow and prosper, the emergence of behaviorally related chronic diseases stands out as a "joint totem" of success.[24]

"It makes little sense to expect individuals to behave differently from their peers," wrote Geoffrey Rose in 1992.[25] The problem is that one's peers used to be neighbors, and so behavior varied across places according to cultural norms. Today the influences on behavior are broad and diffuse. In the age of the Internet, cable television, multinational corporations, and global markets, it is rarely possible to change behavior solely through action at a local, state, or even national level. Governments cannot meaningfully effect behavior change without global cooperation and solutions based on a shared commitment to health.[26] It is for this reason that public health law must transcend frontiers.

Global Governance for Health

Globalization, as the previous section demonstrates, is a powerful force, propelling people, pathogens, goods, and even cultures to far-off places. Consequently, there is a demonstrable need for global cooperation and governance in world health.[27] The very purpose of international law is to address grave problems of transnational significance that no single country can solve on its own. International health law, however, has a number of structural weaknesses—e.g., vague standards, ineffective monitoring, weak enforcement—and a "statist" approach that insufficiently harnesses the creativity and resources of nonstate actors and civil society, including businesses, charitable foundations, and NGOs. The question of whether international law can, or should, govern the diverse entities that influence global health is a subject of intense debate in the field.[28] Indeed, modern cutting-edge global health governance initiatives, such as the Global Fund, Global Health Security Initiative (GHSI),[29] International Drug Purchase Facility (UNITAID),[30] and International Finance Facility for Immunization (IFFIm),[31] eschew formal international legal regimes.

INTERNATIONAL HEALTH LAW: WHO'S "THIN" RECORD OF LAWMAKING

Global health should be a major focus of international law, but that has not been the case. The WHO Constitution envisaged a normative institution that would use law, and exercise powers, to proactively promote the attainment of "the highest possible level of health." But the agency has never met these key expectations, although it is beginning to do so.

The WHO Constitution grants the agency extensive normative powers to adopt conventions (Art. 19), promulgate regulations (Art. 21), make recommendations (Art. 23), and monitor national health legislation (Art. 63) (see figure 26).[32] WHO's treaty-making and regulatory powers are noteworthy. The agency can adopt binding conventions or agreements under Article 19, which, unlike normal treaties, affirmatively require states to "take action"—submitting the convention for ratification and notifying the Director-General of the action taken and state's

The World Health Organization

A specialized U.N. agency established in 1946 for the coordination of international health activities.

Mission: "Attainment of the highest possible level of health for all people."

Definition of Health: "A state of complete physical, mental, and social well-being and not merely the absence of disease or infirmity."

Powers

Article 19: Adopt resolutions and agreements pertaining to health

Article 21: Adopt regulations concerning sanitary, diagnostic, and labeling standards

Article 23: Disseminate recommendations, which are nonbinding but scientifically authoritative

Article 63: Member states must notify WHO of important health laws

Activities

The Framework Convention on Tobacco Control (2005) is the first convention adopted by the WHO

International Health Regulations (adopted 1951, revised 2005)

International Code of Marketing of Breast-Milk Substitutes (1981)

Manual of the International Statistical Classification of Disease, Injuries, and Causes of Deaths (1957)

Int'l Digest of Health Legislation (1948)

Major Initiatives

Health for All emphasizes accessible and equitable primary health care as a main priority of the WHO.

The Global Outbreak Alert and Response Network is a technical collaboration for rapid identification and response to outbreaks of international importance.

Global Strategy for Diet, Physical Activity, and Health

3 by 5 was a global target to provide 3 million people worldwide living with HIV/AIDS with antiretroviral medication by 2005.

Figure 26. The World Health Organization.

reasons within eighteen months.[33] WHO's quasi-legislative powers under Article 21 empower the agency to adopt regulations on a broad range of health topics—e.g., international epidemics; the safety, potency, and advertising of biologicals and pharmaceuticals; and a nomenclature for diseases, causes of death, and public health practices. WHO regulations, unlike most international law, are binding on member states unless they proactively "opt out." Once adopted by the World Health Assembly (WHA), the regulations apply to all WHO member countries, even those that voted against it, unless the government specifically notifies WHO that it rejects the regulation or accepts it with reservations.

WHO's normative powers, therefore, are extraordinary. It possesses the authority to oblige states to take health treaties seriously by submitting them to a national political process and informing the international community of the result. Its regulatory powers are even more far-reaching, as states can be bound by health regulations without the requirement to affirmatively sign and ratify. States, moreover, have ongoing duties to make annual reports to the agency on actions taken pursuant to recommendations, conventions, and regulations, as well as to provide annual reports.[34]

Despite WHO's impressive normative powers, modern international health law is remarkably thin—two of the three existing international health instruments predate the agency. The WHA, at its first session in 1948, adopted World Health Regulation No. 1, Nomenclature with Respect to Diseases and Causes of Death, which formalized a long-standing international process on the classification of disease.[35] By providing standardized nomenclature, the regulation facilitates the international comparison of morbidity and mortality data. The Nomenclature Rule was modest at its onset, but subsequently became merely advisory and is now known as the International Classification of Diseases. The Rule is, therefore, technical, rather than normative, and recommended rather than obligatory.

World Health Regulation No. 2, the International Health Regulations (IHR), discussed below, dates back to a series of European sanitary conferences held in the second half of the nineteenth century. Before the IHR were fundamentally revised in 2005, they applied to a limited number of infectious diseases.

The WHO did not create a health convention until 2003, when the WHA adopted the Framework Convention on Tobacco Control (FCTC) (see below).[36] Although a laudable achievement, the FCTC is almost sui generis because it regulates the only lawful product that is uniformly

BOX 14
SOURCES OF INTERNATIONAL LAW

The most authoritative statement of the sources of international law is found in Article 38 of the Statute of the International Court of Justice (ICJ),[1] or World Court.[2] Article 38 lists three primary sources: treaties, custom, and general principles. Judicial decisions and scholarly publications are secondary.[3]

Treaties[4] are international agreements between states and are governed by international law.[5] Treaties primarily govern the conduct of states and concern critical (and sometimes more mundane) national interests, such as security and commerce. However, treaties often also have a significant impact on private parties, such as corporations (e.g., trade law) and individuals (e.g., human rights). Treaties are often analogized to contracts because parties give their consent to be bound and the rules do not legally bind those who do not accept the treaty.[6] However, multinational treaties have important regulatory effects beyond the signatory parties.[7] Although treaties are far from perfect, they help bring order to relationships among IGOs, states, and citizens; provide some stability and predictability in international relations; and institutionalize norms of ethical global conduct in such vital areas as trade, human rights, health, and the environment.[8]

Customary International Law (CIL) refers to unwritten rules of international law generated by a process different from treaties.[9] A rule of CIL forms as a result of widespread repetition by states of similar international acts (state practice); acts taken, and not rejected, by a significant number of states; and acts that occur out of a sense

[1] The ICJ is the principal judicial organ of the United Nations. The court has a dual role: to settle in accordance with international law the legal disputes submitted to it by states, and to give advisory opinions on legal questions referred to it by duly authorized international bodies. UN Charter, Arts. 92-96. However, decisions of the ICJ have no binding force except between the parties to the case. Statute of the Court of the I.C.J., art. 59.

[2] Article 38 of the Statute of the ICJ states that in disputes submitted to it, the court shall apply: (a) international conventions establishing rules expressly recognized by contesting states; (b) international custom, as evidence of a general practice accepted as law; (c) general principles of law recognized by civilized nations; and (d) judicial decisions and the teachings of the most highly qualified publicists of the various nations, as a subsidiary means for the determination of rules of law. Article 38 does not indicate a hierarchy, but for most purposes the ICJ gives precedence to sources in the order in which they appear: treaties, customs, and general principles.

[3] Ian Brownlie, *Principles of Public International Law*, 6th ed. (Oxford: Oxford University Press, 2003): 5.

[4] Multinational treaties, the primary expression of international law, are given many names: treaties, pacts, international agreements, covenants, conventions, etc.; the same rules apply regardless of what the treaty is called. (In the United States, the term *treaty*, as contrasted with an "international executive agreement," has a particular constitutional significance.)

[5] The international rules governing adoption, interpretation, and validity of treaties are codified in the 1969 Vienna Convention on the Law of Treaties (VCLT).

[6] Treaties may also explicitly permit states to make "reservations" (qualifications, conditions, or exceptions) to provisions with which they disagree, thus sacrificing uniformity of obligation for more widespread adherence. Henry J. Steiner and Phillip Alston, *International Human Rights in Context* (Oxford: Oxford University Press, 2000). The IHR, for example, permit reservations whereas the FCTC unusually does not.

[7] John H. Jackson, *The World Trading System: Law and Policy of International Economic Relations*, 2d ed. (Cambridge, MA: MIT Press, 1997): 24-34 ("Notions of reciprocity and a desire to depend on other nations' observance of rules lead many nations to observe rules even when they do not want to").

[8] Steiner and Alston, *International Human Rights*.

[9] *Restatement (Third) of Foreign Relations Law of the United States* § 102 (1987) ("Customary international law results from a general and consistent practice of states followed by them from a sense of legal obligation").

of legal obligation.[10] A rule of CIL is binding on all states, except those that persistently object. Customary rules can be fundamental but also controversial. They are fundamental because of their universal character, sometimes rising to a level of compelling international law *(jus cogens)*. *Jus cogens* is a peremptory norm of international law such as the prohibition of genocide or the slave trade.[11] CIL can be controversial because scholars cannot easily determine when conduct attains customary status. What exactly is "consistent," a "practice," or a sense of "legal obligation"? Despite the conceptual and pragmatic difficulties, CIL is an essential aspect of international law, because it represents the norms of communities and nations.

General Principles of Law are rules of domestic law recognized widely by different national legal systems, which prove useful in international relations in the absence of treaty law or CIL. To become a general principle, a rule must be recognized in most of the world's legal systems–i.e., common law, civil law, and significant religious law (e.g., Sharia, or Islamic law)[12] and ideological (e.g., socialist law) legal cultures. The most frequent use of this source of international law occurs when international tribunals apply general principles of domestic law to resolve legal questions not answered by applicable treaty law or CIL. States and international tribunals are reluctant to apply general principles of law because most of these principles were not generated to apply directly to international relations.[13]

[10] A rule of CIL therefore requires a showing that it has been followed as "general practice" and has been "accepted as law." The "general practice" element is an objective inquiry: Have international actors followed the rule, and has compliance been consistent and for a sufficient period of time? The "accepted as law" element is more subjective: Have international actors observed the practice out of a sense of legal obligation or merely out of courtesy or expediency? David J. Bederman, *International Law Frameworks* (New York: Foundation Press, 2001).

[11] *Jus cogens* is a peremptory norm of general international law accepted and recognized by the international community as a "norm from which no derogation is permitted and which can be modified only by a subsequent norm of general international law having the same character." Vienna Convention on the Law of Treaties, art. 53, May 23, 1969, 1155 U.N.T.S. 331, 8 I.L.M. 679.

[12] Sharia (also Sharīʻah, Shari'a, Shariah, or Syariah) is traditional Islamic law, also known as Allah's Law. Islam classically draws no distinction between religious and secular life. Hence, Sharia covers not only religious rituals, but many aspects of day-to-day life. "Shari'ah," *Encyclopedia Britannica* (2005), http://search.eb.com/eb/article-9105857.

[13] *Restatement (Third) of Foreign Relations Law of the United States* § 102, comment 1 (1987).

harmful. The FCTC was politically feasible because the industry was vilified for denying scientific realities, engineering tobacco to create dependence, engaging in deceptive advertising, and targeting youth, women, and minorities.[37]

Prominent scholars have chastened WHO for its reluctance to create binding norms, despite the bold mission and sweeping powers granted in its constitution.[38] At the turn of the twenty-first century, more than fifty years after its founding, the agency had failed to adopt a single treaty. And its two regulations—on disease classification and epidemic control—were largely historical, limited in scope, and lacking in real-world impact. Since that time, WHO has been far more proactive, suggesting that it may be prepared to exercise political power when necessary to avert global health crises. The evolution in thinking can be traced to the SARS outbreaks when WHO issued politically controversial travel advisories with severe economic impacts. In the FCTC, the agency demonstrated a willingness to take on a powerful industry. And the revised IHR were, in many respects, the high-water mark for the exercise of normative power, as the agency exerted its influence on matters ranging from capacity building and global surveillance to trade and human rights. The critical question, however, is whether the WHO can build on these recent achievements to deal with the most important, and intractable, health problems in the poorest regions of the world.

There are a number of important areas of international law that influence global health, even if they do not achieve fully effective global health governance. The remainder of this chapter explores major advances in the fields of infectious disease control, tobacco, trade, and human rights. To better understand these global initiatives, it will be helpful to review the principal sources of international law in box 14.

INTERNATIONAL HEALTH REGULATIONS: A HISTORIC DEVELOPMENT IN GLOBAL GOVERNANCE

The origins of the International Health Regulations (IHR)—the only global rules governing the international spread of infectious disease—date back to the first International Sanitary Conference, held in Paris in 1851 to address the European cholera epidemics.[39] During the latter half of the nineteenth century, ten sanitary conferences were held and eight conventions negotiated (though most did not come into force) to address the transboundary effects of infectious diseases.[40] The International Sanitary Convention dealing with cholera, plague, and yellow fever was adopted in Venice in 1892, followed by a convention dealing with plague in 1897.[41] In 1903, a new International Sanitary Convention replaced the conventions of 1892 and 1897.[42]

At the turn of the twentieth century, the international community established regional and international institutions to enforce these conventions. American states set up the International Sanitary Bureau (ISB) in 1902, which became the Pan American Sanitary Bureau (PASB), a precursor to the Pan American Health Organization (PAHO).[43] In 1907 European nations developed their own multilateral institution, the Office International d'Hygiène Publique (OIHP).[44] The Health Organization of the League of Nations (HOLN) was formed in 1923, between the two world wars. Article 23 of the League of Nations Covenant meekly stated that members would "endeavor to take steps in matters of international concern for the prevention and control of disease."[45] The ISB, OIHP, and HOLN were separate institutions, without harmonization in goals or practices.

The United Nations was established after the horrors of World War II, and one of its primary functions was the protection of global health.[46] The World Health Organization (WHO) was the first international agency established by the United Nations.[47] Its preamble expresses universal aspirations,[48] stating that its "principles are basic to the happiness, harmonious relations and security of all peoples."[49]

Pursuant to the agency's Article 21 power, WHO member states adopted the International Sanitary Regulations (ISR) on July 25, 1951. The ISR were renamed the International Health Regulations (IHR) in 1969. The IHR initially applied to six diseases—cholera, plague, relapsing fever, smallpox, typhus, and yellow fever—but were slightly modified in 1969[50] (to exclude louseborne typhus and relapsing fever) and again in 1981[51] (to exclude smallpox, in view of its global eradication). By the early 1980s the IHR applied only to cholera, plague, and yellow fever—the same diseases originally discussed at the first International Sanitary Conference in 1851. Thus, before the IHR were fundamentally revised in 2005,[52] their scope and approach were similar to that of the ISR in the mid–twentieth century.

The fundamental reform of the IHR that took place in 2005 would not have been possible were it not for a confluence of events that raised infectious diseases to the realm of "high politics."[53] The WHA resolved in 1995 to revise the IHR in response to frightening outbreaks of cholera in Peru, the plague in India, and Ebola hemorrhagic fever in Zaire.[54] During this time, the world was also facing one of the greatest pandemics in global history, HIV/AIDS,[55] as well as the looming threats of SARS,[56] avian influenza,[57] Marburg,[58] and bioterrorism.[59] The potentially drastic economic and security consequences of these health threats made it politically difficult to oppose an ambitious reform of international infectious disease law.

The IHR (2005) contain sixty-six articles organized into ten parts, with nine annexes. The rules expand WHO jurisdiction beyond a narrow band of infectious diseases to the entire spectrum of public health risks of international importance. The IHR focus on key aspects of global preparedness, ranging from surveillance and capacity building to public health response and border control. The cumulative effect of reforms could transform WHO's role and stature in international law and establish a coherent structure for systematic detection and intervention in the face of global health threats.[60]

Purpose, Scope, and Principles: Health, Trade, and Human Rights

The IHR are expansive in scope, covering "public health risks"[61] and "public health emergencies of international concern."[62] Consequently, WHO has authority to act in most contexts where an event has health-related transnational dimensions, which include biological, chemical, and radio-nuclear health risks. Since the source of the hazard is immaterial, WHO possesses jurisdiction for events that are naturally occurring, accidental, and intentional.[63]

The purpose of the IHR is "to prevent, protect against, control and provide a public health response to the international spread of disease in ways that are commensurate with and restricted to public health risks, and which avoid unnecessary interference with international traffic and trade" (Art. 2). The IHR therefore balance the need for health regulation with trade interests. Health measures cannot be more stringent than what is needed to avert or ameliorate the public health risk; state action must be rooted in scientific evidence.[64] The IHR interact with international trade law in interesting, important ways, with both areas of law focusing on the legitimacy of state health measures that adversely affect international commerce.

The IHR balance not only health with trade, but also health with human rights.[65] The IHR have "universal application for the protection of all people of the world," and States Parties must have "full respect for the dignity, human rights and fundamental freedoms of persons" (Art. 3). Health measures taken must be applied in a transparent and nondiscriminatory manner (Art. 42). States Parties must, in particular, treat international travelers with "respect for their dignity, human rights and fundamental freedoms and minimize any discomfort or distress"; respectful treatment requires consideration of travelers' gender, culture, ethnicity, and religion (Art. 32).

The balancing dynamic in the IHR, then, includes adherence to scientific methodologies, the flow of trade and travel, and respect for human rights (see figure 27). In each of these realms, there are difficult trade-offs:

- When can countries act in the face of scientific uncertainty?
- How much interference with economic freedom can be tolerated

Trade and Travel	Scientific Methodologies	Human Rights
• Consider risk of interfering with international traffic when determining if an event is a public health emergency (Art. 12) • No ship or aircraft shall be prevented from calling at a port of entry for public health reasons unless the point of entry is unable to apply health measures (Art. 28) • Unless otherwise authorized, goods in transit without transshipment that are not live animals will not be subject to IHR health measures or detained for public health purposes (Art. 33) • Health measures shall not be more restrictive to international traffic than reasonably available alternatives that would achieve the appropriate level of health protection (Art. 43) • States implementing additional health measures that significantly interfere with international traffic shall provide WHO with rationale and relevant scientific information (Art. 43)	• Determination of a public health emergency of international concern based on scientific principles, available scientific evidence and other relevant information (Art. 12) • Determination of whether to implement health measures based on scientific principles and available scientific evidence of risk to health (Art. 43) • Consultation between states impacted by an emergency and states implementing health measures to clarify scientific information and public health rationale underlying implemented health measures (Art. 43)	• IHR implementation shall be with full respect for the dignity, human rights and fundamental freedoms of persons (Art. 3) • No IHR medical examination, vaccination, prophylaxis or health measure will be performed on travelers without prior informed consent, except as otherwise noted (Art. 23) • States shall minimize discomfort or distress from IHR measures by treating all travelers with courtesy and respect and taking into consideration gender, sociocultural, ethnic or religious concerns of travelers (Art. 32) • Health measures pursuant to the IHR shall be applied in a transparent and non-discriminatory manner (Art. 42) • Health information collected or received under the IHR referring to an identifiable person shall be kept confidential and processed anonymously, unless otherwise mentioned (Art. 45)

Figure 27. The International Health Regulations' (IHR) balancing dynamic.

in the name of health? And who should bear the financial cost of health regulation?

- When should personal autonomy, privacy, and liberty yield for the sake of the public's health and safety?

Core National Capacities for Public Health Preparedness

States Parties have the duty to develop, strengthen, and maintain core public health capacities to detect, assess, notify, and report events; and to respond promptly and effectively to public health risks and emergencies of international concern (Arts. 5[1], 13(1), and Annex 1). Global health protection relies on the ability of national and subnational governments to engage in speedy and accurate surveillance and response to health threats.

The mandate to build public health infrastructures is powerless, however, without adequate resources for poor countries, where in some cases the per capita annual spending on health is unconscionably low. The least developed countries spend between $1 and $25 per capita per year on health care; in contrast, developed nations spend between $1,500 and $4,500.[66] The World Health Assembly urged member states to "mobilize the resources necessary" and to provide support upon request "in the building, strengthening and maintenance of public health capacities."[67] Although the IHR ask States Parties to provide financial and technical resources, these provisions are either nonbinding[68] or weak;[69] they require states to comply only "to the extent possible." Similarly, WHO duties to provide surveillance and response assistance[70] do not address WHO's own shortage of funds and personnel. Given the financial demands created by other global health problems, such as the need to increase access to HIV/AIDS treatment[71] and meet the health-related Millennium Development Goals,[72] the IHR's silence on how the economic demands of the core-capacity objectives will be met is a serious problem for which the IHR provide no apparent answers or strategies.

Surveillance

The IHR, cognizant of past recalcitrance of member states to communicate promptly and fully events that pose health risks, provide detailed requirements for data dissemination. The new approach is radical because it does not limit surveillance and reporting requirements to a narrow list

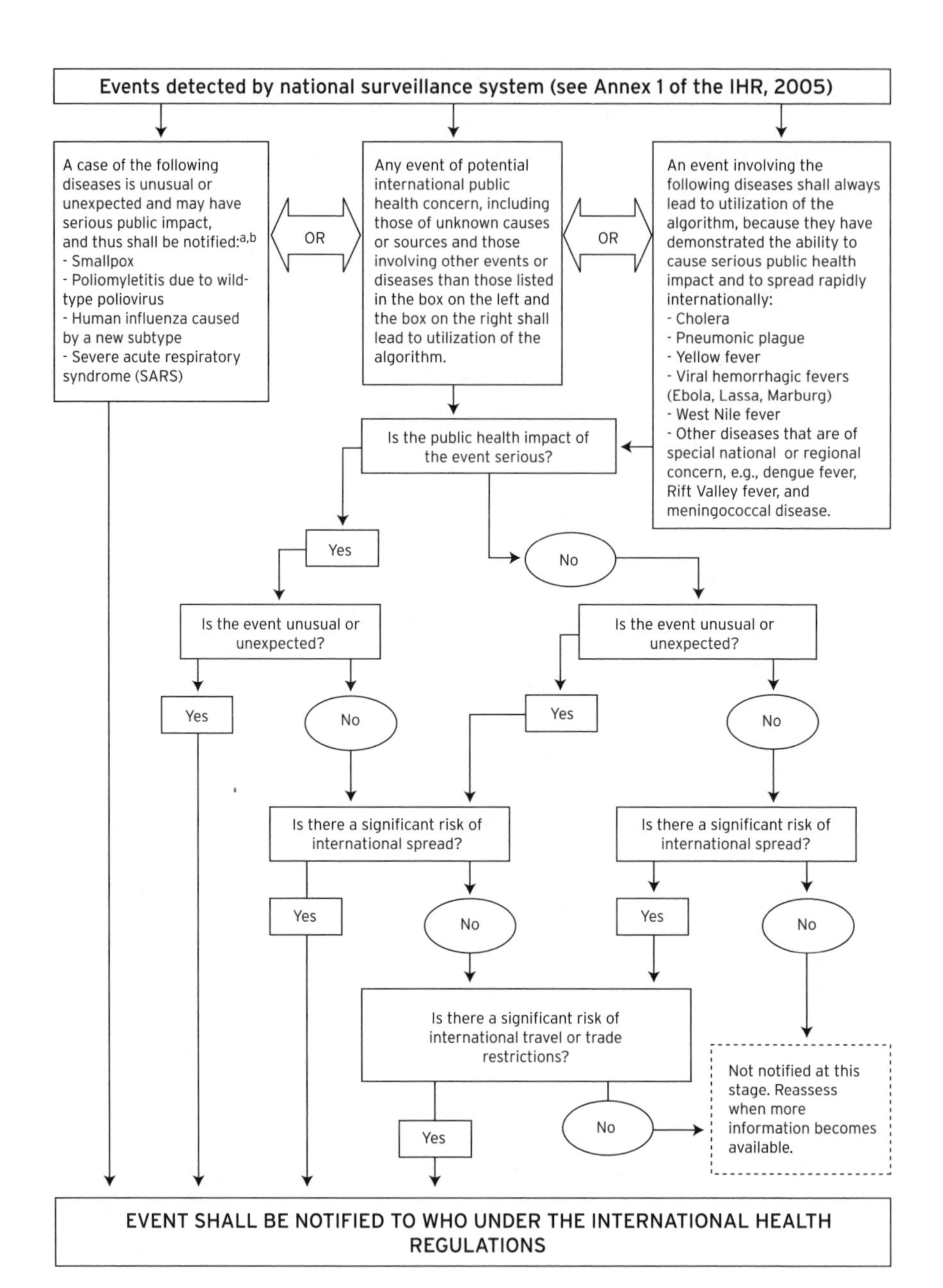

[a] As per WHO case definitions.
[b] The disease list shall be used only for purposes of these Regulations.

Figure 28. Decision instrument for the assessment and notification of events that may constitute a public health emergency of international concern. *Source:* World Health Organization, "Decision Instrument for the Assessment and Notification of Events That May Constitute a Public Health Emergency of International Concern," February 22, 2005, www.who.int/gb/ghs/pdf/IHR_IGWG2_ID4-en.pdf.

of diseases, but instead requires States Parties to *notify* WHO within twenty-four hours of all events in their territory[73] that may constitute a "public health emergency of international concern" (Art. 6) (see figure 28).[74] States Parties must *share all relevant public health information* during an unexpected or unusual public health event, irrespective of origin or source, that may constitute a public health emergency of international concern (Art. 7). This power implies a state obligation to share data about accidental or intentional health hazards,[75] an obligation that became highly politicized in intergovernmental negotiations.[76] States Parties must also *consult and keep WHO apprised* of events that may not be notifiable due to incomplete scientific information (Art. 8).

The IHR authorize WHO to take into account unofficial sources of information (e.g., NGOs and independent scientists), which must be assessed according to established epidemiological principles (Arts. 9, 10). This power enables WHO to utilize the broad network of potentially important surveillance data available in the age of the Internet and other electronic information systems. The Global Outbreak Alert and Response Network (GOARN), based on this concept, is a collaboration of institutions and networks that pool human and technical resources for the rapid identification, confirmation, and response to outbreaks of international importance. This network is central to the functioning of the IHR.[77]

The regulations require WHO to share nongovernmental information with States Parties, "and only where it is duly justified may WHO maintain the confidentiality of the source" (Art. 9[1]). This requirement to disclose the source of nongovernmental information might deter nonstate actors from supplying the WHO with information, particularly in authoritarian regimes. The IHR provide no express guidance for determining under what circumstances WHO would be justified in maintaining the confidentiality of nonstate sources.

Dissemination of Health Information: Privacy

States Parties must keep personally identified or identifiable information "confidential and processed anonymously as required by national law" (Art. 45[1]). Some states and regional alliances, including the United States[78] and the European Union,[79] have data protection laws, but many others do not, which could considerably weaken the IHR's privacy mandate. States may disclose and process personal data where "essential for the purposes of assessing and managing a public health risk," but must follow fair information practices. These practices require that personal data be relevant and not excessive; be accurate and current; be processed fairly and lawfully; and not be kept longer than necessary. WHO must also, as far as practicable, provide individuals with their personal data in an intelligible form and allow for correction of inaccuracies (Art. 45).

WHO Recommendations

WHO has the power to issue temporary and standing recommendations. The Director-General must issue temporary recommendations upon determining that a public health emergency of international concern is occurring (Art. 15). WHO may also make standing recommendations on the appropriate health measures to be applied routinely or periodically in relation to specific ongoing public health risks (Art. 16). Article 18 contains applicable health measures for persons (e.g., medical examinations, vaccination, contact tracing, isolation, and exit screening), as well as for baggage, cargo, containers, conveyances, and goods (e.g., review of the manifest and routing documents, inspections, safe handling, seizure and destruction, and refusal of departure or entry).[80]

International Travelers

International travel is one of the primary means by which pathogens spread across frontiers. A health measure directed at travelers can be an effective means of containing an outbreak or it can overreach, causing adverse effects on trade, tourism, and human rights (Arts. 23, 30–32, 43). A "suspect" traveler, who may have been exposed to infection[81] and is placed under "public health observation," can continue an international voyage only if he or she does not present an imminent public health risk. Despite the duty to be respectful to travelers and allow their passage (Art. 30), States Parties may require, for public health purposes, information about the traveler's destination and itinerary, and a *noninvasive* medical examination that is the least intrusive necessary to achieve the public health objective (Art. 23). Upon evidence of a public health risk, States Parties may conduct the least intrusive and invasive medical examination or other health measure necessary to achieve the objective of preventing the international spread of disease. Travelers, or their parents or guardians, must be informed of any health risk associated with vaccination or other prophylaxis, and physicians must be educated about this requirement. Similarly, medical examinations and procedures must conform to established national or international safety standards (see further, chapter 11).

A New Paradigm for Global Health Governance

The IHR offer an opportunity to improve global health governance, overcoming the problems of sovereignty and entrenched power. An innovative governance paradigm, based on the new IHR, would include:

The salience of health over trade. WHO should dedicate itself to the protection and promotion of global health, respecting travel and trade wherever possible. That is the vision of the WHO Constitution, which does not mention the protection of commerce.

Wide jurisdiction. The expansive scope of the new IHR is preferable because it is flexible, prospective, and covers all hazards (radiological, chemical, and biological), whether naturally occurring, accidental, or intentional.

Comprehensive data collection. The WHO could dramatically improve global surveillance by establishing standards for uniform data sets, core informational requirements, and timely monitoring and reporting; creating "small-world networks" consisting of scientists, health professionals, and NGOs to broaden the sources of health information; and using modern technology (e.g., electronic health records and the Internet) to gather and analyze surveillance data.[82]

National public health preparedness. To improve national competencies, WHO should set minimum standards for laboratories, data systems, and response capabilities. The international community should substantially increase technical and financial assistance for health system improvement in developing countries. Not only will this kind of commitment allow progressive development of higher health standards in resource-poor countries, but it is also in the interests of the industrialized world.

Human rights safeguards. The new IHR go a long way to respecting human rights but leave out important safeguards. The WHO could demonstrate even greater respect for human rights by applying the internationally accepted norms contained in the Siracusa Principles (discussed below), which require health measures to be necessary, proportionate, and fair.[83] Health measures should be based on the rule of law and provide due process for persons whose liberty is placed in jeopardy.

Sound public health governance. WHO member states have not always followed basic principles of good public health governance, such as openness, nondiscrimination, and compliance with scientific methods. The WHO should set an example by establishing its policies and recommendations in an open manner, basing them on scientific evidence, and exercising power equitably. The agency gains credibility by its adherence to science, the truthfulness of its disclosures, and its fair dealings with all countries, rich and poor alike.

The future of global health governance. The new IHR will not assure capable leadership and sound governance by the WHO. Yet the revision offers an opportunity for a renewed commitment by the international community to a shared vision of global health. The revision gives the WHO a clear mission, significantly enhanced jurisdiction, and formal power to set standards and make recommendations. By assenting to a far-reaching revision of the IHR, member states are ceding some control over global health threats and have taken a vital step toward better protection against the biological, chemical, and radiological hazards posed in the modern age.

FRAMEWORK CONVENTION ON TOBACCO CONTROL: GLOBAL STRATEGIES TO REDUCE SMOKING

The WHO has turned to international law solutions in the area of chronic disease as well as infectious disease. Particularly remarkable is the adoption of the Framework Convention on Tobacco Control (FCTC).[84] The FCTC, the first treaty negotiated under WHO auspices, was a decade in the making:[85] The convention was initiated in 1995[86] and adopted by the World Health Assembly in 2003,[87] and it entered into force on February 27, 2005.[88]

The FCTC arose in response to the human, social, and economic costs of the tobacco pandemic. More than 1.25 billion smokers inhabit the earth today, representing approximately one-third of the adult population.[89] Cigarette smoking is a leading cause of preventable death and disability worldwide, killing around 4.9 million people each year; smoking is projected to kill about 10 million people annually by 2020, with two-thirds in developing countries.[90] Once confined largely to industrialized nations, the burden of disease and death is rapidly shifting to low- and middle-income countries, as a result of rising incomes, trade liberalization, the emancipation of women, and global marketing and communications.[91] Compounding the immense death toll are the economic implications of cigarette and passive smoking. In the United States, the social cost of smoking (i.e., costs shared by the public) is an average of $106,000 for every woman and $220,000 for every man who smokes; this price includes the cost of health care related to secondhand smoking, and increased Medicare, Medicaid, and Social Security payments.[92]

The FCTC's global strategy was also thought necessary to counteract an economically and politically powerful multinational industry.[93] The tobacco industry for decades denied the reality of addiction, disease, and death; engineered the product to create and maintain dependence; engaged in deceptive advertising; targeted youth, women, and minorities; and aggressively blocked national legislation.[94] Consider Philip Morris's opposition to tobacco regulation in the Czech Republic, arguing that smoking had saved the government $147 million due to smokers' early deaths.[95] The company itself later conceded that the report exhibited "terrible judgment [and] disregard of basic human values."[96] Undeterred, the industry has aggressively pursued new markets in Latin America, Eastern Europe, Africa, and newly industrializing economies in Asia such as China, India, Indonesia, and Thailand.[97]

Objectives, Principles, and Legal Force

The FCTC's declared objective is to protect present and future generations from "the devastating health, social, environmental and economic consequences of tobacco consumption and exposure to tobacco smoke (Art. 3)." It aims to keep citizens informed of the health hazards and to facilitate political commitment, international cooperation, and financial assistance (Art. 4). It mandates that States Parties develop and implement comprehensive multisectoral national tobacco control strategies (Art. 5).

Although it requires national tobacco control strategies, the FCTC rarely contains specific standards that countries must meet. Framework conventions typically establish broadly stated goals and avoid the more onerous commitments normally embodied in a conventional treaty. This has the distinct advantage of helping to build a global consensus on a politically charged public health issue. However, the framework convention approach is vulnerable to the critique that it uses "hortatory rather than legal statements, soft rather than hard law, and denies [the FCTC] of any self-executing requirements."[98] The FCTC expresses non-obligatory legal language throughout: "recognize," "consider," "guidelines," "endeavor to," and "without prejudice to the sovereign right of the Parties." Consequently, signing the treaty can be seen as relatively cost-free because states become bound by more rigorous commitments only if they consent subsequently to negotiated protocols.[99] It is perhaps because the rules established were so elastic that President George W. Bush signed the FCTC. Even so, the United States has not ratified the treaty.[100]

Despite its deficits in standard setting, implementation, and monitoring, the FCTC establishes a blueprint for comprehensive tobacco control activities that nations can emulate. The FCTC adopts several strategies: demand reduction, supply reduction, and tort litigation.

Reduction of Demand for Tobacco

Articles 6–14 of the FCTC establish core demand-reduction strategies, including price and tax measures, as well as nonprice measures. Tax and price policies are designed to reduce demand for cigarettes. Data show that taxation and high prices reduce smoking, particularly among consumers without significant disposable income, such as children and adolescents.[101] States Parties are required to report cigarette tax rates and tobacco consumption trends (Arts. 6, 21). Countries are also urged to restrict or prohibit duty-free tobacco sales to prevent importation and smuggling (Art. 6(3)). Nonprice measures include protection from exposure to tobacco smoke (e.g., workplaces, indoor public places, and public transport); regulation of the contents of tobacco products; and disclosure requirements for manufacturers (Arts. 6–10). These measures are designed to inform consumers about the risks and reduce exposure to environmental tobacco smoke.

The FCTC regulates the packaging, labeling, advertising, and promotion of tobacco products (Arts. 11–13). Packaging and labeling regulation is designed to deter false, misleading, or deceptive messages that create an erroneous impression (e.g., "low tar," "light," "ultra light," or "mild"). The treaty obliges States Parties to adopt and implement large, clear, visible, legible, and rotating health warnings and messages on tobacco products, occupying at least 30 percent of the principal display areas. (See, e.g., the graphic images on cigarette packets in Australia.)

Tobacco products are advertised and promoted through sports events, music festivals, films, and fashion—in fact, anywhere the tobacco industry can target potential new smokers. Cigarettes are often associated with ideas and images that convey adventure, glamour, and vitality. Tobacco advertisements frequently target minorities, women, and young people. Recognizing the pervasive effects of marketing, the FCTC calls for a comprehensive ban on tobacco advertising, promotion, and sponsorship. In deference to politically powerful countries, however, the FCTC states that such regulation should be in accordance with the country's constitutional principles (Art. 13). The U.S. Supreme Court, for example, has strongly defended commercial speech (see chapter 9), and to a lesser extent, one can see similar constitutional arguments in Canada[102] and Europe.[103]

Reduction of Supply of Tobacco

Articles 15–17 of the FCTC establish core supply-reduction strategies, including measures to control illicit trade and sales to minors, as well as to create economically viable alternatives to tobacco production. The illicit trade in cigarettes—smuggling, unlawful manufacturing, and counterfeiting—is found throughout the world. The illicit trade makes international brands more affordable and enables smugglers to evade health regulations. Measures in the FCTC include marking unit packets with the product's origin and, for domestic sales, a statement that they can be sold only in that country. Countries are required to monitor and collect data on cross-border trade and enact penalties for unlawful purchase, sale, and transport (Art. 15).

Tobacco use among young people is pervasive. Most tobacco use starts during childhood and adolescence, and statistics indicate an upward trend in tobacco initiation and use among young persons.[104] Tobacco is available to children in many countries, even countries with legal prohibitions. Young people's access to tobacco is a serious problem due to the addictive and psychosocial effects of smoking.[105] Recognizing these adverse effects, the FCTC requires States Parties to prohibit sales to minors and ensure effective implementation. The treaty, for example, calls for prominent signs at the point of sale, bans on sweets and toys in the form of cigarettes, and inaccessibility of vending machines to young people (Art. 16).

The FCTC requires States Parties to promote economically viable alternatives for tobacco workers, growers, and sellers (Art. 17). The purpose is to create economic incentives for the workforce to discontinue tobacco production in favor of more socially beneficial activities.

Civil and Criminal Liability

Tobacco litigation strategies in the United States were influential in the negotiations on the FCTC. Although not entirely successful, litigation changed the social and political culture of tobacco and had a deterrent effect on the most egregious industry practices.[106] Most regions of the world are not as litigious as the United States. Still, Article 19 asks States Parties to consider criminal and civil liability for the tobacco industry. Because the industry is so powerful and skilled at defending against liability, the FCTC promotes international cooperation such as information exchange and legal assistance. More generally, the FCTC contains provisions encouraging reporting, scientific and technical cooperation, and communication of information (Arts. 20–22).

The FCTC's Future Effectiveness

The future effectiveness of the FCTC is difficult to predict. Certainly, the treaty was a momentous achievement in global health governance. It forged a global consensus to combat a devastating health hazard—a rare event in international relations. Even without enforceable norms, the FCTC sets out a comprehensive program for smoking prevention and cessation.[107]

At the time of its adoption, the rate of smoking in the industrialized world was already abating—the result of a decades-long campaign of legislation, litigation, and health education. The same dynamic could occur in low- and middle-income countries as they follow the FCTC's core strategies. To achieve this global public good for health will require considerable political will and economic resources from the international community.

WORLD TRADE AND WORLD HEALTH

Too much of this century was marked by force and
coercion. Our dream must be a world managed by
persuasion, the rule of law, the settlement of differences

> peacefully within the law and cooperation. It's a good thing that all our living standards are now based on the ability of our neighbours to purchase our products. That's where the WTO can do splendid work and advance the progress of the human species.
>
> Mike Moore, speech to the Transatlantic Business Dialogue, Oct. 29, 1999

> What is called "globalization" is a specific form of international integration, designed and instituted for particular purposes. There are many possible alternatives. This particular form happens to be geared to the interests of private power, manufacturing corporations and financial institutions, closely linked to powerful states. Effects on others are incidental. Sometimes they happen to be beneficial, often not.
>
> Noam Chomsky, interview with *Washington Post* readers: "Globalization and Its Discontents with Noam Chomsky," May 16, 2000

The trading of goods and services from one area to another, across political and geographic boundaries, is pervasive.[108] The movement of products and knowledge along routes of trade is the engine that drives economies, but it is also the means by which disease is spread and cultures are homogenized. Trade can provide nations with resources or technological advances to which they would not otherwise have access. It opens markets to life-saving products such as medicines or medical equipment, and to life-threatening products such as tobacco or asbestos. It also can make essential medicines, such as antiretroviral medication for HIV/AIDS, so expensive that they are out of reach for the poor. Trade in services can reallocate expertise where it is needed or drain an area of its human capital. International trading systems can (for better or worse) change the way nations regulate their products. Trade may also provide an avenue for the exchange of ideas, information, and culture.[109]

In short, the effects of trade on prosperity and health are deeply complex.[110] To those who embrace capitalism and competitive markets, trade is the answer to many socioeconomic problems. To those who prefer equity and social distribution, trade liberalization places the interests of rich countries and multinational corporations ahead of the health and lives of the world's poor.

Like it or not, trade is a social, political, and economic reality. In the late twentieth century, countries joined together to form the World Trade Organization (WTO), setting trade into a global system of governance. The current trade system has as its goals providing predictability and stability and reducing barriers to trade so as to increase the standard of living for all.[111] The WTO's principal mission is the reduction of trade barriers, but it cannot escape the inexorable links between commerce and health. The goal of a rational trade system should be to find a balance between economic prosperity and health protection.

The World Trade System: Origins and Objectives

The framework for the modern world trade system originated after World War II with the Bretton Woods Accord, which led to the creation of the International Monetary Fund (IMF), the World Bank, and the General Agreement on Tariffs and Trade (the GATT). The GATT, developed in 1947 and superseded by GATT 1994, was designed to liberalize trade by reducing tariff (e.g., import and export duties) and nontariff (e.g., import quotas, licensing, and health and safety standards) trade barriers.

Under the auspices of the GATT, the contracting parties agreed to hold periodic multinational negotiations ("Rounds"). The Uruguay Round, in 1986–94, culminated in the establishment of the WTO on January 1, 1995.[112] The WTO Agreement sets forth its objectives:

> Raising standards of living, ensuring full employment, . . . and expanding the production of and trade in goods and services, while allowing for the optimal use of the world's resources [for] sustainable development . . . [and ensuring] that developing countries . . . secure a share in the growth in international trade.[113]

The WTO founders, therefore, intended trade expansion to be environmentally sound, and aspired not to leave the least developed countries behind. Yet, more than a decade later, there still exists bitter controversy over the effects of trade on health, the environment, and economic development for the poor.

The WTO includes a package of agreements, notably GATT 1994[114] and the General Agreement on Trade in Services (GATS).[115] The WTO agreements most relevant to health include:[116] the GATT 1994; Sanitary and Phytosanitary Measures (SPS); and Trade-Related Aspects of Intellectual Property Rights (TRIPS) (see table 9).[117] Regional trade pacts such as the North American (NAFTA) and Central American (CAFTA) Free Trade Agreements also affect commerce and health.[118]

TABLE 9. WTO agreements relevant to health

WTO Agreement	Mission	Health Area	Enforcement
1994 General Agreement on Tariffs and Trade (GATT 1994)	Liberalize trade and increase market access by decreasing tariffs and other trade barriers	Article 20(b): exception allowing imposition of trade restrictions to protect the health of humans, animals, and plants, e.g., cigarettes, air pollution, asbestos	"The provisions of this Agreement shall apply to the metropolitan customs territories of the contracting parties" (Art. 24) Contracting parties "may authorize a contracting party or parties to suspend the application to any other contracting party or parties of such concessions or other obligations under this Agreement as they determine to be appropriate in the circumstances" (Art. 23)
Sanitary and Phytosanitary Measures (SPS)	Harmonize sanitary and phytosanitary measures internationally to protect human, animal, and plant health	Regulation of goods that may carry disease or disease-causing organisms and consumables that contain contaminant additives, contaminants, or toxins creating a risk to health, e.g., beef hormones, genetically modified foods	"Members are fully responsible under this Agreement for the observance of all obligations set forth herein" (Art. 13) Articles 22 and 23 of GATT 1994 govern dispute settlements and consultations (Art. 11)
Trade-Related Aspects of Intellectual Property Rights (TRIPS)	Promote effective intellectual property rights protection, especially patenting and licensing	Article 31: compulsory licensing in national emergencies, e.g., HIV/AIDS anti-retrovirals	"Members shall give effect to the provisions of this Agreement" (Art. 1). Articles 22 and 23 of GATT 1994 govern dispute settlements and consultations (Art. 64) "Members shall ensure that enforcement procedures . . . are available under their law so as to permit effective action against . . . infringement of intellectual property rights" (Art. 41)

BOX 15
WTO STRUCTURE

Membership

WTO membership is not automatic. Countries must negotiate their entry into the WTO system with existing members. Currently, there are 148 member states, accounting for more than 90 percent of world trade.[1]

Decision Making

WTO decisions are made by various bodies.[2] The Ministerial Conference, which meets at least biennially and comprises all WTO members, is the highest decision-making body. The General Council has executive authority over day-to-day operations of the WTO. Its members also meet as the Dispute Settlement Body.

Dispute Settlement

Member states that believe they have been injured by other members' violation of WTO obligations can seek redress before the Dispute Settlement Body. The Dispute Settlement Body then convenes a panel to hear and decide the case. Panel decisions can be appealed to the Appellate Body (AB), a standing body of seven members with expertise in law and international trade.[3] Decisions of the AB become final and binding, unless the Dispute Settlement Body unanimously decides otherwise.

[1] WHO Secretariat and WTO Secretariat, *WTO Agreements and Public Health* (Geneva: World Trade Organization, 2002): 28.

[2] Marrakesh Agreement, Art. 9. Decision-making bodies are technically comprised of representatives from all member states, who can be government officials or representatives of observer organizations.

[3] AB members are elected by the Dispute Settlement Body for terms of four years. Usually, three members of the AB hear a controversy.

Basic Principles of International Trade: Nondiscrimination

The general principles of "most favored nation" (MFN) and "national treatment" guide the substance of WTO agreements. These principles are designed to prevent discrimination between trading partners and avert protectionist trade measures. Under the MFN principle, a benefit granted to one country in regard to a product must be granted to all WTO members in regard to "like" products.[119] For example, if a country offers a lower customs tariff on cigarettes for one country, this lower tariff must be applied to cigarettes from any other WTO member. WTO members thus cannot unjustifiably discriminate among their trading partners.

The general principle of "national treatment" prohibits discrimination in taxes and regulations between domestic and foreign (imported) goods.[120] A country may, for example, restrict pesticide use on fruit because of the risk to health. However, if that country applied the pesticide regulation to imported fruit but not domestic fruit, the policy would violate the national treatment principle because the risk to consumers is the same irrespective of the fruit's country of origin.

The WTO Appellate Body (see box 15) has made it clear that health concerns are relevant in interpreting and applying the basic principles of international trade. In the *EC-Canada Asbestos Case* (2001), it upheld a French regulation prohibiting the manufacture, domestic sale, and import of asbestos-containing products. The Appellate Body stressed that human health is "important to the highest degree" and noted the strong scientific evidence that asbestos fibers were toxic, whereas similar fibers were not. Based on this distinction, they held that products containing asbestos were not "like" similar products containing other fibers and could properly be excluded.[121]

National Health Regulation: Necessity and Less Trade-Restrictive Alternatives

The drafters of the GATT were concerned that the nondiscrimination principles could interfere with states' sovereign rights to protect the health and safety of their citizens. Article XX(b) of the GATT states that nothing in the agreement shall be construed to prevent members from adopting and enforcing measures "necessary to protect human, animal or plant life or health."[122] Although countries have sovereignty to protect the health and safety of their populations, they cannot arbitrarily or unjustifiably discriminate between countries where the same conditions prevail or adopt measures as a subterfuge for discrimination.

The WTO often grants countries deference in determining the necessity of a public health regulation.[123] The Dispute Settlement Body panel does not inquire as to the necessity of underlying public health goals.[124] Thus, national health officials may set health policy goals. However, international trade law does review the means by which countries achieve health goals. The means must be science-based, although countries can rely on minority opinions that nonetheless represent a respected scientific authority.[125]

Despite the deference afforded to member states, the WTO will examine "reasonably available" alternatives in evaluating the necessity of a trade-restrictive health measure: "Import restrictions . . . [are] considered to be 'necessary' . . . only if there were no alternative measure consistent with the General Agreement . . . [which a country] could reasonably be expected to employ to achieve its health policy objectives."[126] In the *Thailand-Cigarette Case,* decided under the health exception to the GATT 1947, the United States challenged Thailand's decision to ban the importation of cigarettes while permitting the sale of domestic cigarettes. Thailand argued that U.S. cigarettes contain chemicals and other additives that make them more harmful than Thai cigarettes, a claim affirmed by the WHO. The GATT dispute panel, however, found that Thailand's import ban was unnecessary because less trade-restrictive alternatives existed—e.g., warning labels, ingredient lists, and bans on certain additives. The panel did uphold Thailand's internal cigarette taxes and the ban on advertising and point-of-sale promotion.

Sanitary and Phytosanitary Measures (SPS)

The SPS Agreement covers sanitary and phytosanitary measures, which are defined to include any measure applied to protect human life or health from "risks arising from additives, contaminants, toxins or disease-causing organisms in foods, beverages or feedstuffs" or "arising from diseases carried by animals, plants or products thereof, or from the entry, establishment or spread of pests" (Annex A, paragraphs 1[b])–[c]). The SPS Agreement affords members the sovereign right to protect the life and health of their human, animal, and plant populations, provided that such measures are "based on scientific principles" and do not constitute arbitrary, unjustifiable discrimination or a disguised restriction on international trade (Preamble, Art. 2[1]). National health measures that conform to the SPS Agreement are deemed to fulfill the country's obligations under the umbrella WTO agreement and specifically the GATT 1994 (Art. XX) (SPS, Art. 2[4]).

International Standards. The SPS Agreement reflects a preference for the adoption and use of international SPS standards to harmonize national measures. Members that adopt measures in conformity with such standards are automatically presumed to be in compliance with the SPS Agreement. In the area of food safety, the SPS Agreement explicitly recognizes the international standards developed by the joint FAO/WHO Codex Alimentarius Commission.[127] Thus, if a government bases its regulation (such as a maximum residue level for a pesticide in food) on Codex, it is presumed to meet WTO obligations. Members retain the sovereign authority to choose measures that result in a higher level of protection than would be achieved under international standards (Art. 3.3). A member choosing a stricter standard will, if challenged, have to demonstrate that there is scientific support for its position and that it has conducted a risk assessment (Art. 5).

Necessity and Science. National SPS measures can be applied only to the extent necessary to protect human, animal, or plant life or health. They must be based on scientific principles and maintained only while justified by science (Art. 2[2]). There must be an "objective" or "rational" relationship between the SPS measure and the scientific evidence.[128]

Risk Assessments. National SPS measures must be based on objective risk assessments. Risk assessments must take into account available scientific evidence and public health methods, as well as economic costs. As explained in chapter 2, public health decisions often must be made under conditions of scientific uncertainty, and some argue for the application of the precautionary principle. The SPS Agreement permits the adoption of provisional measures based on the available data. Provisional measures, for example, could be taken in response to a novel outbreak of foodborne disease. Where this provision is invoked, members are required to seek the additional data needed to make a valid risk assessment, and while such investigations are pending, they must periodically review sanitary measures (Art. 5.7).

The European Community Beef Hormone Case (1998) examined the concepts of international standards, necessity, and risk assessments in the SPS Agreement.[129] The European Community (EC), in response to consumer concerns, banned imports of beef from cattle treated with one of six growth hormones. Five of these six hormones were governed by applicable international standards (Codex), but the EC argued that the import ban was permitted as a more stringent SPS measure designed to avert health risks. The risk assessment, however, failed to show that the hormones posed a significant risk to humans. The import ban violated the SPS Agreement because the EC did not conduct a risk assessment.[130]

The European Community Biotech Products Case, currently before the WTO, similarly concerns the adequacy of scientific data to support domestic health measures.[131] Despite the absence of scientific evidence that genetically modified (GM) food is harmful to humans,[132] European consumers sought the right to make informed choices. EU regulations require labeling and traceability, as well as authorization for placing GM ingredients on the market.[133] In 1999, the EU issued a four-year ban on new genetically modified crops. This resulted in three complaints to the WTO (from the United States, Canada, and Argentina). These cases were consolidated, and in 2006 an expert panel of the WTO Dispute Settlement Body held that the EU moratorium on genetically modified organisms violated the SPS Agreement and the Agreement on Technical Barriers to Trade. The panel found insufficient scientific evidence to support the moratorium.[134] The EU plans to appeal this ruling to an Appellate Body set up by the WTO Dispute Settlement Body.

The GMO case is fascinating because it raises the question of whether the EU moratorium could be justified under the precautionary principle. The EU cited consumer apprehension about food safety, eroded public trust in government oversight of the food industry, and concern about environmental effects, particularly biodiversity. Consumers are often unwilling to consider science to be a guarantee of quality. Should countries be permitted to require strict labeling and traceability, or restrict sale of GM products, despite the trade-restrictive effects? Does human health require the right to know about potential risks to people or the environment?

The *Beef Hormone* and *Biotech Products* cases raise the question of why states must base their regulations on demonstrable health effects. Should the precautionary principle apply, so that industry carries the burden of proving that their products do *not* cause harmful effects? Should governments be permitted to consider " nonhealth" interests, such as potential effects on the ecosystem or even consumer preferences? Suppose the EU had simply required manufacturers to label their products as containing GM organisms; the outcome could be just as "trade-restrictive" because consumers might not buy the product. How should the trade system deal with consumer preferences and the "right to know"?[135]

Trade-Related Aspects of Intellectual Property Rights (TRIPS): Compulsory Licensing

The TRIPS Agreement introduced intellectual property (IP) rules into the multilateral trading system. Ideas and knowledge are an increasingly important part of trade. Most of the value of new medicines, vaccines, and other high technology products lies in the invention, innovation, research, design, and testing. The TRIPS Agreement establishes minimum levels of IP protection that each WTO member must afford to creators, thus assuring more uniformity and bringing national policies under international rules with a dispute settlement system.

The central mission of the TRIPS Agreement is to protect and enforce IP rights "to the promotion of technological innovation and to the transfer and dissemination of technology, to the mutual advantage of producers and users of technological knowledge and in a manner conducive to social and economic welfare" (Art. 7). Whether the TRIPS Agreement is fair and effective, however, is still subject to bitter dispute and ongoing negotiation.[136]

Affording IP protection gives creators incentives to generate ideas to benefit society as a whole. At the same time, by giving creators exclusive rights to their inventions, designs, or other ideas, IP protection can make products unaffordable. It is for this reason that IP rights are so politically charged.[137] To entrepreneurs, IP protection is indispensable to scientific innovation and the long-term public good. They argue that exclusive rights to a drug or vaccine are necessary to recoup the high costs of research and development. To consumer advocates, however, IP protection can make essential medicines so expensive as to be inaccessible to the world's poorest people. Certainly, access to essential medicines is affected by many economic and noneconomic factors beyond IP protection. However, advocates believe that it is intolerable when countless people die of treatable diseases while pharmaceutical and biotech companies are enriched.

The TRIPS Agreement, in particular, has stirred intense debate about its effects on developing countries.[138] Arguably, poor countries do not have the systems of education, manufacturing, and marketing to innovate and gain the benefits of IP protection.[139] To these nations, TRIPS may afford little advantage because they possess few, if any, patentable products. At the same time, the TRIPS Agreement can make it difficult to produce or purchase affordable generic medications that countries need desperately. Some economists estimate that a transfer of $60 billion per year from poor to rich countries would occur if the TRIPS Agreement were fully implemented—caused mainly by increased patent and royalty payments as well as higher prices.[140]

The TRIPS Agreement affords protection to a variety of IP rights, including trademarks, copyrights, and designs.[141] Patent protection is perhaps most important in matters of health. The agreement requires patents for inventions to last at least twenty years (Art. 33). Patent protection must be available for both products (e.g., medicines) and processes (e.g., methods of producing chemical ingredients for medicines) in almost all fields of technology, with certain exceptions (Art. 27).[142] The agreement allows countries to adopt measures necessary to protect the public's health, provided that they are consistent with the provisions of the agreement (Art. 8).

The TRIPS Agreement allows countries to issue a compulsory license:

a legal vehicle whereby a government grants to itself or to a third party the right to produce or import a patented product without authorization from the patent holder (Art. 31). Compulsory licenses are subject to conditions: (1) the government must first attempt to negotiate a voluntary license from the right-holder on reasonable commercial terms; (2) the government need not seek a voluntary license in a national emergency or other urgent circumstance; (3) adequate remuneration must be paid to the right-holder, taking into account the economic value, if a compulsory license is issued; and (4) the compulsory license must be "predominantly for the supply of the domestic market."

In the aftermath of TRIPS, many developing countries began resisting the restrictive concessions required by the agreement.[143] As a result, the international community gradually became more sensitive to the public health concerns of developing nations, lessening international support for the harsh intellectual property demands of the United States and other industrialized nations. Accordingly, the U.S. government adopted a new strategy of negotiating bilateral or regional agreements with individual countries in an attempt to implement a U.S.-type intellectual property regime that does not recognize the tension between public health and intellectual property.[144] These so-called TRIPS-plus agreements further undermine the ability of developing nations to protect the public health of their citizens, beyond the restrictive levels already achieved by the TRIPS Agreement.[145]

The Doha Declaration

Although compulsory licensing was designed to provide the flexibility necessary to protect the public's health, the HIV/AIDS pandemic brought its shortcomings into stark contrast with its goals. Patented drugs cost anywhere from three to fifteen times that of their generic equivalents, although the cost of "front-line" drugs has been sharply reduced. Developing countries cannot afford to pay the high costs of combination drug therapy for HIV/AIDS—even when UNAIDS can negotiate a significantly lower cost. Highly active antiretroviral therapy reaches only 7 percent of people living with HIV/AIDS in low- and middle-income countries.

To ensure greater access to life-saving medications for resource-poor countries, the WTO Ministerial Conference promulgated the Declaration on the TRIPS Agreement and Public Health in November 2001.[146] The declaration explicitly recognized the public health problems facing resource-poor countries, especially HIV/AIDS, tuberculosis, and malaria. The declaration called for the TRIPS Agreement's "flexibilities" to be used to protect the public's health by promoting access to essential medicines: Countries have the right to determine what constitutes a national emergency and the grounds on which compulsory licenses are granted.

Countries with manufacturing capacity, such as Brazil, India, and Thailand, can produce generic antiretroviral medications for their populations. Domestic production of generic drugs can yield dramatic health benefits. Brazil, for example, was able to reduce AIDS deaths by 50 percent over a four-year period.[147] Countries manufacturing generic drugs faced intense pressure from the United States and pharmaceutical companies to respect existing patents. Indeed, in 2001, thirty-nine drug companies sued the South African government to block the production of generic anti-HIV drugs on the grounds that it breached patent protection. The suit was dropped when the public and NGOs protested vehemently.[148]

The Doha Declaration left an important problem unresolved. It recognized that "WTO Members with insufficient or no manufacturing capacities in the pharmaceutical sector could face difficulties in making effective use of compulsory licensing under the TRIPS Agreement." Industrialized countries could not help by exporting generic drugs because of the TRIPS Agreement requirement that compulsory licenses be primarily to supply the domestic market. The ministers charged the TRIPS Council to find "an expeditious solution to the problem" (Doha Declaration, paragraph 6).

A decision was nearly reached in December 2002, when 143 of 144 countries agreed to a waiver that would have allowed developed countries to export generic drugs made under compulsory license to countries that lacked manufacturing capacity. The United States was the only dissenter. Finally, in August 2003, all WTO members agreed to allow export of generic drugs under specified conditions.[149] Although the WHO has encouraged implementation of the August 2003 agreement,[150] progress has been painstakingly slow.[151]

The Doha Declaration was intended to prevent international trade rules from becoming a barrier to the provision of essential drugs.[152] Many problems remain, however, such as poor health care infrastructures in developing countries, making it difficult to deliver medicines to a large population and provide appropriate medical supervision. In retrospect, it is difficult to understand why politically and economically powerful countries would seek to use trade rules to prevent access to affordable treatments for the world's poor. It seems particularly incomprehensible that some members of the U.S. government argued for compulsory licensing of Ciprofloxacin Hydrochloride (Cipro) after the anthrax attacks in 2001 (which killed only a handful of people), while they opposed licensing of antiretrovirals for African nations burdened by millions of AIDS deaths.[153]

HUMAN RIGHTS: ADVANCING DIGNITY, JUSTICE, AND SECURITY IN HEALTH

> Where after all do universal human rights begin? In small places, closest to home—so close and so small that they cannot be seen on any map of the world. Yet they are the world of the individual person: The neighborhood he lives in; the school or college he attends; the factory, farm or office where he works. Such are the places where every man, woman, and child seeks equal justice, equal opportunity, equal dignity without discrimination. Unless these rights have meaning there, they have little meaning anywhere. Without concerted citizen action to uphold them close to home, we shall look in vain for progress in the larger world.
>
> Eleanor Roosevelt (1953)

International human rights law originated in response to the egregious affronts to peace and human dignity committed during World War II. The National Socialist German Workers Party (the Nazi Party of 1933–45) led by Adolf Hitler committed unspeakable atrocities, including genocide (Jews, the Roma, gays, people with disabilities) and human experimentation (sterilization, methods of execution, typhus, the effects of decompression and freezing water). The international community, after turning a blind eye to the events taking place during the Third Reich, was horrified when it realized the full extent of the wretchedness of the Nazi regime. Photographs of mass graves, piles of skeletons, and countless maltreated and emaciated prisoners were seared into the world's memory.

In the aftermath of the war, delegates of fifty nations signed the UN Charter at the San Francisco Conference on International Organization in 1945.[154] The U.S. representative, Eleanor Roosevelt, stressed the fundamental importance of human rights to a civilized world: "I know that we will be the sufferers if we let great wrongs occur without exerting ourselves to correct them."[155] In its preamble, the charter articulates the international community's determination "to reaffirm faith in fundamental human rights, [and] in the dignity and worth of the human person." The charter, as a binding treaty, pledges member states to promote "universal respect

BOX 16

THE UNITED NATIONS HUMAN RIGHTS COUNCIL

On March 15, 2005 the UN General Assembly voted to replace (effective June 2006) the Commission on Human Rights with the Human Rights Council. The council is a standing body with a generally elected membership, which meets no less than three times a year to address human rights concerns and evaluate the fulfillment of each UN member state's human rights obligations.

The council has been heralded as a bold move toward effective international protection for human rights and a significant improvement over the old commission, which met for one six-week session each year, and which suffered from a lack of credibility in recent years as it failed to adopt resolutions on the gross human rights violations in Iraq, Chechnya, and Darfur. The council gives any member the power to propose a country-specific resolution, and the frequency of meetings allows for faster action.

The old commission was frequently criticized for giving seats to member states with poor domestic human rights records, such as Zimbabwe, Libya, and Sudan; these states successfully thwarted action on their own human rights violations. The first set of member countries elected to the new council, however, has been controversial, and its actions have been criticized by human rights advocates. Six elected member states—China, Cuba, Pakistan, Russia, Saudi Arabia, and Azerbaijan—have been cited by human rights NGOs as not deserving membership. The United States (along with the Marshall Islands, Palau, and Israel) voted against the council's creation, claiming that it will have insufficient safeguards against membership of and control by rights-abusing nations; the United States did not seek a seat on the new council.

The General Assembly resolution establishing the council reaffirmed that "all human rights are universal, indivisible, interrelated, interdependent and mutually reinforcing and that all human rights must be treated in a fair and equal manner, on the same footing and with the same emphasis."[1] The resolution makes no mention of health but does reaffirm commitment to political, cultural, and socioeconomic rights, as well as the importance of development in the realization of human rights.

[1] G.A. Res. 60/521, U.N. Doc. A/60/L.48 (Mar. 15, 2006).

for, and observance of, human rights and fundamental freedoms for all without distinction as to race, sex, language, or religion" (Arts. 55, 56).

The charter established the Economic and Social Council (ECOSOC) as the principal organ to coordinate the economic and social work of the United Nations, notably international health and universal respect for human rights. ECOSOC created the Commission on Human Rights in 1946, and the Sub-Commission on Promotion and Protection of Human Rights the following year. (The Council on Human Rights replaced the Commission on Human Rights in 2005—see box 16.) The UN High Commissioner on Human Rights (UNHCHR), created in 1993, is the principal UN official with responsibility for human rights. The two international covenants created their own monitoring and compliance mechanisms: The International Covenant on Civil and Political Rights

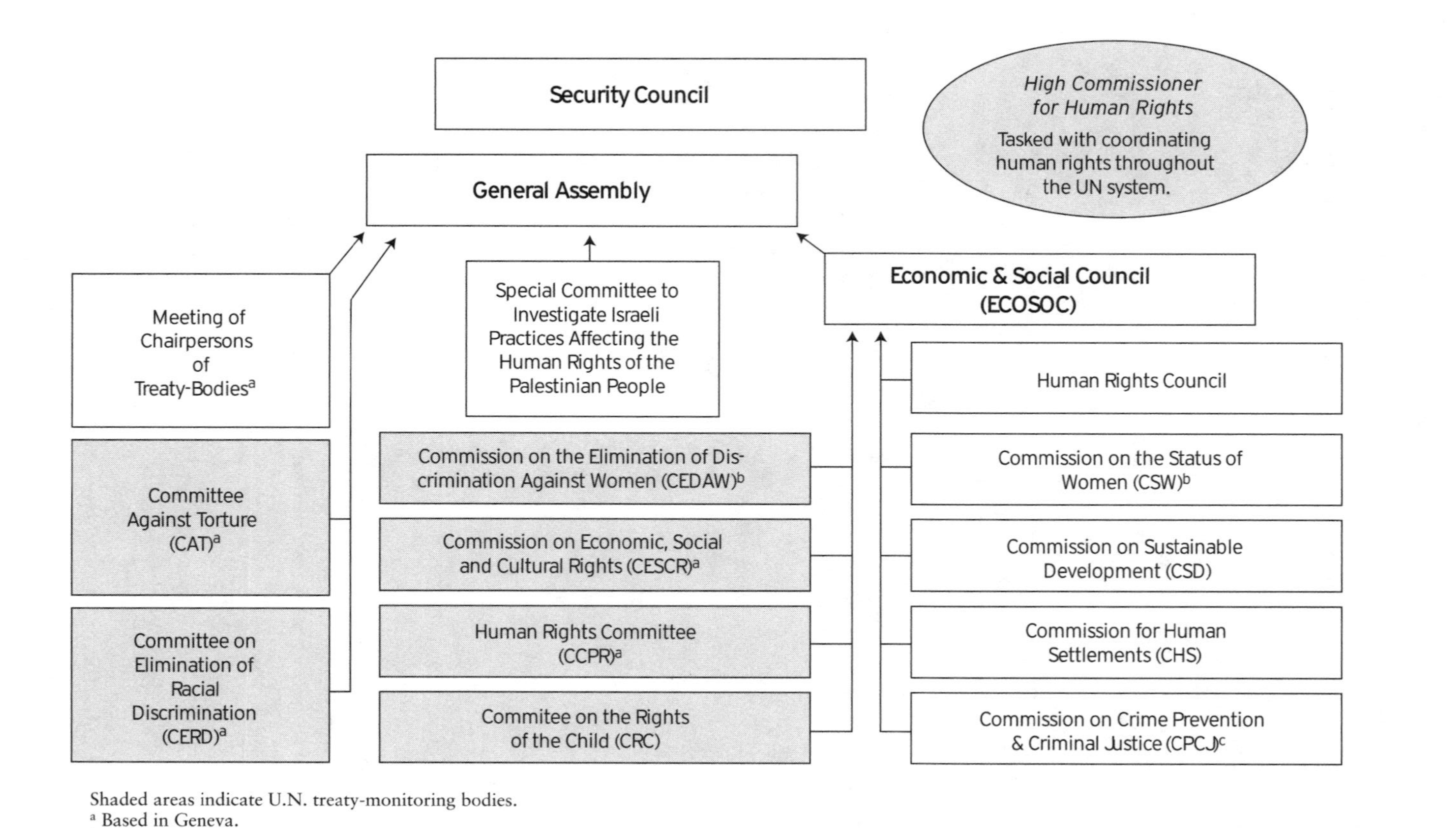

Shaded areas indicate U.N. treaty-monitoring bodies.
[a] Based in Geneva.
[b] Based in New York.
[c] Based in Vienna.

Figure 29. United Nations human rights bodies.

(ICCPR) established the Human Rights Committee, and the International Covenant on Economic, Social, and Cultural Rights (ICESCR) established the Committee on Economic, Cultural and Social Rights (see figure 29).

The basic characteristics of human rights are that they inhere in all people because all people are human; they are universal, hence people everywhere in the world are "rights-holders"; and they impose robust duties on the state.[156] State duties, particularly applicable to economic, social, and cultural rights, encompass the obligation to *respect*—states do not interfere directly or indirectly with the enjoyment of human rights; *protect*—states take measures to prevent private actors from interfering with the right; and *fulfill* or facilitate—states take positive measures (e.g., legislative, budgetary, and promotional) to enable and assist individuals and communities to enjoy rights. Human rights are protected under international law, so that a state can no longer assert that systematic maltreatment of its own nationals is exclusively a domestic concern.[157]

The main source of human rights law within the UN system is the International Bill of Human Rights, comprising the UN Charter, the Universal Declaration of Human Rights, two international covenants on human rights, and an optional protocol. The United Nations has promulgated numerous treaties dealing with specific human rights violations, including racial and gender discrimination, the rights of the child, genocide, and torture.[158] Human rights are also protected under regional systems, including those in the Americas, Europe, and Africa.[159]

The Universal Declaration of Human Rights (UDHR)

The UDHR, adopted in 1948, built upon the promise of the UN Charter by identifying specific rights and freedoms that deserve promotion and protection. The UDHR was the organized international community's first attempt to establish "a common standard of achievement for all peoples and all nations" to promote human rights (Preamble). The UDHR represents a milestone in the struggle of humanity for freedom and human dignity, stating that human rights are self-evident, the "highest aspiration of the common people" (Preamble). Article 1 proclaims: "All human beings are born free and equal in dignity and rights." The Universal Declaration is not a treaty but rather a resolution with no force of law. Nevertheless, its key provisions have so often been applied and accepted that they are now widely considered to have attained the status of customary international law.[160]

The adoption of the UDHR set the stage for a binding, treaty-based scheme to promote and protect human rights. The ICCPR and the ICESCR were adopted in 1966 and entered into force in 1976.[161] The United States has ratified the ICCPR but not the ICESCR. The division of human rights into separate treaties perhaps symbolizes an ideological division between liberal democracies, which view personal autonomy and freedom as salient values, and countries with social welfare traditions, which view socioeconomic needs and equality as salient values. Although there are differences, it is important to emphasize that all rights are interdependent, interrelated, and of equal importance.

The ICCPR and the Optional Protocol

The ICCPR imposes an immediate obligation "to respect and to ensure" civil and political rights (see table 10). The principal compliance mechanisms of the ICCPR are reporting and complaints systems.[162] States Parties are required to report to the Human Rights Committee (HRC), established by the ICCPR, on the measures adopted and progress made in the enjoyment of civil and political rights (Art. 40[1]). The ICCPR also empowers a State Party to charge another with a violation of the treaty, but the enforcement is weak (Arts. 42, 43). The interstate complaints system is available only if the state has acceded to the committee's jurisdiction, and there is no formal adjudication procedure. Private parties may submit individual complaints, but only if the State Party has separately ratified the First Optional Protocol to the ICCPR. Individuals must first exhaust all available domestic remedies. The decisions or "views" of the HRC represent an important body of human rights case law. There is no specific enforcement, but the HRC has established a special rapporteur for follow-up and requires states to report their conformance measures.

The ICESCR

The UDHR characterizes economic, social, and cultural rights as "indispensable for [a person's] dignity and the development of his personality" (Art. 22) (see table 11). Yet, unlike the ICCPR, States Parties are not obliged to immediately implement the ICESCR but rather undertake:

> to take steps, individually and though international assistance and co-operation, especially economic and technical, to the maximum of its available resources, with a view to achieving progressively the full realization of the rights recognized . . . by all appropriate means, including particularly the adoption of legislative measures. (Art. 2)

TABLE 10. International Covenant on Civil and Political Rights (ICCPR)

Nonderogable Rights[a]	Derogable Rights
Article 6: Freedom from arbitrary deprivation of life; inherent right to life	Articles 1, 25: Right to self-determination of the pursuit of economic, social, and cultural development
Article 7: Freedom from torture and cruel, inhuman, or degrading treatment or punishment and freedom from subjection without free consent to medical or scientific treatment	Article 9: Right to liberty and security of person; freedom from arbitrary arrest or detention
Article 8: Freedom from being held in slavery and servitude	Article 10: Right to be treated with humanity and with respect for the inherent dignity of the human person if deprived of liberty
Article 11: Freedom from imprisonment merely for an inability to fulfill contractual obligation	
Article 14: Right to be equal before courts and tribunals	
Article 15: Freedom from being convicted of an act that was not a criminal offense at the time of the action and freedom from imposition of heavier penalties than those imposed for the offense	Articles 17, 23: Freedom from arbitrary or unlawful interference with one's privacy, family, or reputation
Articles 16, 26: Right to recognition everywhere as a person before the law	Articles 21, 22: Right to peaceful assembly and association with others
Articles 18, 19: Freedom of thought, conscience, and religion	Article 24: Right of child to protection

NOTE: Adopted by General Assembly resolution 2200A (XXI) on December 16, 1966, entered into force March 23, 1976. The ICCPR supplements the Universal Declaration of Human Rights and enumerates fundamental civil and political rights that states must recognize and protect.

[a] Article 4, paragraph 2, lists seven nonderogable rights, rights that cannot be altered or suspended during public emergencies.

The language of "progressive realization" and "maximum resources" may have been inserted because economic and social rights typically require greater funding and more complex solutions than civil and political rights. Still, the Committee on Economic, Social and Cultural Rights, established by the ICESCR, made clear that States Parties do have immediate obligations. "Steps" toward the goal of full realization "must be taken within a reasonably short time." States Parties have "a mini-

TABLE 11. International Covenant on Economic, Social and Cultural Rights (ICESCR)

Right[a]	Article
Right of self-determination to freely pursue economic, social, and cultural development	1
Right to work and to the opportunity to gain a living by freely chosen and accepted work	6
Right to the enjoyment of just and favorable conditions of work	7
Right to form and join trade unions of choice	8
Right to social security and social insurance	9
Protection of family, of mothers before and after childbirth, and of children from economic and social exploitation	10
Right to an adequate standard of living for self and family and to be free from hunger	11
Right to the enjoyment of the highest attainable standard of physical and mental health	12
Right to education	13
Right to take part in cultural life	15
Right to enjoy the benefits and applications of social progress	15
Right to benefit from the protection of moral or material interests resulting from one's own products	15

NOTE: Adopted by General Assembly resolution 2200A (XXI) on December 16, 1966, entered into force January 3, 1976. The ICESCR supplements the Universal Declaration of Human Rights and enumerates fundamental economic, social, and cultural rights that states should recognize and protect.

[a] The ICESCR does not recognize any rights as nonderogable. However, Article 4 specifies that these rights can only be limited by law, as long as the limitations are "compatible with the nature of these rights and solely for the purpose of promoting the general welfare in a democratic society."

mum core obligation to ensure the satisfaction of . . . each of the rights." The committee also said that States Parties should immediately implement legislation and judicial remedies to ensure nondiscrimination in the exercise of economic and social rights (Art. 2[1]).[163]

The ICESCR does not establish a formal complaints system, but requires States Parties to submit reports to ECOSOC. The council has delegated the task of reviewing state reports to the Committee on Economic, Social and Cultural Rights.[164]

Valid Public Health Limitations on Human Rights

Human rights have transcending value, but international law does allow restrictions when necessary for the public good. Under the UDHR, the sole purpose for the limitation of rights is to secure "due recognition and respect for the rights and freedoms of others and of meeting the just requirements of morality, public order and general welfare in a democratic society (Art. 29[2])." States may not "perform any act aimed at the destruction of any of the rights and freedoms" proclaimed in the declaration (Art. 30).

The two covenants diverge in their treatment of permissible derogations and limitations. The ICCPR's most fundamental guarantees are so essential as to be absolute, and no state, even in a time of emergency, may derogate from them. The ICCPR, however, allows States Parties "in time of public emergency that threatens the life of the nation" to suspend most other civil and political rights (Art. 4) (see table 10). The state must officially proclaim the public emergency and cannot engage in discrimination. The principal conditions for restraints on civil and political rights are that they must be prescribed by law; be enacted within a democratic society; and be necessary to secure public order, public health, public morals, national security, public safety, or the rights and freedoms of others.[165] However, States Parties may not impose restrictions aimed at the destruction of rights or their limitation to a greater extent than provided in the covenant (Art. 5[1]).[166]

The Siracusa Principles, conceptualized at a meeting in Siracusa, Italy, in 1985, are widely recognized as a legal standard for measuring valid limitations on human rights.[167] The principles make clear that even when the state acts for good reasons, it must respect human dignity and freedom. Echoing the language of the ICCPR, the Siracusa Principles require that state limitations must be: in accordance with the law; based on a legitimate objective; strictly necessary in a democratic society; the least restrictive and intrusive means available; and not arbitrary, unreasonable, or discriminatory. International tribunals have relied on the Siracusa Principles to require states to use the least restrictive measure necessary to achieve the public health purpose.[168]

It is far more difficult to think about legitimate limitations on economic, social, and cultural rights. The ICESCR permits "such limitations as are determined by law only in so far as this may be compatible with the nature of these rights and solely for the purpose of promoting the general welfare in a democratic society (Art. 4)."[169] Since the ICESCR includes a "right to health," it is best to conceptualize valid "limitations" as those measures necessary to attain health protection for the population. For example, the covenant requires States Parties to prevent, treat, and control epidemic, endemic, and occupational diseases

(Art. 12[2][c]). Thus, compulsory measures such as vaccination, treatment, or isolation would be permitted only if necessary to protect the public's health.

The "Right to Health"

Human rights constitute perhaps the most important social movement of the twentieth century. In the latter part of that century and up to the present day, the theory and practice of human rights have been applied to another transcending human value: the health and safety of the world's population.[170] The International Bill of Human Rights, as well as numerous UN and regional human rights treaties, proclaims the right to health. Many countries also have incorporated a right to health or health care under domestic law[171] (see table 12).

The widespread recognition of health as an entitlement demonstrates its normative value in international law, even though states do not always safeguard the right to health. Viewing health as a fundamental right, part of the fabric of democracy and justice, transforms the social and political discourse.[172] The language of "rights" suggests that states have obligations and can be held accountable for violations.[173] The states' obligations, moreover, are not limited to medical care but extend to insurance of the socioeconomic conditions necessary for people to lead healthy and safe lives (e.g., nutrition, housing, uncontaminated drinking water, sanitation, safe workplaces, and a clean environment).

The basic mission of the United Nations includes the creation of conditions that support the world's health. The UN Charter pledges to find "solutions of international economic, social, [and] health problems" (Art. 56). Article 25 of the UDHR proclaims: "Everyone has the right to a standard of living adequate for the health and well-being of himself and his family, including food, clothing, housing and medical care and necessary social services, and the right to security in the event of unemployment, sickness, disability, widowhood, old age or other lack of livelihood in circumstances beyond his control." Thus, the UDHR constructs the right to health as encompassing the basic necessities of life and a state-supported safety net of services.

The ICESCR recognizes "the right of everyone to the highest attainable standard of physical and mental health." Article 12 defines the steps needed to achieve full realization of the right to health: reduction of the stillbirth rate and infant mortality, and healthy development of the child; improvement in environmental and industrial hygiene; prevention,

TABLE 12. Sources for the human right to health

Document	Provision
International Agreements	
Universal Declaration on Human Rights	Everyone has a right to a standard of living adequate for the health and well-being of himself and of his family. (Art. 25)
International Covenant on Economic, Social and Cultural Rights	The States Parties to the present Covenant recognize the right of everyone to the enjoyment of the highest attainable standard of physical and mental health. (Art. 12)
UN Declaration on the Rights of the Child	The child shall enjoy special protection, and shall be given opportunities and facilities . . . to enable him to develop physically, mentally, morally, spiritually and socially in a healthy and normal manner and in conditions of freedom and dignity. (Prin. 2)
Convention on the Elimination of All Forms of Discrimination against Women	States Parties shall take all appropriate measures to eliminate discrimination against women in the field of health care in order to ensure, on a basis of equality of men and women, access to health care services, including those related to family planning. (Art. 12)
Convention on the Elimination of All Forms of Racial Discrimination	States Parties undertake to prohibit and to eliminate racial discrimination in all its forms and to guarantee . . . the right to public health, medical care, social security and social services. (Art. 5)
Regional Accords	
European Social Charter	With a view to ensuring the effective exercise of the right to protection of health, the Contracting Parties undertake . . . to remove as far as possible the causes of ill-health, to provide . . . facilities for the promotion of health and the encouragement of individual responsibility in matters of health, [and] to prevent as far as possible epidemic, endemic and other diseases. (Art. 11)
African Charter on Human and Peoples' Rights	Human beings are inviolable. Every human being shall be entitled to respect for his life and the integrity of his person. No one may be arbitrarily deprived of this right. (Art. 4)
American Convention on Human Rights: Protocol of San Salvador	Everyone shall have the right to health, understood to mean the enjoyment of the highest level of physical, mental and social well-being. (Art. 10)

TABLE 12. *(continued)*

Document	Provision
Major Initiatives	
Declaration of Alma Ata	Governments have a responsibility for the health of their people which can be fulfilled only by the provision of adequate health and social measures. (Decl. V)
Vienna Declaration	The World Conference on Human Rights calls upon States to refrain from any unilateral measure . . . that creates obstacles to . . . the rights of everyone to a standard of living adequate for their health and well-being. (Decl. 31)
Rio Declaration on Environment and Development	Human beings are . . . entitled to a healthy and productive life in harmony with nature. (Prin. 1)
Copenhagen Declaration on Health Policy	We, the delegations of the Member States in the European Region of the World Health Organization, . . . pledge ourselves to promote and protect the health of our peoples as a fundamental value of our societies. (Opening)
Beijing Declaration	The explicit recognition and reaffirmation of the right of all women to control all aspects of their health, in particular their own fertility, is basic to their empowerment. (Decl. 17)
National Constitutions	
Constitution of South Africa	Everyone has the right to have access to health care services, including reproductive health care. (Bill of Rights, § 27(1))
Constitution of the Russian Federation	Everyone shall have the right to health care and medical assistance. (§ 1, Ch. 2, Art. 41)
Constitution of the Great Socialist People's Libyan Arab Jamahiriya	Health care is a right guaranteed by the State through the creation of hospitals and health establishments in accordance with the law. (Art. 15)
Constitution of the Republic of Haiti	The State has the absolute obligation to guarantee the right to life, health, and respect of the human person for all citizens without distinction, in conformity with the Universal Declaration of the Rights of Man. (Ch. 2, § A, Art. 19)
Constitution of the Republic of the Philippines	The State shall protect and promote the right to health of the people and instill health consciousness among them. (Art. II, § 15)

SOURCE: World Health Organization, "Twenty-five Questions and Answers on Health and Human Rights," *Health and Human Rights Publication Series,* 1 (2002): 29–31.

BOX 17

THE RIGHT TO THE HIGHEST ATTAINABLE STANDARD OF HEALTH

General Comment 14, issued by the Committee on Economic, Social and Cultural Rights (CESCR), proclaims that "health is a fundamental human right indispensable for the exercise of other human rights. Every human being is entitled to the enjoyment of the highest attainable standard of health conducive to living a life in dignity." The CESCR categorizes the right to health in terms of norms, obligations, violations, and implementation, and encourages states to "respect, protect, and fulfill" the right to health.

Norms

The normative content of the right to health is expressed in terms of "availability, accessibility, acceptability, and quality" of public health and health care services. "Availability" requires healthy conditions (e.g., safe and potable drinking water and sanitation) and functioning health services (e.g., hospitals, clinics, trained health care professionals, and essential drugs). "Accessibility" requires health services to be accessible to the entire population, without discrimination or physical, geographical, or economic barriers. "Acceptability" requires adherence to medical ethics and culturally appropriate health services. "Quality" requires health services to be scientifically and medically appropriate and of good quality.

Obligations

General Comment 14 imposes "core obligations" to ensure minimum services, including: (i) access to health on a nondiscriminatory basis, especially for vulnerable or marginalized groups; (ii) essential food that is nutritionally adequate and safe; (iii) basic shelter, sanitation, and safe and potable water; and (iv) essential drugs. The CESCR gives priority to the following services: reproductive and maternal, immunization, infectious disease control, and health information.

Violations

In determining which actions or omissions violate the right to health, it is important to distinguish between a state's inability to comply (due to lack of resources) and its unwillingness to comply. Violations through *acts of omission* include failure to take appropriate steps to realize everyone's right to the enjoyment of the highest attainable standard of physical and mental health. Violations through *actions* include state policies that contravene the standards set in the General Comment and are likely to result in injury, disease, or premature mortality (e.g., denial of access to health services or deliberate withholding of information vital to health).

Implementation

The General Comment contains detailed standards for implementing the right to health, including the duty to: (i) adopt framework legislation (e.g., a national strategy and plan of action, with sufficient resources); (ii) identify appropriate right to health indicators and benchmarks (e.g., to monitor improvements in community health); and (iii) establish adequate remedies and accountability (e.g., access to courts, ombudsmen, or human rights commissions).

BOX 18

THE SPECIAL RAPPORTEUR ON THE RIGHT TO HEALTH

The Commission on Human Rights created a Special Rapporteur on the Right to Health in 2002 with a mandate to form an understanding of "the right of everyone to the enjoyment of the highest attainable standard of physical and mental health."[1] The Rapporteur's work includes gathering and sharing information, reporting on the status of the right to health, and proposing recommendations.

The first Special Rapporteur, Paul Hunt, was appointed in August 2002. He focused on themes relating to vulnerable populations: poverty, discrimination, and stigma.[2] He offered leading indicators (measures for evaluation) for the right to health: structures, processes, and outcomes. Structural indicators inquire whether adequate systems that affect health are in place (e.g., does the state include the right to health in its constitution?). Process and outcome indicators measure progress over time, consistent with the idea of the progressive realization (e.g., benchmarks or targets). Process indicators monitor effort (e.g., the proportion of women receiving prenatal care) and outcome indicators measure results (e.g., infant mortality and life expectancy).

The Special Rapporteur has issued reports on the elements of the right to health, reproductive rights, mental disabilities,[3] and the effects of trade on health.[4] By opening a dialogue between governments, civil society organizations, and international bodies, the Special Rapporteur has increased the visibility of the right to health while clarifying its meaning.

[1] UN Commission on Human Rights, Res. 2002/31, U.N. Doc. E/CN.4/2002/20 (Apr. 22, 2002).
[2] Hunt, U.N. Doc. E/CN.4/2005/51, ¶ 41.
[3] See also Lawrence O. Gostin and Lance Gable, "The Human Rights of Persons with Mental Disabilities: A Global Perspective on the Application of Human Rights Principles to Mental Health," *Maryland Law Review*, 63 (2004): 120-21.
[4] Hunt, U.N. Doc. E/CN.4/2004/49.

treatment, and control of epidemic, endemic, and occupational diseases; and the creation of conditions to assure medical services in the event of sickness. The ICESCR, therefore, defines the right to health as encompassing both physical and mental health and offers concrete tasks to achieve the goal. The covenant refers to the "highest attainable" standard of health because many aspects of health are not within the state's exclusive control—e.g., genetics, accidents, and socioeconomic class.

The meaning of the right to health is not inherent in the text. Work, therefore, is needed to clarify state obligations, identify violations, and establish criteria and procedures for enforcement. The contours of the right to health have been richly developed by the Committee on Economic, Social and Cultural Rights in General Comment No. 14[174] and by the Special Rapporteur on the Right to Health appointed by the General Assembly[175] (see boxes 17 and 18).

The International Bill of Human Rights has become a powerful tool in public discourse and international law. Certainly, there are marked deficiencies in the clarity and enforcement of human rights. Nevertheless, a growing body of case law and commentary is advancing the theory and practice of international human rights. Just as important, the language of human rights is being employed in every region to assert fundamental claims of human dignity, inspire action, and persuade governments to act for the individual and collective good.

This chapter has explained the most basic problem in global health: why health hazards seem to change form and migrate everywhere on earth. States should care about serious health threats outside their borders and realize that solutions cannot be found solely in domestic regulation. Rather, the international community needs to find innovative ways to govern the wide variety of actors in the public and private sectors that powerfully influence global health. International law can play an important role in global needs for health protection. International instruments in a wide variety of health contexts have been created, but this chapter has only been able to discuss a few of the more important ones: the IHR, FCTC, WTO agreements, and international bill of human rights. This body of international law is certainly helpful, but much more needs to be accomplished to ensure adequate capacities to protect global health, as well as to foster greater cooperation among states and civil society more generally.

Amelioration of the enduring and complex problems of global health is virtually impossible without a collective response. No state or stakeholder, acting alone, can avert the ubiquitous threats of pathogens, and even unhealthy lifestyles, as they rapidly migrate. Truly effective global health governance could significantly improve life prospects for the world's population.

Given the pervasive health hazards faced by global society, perhaps we are coming to a tipping point where the status quo is no longer acceptable and it is time to take bold action. Global health, like global climate change, may soon become a matter so important to the world's future that it demands international attention, and no state can escape the responsibility to act.[176]

PART THREE

Public Health and Civil Liberties in Conflict

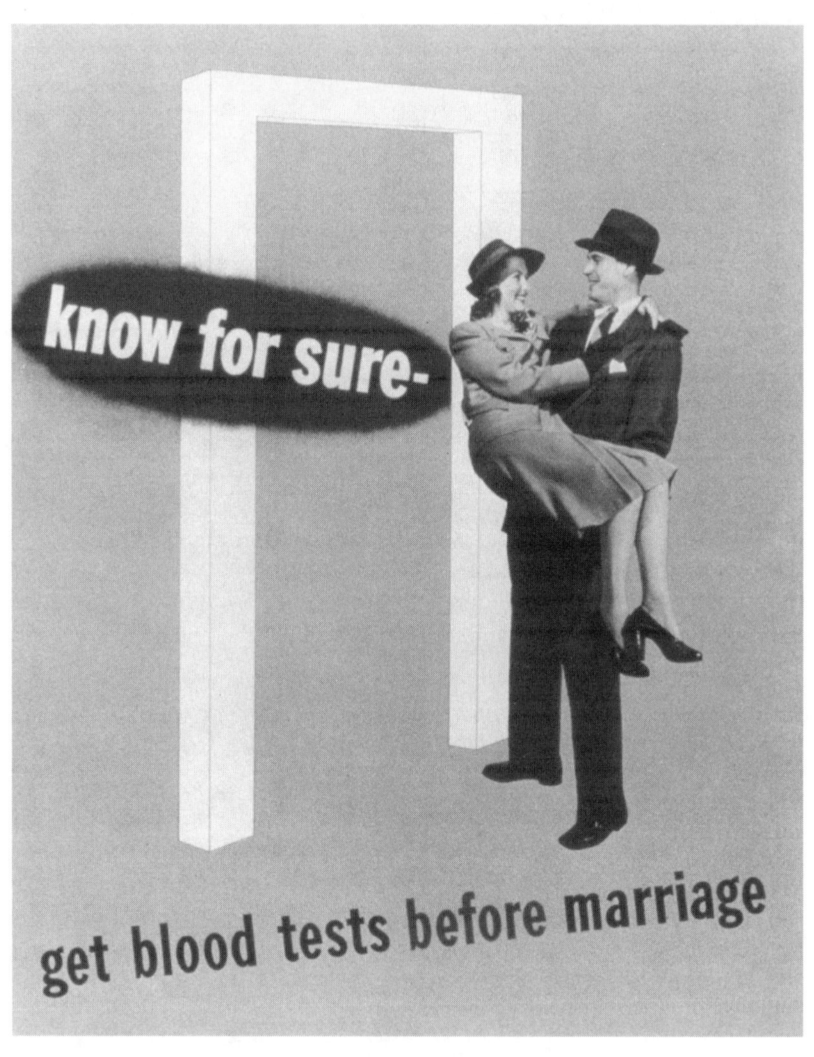

Photo 15. Public Health Service campaign encouraging premarital blood tests. This 1940s poster was part of a Public Health Service campaign to encourage testing for syphilis before marriage. Many states enacted laws requiring premarital screening for sexually transmitted diseases. Courtesy of the National Library of Medicine.

CHAPTER 8

Surveillance and Public Health Research

Personal Privacy and the "Right to Know"

> Half the life is passed in infancy, sickness and dependent helplessness . . . in exhibiting the high mortality, the diseases by which it is occasioned and the exciting causes of disease, the abstracts of the registers will prove that while a part of the sickness is inevitable and a part may be expected to disappear by progressive social amelioration a considerable proportion may be suppressed by the general adoption of hygienic measures.
>
> William Farr (1838)

One of the core functions of the public health system is to gather health information and deploy those data for the welfare of the community.[1] Information concerning risk factors for—and patterns, trends, and causes of—injury and disease forms the basis for rational public health decision making. Health information is indispensable for virtually all public health activities, including identifying, monitoring, and forecasting health threats; prevention, response, and intervention; program evaluation; and population-based research. It is for this reason that biostatistics and epidemiology are the foundational sciences of public health. Together, they supply the empirical evidence upon which public health judgments are made and upon which public policy should rely.

I define the public health information infrastructure as the acquisition, use, retention, and transmission of data about the population's health that supports the essential functions of the public health system (see tables 13 and 14). The development of population-based information systems in electronic form is not a distant concept, but an emerging

TABLE 13. Essential public health functions

Function	Definition
Assessment	Identify needs, analyze causes, and find cases
Policy Development	Determine priorities, objectives, and means
Assurance	Ensure services to meet health needs

reality.[2] National, regional, and statewide databases are becoming vast reservoirs of public health information. Public health agencies can collect, reconfigure, identify patterns in, and disseminate health information with a speed and efficiency never before possible.[3]

A sound public health information infrastructure can produce many social benefits,[4] including the early detection of naturally occurring (e.g., *Cryptosporidium* or *E. coli*) or intentional (e.g., anthrax or *salmonella*) microbial infections, environmental exposures (e.g., lead poisoning or radon), behavioral risks (e.g., iatrogenic injuries or gunshot wounds), and other health threats (e.g., child abuse). Effective public health information systems can also concentrate resources and focus interventions in the areas of greatest need; promote behavioral, social, and environmental changes by identifying hazards and providing health information to persons at risk; assess public health measures by evaluations of effectiveness and cost; and affect legislation and alter social norms by providing accurate health information to citizens and policymakers. In short, health data enable agencies to identify health risks, inform the public, intervene, and influence funding decisions, all of which are indispensable to the mission of public health.

The systematic acquisition of personal health data, however, poses serious privacy risks to individuals and groups. American society places a high value on individual rights, autonomous decision making, and protection of the private sphere from governmental or other intrusion.[5] Health information can reveal intimate aspects about an individual's or a family's life and may affect the ability to hold a job, maintain custody of children, secure immigration status, or obtain access to insurance or public benefits. As vastly greater quantities of information are collected and transmitted to an increasing number of users, the ability of individuals to control access to personal information is sharply reduced.

Scholars sometimes assume that significant levels of privacy can coexist with the development of a modern public health information infrastructure. To a certain extent, respecting confidences and promoting

TABLE 14. The sciences and practices of public health: Definitions

Public Health Information Infrastructure	The acquisition, use, retention, and transmission of data about the population's health that supports the essential functions of the public health system.
Epidemiology	The discipline concerned with the study of the distribution and determinants of health-related states or events in specified populations, and the application of this study to control health problems. Epidemiologists seek patterns, trends, and causes of morbidity and premature mortality, and proceed from two basic premises: (1) disease is not randomly distributed in populations, and (2) subgroups differ in both disease frequency and contributing factors. (Originally the study of epidemics.)
Biostatistics	The branch of statistics that analyzes data derived from the medical and biological sciences and is concerned with (1) the collection, organization, and summarization of data and (2) the drawing of inferences about a body of data when only part of the data is observed.
Public Health Surveillance	The public health practice of continual watchfuness over the distribution and trends of risk factors, injury, and disease in the population through the systematic collection, analysis, and interpretation of selected health data for use in the planning, implementation, and evaluation of public health practice.

public health are consistent goals. Public health depends on the community's trust and cooperation, and failure to safeguard privacy discourages individuals from participating in programs such as screening, partner notification, and medical treatment. However, we cannot have it both ways; that is, society cannot fully protect privacy while still maintaining all the collective benefits of health information. Because privacy cannot realistically be assured, we confront a hard choice. Should we sharply limit the systematic collection of identifiable health data in order to achieve high levels of informational privacy? Alternatively, we may decide that the value of information is so important to the achievement of societal aspirations for health that government should not impede data flows with strong privacy safeguards.

This chapter first examines the major methods of information gathering undertaken by public health authorities: surveillance, reporting, partner notification, and public health research. Then it takes a hard look at two forms of personal privacy—informational privacy and relational privacy—including major ethical dilemmas faced by health care professionals such as those occasioned by the "duty to warn" and the "right to know." Finally, it presents a model law designed to safeguard personal privacy while not unduly diminishing effective public health action.

PUBLIC HEALTH SURVEILLANCE

The French word *surveillance* was introduced into the English language at the time of the Napoleonic wars and meant "a close watch or guard kept over a person."[6] Today, public health surveillance means the continued watchfulness over the distribution and trends of risk factors, injury, and disease in the population through the systematic collection, analysis, and interpretation of selected health data for use in the planning, implementation, and evaluation of public health practice.[7] Surveillance activities range from case-specific interventions (e.g., reporting, contact tracing, and outbreak investigations), which engender privacy concerns, to statistical methods (collection of aggregate data—e.g., serological and behavioral surveys, and vital statistics).

Historically, surveillance focused on identifying and controlling persons with communicable diseases. Mandatory reporting of diseases predated the founding of the republic. A Rhode Island statute of 1741 required tavern keepers to report to local authorities any patrons known to harbor contagious diseases.[8] Systematic disease reporting at the state level was initiated in 1874, when Massachusetts instituted a voluntary plan for weekly physician reporting. In a letter to physicians, the State Board of Health enclosed a sample notification card to "reduce to the minimum the expenditure of time and trouble incident to the service asked of busy medical men."[9]

The federal government instituted national mortality data collection in 1850, the year of the first decennial census,[10] followed by morbidity data collection on plague, cholera, smallpox, and yellow fever in 1878.[11] The U.S. Public Health Service circulated a model law in 1913 to harmonize reporting requirements, but few states adopted it.[12] It was not until 1925 that all states participated in national morbidity reporting, following the 1916 poliomyelitis and 1918–19 influenza epidemics, which heightened public awareness of infectious diseases.[13]

Infectious disease surveillance assumed critical public health importance in the mid- to late twentieth century. In 1955, acute poliomyelitis among vaccine recipients in the United States threatened the entire vaccination

BOX 19

BIOSURVEILLANCE: NEDSS, BIOSENSE, AND SYNDROMIC SURVEILLANCE

Early detection of novel infections and bioterrorism

Biosurveillance is the systematic monitoring of a wide range of health data of potential value in detecting emerging health threats, whether occurring naturally or as a result of bioterrorism.[1] Data sources can include reportable diseases, medical records (managed care, hospitals, and emergency rooms), pharmacy sales, school and work absenteeism, and calls to nurse hotlines.[2] Public health agencies at all levels of government collect, analyze, and share these data as an early warning system and to monitor ongoing health threats. Since public health agencies collect voluminous data, they must employ sophisticated statistical methods and information technologies. Contemporary biosurveillance activities include the National Electronic Disease Surveillance System (NEDSS), BioSense, and syndromic surveillance, all supported through federal programs.

NEDSS promotes the development of efficient, integrated, and interoperable surveillance systems at federal, state, and local levels.[3] The vision of NEDSS is to have complementary and integrated electronic information systems for public health, laboratory, and clinical data. NEDSS should facilitate data collection on a real-time basis, monitoring community health, analyzing trends and detecting emerging public health problems, and providing information for setting public health policy.[4] NEDSS allows secure transfer of data through the Internet.

BioSense is the national program designed to improve the nation's capabilities for real-time biosurveillance and situational awareness at a time when most health information systems vary in their ability to acquire, use, and share data. By providing access to data from hospitals and health care systems in major metropolitan cities across the nation, BioSense connects existing medical information to public health. It provides immediate, constant, and comparable information needed to inform local, state, and national public health efforts and to support national preparedness.[5]

Syndromic surveillance is the collection, analysis, and use of health-related data that precede diagnosis and signal probability of a case or outbreak sufficient to warrant further public health response.[6] By focusing on symptoms rather than confirmed

[1] Mark A. Hoffman, Tiffany H. Wilkinson, Aaron Bush, et al., "Multijurisdictional Approach to Biosurveillance, Kansas City," *Emerging Infectious Diseases,* 9 (2003): 1281–86.

[2] Association of State and Territorial Health Officers, "Biosurveillance: Position Statement," *Association of State and Territorial Health Officers,* 2006, http://www.astho.org/pubs/BiosurveillancePositionStatementFINAL030706.pdf (biosurveillance systems should be developed with established protocols, including consequence management, system integrity, timeliness of information sharing, and appropriate safeguards).

[3] Nkuchia M. M'ikanatha, Brian Southwell, and Ebbing Lautenbach, "Automated Laboratory Reporting of Infectious Diseases in a Climate of Bioterrorism," *Emerging Infectious Diseases,* 9 (2003): 1053–57.

[4] Centers for Disease Control and Prevention, "An Overview of NEDSS Initiative," *Centers for Disease Control and Prevention,* http://www.cdc.gov/nedss/About/overview.html.

[5] Centers for Disease Control and Prevention, "Public Health Preparedness—Programs In Brief: BioSense," *Centers for Disease Control and Prevention,* December 2004; Council of State and Territorial Epidemiologists, "Coordinated State, Federal and Local Public Health Surveillance Using BioSense for Situational Awareness," *Council of State and Territorial Epidemiologists,* 2006, http://www.cste.org/PS/2006pdfs/PSFINAL2006/06-EC-03FINAL.pdf.

[6] Centers for Disease Control and Prevention, "Syndromic Surveillance: An Applied Approach to Outbreak Detection," *Centers for Disease Control and Prevention,* January 13, 2006, http://www.cdc.gov/EPO/dphsi/syndromic.htm; see also Centers for Disease Control and Prevention, "Annotated Bibliography for Syndromic Surveillance," June 26, 2006, http://www.cdc.gov/epo/dphsi/syndromic/overview.htm; Centers for Disease Control and Prevention, "Syndromic Surveillance: Reports from a National Conference, 2003," *Morbidity and Mortality Weekly Report,* 53 (2004).

diagnoses, syndromic surveillance aims to detect health threats earlier than traditional disease surveillance.[7] The theory is that during an outbreak or attack, people first develop symptoms, then stay home from work or school, attempt to self-treat with over-the-counter medications, and eventually see a physician with nonspecific symptoms, all before a formal diagnosis and report to the health department. To identify such behaviors, syndromic surveillance systems regularly monitor existing data for sudden changes or anomalies that might signal an adverse health event. For example, because lethal agents such as plague, brucellosis, or tularemia initially present with "flu-like" illness, an unexpected increase of individuals with fever, headache, muscle pain, and malaise could be an indication of a bioterrorist attack or natural disease outbreak.

Biosurveillance systems face inherent trade-offs among their levels of sensitivity, timeliness, and false positive rates, which can limit their effectiveness for early notification of novel infections and bioterrorism. There are insufficient data to determine the effectiveness of biosurveillance, so more research is required.[8] At the same time, there are trade-offs between the public health benefits of surveillance and risks to personal privacy, so biosurveillance systems require strict security and privacy standards.[9]

[7] Michael A. Stoto, Matthias Schonlau, and Louis T. Mariano, "Syndromic Surveillance: Is It Worth the Effort?" *Chance*, 17 (2004): 19–24.

[8] Stoto et al., "Syndromic Surveillance"; Dena M. Bravata, Kathryn M. McDonald, Wendy M. Smith, et al., "Systematic Review: Surveillance Systems for Early Detection of Bioterrorism-Related Diseases," *Annals of Internal Medicine*, 140 (2004): 910–22.

[9] Daniel Drociuk, James J. Gibson, and James G. Hodge, Jr., "Health Information Privacy and Syndromic Surveillance Systems," *Morbidity and Mortality Weekly Report*, 53 (2004): 221–25.

program until surveillance data linked the problem to a single manufacturer. Globally, surveillance was the foundation for malaria control and smallpox eradication during the 1960s and 1970s.[14] In 1981, shortly after surveillance led to reports of case clusters of unusual pneumonia and rare cancers among gay men, epidemiologists described acquired immunodeficiency syndrome (AIDS) and determined its likely mode of transmission.[15] Similarly, in 1993, after clusters of deaths among otherwise healthy residents of the Southwest were described, investigators identified a new strain of hantavirus and devised means of prevention.[16] More recently, the international community has rapidly mobilized to identify and respond to novel infections such as the SARS corona virus[17] and influenza A (H5N1).[18] At the start of a new century, surveillance to identify emerging infections and bioterrorism has become a national and global priority, which is a major impetus for biosurveillance (see box 19).

Public health agencies gather data on more than just infectious diseases. In growing recognition of the effects of behavior on personal health, health officials collect and analyze behavioral information regarding, for instance, alcohol and drug use, seat-belt and bicycle helmet use, smoking, eating, exercise, and sexual practices.[19] The Behavioral Risk Factor

BOX 20

ENVIRONMENTAL PUBLIC HEALTH TRACKING

The interaction of hazards, exposures, and disease

The environment plays an important role in human development and health.[1] In 2001, the Pew Environmental Health Commission recommended the creation of a Nationwide Health Tracking Network for disease and exposures.[2] The CDC funded a National Environmental Public Health Tracking (EPHT) program in 2002,[3] and the Institute of Medicine lent its support to the idea in 2004.[4] Most recently, California has initiated a statewide biomonitoring program to measure people's exposure to toxic chemicals.[5] Environmental public health tracking is the ongoing collection, integration, analysis, and interpretation of data about environmental hazards, exposures to those hazards, and health effects of environmental exposures. EPHT monitors risks and provides data to public health agencies to reduce harmful exposures.

Hazard surveillance assesses the occurrence of, distribution of, and trends in levels of hazards—chemicals, physical agents, biomechanical stressors, and biological agents responsible for injury and disease. Exposure surveillance monitors members of the population for the presence of environmental hazards (e.g., pediatric lead, arsenic, radon, and radiation levels). Disease surveillance monitors the population for incidence of illnesses attributable to environmental hazards (e.g., cancers, birth defects, and respiratory disease). EPHT links data about hazards, exposures, and diseases to look for possible associations as part of the surveillance system.[6] The primary goal is to reduce hazards in the environment, rather than facilitate treatment of the individual, so as to reduce overall population risk.[7] EPHT also has value as an early warning system for hidden threats, such as biological, chemical, or radiological terrorism, as occurred in the anthrax attacks in 2001.[8]

[1] For a survey of environmental health issues, see Robert H. Friis, *Essentials of Environmental Health* (Boston: Jones and Bartlett Publishers, 2006).

[2] Jill Litt, Nga Tran, Kristen Chossek Malecki, et al., "Identifying Priority Health Conditions, Environmental Data, and Infrastructure Needs: A Synopsis of the Pew Environmental Health Tracking Project," *Environmental Health Perspectives,* 112 (2004): 1414-18.

[3] Centers for Disease Control and Prevention, "National Public Health Tracking Program," *Centers for Disease Control and Prevention,* http://www.cdc.gov/nceh/tracking/.

[4] Institute of Medicine, *Environmental Health Indicators: Bridging the Chasm of Public Health and the Environment—Workshop Summary* (Washington, DC: National Academies Press, 2004).

[5] Cal. S. B. 1379, Reg. Sess. (Cal. 2006) (creating a biomonitoring program to identify the chemicals present in the bodies of Californians, with the goal of mitigating exposure to contaminants and assessing a fee upon manufacturers or persons who are responsible for identifiable sources of toxic chemicals).

[6] Amy D. Kyle, John R. Balmes, Patricia A. Buffler, et al., "Integrating Research, Surveillance, and Practice in Environmental Public Health Tracking," *Environmental Health Perspectives,* 114 (2006): 980-84.

[7] Beate Ritz, Ira Tager, and John Balmes, "Can Lessons from Public Health Disease Surveillance Be Applied to Environmental Public Health Tracking?" *Environmental Health Perspectives,* 113 (2005): 243-49.

[8] Susan West Marmagas, Laura Rasar King, and Michelle Chuk, "Public Health's Response to a Changed World: September 11, Biological Terrorism, and the Development of an Environmental Health Tracking Network," *American Journal of Public Health,* 93 (2003): 1226-30.

Surveillance System (BRFSS), for example, is the world's largest ongoing telephone health-survey system, tracking health conditions and risk behaviors in the United States every year since 1984.[20]

To assess environmental risks, health agencies collect data on hazards (toxic substances in the air, food, or water), exposures (pediatric blood

TABLE 15. Current data used to monitor health status

Type of Data	Description
Vital Statistics	Registration system from records of live births, deaths, fetal deaths, and induced terminations of pregnancy
Morbidity and Mortality Reporting	Surveillance for selected diseases
National Health Interview Survey	National data on the incidence of acute illness and injury, chronic conditions and disabilities, and the utilization of health care services
National Health and Nutrition Examination Survey (NHANES)	Population-wide data collection by direct physical examination, clinical laboratory tests, and related measurements
National Electronic Injury Surveillance System (NEISS)	Surveillance of hospital emergency departments and investigation of representative cases of injury
Biosurveillance	Systematic monitoring of health data of potential value in detecting emerging health threats, whether occurring naturally or as a result of bioterrorism
Environmental Health Tracking	Ongoing collection, integration, analysis, and interpretation of data about environmental hazards, exposures to those hazards, and health effects of environmental exposures
Disease- or Purpose-Specific Data Collection	Data collection for diseases, such as HIV (serosurveillance) or cancer (tumor registries), or to support functions such as childhood immunization
Genetic Databases	Research on stored tissue samples and systematic collection of population-based generic information

lead levels), and diseases (incidence of cancers, birth defects, and pulmonary illnesses). Environmental public health tracking, for example, links data about hazards, exposures, and diseases to identify possible associations (see box 20).

To assess genetic variations associated with disease, health professionals collect and evaluate genetic data among the population.[21] They are interested, for example, in the susceptibility of subpopulations to behavioral and environmental triggers for disease. The public health system requires reliable information about communicable, behavioral, environmental, and genetic risks in order to reduce morbidity and excess mortality (see table 15).

Basic responsibility for surveillance lies with individual countries.

However, with the contemporary globalization of the world's political economy, as evidenced by the increased movement of people and expansion of international trade and services, surveillance is no longer purely a domestic concern.[22] The SARS outbreaks illustrate how inadequate surveillance and communication in one country can endanger public health security in the entire world.[23] In the current milieu of emerging, adapting, and highly mobile pathogens, the best defense is systematic global health surveillance.[24] The WHO's Global Outbreak Alert and Response Network (GOARN) links existing local, regional, national, and international networks of laboratories and medical centers into a global surveillance system. The International Health Regulations (IHR), described in chapter 7, create a transnational legal structure for global surveillance of "public health emergencies of international concern."[25]

MANDATORY REPORTING OF DISEASES AND OTHER HEALTH CONDITIONS

> Morbidity registration will be an invaluable contribution to therapeutics, as well as to hygiene, for it will enable the therapeutists to determine the duration and fatality of all forms of disease. . . . Illusion will be dispelled, quackery . . . suppressed, a science of therapeutics created, suffering diminished, life shielded from many dangers.
>
> William Farr (1838)

Reporting, or notification, of health conditions to a public health agency is the cornerstone of surveillance. States possess constitutional authority under their police powers to mandate reporting of a wide range of infectious diseases, injuries, behavioral risk factors, and other health conditions (e.g., partner or child abuse, gunshot wounds, and hospital-acquired infections) to public health agencies.[26] The Supreme Court has upheld reporting requirements against challenges that they violate personal privacy, as discussed below.[27] The states effectuate their police powers by enacting legislation enumerating reportable health conditions (or classes of reportable diseases, such as "communicable" and "sexually transmitted") or delegating that task to state or local health agencies.[28] Where legislation delegates authority, courts afford health agencies considerable discretion in deciding how to classify particular diseases. New York's highest court, for example, rejected a challenge by physician organiza-

BOX 21

REPORTING REQUIREMENTS FOR OUT-OF-STATE LABORATORIES

As explained above, states usually require reporting both by the physician and the laboratory. Laboratories are usually more reliable reporters of data and act as a failsafe system. This failsafe system can break down if large health care providers send their tests to laboratories outside the state, as out-of-state laboratories often have no duty to comply with a reporting requirement in the originating state. Certainly, the in-state physician who receives a positive test result from the out-of-state laboratory must furnish a report to the health department, but if she fails to do so, there is no backup system of laboratory reporting. In addition, laboratories often hold only limited patient data, so their reports to public health departments may be incomplete.

There are imaginative state and federal remedies for this jurisdictional problem. At the state level, regulators could require managed care organizations (MCOs) and other providers to contract only with out-of-state laboratories that agree to report. Sanctions for failure to report would be directed at the in-state MCO rather than the out-of-state laboratory. At the federal level, Congress probably has the power under the Commerce Clause to require reporting. Infectious disease control is a problem that crosses state lines, and reportable data may be viewed as articles of commerce. In the absence of some remedy, however, the jurisdictional problem can thwart efforts for complete reporting, particularly in an era of integrated delivery systems that operate regionally or nationally.

tions that insisted the health commissioner classify HIV as an STI; the commissioner refused to do so, and the court upheld his exercise of discretion.[29]

States vary in the diseases that are reportable, the conditions under which reports must be furnished, the time frames for reporting, and the agencies responsible for receiving reports.[30] Statutes also vary in the persons that owe a duty to report, but most impose the obligation on specified health care professionals and laboratories. (For a discussion of the problem of enforcing reporting requirements on out-of-state laboratories, see box 21.)

All states and territories participate in a national morbidity notification system by regularly and voluntarily reporting aggregate or case-specific data to the CDC.[31] Currently, approximately sixty reportable conditions are included in the national morbidity reporting system.[32] The Council of State and Territorial Epidemiologists (CSTE), in conjunction with the CDC, annually proposes additions to and deletions from the list of diseases under national surveillance, and most states conform to these recommendations.[33] The CDC creates standardized case definitions for infectious diseases;[34] it is also developing case definitions for chronic, environmental, and occupational injuries and diseases. Standardized case reports contain extensive information, such as demographics (e.g., patient's name, age, race, and address), laboratory analysis, risk behaviors, and clinical history.

Despite its long traditions and current prevalence, reporting is politically contentious and socially divisive. Reporting is viewed very differently in the fields of public health and medicine.[35] Public health professionals see their first duty as protecting the population, and they justify reporting by invoking science and the ethics of collective responsibility. Private physicians, on the other hand, see their first duty as safeguarding patients; they accord higher priority to the sanctity of their therapeutic relationships.[36] Mandatory duties to report usually require physicians to notify the government of their patients' names and other sensitive information, which is regarded as a breach of confidentiality. Patients and the organizations that represent them also sometimes oppose mandatory reporting because they do not trust the state to maintain sensitive case registries and are concerned about political retribution, invasion of privacy, and discrimination. Perhaps because of the divergent interests in medicine and public health, or perhaps because of a lack of clear communication between the two fields,[37] physician compliance with reporting systems has been variable and often low.[38]

PHYSICIAN AND COMMUNITY RESISTANCE TO NOTIFICATION LAWS: CASE STUDIES ON HIV AND DIABETES SURVEILLANCE

Surveillance activities can be bitterly contested from both sides of the political spectrum. From the conservative perspective, surveillance can appear intrusive and meddlesome: government prying into the lives of individuals, where it has no place. From a liberal perspective, surveillance can invade a sphere of personal privacy, driving individuals away from services for fear of stigma and discrimination. Perhaps the two most controversial surveillance activities are name-based HIV reporting and diabetes surveillance.

Case Study I: Name-Based HIV Reporting

HIV case reporting has generated bitter political controversy and impassioned community resistance.[39] HIV reporting offers many public health benefits, including improved monitoring of the epidemic, more efficient targeting of prevention and support services, and clinical benefits by referring individuals for treatment.[40] Despite the importance of HIV surveillance, advocates fear government misuse of sensitive data.[41] In the late 1990s, for instance, a Florida health official disclosed the names from an HIV registry to a dating service,[42] and Illinois enacted (but never implemented) legislation requiring cross-matching of the state AIDS registry with health care licensure records.[43] Community representatives also express concern that HIV case reporting might deter people from being tested and seeking treatment,[44] although empirical research does not validate this concern.[45]

Because of their fears about privacy and discrimination, community organizations have urged public health authorities to implement a system of unique identifiers as an alternative to named surveillance,[46] yet studies of unique identifier systems have found that data collected sometimes contain incomplete and difficult-to-match records.[47] The CDC recommends named HIV reporting with alternative test sites and strong privacy and security assurances.[48] It took nearly two decades to make HIV reportable throughout the United States.[49] As of April 2006, forty-three states had name-based reporting, five states and the District of Columbia had code-based reporting, and two states had name-to-code reporting (cases initially are reported by name, but are converted to code after public health follow-up and collection of epidemiologic data).[50] Named HIV reporting varies widely in other parts of the world.[51]

Influential public health officials have gone farther, urging the adoption of systematic HIV surveillance, treatment, and case management—e.g., close monitoring of viral loads, CD4 cell counts, and drug-resistant strains of infection, with feedback to patients and health care professionals.[52] Data would be delivered to patients and health care professionals to effectively coordinate a continuum of care. Needless to say, such proposals are politically controversial, with advocates expressing deep concerns about invasion of privacy and the integrity of the physician/patient relationship.

Here we have a classic illustration of strategies that can produce important public health benefits but which engender fear and distrust within the community. Furthermore, less restrictive alternatives, such as unique identifiers, are not fully effective. No easy resolution exists: Policies that meet public health objectives fail to satisfy community representatives, and policies that meet civil liberties objectives fail to satisfy public health officials. Should public health benefits outweigh civil liberties concerns? Should public health agencies be trusted to safeguard personal privacy? The critical unresolved question is whether, in a representative democracy, government should impose its view of the collective good on an unwilling community.

Case Study II: Diabetes Surveillance

> In East Harlem, it is possible to take any simple nexus of people—the line at an A.T.M., a portion of a postal route, the members of a church choir—and trace an invisible web of diabetes that stretches through the group and out into the neighborhood, touching nearly every life with its menace. . . . Human behavior makes dealing with Type 2 diabetes often feel so futile—the force of habit, the failure of will, the shrugging defeatism, the urge to salve a hard life by surrendering to small comforts: a piece of cake, a couple of beers, a day off from sticking oneself with needles.
>
> N. R. Kleinfield (2006)

If anything, diabetes surveillance is more contentious than HIV reporting. After all, HIV is an infectious disease, so surveillance is justified by the imperative of preventing risk to others. Diabetes, as a chronic disease, offers no such justification. It relies on the pure paternalistic assumption that patients, and their physicians, need state supervision in the recognition and management of their disease.[53]

The justification for diabetes surveillance begins with the crushing burden of the interconnected epidemics of obesity and diabetes, especially in indigent and minority populations, where behavior and genetic predisposition place people at alarmingly high risk. Diabetes exacts a staggering toll in acute and chronic illness, disability, and death, as box 22 explains.[54] Public health agencies, however, do not systematically monitor diabetes within the population, even though the majority of patients do not adequately manage the disease or even know their glycosylated hemoglobin values, because they have not been tested, have not been informed about test results, or do not recall them.[55]

In early 2006, the New York City Board of Health implemented a novel response to the diabetes epidemic modeled on the Vermont Diabetes Information System, which uses a network of community laboratories to provide data for reminders, action alerts, and population reports sent to primary care providers and patients.[56] The New York diabetes surveillance initiative entails three interrelated activities: (1) mandatory electronic

BOX 22

DIABETES: MEDICAL EXPLANATION AND PREVALENCE

Diabetes is a chronic disease characterized by high blood glucose levels (hyperglycemia) resulting from defects in insulin secretion or insulin action. The two most common types of diabetes are type 1, accounting for about 5-10 percent of all diabetes, and type 2, accounting for about 90-95 percent of all diabetes. Type 1, which develops most often in children and young adults, is an autoimmune disease characterized by destruction of the pancreas cells, usually leading to absolute insulin deficiency. Type 2 is characterized by insulin resistance and relative insulin deficiency. The risk of developing type 2 diabetes increases with age, obesity, and lack of physical activity.

If not controlled, both types of diabetes can lead to the same set of chronic complications in the eyes (retinopathy), kidneys (nephropathy), peripheral nerve system (neuropathy), and arteries (atherosclerosis). Diabetes can affect nearly every organ system of the body and is a leading cause of blindness, end-stage renal disease, lower extremity amputation, cerebrovascular disease, ischemic heart disease, and peripheral vascular disease. Women with preexisting diabetes who become pregnant are at risk of preventable congenital malformations and perinatal mortality.

Diabetes is a significant contributor to morbidity and mortality—the sixth leading cause of death in the United States, and the leading cause of nontraumatic lower extremity amputations, blindness among working-age adults, and end-stage renal disease. From 1980 through 2004, the number of Americans with diabetes more than doubled (from 5.8 million to 14.7 million). Although the disease affects all demographic and geographic segments of the population, minority populations are disproportionately affected. Prevalence among Latinos is twice as high as that among African Americans and four times as high as that among Whites or Asians. Nationally, the highest rates are found among Native Americans.

Trends in lifestyle (e.g., overeating, low activity, and smoking), an aging population, and a larger percentage of minorities in the population fuel the increase in diabetes. It is reasonable to assume that the burden of diabetes will only grow over the ensuing decades. Regretfully, as the diabetes threat has risen, costing an estimated $132 billion annually, federal funding has shrunk.[1]

Source: Box 22 is derived from the following sources: New York Department of Health, "Diabetes Surveillance in New York State," March 2003, http://www.health.state.ny.us/nysdoh/consumer/diabetes/surv/en/intro.htm; Centers for Disease Control and Prevention, "National Diabetes Fact Sheet: General Information and National Estimates on Diabetes in the United States, 2005," *Centers for Disease Control and Prevention*, Feb. 3, 2006, http://www.cdc.gov/diabetes/pubs/factsheet05.htm; Mary T. Bassett, "Diabetes Is Epidemic," *American Journal of Public Health*, 95 (2005): 1496.

[1] Ian Urbina, "Rising Diabetes Threat Meets a Falling Budget," *New York Times*, May 16, 2006 ("The government has cut diabetes funds in the budgets for this year and next, despite the explosive growth of a disease that now figures in the deaths of 225,000 Americans each year").

reporting of glycosylated hemoglobin by laboratories but not by physicians; (2) best practice recommendations for health care providers and rosters of patients in their practice who are in poor glycemic control; and (3) information and resources on diabetes management for patients with high glycosylated hemoglobin values, sent by the health department through the post. The initiative will create a registry of glycosylated hemoglobin test results—an estimated 1–2 million results annually—that is linked to patients and their physicians, with identifiable information such as name, birth date, and address.[57]

The purposes of the regulatory requirements are, first, to improve diabetes surveillance and epidemiology by describing and characterizing the burden of disease in the population; and, second, to provide individual and aggregate feedback and support to providers and patients.

The New York diabetes initiative has been engulfed in criticism from many quarters since its inception. Clinical laboratories worry about the increase in reporting responsibilities, which include hard-to-find demographic information.[58] Physicians claim that the program impinges on their clinical autonomy and interferes with the therapeutic relationship. And civil libertarians point to the problems of informed consent and confidentiality. The fault lines on informed consent are found in the "opt-out" provisions in the New York regulations, which allow patients to request that the health department not contact them.[59] Patients cannot circumvent the reporting requirement, however, and remain part of the registry. Critics complain that patients may not understand their rights to opt out, and in any case, the opt-out process is complex and itself requires some information disclosure. An opt-in policy would better ensure informed consent, but it would also significantly reduce the number of people served by the program.

The regulations state that hemoglobin test results and other information "shall be kept confidential and shall not be disclosed to any person other than the individual . . . or [her] medical provider."[60] Consequently, the data cannot be used to the person's detriment—for example, to deny him a driver's license, health or life insurance, or employment.[61] Nevertheless, critics believe that the invasion of privacy occurs simply because the government gains access to sensitive personal information.

Advocates also claim that diabetes, as a chronic disease, is unsuitable for mandatory surveillance. Reporting infectious diseases is well established as a measure to prevent harm to the public. Diabetes, however, primarily affects individuals, with no direct spillover effects on public health or safety. The critical unresolved issue is the appropriate role of government in surveillance and case management of a chronic disease with a crippling effect on the well-being of the population. Beyond all this is the question of social justice. Is ongoing, systematic diabetes surveillance unjustified paternalism that overrides individual autonomy? Or is it a social imperative to care for the most disadvantaged, who do not enjoy the benefit of a stable physician-patient relationship?[62]

PARTNER NOTIFICATION: CONTACT TRACING, DUTY TO WARN, AND RIGHT TO KNOW

In no other respect is the [medical] practice in this country more reprehensible than in the failure of physicians, and even of public health clinics, to make diligent inquiry as to sources of infection and to use all available methods to bring these persons under treatment.

Thomas Parran (1931)

Partner notification is a highly complex concept that has at least three distinct, if at times overlapping, meanings:[63] (1) contact tracing—the statutory powers of public health agencies to identify and locate sexual partners and other "contacts" at risk of infection, and to notify them of their exposure; (2) duty to warn—the power or duty of private health care professionals to inform their patient's sexual or other partners of foreseeable risks; and (3) right to know—the common law duty of infected persons to disclose their serological status to a sexual or other partner placed at risk.

Contact Tracing

Sexual contact tracing probably originated in Europe in the sixteenth century with the medical inspection of suspected syphilitic prostitutes through regulations that came to be known as reglementation.[64] The earliest reference to contact tracing in contagious disease law dates to mid-nineteenth-century Europe.[65] "Contact epidemiology" became a central public health strategy in the United States during the syphilis epidemic in the 1930s.[66] The National Venereal Disease Act of 1938 adopted STI control measures proposed by the anti–venereal disease campaigner Surgeon General Thomas Parran.[67] Around the same time, states began enacting STI statutes giving public health authorities wide-ranging powers to control venereal disease.

From its widespread use during the 1930s, the notification of sexual partners has remained an accepted part of the law and practice of STI control.[68] This concept of tracking sexual contacts later would be called "partner notification," which has expanded over the years to include a range of support services, including counseling and medical treatment.[69]

Partner notification, sometimes called partner counseling and referral services (PCRS), is a quintessential state and local function exercised through the police power. State statutes empower public health agencies to implement partner notification as part of STI or HIV prevention programs.[70] The federal government does not require partner notification, but as early as 1918[71] through to the present day,[72] Congress has influenced contact tracing policy through its conditional spending power. Despite being classified as an STI since 1988, Congress has treated HIV separately from other STIs. The Ryan White Act provides grants to states to implement partner notification programs for HIV-infected persons,[73] and now requires states to notify spouses of persons infected with HIV as a condition of the receipt of partner notification funds.[74] The CDC strongly recommends systematic identification of persons with HIV, who should then receive "behavioral risk-reduction interventions": counseling, education, condoms, and PCRS.[75]

Public health authorities utilize two primary models of partner notification: patient referral and provider referral.[76] With patient referral, index patients (infected patients identified in public health clinics or by physician referrals) are asked to contact their partners. Provider referral switches the responsibility for notification to trained public health personnel, who inform contacts and offer counseling and treatment. Public health professionals protect confidentiality by declining to reveal the index patient's name (although contacts can often deduce the patient's identity).

Partner notification, like reporting, has generated bitter controversy. As members of stigmatized groups, commercial sex workers in the syphilis epidemic of the 1930s and gay men in the AIDS epidemic of the late twentieth century[77] were suspicious of the true intentions of public health officials. These groups believed that partner notification, although nominally voluntary, had coercive elements because vulnerable persons might feel they had no choice but to cooperate with government officials. Providing the names of intimate sexual partners also was thought to be a gross invasion of privacy and left contacts susceptible to discrimination. Persons revealing the names of their partners also faced serious physical, sexual, and emotional abuse.[78] For example, a woman trapped in an abusive relationship might reasonably fear that she would be subject to a violent reaction if her partner discovered she was HIV-infected.

While many in the community have opposed partner notification because of its intrusive qualities, persons in relationships with an infected person have claimed a right to be informed of the risk. Armed with adequate knowledge, the partners of infected persons could make reasoned judgments about sex and sharing drug injection equipment. Think about the situation of a woman who has been in a long-term sexual relationship and has never been apprised of the fact that her partner has an STI. She may feel genuinely wronged if health officials are aware of the risk but fail to disclose it.

Partner notification programs have sought mightily to straddle a fine line between the interests of infected persons and those of their partners. Partner notification, in theory, is warranted because only persons who are informed of their infected status can take steps to reduce risks and ameliorate harms. Though partner notification is unexceptional in theory, empirical evidence of its cost-effectiveness is decidedly mixed.[79] On balance, however, partner notification remains a viable strategy for connecting asymptomatic partners to counseling and treatment resources. The traditions of voluntary cooperation, nondisclosure of names, and the provision of support services minimize social harms while still recognizing legitimate public claims to protection against undisclosed risks of infection.

Health Care Professionals' "Duty to Warn"

> In early shades of feminist theory, an ethical conundrum between medical secrecy and warning of risk was evident in the views of a female physician: we have seen the wife murdered by syphilis contracted from an unfaithful husband and an innocent woman its victim for life.
>
> Marion C. Potter (1907)

The duty of confidentiality poses a powerful dilemma for physicians and other health care professionals[80] when their patients pose a significant risk to others (for example, if the patient discloses an intention to harm a third party). If the physician reveals the risk, she breaches patient confidentiality; if she fails to disclose, she subjects known persons to danger.[81] Most states impose on physicians a *duty* to protect third parties at risk, which may include a duty to warn. In such cases, physicians are held liable if they do not take reasonable care to protect third parties. Other states *permit* disclosures to protect third parties without creating a legal obligation. This approach creates a "privilege" but not a "duty" to inform third parties at risk.[82] In such cases, physicians have discretion to maintain confidentiality or to reveal a known risk; in either case, they do not face liability. These duties and privileges are created by statute or by court decision.[83]

The duty to protect was famously recognized in *Tarasoff v. Regents of the University of California* (1976),[84] where a therapist was held liable for failing to warn a woman of the patient's intent to kill her.[85] Under *Tarasoff*, the duty to protect requires (1) foreseeability—the therapist must have determined, or reasonably should have determined, that her patient poses a risk to another;[86] (2) a serious risk—the risk posed to the third party must be genuine and not merely speculative or remote;[87] and (3) an identifiable victim—the person endangered should be known to the patient and therapist.[88] The *Tarasoff* line of cases is said to establish a "duty to warn," but this is technically incorrect. Rather, the physician has an obligation to use reasonable care to protect the third party placed in danger. This may require a "warning," but not in every case.

The duty to protect applies not only when patients pose a threat of physical harm but also when they risk transmission of an infectious or sexually transmitted disease.[89] Courts usually require protection of an identifiable person who faces a serious risk of contracting a disease, such as a known sexual or needle-sharing partner of a patient with HIV infection. For example, in *Gammill v. United States* (1984), a court held that an army physician had no duty to inform a nearby community of an outbreak of hepatitis B because he was not aware of specific risks to particular persons.[90]

The physician still may have duties to protect the public from an infectious disease, even if there is no identifiable victim. Some courts hold physicians liable for failing to diagnose an infectious condition[91] or, if they do diagnose the condition, for failing to "instruct and advise" patients about the public risks they present.[92] Thus, physicians should advise patients of the nature of the infection, how it is spread, and precautions that can be taken. This may require explaining safer sex to persons with HIV infection or the importance of treatment and isolation for a person with infectious TB.[93]

The Duty of Infected Persons to Inform: The "Right to Know"

Persons who know they have an infectious condition have a duty to protect their close contacts or partners.[94] This duty ordinarily means abstaining from sexual relations or from sharing drug injection equipment. If a contagious person does expose another to infection, he may have to disclose the risk. For example, in the widely publicized case of *Christian v. Sheft* (1989),[95] a jury rendered a verdict against the estate of Rock Hudson because Mr. Hudson had engaged in "high-risk" sex and intentionally concealed his HIV status.[96] The duty to inform only holds if the person knew, or should have known, that he was contagious. For example, a Michigan court found that Earvin "Magic" Johnson had no duty to inform his sexual partners of his HIV infection (of which he was then unaware), even though he had an extensive history of sexual relationships.[97] (As to the duty to inform sexual partners under the criminal law, see chapter 11.)

The California Supreme Court in *John B. v. Superior Court of L.A. County* (2006) wrestled with a series of thorny questions: What duty does a husband have to avoid transmitting HIV to his spouse? What level of awareness should be required before a court imposes such a duty? And what responsibility does the wife have to protect herself against exposure?[98] Although the court did not answer all these questions, in a 4–3 opinion it ruled that a wife could proceed with legal discovery into her husband's sexual history for the purpose of determining whether he transmitted the infection to her. The court decided that even if the husband did not have actual knowledge of his HIV status, he could be held liable if he had "constructive knowledge"—i.e., the husband had reason to believe he was infected. The ruling is limited to married or monogamous couples, not those engaged in casual sex.

The duty of physicians and infected persons to protect individuals at foreseeable risk raises fascinating public policy issues. Most people would not dispute that, at least in some circumstances, individuals have a valid claim to be informed of the risks they face. Whereas a person who visits a bathhouse for casual or anonymous sex may be said to assume the risk, the same probably cannot be said of a person in a stable long-term relationship who is kept in ignorance. The so-called right to know is grounded on a person's need to make informed decisions and to take steps to protect himself against infection.

Although individuals may have legitimate interests in knowing the risks they face, disclosure policies have heavy social costs. In the context of contact tracing, notifying partners that they have been infected may involve admission of a criminal offense.[99] In the context of a physician's duty to warn, the consequence may be that patients are less likely to divulge their intimate secrets. In the context of a patient's duty to inform, the consequence may be that individuals refrain from getting tested for infectious conditions. (If there is liability only when a person knows his serological status, the law may create incentives not to know, which is one reason why the court in *John B.* extended liability to constructive knowledge.) The duty to inform also presupposes that the infected person is solely "responsible" for ensuring safety. Public health authorities, however, prefer to counsel that both infected and uninfected persons are responsible for safety (e.g., by using condoms and sterile drug injection equipment).

In thinking about the duty to warn, therefore, policymakers have to balance the right to confidentiality against the "right to know." Beyond this conflict is the broader issue of the effects on seeking access to testing, counseling, and treatment once the community realizes that health care professionals will disclose confidences. One way to balance these interests would be to create a narrow power, but not a duty, to inform. The power could be exercisable only where necessary to avoid serious, prospective harm to an identifiable person, and when no less intrusive measure could ameliorate the risk (e.g., the patient making the disclosure himself).

PUBLIC HEALTH RESEARCH

Public health research is characterized by a multidisciplinary approach to addressing questions involving the health of populations, often to identify the determinants of community health or to evaluate the effectiveness of interventions. Public health researchers want to understand the nature and extent of health hazards, the burdens on communities, and interventions of a complex nature. Specific methodologies range from large field trials of candidate vaccines and pharmaceuticals to epidemiological or biostatistical studies and population surveys.[100] Without a systematic agenda for rigorous research, public health officials would lack the scientific evidence needed for developing policies and programs, as well as for allocating health resources.

Despite its undoubted importance, public health research poses important ethical and legal questions. Box 23 briefly describes illustrations of controversial public health research, while box 24 explains the ethical principles and legal rules that guide research on human subjects. This section addresses two questions of contemporary importance: (1) What is public health research and how does it differ from routine public health practice? (2) How can the benefits of research be balanced with risks to privacy?

BOX 23

ETHICS AND TRUST IN PUBLIC HEALTH RESEARCH

From the Tuskegee syphilis study to the Kennedy Krieger lead paint study

Public health professionals rely so heavily on population-based research that it is critical to maintain the trust of participating communities and to ensure that research is conducted ethically. The trust of vulnerable communities has been strained by unethical research studies, such as the CDC-supported Tuskegee study initiated in the early 1930s to observe the natural course of syphilis among African American men in Alabama. The men were not informed that they were research subjects and were not offered penicillin (a known cure for syphilis) until the study became public in 1972.[1] Similarly, during the Cold War (1944–74), vulnerable human subjects were exposed to radiation without their knowledge or consent. The experiments resulted in significant harms to research subjects.[2] The research subjects in both the Tuskegee[3] and human radiation experiments[4] received presidential apologies. President William J. Clinton said, "The American people . . . must be able to rely upon the United States to keep its word, to tell the truth, and to do the right thing," and that "when the government does wrong, we have a moral responsibility to admit it."[5]

Modern research has been compared with these infamous studies, sometimes unfairly. During the 1990s, the Kennedy Krieger Institute (KKI) lead paint study divided impoverished, mostly African American children living in Baltimore homes into three treatment groups (homes receiving lead abatement procedures costing $1,650, $3,500, and $6,500) and two comparison groups (homes abated by the City of Baltimore and homes built after 1978 presumed to be lead-free). In *Grimes v. Kennedy Krieger Institute, Inc.* (2001),[6] Maryland's highest court issued a scathing ruling comparing the research to the Tuskegee syphilis study and Nazi prisoner research. The court called it a callous scientific experiment that used children as "measuring tools." It remanded the case to determine three main issues: informed consent, declaring that parents cannot give consent for their children to enroll in "non-therapeutic" research, the duty to warn research subjects of the risks, and the inadequacy of the IRB review at Johns Hopkins.

The KKI lead paint study stirred controversy about whether research designed to develop less expensive interventions that are not as effective as existing treatments can be ethically warranted.[7] Similar ethical issues arise in the context of international collaborative research conducted in developing countries.[8] In 1997, the CDC and NIH

[1] James H. Jones, *Bad Blood: The Tuskegee Syphilis Experiment* (New York: Free Press, 1993).

[2] Advisory Committee on Human Radiation Experiments, *Final Report* (Washington, DC: U.S. Government Printing Office, 1996).

[3] Allison Mitchell, "Clinton Regrets 'Clearly Racist' U.S. Study," *New York* Times, May 17, 1997.

[4] William J. Clinton, "Remarks in Acceptance of Human Radiation Final Report," Washington, DC, October 3, 1995.

[5] Clinton, "Remarks in Acceptance."

[6] *Grimes v. Kennedy Krieger Inst., Inc.*, 782 A.2d 807 (Md. 2001).

[7] Institute of Medicine, *Ethical Considerations for Research on Housing-Related Health Hazards involving Children* (Washington, DC: National Academies Press, 2005); David R. Buchanan and Franklin G. Miller, "Justice and Fairness in the Kennedy Krieger Institute Lead Paint Study: The Ethics of Public Health Research on Less Expensive, Less Effective Interventions," *American Journal of Public Health*, 96 (2006): 781–87 (contending that the failure to conduct such research causes greater harm, because it deprives disadvantaged populations of the benefits of imminent incremental improvements in their health conditions).

[8] Alex J. London, "Justice and the Human Development Approach to International Research," *Hastings Center Report*, 35 (2005): 24–37; Winston Chiong, "The Real Problem with Equipoise," *American Journal of Bioethics*, 6 (2006): 37–47 (critiquing the traditional ethical obligation of equipoise,

sponsored placebo-controlled trials of zidovudine (AZT) among pregnant women in Africa. A placebo-controlled trial would have been unethical if performed in developed countries because AZT is known to be highly effective in preventing mother-to-infant transmission of HIV (see chapter 7). Comparing the African trials to the Tuskegee study, commentators argued that researchers knowingly permitted babies in their care to be born with preventable HIV infection.[9] However, the CDC and NIH observed that, far from harming African women, they were engaged in a search for an affordable regimen of AZT that could save hundreds of thousands of African children in the future.[10]

---

which requires genuine uncertainty about the relative therapeutic merits of two arms of a clinical trial, because it is poorly suited to research on sustainable and desperately needed therapies for use in poor countries).

[9] Marcia Angell, "The Ethics of Clinical Research in the Third World," *New Eng. J. Med,.* 337 (1997): 847; Peter Lurie and Sidney M. Wolfe, "Unethical Trials of Interventions to Reduce Perinatal Transmission of the Human Immunodeficiency Virus in Developing Countries," *New Eng. J. Med.*, 337 (1997): 853. For a more recent ethical discussion of a clinical trial in rural Uganda, see Marcia Angell, "Investigators' Responsibilities for Human Subjects in Developing Countries," *New Eng. J. Med.*, 342 (2000): 967.

[10] Harold Varmus and David Satcher, "Ethical Complexities of Conducting Research in Developing Countries," *New Eng. J. Med.*, 337 (1997): 1003.

Distinguishing Human Subject Research from Public Health Practice

> Surveillance is not research. Public health surveillance is essentially descriptive in nature. It describes the occurrence of injury or disease and its determinants in the population. It also leads to public health action. . . . If we confuse surveillance with research, we may be motivated to collect large amounts of detailed data on each case. The burden of this approach is too great for the resources available.
>
> World Bank (2002)

State and local health departments routinely engage in a broad range of activities, including surveillance (e.g., reporting, disease registries, and sentinel networks), epidemiological investigations (e.g., outbreak investigations and emergency response), and evaluation and monitoring (e.g., program evaluation and oversight). Scholars have been wrestling with the problem of when these routine practices become a form of population-based research. This is a vexing and important problem, because if routine public health practices were classified as "research," health departments would have to submit this activity for review by institutional review boards (IRBs) and obtain informed consent from participants. Classification of practice as research, therefore, could impede rapid and effective responses to community health threats.

At the outset, it is important to recognize that the source of legal and

BOX 24

ETHICS AND REGULATION OF HUMAN SUBJECT RESEARCH

Ethical principles and regulation of human subject research in the United States favor the inherent worth and dignity of the individual over the benefits to communities. Under conventional theories, researchers should show respect for persons, which requires strict conformance with the choices made by competent and fully informed persons and protection of vulnerable persons.[1] Beneficence (do good) and nonmaleficence (do no harm) impose affirmative duties on researchers to maximize benefits for subjects and minimize risks. Justice requires that human beings be treated equally unless there is a strong ethical justification for treating them differently. Thus, the selection of subjects and the distribution of benefits and burdens in research should be equitable.

These ethical principles have found expression in guidelines for the conduct of research, notably, in the United States in the Belmont Report[2] and internationally in the Nuremberg Code,[3] the Declaration of Helsinki,[4] and the Council of International Organizations of Medical Sciences' (CIOMS) Ethical Guidelines for Biomedical Research[5] and Epidemiological Studies.[6] Most of these ethical guidelines apply specifically to biomedical research and do not carefully consider population-based research.[7] However, there has been a growing awareness of the need for more flexible ethical norms that do not unduly inhibit novel research methodologies,[8] and which grapple with the complex problems of applying conventional ethics to population-based research.[9]

Current legal regulations governing federally sponsored research adopt a biomedical approach. The Department of Health and Human Services (DHHS) issued human subject regulations based on the Belmont Report in 1981, and in 1991 DHHS and sixteen additional executive branch agencies adopted a revised Federal Policy for the

[1] National Commission for the Protection of Human Subjects of Biomedical and Behavioral Research, *Belmont Report: Ethical Principles and Guidelines for the Protection of Human Subjects of Research* (Washington, DC: DHEW, 1979).

[2] National Commission, *Belmont Report*; see James F. Childress, Eric M. Meslin, and Harold T. Shapiro, eds., *Belmont Revisited: Ethical Principles for Research with Human Subjects* (Washington, DC: Georgetown University Press, 2005).

[3] Nuremberg Code 1947, reprinted in *Trials of War Criminals before the Nuremberg Military Tribunals under Control Council Law No. 10* (Washington, DC: U.S. Government Printing Office, 1949): 2: 181-82 ("The voluntary consent of the human subject is absolutely essential").

[4] World Medical Association, *Declaration of Helsinki: Recommendations Guiding Medical Doctors in Biomedical Research Involving Human Subjects,* adopted by the Eighteenth World Medical Assembly (WMA), Helsinki, Finland, 1964; amended by the 29th WMA, Tokyo, Japan, 1975; 35th WMA in Venice, Italy, 1983; the 41st WMA in Hong Kong, 1989; the 48th WMA, Somerset West, Republic of South Africa, 1996; and the 52d WMA, Edinburgh, Scotland, October 2000 ("In research on man, the interest of science and society should never take precedence over considerations related to the wellbeing [*sic*] of the subject"). See Medical Ethics Committee, *Proposed Revision of the World Medical Association Declaration of Helsinki* (WMA Document 17.C/Rev. 1/98, 1999); Robert J. Levine, "The Need to Revise the Declaration of Helsinki," *New Eng. J. Med.*, 341 (1999): 531.

[5] Council of International Organizations of Medical Sciences, *International Guidelines for Biomedical Research Involving Human Subjects* (Geneva: CIOMS, 2002).

[6] Council of International Organizations of Medical Sciences, *International Guidelines for Ethical Review of Epidemiologic Studies* (Geneva: CIOMS, 1991).

[7] Lawrence O. Gostin, "Ethical Principles for the Conduct of Human Subject Research: Population-Based Research and Ethics," *Law, Medicine and Health Care,* 19 (1991): 191-201.

[8] Bartha Maria Knoppers and Alastair Kent, "Ethics Watch: Policy Barriers in Coherent Population-Based Research," *Nature,* 7 (2006): 8.

[9] Steven S. Coughlin, ed., *Ethics in Epidemiology and Public Health Practice: Collected Works* (Columbus, GA: Quill Publications, 1997); Steven S. Coughlin and Tom L. Beauchamp, eds., *Ethics and Epidemiology* (New York: Oxford University Press, 1996); Alexander M. Capron, "Protection of Research Subjects: Do Special Rules Apply in Epidemiology?" *Journal of Clinical Epidemiology*, 44 (1991): 81-89.

Protection of Human Subjects (the "Common Rule").[10] The Common Rule, which applies to human subject research conducted or supported by a federal agency, requires review and approval by an institutional review board (IRB) and the informed consent of human subjects. Despite providing important protection for research subjects, the Common Rule has significant gaps. It applies only to federally funded studies, so purely private research remains unregulated.[11] Furthermore, even with federally funded studies, the rigor with which IRBs review research protocols varies considerably.[12] Finally, the Common Rule's emphasis on individual autonomy (expressed through stringent requirements for informed consent)[13] may limit researchers' ability to realize health gains from large-scale population-based research.

[10] *Protection of Human Subjects,* 45 C.F.R. §§46.101-404 (1993) (also known as the "Common Rule"). The federal Food and Drug Administration (FDA) operates under its own rules for protection of human subjects, which are similar but not identical to the Common Rule.

[11] Institute of Medicine, *Ethical Considerations for Research Involving Prisoners* (Washington, DC: National Academies Press, 2006).

[12] Department of Health and Human Services, Office of Inspector General, *Institutional Review Boards: Their Role in Reviewing Approved Research* (OEI-01-97-00190,1998); Department of Health and Human Services, Office of Inspector General, *Institutional Review Boards: The Emergence of Independent Boards* (OEI-01-97-00192, 1998); Department of Health and Human Services, Office of Inspector General, *Institutional Review Boards: A Time for Reform* (OEI-01-97-00193, 1998); National Bioethics Advisory Commission, *Ethical and Policy Issues in Research Involving Human Participants* (Bethesda, MD: NBAC, 2001).

[13] 45 C.F.R. 46 § 116.

moral authority for public health practice and that for research differ significantly.[101] The former traditionally has been viewed as the historic and constitutionally recognized exercise of state police powers, supported by state statutes that often mandate surveillance and response. Federal restraints on the exercise of public health powers squarely raise problems of federalism, because states are sovereign governments with inherent authority to safeguard their population's health.[102] By contrast, there is no "right" to conduct human subject research either under the Constitution or by statute.[103] The federal government is well within its power to create and enforce safeguards against abuse of human subjects, particularly if it is funding the research. Moreover, the moral authority to conduct research depends largely upon the subject's consent, whereas the moral authority to safeguard the public's health is not reliant on individual consent. Rather, public health law can compel individuals to do, or refrain from doing, certain activities for the common good. This distinction between public health practice and research suggests that there are public health activities that can be legitimately carried out without the willing participation of affected persons—but what are they?

Defining Human Subjects Research. The framers of the Common Rule (defined in box 24) never directly addressed the broad range of activities undertaken by health departments. In reading the Common Rule, therefore, it can be difficult to tell when state agencies must comply with federal research regulations. The Common Rule and the HIPAA Privacy Rule (see below) define human subjects research as "a systematic investigation, including research development, testing, and evaluation, designed to develop or contribute to generalizable knowledge."[104] This definition focuses on research design—testing a hypothesis and drawing conclusions from data collected, and thereby contributing to generalizable knowledge.

Unfortunately, the Common Rule's definition does not always help distinguish public health practice from research. Routine public health practice often utilizes scientific methodologies and evidence similar to those used in research. Many public health activities are "systematic" in that they use rigorous scientific procedures to monitor and respond to health threats. Much public health practice similarly is designed to contribute to "generalizable knowledge," since agencies want to extrapolate knowledge gained in public health activities to general understanding of health threats now and in the future. Indeed, the National Bioethics Advisory Commission criticized the ambiguity of this regulatory language, noting that it offers little guidance to distinguish research from public health practice.[105]

National Guidance. In an attempt to clarify the issue, the CDC has relied upon the intent of the actor to determine whether a given public health activity constitutes "research."[106] Following this logic, the public health researcher intends to generate new information with relevance beyond her particular study or program, whereas the public health practitioner intends primarily to prevent or control disease or injury in a given population.[107] The CDC points out that in public health practice, the primary purpose is to benefit communities and protect the health of populations. This view is similar to that taken in the Belmont Report, which defines "practice" as interventions designed to enhance human well-being; in the case of public health, well-being is measured from a community-based perspective.[108] The CDC approach, however, has been criticized as overly subjective, creating incentives for researchers to characterize their work as public health practice in order to avoid IRB review.[109]

The Council of State and Territorial Epidemiologists (CSTE) has proposed enhanced guidelines for distinguishing practice from research.[110] These guidelines focus on (1) *legal authority*—public health practice is authorized by law with a corresponding duty on the agency to conduct the activity; (2) *specific intent*—a practitioner's intent is primarily aimed at ameliorating health threats in the affected community, whereas a researcher's intent is to test a hypothesis and seek generalized findings beyond the activity's participants; (3) *participant benefits*—public health practice aims to provide benefits to the community, whereas research aims primarily to benefit society more generally through advancements in scientific knowledge; and (4) *methodology*—practice is dominated by standard, accepted, and proven interventions to address a public health problem, whereas research often has an experimental design, such as random selection.[111] These guidelines do not solve the dilemma, of course, but they do provide additional tools to make differentiations. It is also apparent that even if public health activities begin as forms of practice, they can evolve into research.

CSTE resists federal oversight of routine public health practices, asserting that state officials already are legally and politically accountable. Still, if federal oversight of public health practice is inappropriate, should each state then mandate quite specific processes and standards for independent ethical review? Some ethicists argue that even if routine public health practices are not classified as research, they should nonetheless be subjected to careful, dispassionate review to ensure that participants are treated with dignity and respect.[112] This could take the form of specific state accountability or, minimally, a code of public health research ethics with a well-articulated statement of principles. Although the ethics of public health research and practice has received increased attention from scholars and government agencies, an authoritative articulation of workable principles has yet to be promulgated.

Privacy and Confidentiality in Research

Public health investigators collect a great deal of sensitive personal health information, often in identifiable form. It is, therefore, important to understand the privacy safeguards that apply to research. The Common Rule, the HIPAA Privacy Rule, and Certificates of Confidentiality are the three primary ways in which the privacy of research subjects is protected.

The Common Rule. The Common Rule surprisingly does not set minimum privacy standards. It does require IRBs to ensure that "when appropriate, there are adequate provisions to protect the privacy of subjects."[113] Furthermore, in seeking informed consent, the investigator must provide the subject with "a statement describing the extent, if any, to which confidentiality of records identifying the subject will be maintained."[114] Even if IRBs do take privacy seriously, the regulations themselves merely require safeguards when "appropriate." Although subjects must be informed whether their data are to be held confidentially, the regulations do not require researchers to develop particular safeguards. The model for privacy under the Common Rule therefore depends on consent and independent review rather than on identifiable forms of protection.

The HIPAA Privacy Rule. Confidentiality protections are now supplemented by the requirements of the HIPAA Privacy Rule, discussed in greater detail below.[115] Under the provisions of this rule, covered entities (such as health care providers and insurers) may use or disclose identifiable health information for research without the person's permission only if they obtain a waiver from an IRB or privacy board. Privacy boards must have members with varying backgrounds and appropriate competencies. The waiver criteria include findings that (1) the disclosure involves no more than minimal risk; (2) the research could not practicably be conducted without the waiver; (3) the privacy risks are reasonable in relation to the anticipated benefits, if any, to the individual and the importance of the research; (4) a plan to destroy the identifiers exists unless there is a health or research justification for retaining them; and (5) there are written assurances that the data will not be reused or disclosed to others, except for research oversight or additional research that would also qualify for a waiver.[116] The increased protections in the Privacy Rule have created discontent among researchers. Many contend that its burdens are not sufficiently justified by increased privacy benefits for subjects.[117]

Certificates of Confidentiality. A "confidentiality assurance" (or Certificate of Confidentiality) under section 301(d) of the Public Health Service Act authorizes investigators to withhold the names or other identifying characteristics of research subjects.[118] Investigators who receive a Certificate of Confidentiality cannot be compelled to identify research subjects in any civil, criminal, administrative, or legislative proceeding.[119] The Certificate also appears to relieve researchers from the obligation to comply with state reporting requirements.[120] Although confidentiality assurances provide strong privacy protection, they are subject to important limitations. Their protection is not automatic but must be obtained through a potentially lengthy application process.[121] In addition, although the National Institutes of Health (NIH) has promoted use of Certificates of Confidentiality,[122] researchers remain unaware of their availability.[123] Finally, Certificates of Confidentiality have not been thoroughly tested

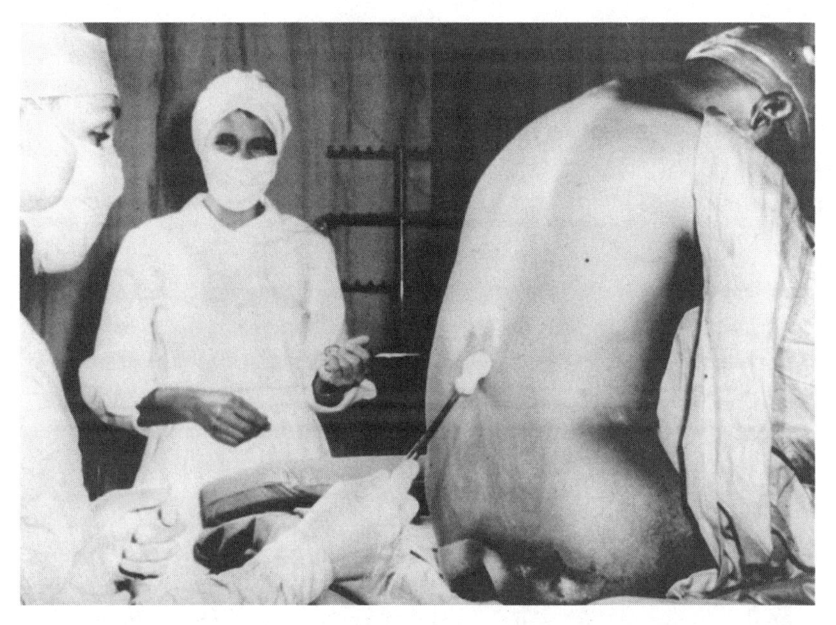

Photo 16. The Tuskegee experiments: A scar on the history of American public health research. The syphilis study in Tuskegee, Alabama, is perhaps the most prominent example of unethical government-sponsored research on human subjects in U.S. history. Spinal taps, such as this one on an unidentified man in 1933, were performed to diagnose neural syphilis. Side effects of the procedure included painful headaches and, in rare cases, paralysis or death. Courtesy of the National Library of Medicine.

in court, so the ultimate value of their protection is uncertain. In the sole documented challenge, the New York Court of Appeals permitted the director of a methadone clinic to resist disclosure of identifiable research data in a murder trial. The court reasoned that research was important, and the agency's interpretation of the legislation is entitled to considerable weight.[124]

Having discussed the ethics and privacy of public health research, the next section discusses health information privacy more generally by defining the concepts, exploring the ethical dimensions, and explaining the legal safeguards.

PRIVACY, CONFIDENTIALITY, AND SECURITY: DEFINING CONCEPTS

Disease provokes enormous fear. Dread of sickness and death is often matched by anxiety about the loss

> of privacy, which can transform a threat to the body
> into something that places one's reputation, resources,
> and even autonomy and liberty at risk. These two
> deeply rooted apprehensions come together as the State
> seeks to monitor diseases in the name of public health.
> Amy L. Fairchild, Ronald Bayer, and James Colgrove (2007)

Public health professionals and researchers collect a great deal of personal information that invades the private sphere of human life. Here, I explore this private sphere, its philosophical underpinnings, and its legal status.[125] Privacy, confidentiality, and security are sometimes thought to be identical concepts, but they are not.[126] Before examining privacy more closely, it will be helpful to offer definitions of these terms (see table 16).

Privacy. The term *privacy*—an individual's claim to limit access by others to some aspect of her personal life—has acquired several different meanings in ethical discourse. This chapter is not concerned with "decisional" privacy—the freedom claimed by individuals to make intimate decisions about their bodily integrity without interference. (Decisional privacy, asserted in contexts of medical treatment, is examined in chapter 10.) It is also not concerned with Samuel Warren and Louis Brandeis's conception of privacy as the "right to be let alone"—the freedom claimed by individuals not to be viewed, photographed, or otherwise inspected without their knowledge.[127] This chapter refers primarily to "informational" privacy and secondarily to confidentiality (sometimes called "relational" privacy). I define health informational privacy as an individual's claim to control the circumstances in which personal health information is collected, used, stored, and transmitted.[128] Informational privacy, then, is concerned with an individual's claim to determine those persons or organizations that may access an identifiable health record (see box 25).

Confidentiality. Confidentiality is a form of health information privacy that focuses on maintaining trust between two individuals engaged in an intimate relationship, characteristically a physician-patient relationship. Confidentiality is a person's claim to keep private the secrets exchanged in the course of that relationship, enforced not simply to respect the person whose confidences are divulged but also to underscore the importance of relationships of trust.

Security. I define security as the technological, organizational, and administrative safety practices, policies, and procedures designed to protect

TABLE 16. The nature of privacy: Defining relevant terms

Privacy	An individual's claim to limit access by others to some aspect of her personal life
Health Informational Privacy	An individual's claim to control the circumstances in which personal health information is collected, used, stored, and transmitted
Confidentiality	A form of health informational privacy that focuses on maintaining trust between two individuals engaged in an intimate relationship, characteristically a physician-patient relationship
Security	The technological, organizational, and administrative safety practices designed to protect a data system against unwarranted disclosure, modification, or destruction and to safeguard the system itself

BOX 25

THE NATURE OF THE PRIVACY INTEREST

Personally identifiable, coded, or anonymous data

A claim to informational privacy is generally valid only if the health record reveals private information about the subject of that record. Consequently, standards for disclosure should vary according to whether the record can be associated with a particular person (see table 17). The most serious privacy concern arises when public health authorities use personally identifiable data, meaning that the person can be identified either by information contained in the record alone or with other information that is available to the record holder.[1] The inclusion of any uniquely identifiable characteristic, such as a name, social security number, fingerprint, or phone number, classifies data as identifiable. Even without a unique identifier, the data may provide sufficient evidence to make a connection to a specific person. Information about location, race, sex, date of birth, and other personal characteristics may make it possible to identify individuals within a small population (e.g., an STI study in a small, predominantly white school that identifies a cluster of syphilis infections among African American females).

The HIPAA Privacy Rule, which applies only to individually identifiable data, specifies two ways a covered entity can determine that health information is nonidentifiable: (1) if an expert applying scientific and statistical principles finds "that the

[1] There is no settled view as to how difficult it must be to determine the person's identity in order to classify the record as "identifiable." Human subject regulations, for example, exempt research involving data recorded in such a manner that "subjects cannot be identified, directly or through identifiers linked to the subjects." *Protection of Human Subjects,* 45 C.F.R. §46.101(b)(4) (1993). A record is "individually identifiable" if "the identity of the subject is or may readily be ascertained by the investigator or associated with the information." 45 C.F.R. § 46.102(f). See Secretary of Health and Human Services, *Confidentiality of Individually Identifiable Health Information: Recommendations of the Secretary of Health and Human Services, Pursuant to Section 264 of the Health Insurance Portability and Accountability Act of 1996* (Sept. 11, 1997) (defining "covered" information as that which "identifies the individual, or with respect to which there is a reasonable basis to believe that the information can be used to identify the patient").

risk is very small that the information could be used, alone or in combination with other reasonably available data, to identify an individual," or (2) if the entity deletes from the record a list of identifiers such as name, geographic designators, dates, telephone numbers, and social security numbers (the "safe harbor").[2]

The HIPAA Privacy Rule does not cover anonymous information—data that have all identifiers stripped, with no reasonable means to associate the record with a specific person. Release of anonymous data does not entail significant privacy concerns because individuals cannot realistically be known. Epidemiologic research and statistical applications involving aggregate data provide illustrations of anonymous research that affords substantial public health benefits with negligible effects on individual privacy. For example, collection and analysis of blood samples or other tissue that cannot be linked to any individual are anonymous; few, if any, restrictions need to be placed on research of this kind.[3]

Anonymous data can raise concerns about "group" privacy—the contested idea that ethnic, racial, or religious groups possess privacy interests. Suppose that a researcher does not collect personally identifiable data but publishes information that stigmatizes a particular group, such as data associated with genetics research on sickle cell anemia (African Americans) or Tay-Sachs disease (Ashkenazi Jews). Or think about a study in a small Native American village finding that the population has extraordinarily high rates of drug abuse, mental illness, or STIs. In each of these cases, members of the group may feel that their reputation and social standing have been diminished.[4]

Linkable data present an intermediate level of privacy concern. These data are not immediately identifiable but can be linked to a named person with the use of a highly secret code. Linkable, or coded, data are not all the same for privacy purposes. If the data holder can readily obtain the key to decode the data, then privacy concerns are heightened; in this case, coded data can be viewed virtually as personally identifiable. However, if the holder cannot realistically decode the data to discover identifiable characteristics, then for all practical purposes, these data may be viewed as anonymous. The major issue becomes whether the firewall between the holder of the data and the holder of the key is penetrable. For example, states send AIDS case reports to the CDC using a "soundex" code that the federal agency cannot decipher. The data held by the state health department are personally identifiable, but the data held by the CDC can be treated as anonymous for privacy purposes.

Public health professionals claim that identifiable, or linkable, data are often necessary for quality surveillance and research in order to assure accurate and complete records, avoid duplication of cases, and conduct follow-up investigations. Anonymous data complicate the task of obtaining useful information about risk behavior and natural history—the type of information that is available from interviews with physicians and patients and from medical record reviews that are currently accessed through the patient's name.[5]

Decisions to use identifiable, anonymous, or coded surveillance also can be controversial. In the mid-1990s, CDC's anonymous HIV seroprevalence study of newborns

[2] 45 C.F.R. §164.514 (2001).

[3] National Bioethics Advisory Commission, *Research Involving Human Biological Materials: Ethical Issues and Policy* (Bethesda, MD: NBAC, 1999).

[4] James G. Hodge, Jr., and Mark E. Harris, "International Genetics Research and Issues of Group Privacy," *Journal of Biolaw and Business,* Special Suppl. (2001): 15–21; Madison Powers, "Justice and Genetics: Privacy Protection and the Moral Basis of Public Policy," in *Genetic Secrets: Protecting Privacy and Confidentiality in the Genetic Era,* ed. Mark A. Rothstein (New Haven, CT: Yale University Press, 1997): 355.

[5] Lawrence O. Gostin and Jack Hadley, "Editorial: Health Services Research—Public Benefits, Personal Privacy, and Proprietary Interests," *Annals of Internal Medicine,* 129 (1998): 833–35.

provided scientifically valid, critically important surveillance data with negligible privacy risks. Nevertheless, this important study was criticized by Congress and ultimately withdrawn because, with anonymous records, health authorities lacked the capacity to inform mothers of an infant's infection status and need for treatment.[6]

[6] Howard Minkof and Anne Willoughby, "Pediatric HIV Disease, Zidovudine in Pregnancy, and Unblinding Heelstick Surveys: Reframing the Debate on Prenatal HIV Testing," *JAMA*, 274 (1995): 1165.

TABLE 17. The nature of personally identifiable information

Personally Identifiable Data	Person can be identified either by information contained in the record or by other information that is available to the record holder
Anonymous Data	Data with all identifiers stripped, with no reasonable means to associate the information with a specific person
Linkable Data	Data that are not immediately identifiable to the record holder, but where the "key" unlocking the person's identity can be ascertained from a third party

a data system against unwarranted disclosure, modification, or destruction and to safeguard the system itself. For example, secure data systems require passwords or "keys" to access information, perform audit trails to monitor system users, and use encryption to scramble access codes. A secure data system protects health records from unauthorized use. Invasions of privacy certainly occur when, due to inadequate security, personal records are accessed without permission. No security measure, however, can prevent invasion of privacy by those who have authority to access the record. And many privacy scholars believe that the most serious threats to privacy come from authorized systemic data uses rather than from unauthorized users who "hack" into the system. Consequently, even the most technologically secure data systems do not ensure privacy.

HEALTH INFORMATION PRIVACY: ETHICAL UNDERPINNINGS

Ethical justifications for privacy rely on the intimate nature of health data, the potential harm to persons, and the overall effect on the public health system if privacy is eroded. Public health records contain significant amounts of sensitive information: Public health officials are concerned about an individual's behavior (e.g., sexuality, smoking, and alcohol or drug use), genetic profile (e.g., genetic carrier states, predispositions, and disease), and social/racial/economic status (e.g., poverty, nutrition, and social relationships). Consequently, public health records contain a vast amount of personal information with multiple uses: demographics, public benefit eligibility, disabilities, sexual relationships, lifestyle choices, current and predictive health status, and much more. This information is frequently sufficient to provide a detailed individual profile. In addition, traditional public health records are only a subset of the records containing substantial health or personal information held by government agencies such as social services, immigration, law enforcement, and education.

A variety of harms may result from unwanted disclosure of these sensitive health data. Intrinsic harms (sometimes called "wrongs") result merely from unwanted or unjustified disclosure of personal information.[129] Many moral views recognize the desirability of protecting individuals against the insult to dignity and lack of respect for the person evidenced by such disclosures. Furthermore, a breach of privacy can result in economic harm, such as loss of employment, insurance, or housing. It can also result in social or psychological harm; disclosure of some conditions (e.g., HIV and other STIs) can be stigmatizing and may cause embarrassment, social isolation, and a loss of self-esteem. These risks are especially great when the perceived causes of the health condition include the use of illegal drugs, socially disfavored forms of sexual expression, or other behavior that engenders social disapproval. Family members, neighbors, and work associates may withdraw social support from individuals known to have certain socially disfavored diseases.

Privacy is important to the effective functioning of the health system. Persons at risk of disease may not come forward for testing, counseling, and treatment if they are not assured that their confidences will be respected. They are also less likely to divulge sensitive information to health professionals. Failure to divulge communicable diseases may pose a risk to the health of sexual, needle-sharing, or other contacts. Informational privacy, therefore, is valued to protect not only patients' social and economic interests but also their health and the health of the wider community.

HEALTH INFORMATION PRIVACY: LEGAL STATUS

Thus far, I have suggested that health information affords meaningful public health benefits but also poses privacy risks. Legal protection of health information should, to the extent possible, facilitate use of health information to gain public benefits while still furnishing reasonable privacy protection.[130] Unfortunately, existing law—constitutional and legislative—neither promotes the public good nor satisfactorily protects privacy.

The Constitutional Right to Informational Privacy

Judicial recognition of a constitutional right to informational privacy is particularly important, since the government is the principal collector and disseminator of public health information.[131] Citizens should not have to rely on the government's choice to protect their privacy interests. Rather, individuals need protection from the government itself, and an effective constitutional remedy is the surest method to shield them from unauthorized government acquisition or disclosure of personal information. The problem with this approach is that the Constitution does not expressly provide a right to privacy.

Despite the absence of express constitutional language, the Supreme Court has found a qualified right to health informational privacy. In *Whalen v. Roe* (1977),[132] the Court squarely faced the question of whether the constitutional right to privacy encompasses the collection, storage, and dissemination of health information in government data banks. At issue was a New York statute requiring physicians to report to the state information about certain dangerous prescription drugs and to store the data in a central computer. The Court acknowledged "the threat to privacy implicit in the accumulation of vast amounts of personal information in computerized data banks or other massive government files."[133] It further noted that the supervision of public health activities "requires the orderly preservation of great quantities of information, much of which is personal in character and potentially embarrassing or harmful if disclosed."[134] However, the Court found no violation in *Whalen* because the state had adequate standards and procedures for protecting privacy: Computer tapes were kept in a locked cabinet, the computer was run off-line to avoid unauthorized access, and the data were disclosed to a limited number of officials.

Lower courts have read *Whalen* as affording a narrow right to informational privacy or have grounded the right in state constitutional law.[135] Courts have employed a flexible test balancing the invasion of privacy against the strength of the government interest. For example, the Third Circuit in *United States v. Westinghouse Electric Corporation* (1980)[136] enunciated five factors to be balanced in determining the scope of the constitutional right to informational privacy: (1) the type of record and the information it contains, (2) the potential for harm in any unauthorized disclosure, (3) the injury from disclosure to the relationship in which the record was generated, (4) the adequacy of safeguards to prevent nonconsensual disclosure, and (5) the degree of need for access (i.e., a recognizable public interest).

Judicial deference to government's express need to acquire and use information is an unmistakable theme running through case law. Provided that the government articulates a valid societal purpose, such as protection of the public's health, and employs reasonable privacy and security measures, courts are unlikely to interfere with traditional surveillance activities.[137]

The HIPAA Privacy Rule

Electronic communication of individually identifiable health information is essential to modern medicine and public health, but the systematic acquisition, use, and disclosure of health data also gives rise to substantial privacy risks.[138] To address these risks, the Secretary for Health and Human Services promulgated privacy regulations pursuant to the Health Insurance Portability and Accountability Act of 1996 (HIPAA),[139] with an implementation date of April 14, 2003, for most entities.[140] The regulations provided the first systematic nationwide privacy protection for health information. The Privacy Rule is so important to public health practice that it will be helpful to cover it in some detail by explaining, first, its basic provisions and, second, its application to public health. (The application of the Privacy Rule to human subject research is covered above.) Except in relation to public health (see below), the Privacy Rule supersedes all state and local laws that provide less privacy protection, a concept known as "floor preemption."

BASIC PROVISIONS OF THE PRIVACY RULE

To understand the Privacy Rule, it is necessary to explain who is covered, the types of data that are protected, and the safeguards that are afforded.

(1) *Covered entities.* The Privacy Rule applies only to a defined set of "covered entities," which include health plans (e.g., health insurers, managed care organizations), health care providers (e.g., physicians, hospitals, clinics), and health clearinghouses (e.g., billing services). Business associates of covered entities, such as lawyers, accountants, and other contractors, are also covered. The Privacy Rule does not cover other entities that

routinely handle sensitive health information, such as certain insurers (life, auto, and workers' compensation) or public agencies that deliver security or welfare benefits.

(2) *Protected health information (PHI).* The Privacy Rule applies only to PHI, which is individually identifiable health data that are transmitted or maintained in electronic form. PHI must relate to past, present, or future physical or mental health, health care, or payment. The regulations have detailed specifications for determining whether data are personally identifiable (see box 25).

(3) *Authorized disclosures for treatment, payment, or health care operations.* The Privacy Rule requires covered entities to obtain the individual's written consent (except in emergencies or other limited circumstances) for "routine" uses and disclosures of PHI for treatment, payment, or health care operations (e.g., quality assurance or utilization review). The consent model for routine uses is not rigorous; it permits, for example, a signed form in the first physician visit authorizing all future disclosures. The consent is not truly voluntary either, because the provider can condition treatment, and the health plan can condition enrollment, on signing the consent.

(4) *Authorized disclosures not related to health care.* The Privacy Rule, however, has strong and meaningful safeguards for non-routine data uses—that is, for purposes unrelated to health care (e.g., employment, insurance, or housing). Covered entities may not use or disclose health information for nonroutine purposes without explicit patient authorization, which must be informed and voluntary. Even with authorization, covered entities must limit disclosures to the minimum necessary to achieve the purposes of the use or disclosure.

(5) *Unauthorized disclosures.* The Privacy Rule allows covered entities to use and disclose PHI for the following purposes or as required by law: abuse, neglect, or domestic violence, law enforcement, judicial and administrative proceedings, agency oversight activities, and workers' compensation. Unauthorized disclosures for public health (see below) and health research (see above) are discussed separately.

(6) *Privacy and security policies.* The Privacy Rule requires covered entities to: notify individuals of their privacy rights and how their PHI is used or disclosed; adopt and implement privacy policies and procedures; train members of the workforce; designate a privacy official responsible for policies and procedures; and accept inquiries or complaints from patients.

THE PRIVACY RULE AND PUBLIC HEALTH

Public health agencies rely heavily on access to identifiable health information to accomplish their core functions of monitoring health threats and responding to injury, disease, and disability among populations.[141] Health information is vital to routine public health activities such as surveillance, program evaluation, terrorism preparedness, and outbreak investigations.

(1) *Disclosures to public health authorities.* The Privacy Rule permits unauthorized disclosures of PHI to public health authorities for specified public health activities, including reporting (disease, injury, child abuse or neglect, and vital statistics); surveillance, investigations, and interventions; activities under FDA jurisdiction (adverse events, product recalls, and postmarketing surveillance); notification of persons at risk of communicable disease; and medical surveillance in the workplace. Consequently, the rule permits public health authorities to engage in the full range of public health activities authorized by law (see below).

(2) *Preemption.* Although the Privacy Rule supersedes state and local law in other venues, it expressly does not preempt state and local law for public health reporting, surveillance, investigation, or intervention.[142]

(3) *Accounting for public health disclosures.* Covered entities must comply with certain requirements related to disclosures of PHI to public health authorities. Most importantly, covered entities must provide individuals, upon request, with an accounting of how their information was shared. To ease the burden on covered entities and to encourage disclosure, the Office of Civil Rights has clarified that multiple public health disclosures need only be accounted for generally, such as by informing patients of the kind of information, the recipient, and the public health purpose.[143]

(4) *Definition of public health authority.* A public health authority is defined widely as a federal, tribal, state, or local agency, or person or entity acting under a grant of authority or contract with the agency.[144] However, a public health agency may also be a covered entity with responsibility for complying with the Privacy Rule. For example, an agency operating a health clinic and providing medical care, such as STI, HIV, or TB treatment, is covered under the Privacy Rule.

(5) *Authorized by law.* The Privacy Rule allows covered entities to disclose PHI to public health authorities when authorized by federal, tribal, state, or local laws. [145] Although it is not a defined term, the Secretary has interpreted "authorized by law" to mean that a legal basis exists for the activity, including actions that are permitted and those that are required by law.[146] Public health authorities, therefore, may operate under broad mandates to protect the health of their constituent populations.

(6) *Ongoing controversies.* Despite the broad authority afforded to public health agencies to carry out their mission, there remain questions and controversies about the application of the Privacy Rule to public health activities. Covered entities are authorized but not required to disclose data to public health authorities under the Privacy Rule, although state law may mandate certain disclosures. Health care providers, for example, may resist sharing large-scale medical data for syndromic surveillance, outbreak investigations, or even in public health emergencies such as bioterrorism. These providers express concerns about the privacy of data uses, the security of data systems, and the increased administrative burdens of accounting to patients for the ways in which their records have been shared.[147]

The Federal Privacy Act and the Freedom of Information Act

Although the HIPAA Privacy Rule affords by far the most important safeguard of health informational privacy, there are additional protections for federal record systems under the Privacy Act of 1974 and the Freedom of Information Act of 1966 (FOIA).

The Privacy Act of 1974 requires federal agencies to utilize fair information practices with regard to "any record" contained in "a system of records."[148] The statute gives individuals the right to consent to the disclosure of information and to review and correct inaccuracies in the record. Agencies can keep only relevant information and cannot "match" files through the use of a personal identifier. The Privacy Act, however, permits agencies to disclose information for "routine uses," meaning that they can use health records for any "purpose which is compatible with the purpose for which [the information] was collected."[149]

The FOIA requires the disclosure of records that would otherwise have to be kept confidential under the Privacy Act.[150] However, the act contains several exemptions that permit agencies to withhold disclosure. The exemptions most important to public health are specific statutory exclusions from FOIA disclosure requirements (e.g., identifiable health statistics, drug abuse treatment records, and venereal disease records);[151] "privileged or confidential" data (federal health agencies rely on this exemption to resist judicial discovery of confidential patient or research records—for example, in cases involving toxic shock, Reyes syndrome, and cancer registry data);[152] and personnel and medical files (federal agencies can use this exemption to protect individuals from injury and embarrassment).[153]

State Privacy Laws

States have enacted health information privacy protection in highly diverse ways, including statutes modeled after the federal Privacy Act and FOIA. A careful examination of the myriad state law protections of public health data is beyond the scope of this text, but national surveys are reported in the literature.[154] All states provide some statutory protection for government-maintained health data—public health data in general, and communicable or sexually transmitted diseases in particular. Many states provide specific protections for data reported to the health department or data held in state registries or databases (e.g., congenital birth defects, cancers, or childhood immunizations). Virtually all states permit disclosure of public health information for various purposes, including statistics, partner notification, epidemiologic investigations, subpoena, and court order.

Although many states have reasonably consistent standards for government-held health information, the privacy protection afforded to privately held data is widely regarded as inadequate. The law is fragmented, highly variable, and at times weak. Some states have comprehensive medical information statutes, others regulate the use of information by licensed professionals or hospitals, and still others regulate the use of insurance information.[155] The Department of Health and Human Services described this body of privacy legislation as "a morass of erratic law."[156]

Federal and state law frequently single out particular diseases for special status; as a result, data relating to these health conditions receive high levels of privacy. For example, the law often affords extraordinary privacy protection for data relating to drug and alcohol treatment,[157] HIV/AIDS,[158] or genetic conditions.[159] These disease-specific privacy statutes create inconsistencies in the rules governing the use of health information: Different standards apply to data held by the same institutions depending on whether the patient is receiving treatment for a protected disease. More important, the argument that certain diseases deserve special status rests on a weak foundation because many other health conditions raise similar issues of sensitivity and intimacy.

TOWARD A MODEL PUBLIC HEALTH INFORMATION PRIVACY LAW

The collection of vast amounts of information in the course of public health practice and research yields substantial collective benefits for the public's health and well-being. At the same time, personally identifiable data pose serious privacy risks. As hard as they may try, policymakers cannot design a perfect method for reconciling these interests. Inevitably, individuals will have to give up some privacy in the interest of the public good, and society will have to forgo some benefits to afford individuals respect for their privacy. Despite these complex trade-offs, rational policy could be formulated to improve informational privacy and security while still facilitating legitimate uses of public health data. Elsewhere, my colleagues and I have proposed a Model State Public Health Privacy Act that balances collective and individual interests.[160] This section offers an abbreviated description of that proposed statute (see figure 30).

The Model Act's approach is to maximize privacy safeguards where they matter most to individuals and facilitate data uses where necessary to promote the public's health. Consider the sequence of events when government collects, uses, and discloses public health data. First, the agency collects the data; for data that has a strong public health purpose, most people believe that individuals should forgo this small privacy invasion for the communal good. For example, the reporting of infectious

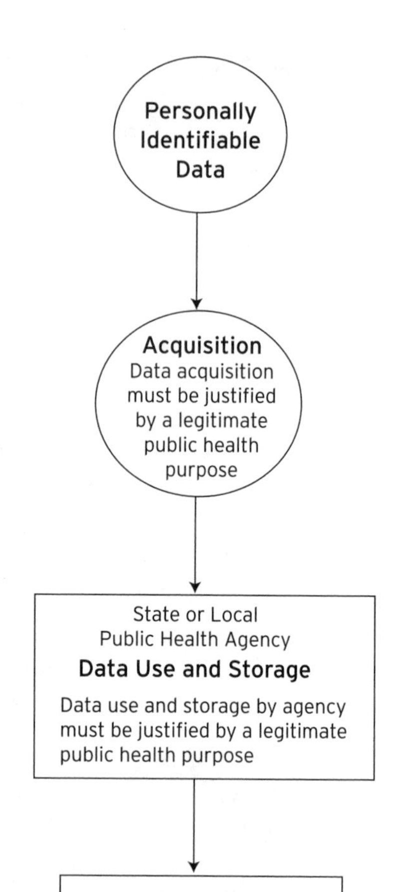

Note: A "legitimate public health purpose" is a population-level activity or individual effort primarily aimed at the prevention of injury, disease, or premature mortality or the promotion of community health.

Figure 30. Model State Public Health Privacy Act.

diseases and injuries by name is indispensable to the public's health, and many believe that chronic disease surveillance can be just as important.

Second, the agency uses the data strictly within the confines of the public health system (i.e., within the agency itself or with other state or local public health agencies). Again, provided the agency has a strong public health purpose and the data are shared only with public health officials who have a need to know, data uses should prevail over privacy. The reason for this conclusion is that when public health authorities acquire and use data strictly within the public health system, health benefits are at their highest and privacy risks are at their lowest. Public health authorities need the freedom to use the data to monitor and prevent health risks. If these data remain inside the public health system, patients face few social risks.

Third, the agency may seek to disclose the information to persons outside the public health system (e.g., employers, insurers, commercial marketers, police, family, or friends). These kinds of disclosures are not very important for the public's health, but they do place patients at considerable risk of embarrassment, stigma, and discrimination. For these reasons, the law ought to provide maximum privacy protection. The Model Act would impose significant civil and criminal penalties for unauthorized disclosures to individuals or businesses outside the confines of the public health system.

In sum, the Model Act's approach is to give government the flexibility to acquire and use data strictly within the confines of the public health system, providing it can demonstrate an important public health purpose. However, the Model Act affords public health authorities very little discretion to release data outside the public health system and imposes serious penalties for unauthorized disclosures without the patient's informed consent.

The Model Act also requires public health agencies to adopt a set of fair information practices with the following components:

- *Data protection review.* An independent data protection authority should be established to carefully review privacy and security protocols and practices.
- *Data collection justification.* Acquisition of health information cannot be regarded as an inherent good, so agencies should demonstrate that identifiable information is necessary to achieve an important public health purpose.

- *Information for persons and populations.* Individuals and populations are entitled to basic information, such as the purposes of data collection and how personal information will be used, the length of time data will be stored, and procedures for disclosure.
- *No secret data systems.* Agencies should inform the public about all record systems maintained by the agency.
- *Access to and correction of information.* Persons should have access to information about themselves, and there should be fair procedures for correcting and amending their records.
- *Security measures.* Agencies should develop and distribute written security plans requiring physically and technologically secure informational environments.

These proposals, while not perfect, provide a balance between the social good of data collection (recognizing its substantial value to community health) and the individual good of privacy (recognizing the normative value of respect for persons). Perhaps citizens do not desire absolute privacy, but rather require only reasonable assurances that public health authorities will treat personal information with respect, store it in an orderly and secure manner, and use it only for important health purposes and in accordance with publicly accountable principles of fairness.

Having examined the multiple ways in which public health agencies collect personal information and the effects on privacy, the next chapter turns to the powers of agencies to regulate the use of information in the private sector. The aim of such regulation, as we will see, is to control the informational environment to encourage healthier and safer behaviors in the population.

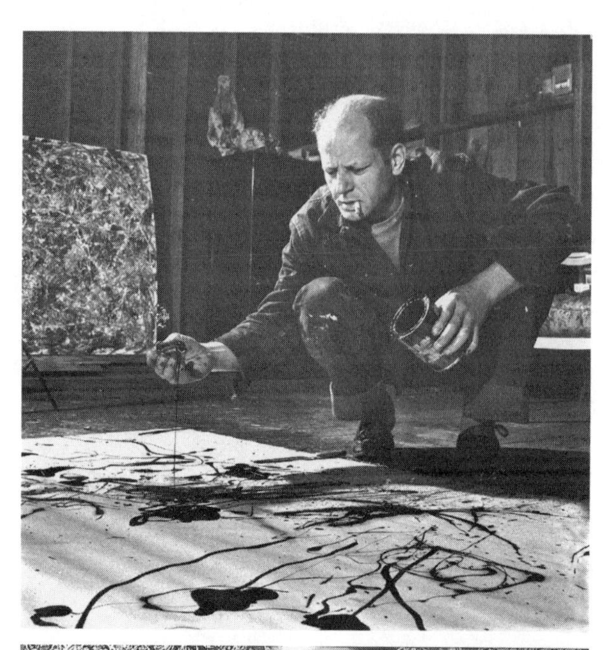

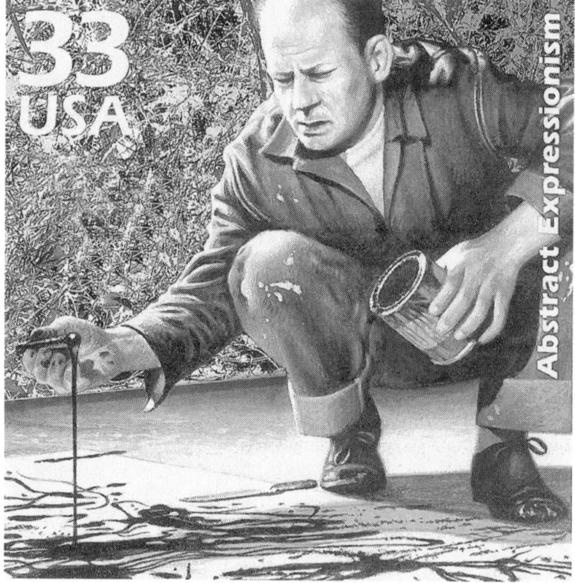

Photo 17. Jackson Pollock photo and corresponding postage stamp image with cigarette removed. This 1960s image of Jackson Pollack was used by the U.S. Postal Service for a stamp issued in 1999. Note that the Postal Service removed the cigarette from the original image. Martha Holmes/Getty Images.

CHAPTER 9

Health, Communication, and Behavior

Freedom of Expression

I met with several kinds of associations in America of which I confess I had no previous notion; and I have often admired the extreme skill with which the inhabitants of the United States succeed in proposing a common object for the exertions of a great many men and in inducing them voluntarily to pursue it. . . . Among the laws that rule human societies there is one which seems to be more precise and clear than all others. If men are to remain civilized or to become so, the art of associating together must grow and improve in the same ratio in which the equality of conditions is increased.

Alexis de Tocqueville (1840)

The field of public health is deeply concerned with the communication of ideas. Human behavior is a powerful contributor to injury and disease, so public health strives to influence behavioral choices. Many factors influence behavior, but information is a prerequisite for change.[1] The population must at least be aware of the health consequences of risk behaviors to make informed decisions. The citizenry is bombarded with behavioral messages that affect its health—by the media and entertainment, trade associations and corporations, religious and civic organizations, and family and peers.[2] Public health officials strive to be heard above the din of conflicting and confusing communications. Consequently, the field of public health is a virtual battleground of ideas.

Public health agencies deliver messages to promote healthy behavior and restrict messages that encourage risk taking. The fields of medicine and public health exert influence on behavior at various levels of intervention: At the individual level, they counsel individuals at risk for injury and disease (e.g., HIV prevention, genetic disease, or reproductive choice); at the group level, they inform and promote behavior change (e.g., hospital or managed care newsletters, or support groups); at the population level, they educate the public and market healthy lifestyles (e.g., public-service advertisements, health communication campaigns, or school-based health education).

Public health agencies not only deliver health messages but also regulate private sector communications. The state suppresses commercial messages deemed hazardous to the public's health and compels messages deemed essential to the public's health. However, governmental control of the informational environment raises profound social and constitutional questions. Substantial public health benefits can be achieved by reducing risk behavior, but regulation of communication can stifle freedom of thought, expression, and association. It is for this reason that government control over the informational environment can be deeply controversial in a modern liberal democracy.

TWO ANTITHETICAL THEORIES OF HEALTH COMMUNICATION

> The ultimate good desired is better reached by free trade in ideas—that the best of truth is the power of the thought to get itself accepted in the competition of the market, and that truth is the only ground upon which their wishes safely can be carried out. That at any rate is the theory of our constitution.
>
> Oliver Wendell Holmes (1919)

The First Amendment, as written, is simple and unqualified—but it is far from easy and certainly not absolute: "Congress shall make no law . . . abridging the freedom of speech, or of the press." First Amendment and public health theorists offer two antithetical visions of government's role in health communication: a "free marketplace of ideas" vision in which individuals are free agents with the ability to assess health messages and make decisions in their own interests, and a "consumer protection" vision in which the government actively intervenes to convey messages conducive to population health and constrain messages detrimental to that goal.[3]

First Amendment theory is grounded in both intrinsic and instrumental values.[4] Free expression is an end in itself, for it is essential to autonomy, self-fulfillment, and personhood. Free expression has intrinsic value because it provides a vehicle for self-realization in which individuals and groups define and proclaim their identity.[5]

Beyond its intrinsic value, the most familiar theories hold that free expression has instrumental value in that it enhances democracy or self-governance and advances truthful ideas. Freedom of expression is necessary for representative government. Without the free exchange of ideas, the electorate cannot become informed, public officials cannot arrive at wise policy choices, and the public cannot exercise democratic control or insist on political accountability.[6] The self-governance theory emphasizes the importance of political speech,[7] which, in turn, may insufficiently value artistic, scientific, and other forms of expression.

Finally, and most important for our purposes, freedom of expression is thought necessary for the discovery of truth. On this theory, a robust discourse of all potential ideas will ultimately advance knowledge and "truth." Classic statements of the "truth-finding" function of free expression are offered by John Milton[8] and, later, John Stuart Mill,[9] who claimed that suppression of communication is always wrong: "If an idea is true, society is denied the truth; if it is false, society is denied the fuller understanding of truth which comes from its conflict with error; and when the received opinion is part truth and part error, society can know the whole truth only by allowing the airing of competing views."[10] Oliver Wendell Holmes invoked the potent metaphor of the "marketplace of ideas" to capture the notion that truthful expressions will prevail in the competition of a free market.[11]

Public health professionals do not dispute the intrinsic value of free expression in promoting autonomy or personhood, nor do they quarrel with the instrumental value of political speech for enhancing representational democracy. Public health authorities do not, however, abide the theory that "truth" (in this context, a health-promoting idea) will necessarily prevail in a free market of communication. The field of public health, by its nature and design, is interventionist, taking as its starting point the necessity of behavioral change to enhance the well-being of the population.[12] Rigorous scientific investigation of behaviors that are safe, and those that are risky, is the ultimate arbiter of "truth." Therefore, "wise" communications are those that convey the best scientific evidence of health and behavior. For this reason public health agencies seek, more or less, to control the environment of health information—to disseminate health messages, to compel "truthful" (that is, science-based) disclosure of risks and hazards, and to constrain false or misleading statements.

Public health authorities are interventionist because they distrust the free market to inform the public objectively about risk behaviors or to persuade the polity to conform to guidelines for healthy living. A cacophony of explicit and implicit messages and images about health exists. How can the lay public identify science-based messages accurately? More important, the "marketplace" rationale assumes that all competing messages possess a fair chance of being heard. In the real world, though, the managers of mass media and those with economic resources or political power gain disproportionate access to the most effective channels of communication.[13] Laurence Tribe asks, "How do we know that the analogy of the market is an apt one? Especially when the wealthy have more access to the most potent media of communication than the poor, how sure can we be that 'free trade in ideas' is likely to generate truth?"[14]

How does the Constitution mediate between these antithetical visions of health, communication, and behavior? In this chapter, I explore the parameters of government's role in controlling the informational environment: first, in conveying health information (government speech); second, in constraining advertising that adversely affects the public's health (commercial speech); and third, in requiring product health and safety disclosures or counteradvertising (compelled commercial speech).[15] I conclude this chapter with a case study on the pervasive marketing of high-calorie/low-nutrient foods to children.

GOVERNMENT SPEECH: PUBLIC HEALTH COMMUNICATIONS

> "If there is any fixed star in our constitutional constellation, it is that no official, high or petty, can prescribe what shall be orthodox in politics, nationalism, religion, or other matters of opinion." . . . Under the First Amendment the government must leave to the people the evaluation of ideas. Bold or subtle, an idea is as powerful as the audience allows it to be.
>
> Frank H. Easterbrook (1985)
> quoting Robert H. Jackson (1943)

> [As part of the "Celebrate the Century" series, the U.S. Postal Service issued a stamp of one of Jackson Pollock's most important abstract expressionist works.] The image, however, is missing something. In the

> original, . . . Pollock had a cigarette stuck in the left corner of his mouth, and a cloud of smoke hung spectrally over his outstretched hand. They're gone. . . . It's a striking visual image that has been cleansed . . . for the masses to see.
>
> David Brown (1999)

Government, as a health educator, uses health communication campaigns as a major public health strategy. Health education campaigns, like other forms of advertising, are persuasive communications; instead of promoting a product or a political philosophy, public health authorities promote safer, more healthful behaviors.[16] Consider some of the highly developed health education campaigns initiated by the Department of Health and Human Services (DHHS): "Girl Power!" (health information targeted to girls), "Back to Sleep" (SIDS), "Sisters Together: Move More / Eat Better" (obesity control), "Milk Matters" (calcium for tweens and teens), and "Above the Influence" (antidrug messages).

The government is becoming highly sophisticated in its health education campaigns and employs a number of mass media technologies: radio and television (paid and public service advertisements), newspapers and magazines (press releases and briefings), telephone lines ("800" number hotlines and "broadcast" and "auto-response" faxes), and the Internet (Web sites, listservs, and e-mails). Government also subsidizes educational messages through grants and contracts with private and voluntary organizations. Government selects the funding recipient and the messages that the organization will convey. In its HIV prevention grants, for example, the government subsidizes health messages about safer sex and forbids encouragement of drug use or homosexuality.[17]

Health education often is a preferred public health strategy, and in many ways, it is unobjectionable. Through health communication campaigns, the government persuades individuals to alter risk behaviors. The government imparts knowledge to help inform the polity about activities that promote health and well-being. When the government speaks, citizens may choose to listen and adhere to the health messages or to reject what the government has communicated.[18]

We like to think that public health's concern with "healthy messages" is an inherent good, and we are prepared to give government considerable leeway in constructing a "favorable" informational environment. But the state's concern with health and personal behavior frequently conflicts with other important social values. When public health agencies counsel individuals or educate groups about the government's view concerning unsafe sex, abortion, smoking, a high-fat diet, or a sedentary lifestyle, there is no formal coercion. Yet education conveys more than information; it is also a process of inculcation and acculturation intended to change behavior. Even though they are not always particularly adept or successful, public health agencies routinely construct social norms or meanings to achieve healthier populations. Not everyone believes that public funds should be expended, or the veneer of government legitimacy used, to prescribe particular social orthodoxies.[19]

Although public health campaigns are well intended, they can cause social and psychological harm by making people feel responsibility (or shame) for their disease or associating ill health with socially undesirable characteristics.[20] As to the issue of responsibility, education campaigns can increase resentment of personal lifestyles that impose financial and other costs. The person who fails to lose weight or stop excessive drinking or smoking is burdened not only with health risks but also with a loss of sympathy and support.

As to the issue of socially undesirable characteristics, consider two alternative ways of delivering a comparable health message. In the first, government conveys basic information about risk behaviors (e.g., smoking cigarettes causes cancer, or eating high-fat foods causes heart disease). In the second, government associates the risk behavior with unattractive features (e.g., people who smoke cigarettes have bad breath, develop aging effects of the skin, or may become sexually impotent; or people who eat high-fat foods or live sedentary lifestyles are lazy and unappealing). The first message is socially acceptable but unlikely to effect behavioral change. The latter message is more likely to alter behavior but can exacerbate social and psychological harms, such as stigma (caused by teasing or ostracizing) and low self-esteem (among, for example, overweight girls with a negative body image).[21] Government may, understandably, claim that these messages simply portray the real health effects of risky behaviors, and public health education does counteract misleading advertisements that associate attractive lifestyles with smoking cigarettes, drinking alcoholic beverages, or eating fast foods. Still, there is a line beyond which government should not go in constructing social meanings, especially when messages and images pose psychological risks for vulnerable populations.[22]

Despite their effects on freedom of choice and social relationships, health communication campaigns can be justified in several ways.[23] Arguably, government has a duty to protect and promote the population's health, independent of individual preferences. Certainly, failure to inform citizens of scientific information relevant to their health and safety would be objectionable. Most people want government to educate the public about healthy lifestyles, recognizing that existing information sources may be insufficient, unreliable, or confusing. Health education campaigns can also appeal to third-party interests. For behaviors that are primarily self-regarding (e.g., diet, smoking, and seat belts), the government can emphasize collective harms, such as social and health care costs. And for behaviors that are "other-regarding" (e.g., drunk driving and unsafe sex), the government can also emphasize the harm to the public's health and safety.

Justifications for health communication campaigns are weakest when government health claims are not based solidly on scientific research. Government cannot claim to be objectively informing citizens if the scientific evidence is unpersuasive or contradictory. In some cases, the scientific underpinnings of the public health message are weak or uncertain. Even the most enduring and credible health messages can be based on observed associations rather than clinical trials. The Women's Health Initiative (a long-term national health study focusing on preventing heart disease and cancer in postmenopausal women), for example, refuted government health messages delivered for many years about the value of hormone replacement therapy[24] and low-fat diets.[25] In other cases, experts disagree on the correct health message. The credibility of government pronouncements about obesity (the CDC overestimated annual deaths due to obesity by more than 300,000)[26] or mammography (expert panels disagreed on screening for forty-year-old women)[27] has also been called in question.

Sometimes public health officials face intriguing ethical questions about "truth telling." Suppose government distorts scientific evidence to achieve desirable public health goals. Public health officials may overestimate the risk in order to secure healthy behavior or conceal the degree of behavioral change necessary to promote good health, if full candor might result in noncompliance.[28] Is the government's beneficent intention sufficient to warrant a misleading health message? For example, would it be ethical for public health officials to overstate or mischaracterize the risk of, say, heterosexual transmission of HIV in high-socioeconomic-status neighborhoods or secondhand smoke in public places to promote behavior change or policy reforms? What if the government conceals or suppresses scientific evidence for political or policy reasons, as critics charged the Bush administration was doing (see box 26)?

BOX 26

GOVERNMENT SUPPRESSION OR DISREGARD OF SCIENCE

Executive privilege or concealment of truth?

Science, like any field of endeavor, relies on freedom of inquiry; and one of the hallmarks of that freedom is objectivity. Now more than ever, on issues ranging from climate change to AIDS research to genetic engineering to food additives, government relies on the impartial perspective of science for guidance.
President George H. W. Bush, 1990

- From 1997 until 2000, the White House Office of National Drug Policy (ONDP) scrutinized scripts of prime-time television shows like *ER* and *Beverly Hills 90210* before they ran. The "drug czar" made "recommendations" about programmatic content, urging broadcasters to filter out messages that tacitly condone drug use and reinforce messages that discourage drug use. Broadcasters who complied were exempt from costly obligations to run antidrug public service announcements. Consumers were never informed that federal officials had filtered the scripts in advance or that broadcasters had altered images and content. Responding to protests that the program amounted to "self-censorship in exchange for a fee," the White House ceased reading scripts in advance but continues to reward networks for shows with strong antidrug themes.[1]
- The General Accountability Office (GAO) in 2006 revealed that the Bush administration had spent more than $1.6 billion in public relations over two years, including payments to columnists, media firms, and networks to editorialize in favor of administration policies.[2] The most infamous illustration was a payment to television pundit Armstrong Williams to promote the No Child Left Behind program, but similar examples can be found in health policy. The DHHS, ONDP, and FDA distributed prepackaged news clips that promoted Medicare reform, discouraged drug use, and warned consumers not to buy prescription drugs from Canada. Other reports placed the government in a favorable light on policies ranging from childhood obesity and drunk driving to preservation of the environment.[3] Neither the agencies nor the networks informed viewers that the messages were paid for and created by the government. Prior GAO reports had found that the production of video news releases by federal agencies violated the congressional ban on "covert propaganda" when broadcast without identifying the government's role.[4]
- A DHHS appropriations act in 2006 required that scientific information "prepared by government researchers and scientists shall be transmitted [to Congress] uncensored and without delay."[5] In his "signing statement," President Bush declared that submission of such information would be "in a manner consistent with the

Epigraph Source: President George H. W. Bush, Remarks to the National Academy of Sciences, April 23, 1990.

[1] Don Van Natta, Jr., "Drug Office Will End Its Scrutiny of TV Scripts," *New York Times*, January 20, 2000, A15.

[2] U.S. Government Accountability Office, *Media Contracts: Activities and Financial Obligations for Seven Federal Departments*, GAO-06-305 (Jan. 2006).

[3] David Barstow and Robin Stein, "The Message Machine: How the Government Makes News under Bush: A New Age of Prepackaged News," *New York Times*, March 13, 2005.

[4] U.S. Government Accountability Office, *Prepackaged News Stories*, B-304-272 (Feb. 17, 2005).

[5] *Department of Labor, Health and Human Services, and Education, and Related Agencies Appropriations Act*, H.R. 3010, 109th Cong. (2006).

President's authority to withhold information that could impair [foreign relations, national security, or the workings of the executive branch]."[6]

In 2004-5, the Union of Concerned Scientists (UCS) issued a statement and two reports signed by sixty leading scientists, including twenty Nobel laureates, asserting that the Bush administration systematically distorted scientific fact in the service of policy goals on the environment, health, and biomedical research.[7] Critics charged the administration with suppressing, discrediting, or altering scientific findings that were inconsistent with its policies. Illustrations include the FDA delay in approval of emergency contraceptives against the advice of staff scientists and two independent advisory panels; the DHHS's obscuring of the scientific evaluation of abstinence-only education and pressuring of scientists to promote abstinence; the CDC's alteration of its Web site to raise doubt about the effectiveness of condoms in preventing HIV transmission; the National Cancer Institute's posting of information on its Web site suggesting a link between abortion and breast cancer despite objections from staff scientists; and the EPA's undermining of climate change science by suppression of reports and public misrepresentation of scientific consensus.[8] Health officials even concealed scientific evidence that social and racial disparities affect health care.[9]

In some instances, one might acknowledge the government's benign intentions (e.g., antidrug messages on television), but does beneficence justify deceit? In other instances, the government's suppression or disregard of science seems calculated to buttress its political ideology or favor special interests. Above all, the public expects transparency and honesty in setting and enforcing health policy. The public wants the state to listen carefully, be objective, and promote the common good.[10]

[6] George W. Bush, White House Press Release, Dec. 30, 2005.

[7] Union of Concerned Scientists, *Scientific Integrity in Policy Making: Investigation of the Bush Administration's Abuse of Science* (2004); Union of Concerned Scientists, *Scientific Integrity in Policy Making: Further Investigation of the Bush Administration's Abuse of Science* (2005), both available at www.ucsusa.org/scientific_integrity/interference/.

[8] Robert F. Kennedy, Jr., "The Junk Science of George W. Bush," *Nation*, March 8, 2004; Henry A. Waxman, *False and Misleading Health Information Provided by Federally Funded Pregnancy Resource Centers* (U.S. House Committee on Government Reform: Minority Staff, July 2006); Union of Concerned Scientists, "Scientific Integrity: Specific Examples of the Abuse of Science," http://www.ucsusa.org/scientific_integrity/interference/specific-examples-of-the-abuse-of-science.html; The National Coalition against Censorship, "Political Science: A Report on Science and Censorship," March 2007, http://ncac.org/science/political_science.pdf.

[9] Robert Steinbrook, "Disparities in Health Care—from Politics to Policy," *New Eng. J. Med.*, 350 (2004): 1486-88.

[10] Gia B. Lee, "Persuasion, Transparency, and Government Speech," *Hastings Law Journal* (2005): 983-1057.

Justifications for health communication are also weak if the campaigns are unlikely to alter risk behavior. Government cannot claim to promote the public's health if educational messages do not work, and unfortunately, evaluations of education campaigns are inherently complex and infrequently undertaken.[29] Two related scientific issues, therefore, are important in thinking about health promotion: the scientific evidence underlying the health claim and the campaign's effectiveness in preventing risk behaviors.

Like so many other public health activities, health communication campaigns entail difficult trade-offs between public goods and private choices. Effective communication campaigns reduce risk behaviors and enhance quality of life and longevity but burden free choice and present social risks.

At the same time, despite their complexity, government's public messages pose few problems from a constitutional perspective.

WHEN GOVERNMENT SPEAKS: A CONSTITUTIONAL PERSPECTIVE

Constitutional scholars distinguish government's use of its own voice from government's silencing of others.[30] Generally, the former raises few, if any, serious constitutional concerns, while the latter requires careful reflection. Thus, government can add its own voice to the other opinions that it must tolerate, provided it does not drown out private communication.[31] Given the prolific health information generated in the private sector, government speech is unlikely to dominate the marketplace. The First Amendment, for example, does not prevent the government from promoting the "right to life" over abortion, life-sustaining treatment over the "right to die," or research on adult over embryonic stem cells. Those who object to these controversial positions cannot insist that government articulate their personal views, nor can they legally contest government's expenditure of considerable resources to enunciate controversial opinions.[32] The public's only realistic remedy for government advocacy of "bad" science policy is through the ballot box.[33]

Subsidized Health Speech: The "Unconstitutional Conditions" Doctrine

Government not only conveys health messages itself but also funds private and voluntary organizations to deliver health information. Although it has considerable discretion in the messages it supports financially, government may not grant a benefit on the condition that the recipient perform or forgo a constitutionally protected activity.[34] What is known as the "unconstitutional conditions" doctrine specifies that government cannot punish those who convey disfavored ideas by denying them benefits.[35]

The Supreme Court has not been wholly consistent in its jurisprudence regarding unconstitutional conditions.[36] For example, in *Rust v. Sullivan* (1991), the Court upheld a so-called gag-rule that forbids clinics receiving federal family planning funds from counseling or referring women for abortion and from encouraging, promoting, or advocating abortion. Chief Justice Rehnquist, writing for the Court, said, "The Government has not discriminated on the basis of viewpoint; it has merely chosen to fund one activity to the exclusion of the other. [This] is not a case of the Government 'suppressing a dangerous idea,' but of a prohibition on a project grantee or its employees from engaging in activities outside of the project's scope."[37] Yet the Court subsequently struck down a federal law that prevented recipients of federal Legal Services funds from challenging the validity of welfare laws and regulations.[38]

The cases appear idiosyncratic: In some instances the Court views conditional funding as a permissible choice to subsidize some activities and not others, and in other instances it views those conditions as an unconstitutional burden on free speech. In *Forum for Academic and Institutional Rights, Inc.* (2006), the Court unanimously upheld the Solomon Amendment, which requires universities, as a condition of federal funding, to grant access to military recruiters, in violation of university policy that prospective employers must not discriminate on the basis of sexual orientation. Chief Justice Roberts said that the Solomon Amendment "regulates conduct, not speech": "It neither limits what law schools may say nor requires them to say anything."[39]

In summary, government has near plenary constitutional authority to convey its own health messages or subsidize private health messages. Government, then, may add its own voice and funds to the marketplace of ideas about health and behavior. However, it has considerably less constitutional power to suppress ideas of which it disapproves.

COMMERCIAL SPEECH

> The task of the political sphere in a republican scheme is to oversee the market in order to protect the common welfare. Public health restrictions on liberty and property to limit the promotion of harmful or dangerous products, including restrictions on advertising, are a staple of public policy in a democratic republic.
>
> Dan E. Beauchamp (1988)

> As to the particular consumer's interest in the free flow of commercial information, that interest may be as keen, if not keener by far, than his interest in the day's most urgent political debate.
>
> Harry Blackmun (1976)

No matter how much government educates the public, it is bound to have difficulty changing risk behaviors. The reason is that the private

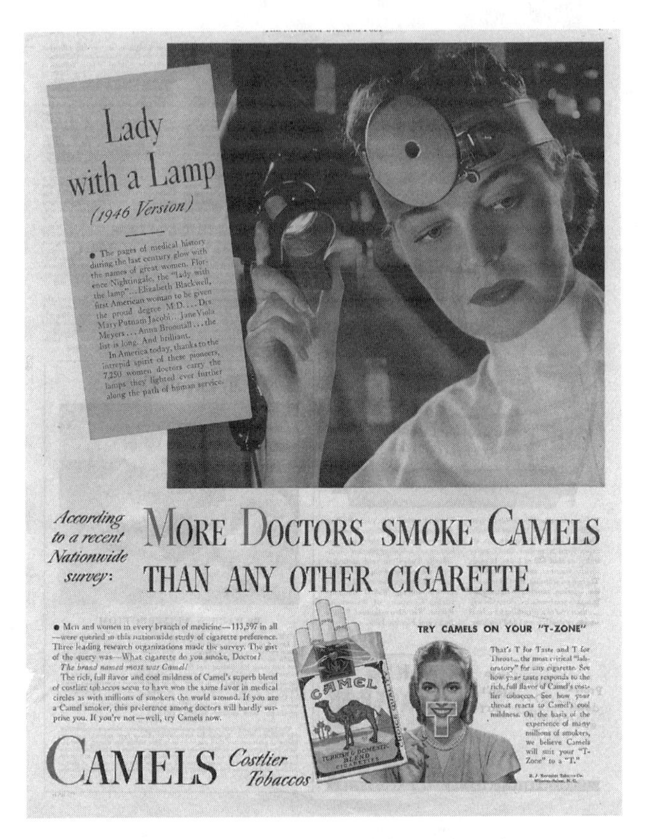

Photo 18. Advertisement depicting doctors' endorsement of Camel cigarettes. Before the detrimental effects of smoking were publicly known, campaigns such as these were prevalent. Doctors often endorsed and advocated smoking; it was perceived as glamorous, fashionable, and trendy. © R. J. Reynolds, 1946.

sector has a strong economic motivation to influence consumer preferences: Manufacturers and retailers desire to sell products, the advertising industry strives to devise alluring campaigns, and the media compete for advertising revenue. Advertising commands ever-increasing resources and engenders ever more creative approaches to stimulate consumer demands.

As a result, government regulation of commercial speech is a vital strategy to safeguard consumer health and safety. First, government is concerned with advertising that increases the use of hazardous products and services, such as cigarettes, alcoholic beverages, firearms, and gambling. For example, advertisements extol the virtues of handguns for home defense and safety, despite scientific evidence of increased risk of suicide, domestic violence, and unintended death.[40] Second, government is concerned with marketing "age-restricted" products to children and adolescents. For example, in 1996 the Distilled Spirits Council lifted its forty-eight-year voluntary ban on hard liquor advertising on radio and television, prompting concern about targeting of young people.[41] Third, government is concerned with industry health claims that mislead the public. Unsubstantiated labeling or advertising by the food, dietary supplement,[42] or pharmaceutical industries can have adverse effects on consumer health and safety. Consider, for example, the influence of ubiquitous direct-to-consumer marketing of prescription drugs.[43] Regulation of commercial speech is becoming even more challenging as government monitors Internet marketing and games, as well as product placement on television and movies. Marketing of high-caloric foods to children illustrates all three of these concerns, and is discussed later in this chapter.

A Legal Definition of Commercial Speech

Commercial speech is an "expression related solely to the economic interests of the speaker and its audience"[44] that "does no more than propose a commercial transaction."[45] The three attributes of commercial speech are that it (1) identifies a specific product (i.e., offers a product for sale), (2) is a form of advertising (i.e., is designed to attract public attention to, or patronage for, a product or service, by paid announcements proclaiming its qualities or advantages), and (3) confers economic benefits (i.e., the speaker stands to profit financially) (see figure 31).[46]

No one of these three factors provides a complete description of commercial speech, but the Supreme Court classifies an expression as commercial if it has a combination of them all. Thus, in *Bolger v. Youngs Drug Products Corp.* (1983), the Court found that "informational pamphlets" with titles such as "Plain Talk about Venereal Disease" and "Condoms and Human Sexuality" were "commercial" because they were advertisements, they referred to a specific product, and the publisher had an economic motivation.[47]

Many speakers stand to gain economically, including publishers, broadcasters, and film producers. The fact that a speaker will profit from

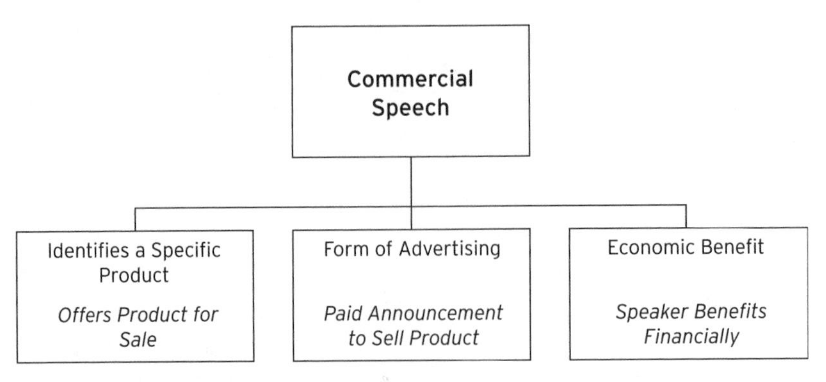

Figure 31. Commercial speech: A definition.

a message is not conclusive, nor is the fact that the speaker must pay for the message definitive.[48] For example, the following advertisement in the *New York Times,* which was paid for by tobacco companies, is political, not commercial, speech: "Can We Really Make the Underage Smoking Problem Smaller by Making the Federal Bureaucracy Bigger? . . . Together We Can Work It Out."[49] The next advertisement, also found in the *New York Times* and paid for by the tobacco industry, is more difficult to classify: "'Of Cigarettes and Science': Why a Federal Study Failed to Prove the Causal Relationship between Smoking and Heart Disease."[50] Both advertisements express an opinion on a matter of public interest rather than propose a commercial transaction.[51] Although the latter message is morally reprehensible, history informs us that it would be a mistake to suppress statements that cast doubt on scientific orthodoxies of the day, because scientific "truths" are rarely stable and certain.

However, what if speech represents a "blending of commercial speech and debate on issues of public importance"?[52] The Nike Corporation, for example, has vigorously defended itself against allegations that it used Third World sweatshops to manufacture its athletic clothing. An activist sued the company in a California court for false advertising. The California Supreme Court ruled that the suit could proceed, and the U.S. Supreme Court dismissed Nike's appeal.[53] The company argued that the publication of press releases and fact sheets about its overseas labor conditions were part of the marketplace of ideas fully protected by the First Amendment, not advertisements. Should industry have a right to defend its corporate image? Would corporate executives be reluctant to talk about product safety, racial discrimination, or environmental concerns if they feared tort liability? Alternatively, should a manufacturer have a legal duty to speak truthfully in defending its corporate image?[54]

The Constitutionalization of Commercial Speech

It is fashionable these days to think that public health regulation of commercial speech poses the "hard" constitutional problem of reconciling two important, incommensurable values—health and free expression. The problem is sometimes framed as having deep historical and constitutional roots. But the truth is that protection of commercial speech, particularly in robust form, is a recent occurrence. Through most of American history, the Supreme Court afforded advertising little, if any, constitutional protection. The Court, in 1942, declared that the Constitution imposes "no such restraint on government as respects purely commercial advertising."[55] It was not until 1975 that the Court first found that commercial speech merited *any* First Amendment protection: "The relationship of speech to the marketplace of products or services does not make it valueless in the marketplace of ideas."[56] The early commercial speech cases, however, involved instances where the message itself had public health value: abortion referral services,[57] advertisements for contraceptives,[58] or the price of pharmaceuticals.[59]

Even today, commercial speech nominally operates as a category of "lower-value" expression, deserving of less constitutional protection than social or political discourse.[60] Recognizing the "commonsense distinction[s],"[61] the Court finds that the Constitution "accords a lesser protection to commercial speech than to other constitutionally guaranteed expression."[62] In reality, though, the level of scrutiny for commercial speech has changed over the years and is still in transition. In fact, the Supreme Court's deferential approach to commercial speech did not evolve into close scrutiny until the mid-1990s.[63] Moreover, with certain forms of commercial speech (e.g., truthful statements about dangerous products), at least four members of the Court would afford it rigorous constitutional protection. Indeed, modern commercial speech doctrine is so uncertain, but still potentially so forceful, that it chills public health regulation (see figure 32).

Given this constitutional history, how much First Amendment protection *should* be afforded to commercial speech? Does the advertising of dangerous products such as tobacco or firearms deserve a level of constitutional protection similar to that of social, artistic, or political dis-

1940
Prior to 1940 there was no discussion of commercial speech.
1942
Valentine
"[N]o restraint on government [for suppressing] purely commercial advertising." Commercial speech deserves no First Amendment protection
1950
For over three decades, the stance on commercial speech remained uncontested in the courts.
1975
Bigelow
Commercial speech is "not valueless in the marketplace of ideas." Commercial speech is afforded First Amendment protection in the advertisement of abortion referrals.
1976
Virginia Pharmacy
Commercial speech advertising the price of pharmaceuticals is protected under the First Amendment.
1977
Carey
Commercial speech advertising contraception is protected under the First Amendment.
1980
Central Hudson
Supreme Court devises "test" that determines the criteria for evaluating commercial speech classes.
1986
Posadas
"The power to ban a product includes the lesser power to regulate advertising." The courts take a permissive approach to government regulation of commercial speech.
1989
Fox
The courts give government "ample scope of regulatory authority" over commercial speech.
1995
Coors Brewing Co.
The "irrationality" of government regulation of commercial speech is more closely scrutinized.
1996
44 Liquormart
Regulation of commercial speech must advance state interest "to a material degree."
1999
New Orleans Broadcasting
Prohibition of commercial speech advertising "private casino gambling" is found unconstitutional.

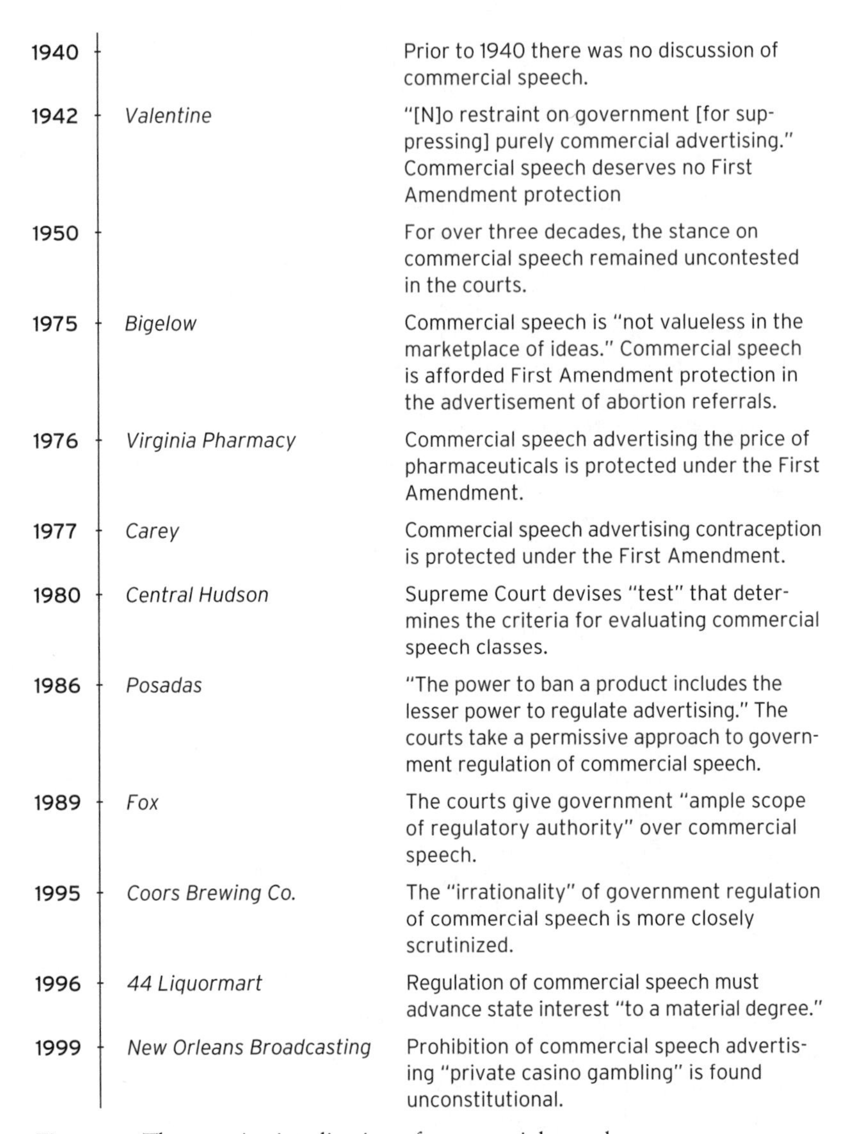

Figure 32. The constitutionalization of commercial speech.

course? And, does it matter that the international community rarely grants advertising the kind of protection found in the United States?[64] The WHO's Framework Convention on Tobacco Control, for example, calls for a comprehensive ban on all tobacco advertisements and promotions, but as a result of American insistence, countries can circumvent the ban based on domestic constitutional principles (see chapter 7).[65]

The "Central Hudson" Test

In *Central Hudson Gas v. Public Service Commission* (1980),[66] the Supreme Court articulated a four-part test for government regulation of commercial speech. First, for commercial speech to be protected by the First Amendment, it must concern a lawful activity and not be false, deceptive, or misleading. Second, the government interest asserted must be substantial. Third, the regulation of commercial speech must directly advance the governmental interest asserted. Fourth, the regulation must be no more extensive than necessary to serve the government's interest. The four parts of the *Central Hudson* test are not discrete but rather interrelated; in particular, the third and fourth parts of the test are complementary.[67] The Court reviews commercial speech under a standard of "intermediate scrutiny,"[68] and the government carries the burden of justification (see figure 33).[69]

STEP 1: IS THE ACTIVITY UNLAWFUL, AND IS THE SPEECH FALSE, DECEPTIVE, OR MISLEADING?

The Court consistently holds that advertisements are not protected by the First Amendment if they promote unlawful activities[70] or if they are false, deceptive, or misleading.[71] The rationale for excluding such commercial expressions from constitutional protection is that they lack value in the commercial or ideological marketplace. False, deceptive, or misleading advertisements distort those markets by leading consumers into error, risk, or a disadvantageous position.[72] Yet it is not always easy to know if a commercial expression fits into one of these categories.[73] The European Union, for example, bans branding cigarettes as "light" or "mild," claiming that it misleads consumers about the dangers of smoking.[74] Until recently, American courts appeared reluctant to make similar findings.[75] In 2006, however, two cases dealing with "light" and "low tar" cigarettes signaled a possible shift in that attitude.[76] (See box 27, p. 358, and chapter 8.)

Unlawful Activities. Government may prohibit commercial speech that promotes or portrays unlawful activities, such as illicit drug use, driving while intoxicated, or underage possession of age-restricted products (tobacco, alcoholic beverages, or handguns). Certainly, a commercial message or image that expressly endorses unlawful behavior (e.g., children smoking cigarettes) is not constitutionally protected. However, it is less clear whether commercial speech that attracts children but also appeals to adults deserves First Amendment protection. Many forms of media

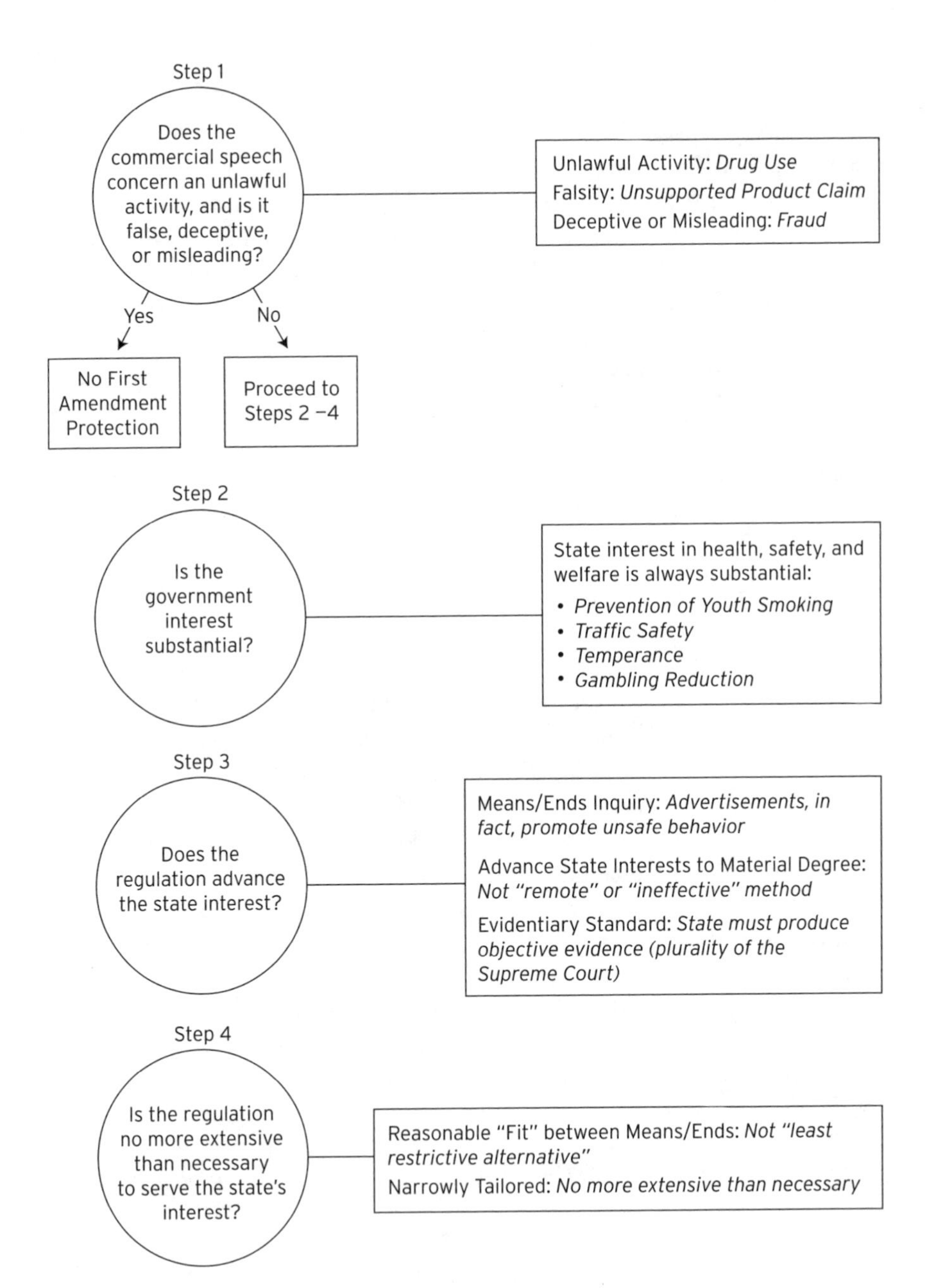

Figure 33. The *Central Hudson* test.

have a mixed viewership, including both adults and children. Should the Court afford First Amendment protection to advertisements that have a clear appeal to children (e.g., cartoons) but also reach an adult audience?[77] Does the determination turn on the company's intent, the percentage of underage viewers, or some other formula? Consider Brown and Williamson's promotion of the Kool MIXX cigarette brand, which focused on hip-hop culture, including DJ competitions, interactive CD-ROMs, and special collectible bags, radios, lighters, and cigarette packs. Copies of the CD were distributed for free in *Spin, Vibe,* and *Rolling Stone,* all of which have high youth readership.[78] Does it matter that empirical evidence suggests that comprehensive advertising bans are most effective in protecting children, who are heavily influenced by the media?[79]

Falsity or Deliberate Concealment. The Supreme Court affords no constitutional protection to commercial messages, such as unsubstantiated health claims, that are false or deliberately conceal or misrepresent the truth.[80] The tobacco industry, for example, cannot assert that cigarettes have no effect on breathing or athletic abilities, or that they pose little risk to health. An advertisement stating that Liggett and Myers filters are "just what the doctor ordered" is unlikely to receive constitutional protection.[81] The problem, of course, is that commercial information is rarely unequivocally either "true" or "false." Rather, there are gradations of truthfulness. An advertisement may state the truth but not the whole truth. Consider a company that informs consumers of a pharmaceutical's benefits but not its significant risks. Alternatively, a company may disseminate messages through prose and images that, although not technically false, convey a false impression. Is the motto for Parliament cigarettes, "Alive with Pleasure," false or misleading? Finally, consider a statement that simply urges consumers to buy the product, which is neither true nor false. Should, for example, McDonald's Corporation be permitted to urge consumers to eat its products daily and in outsized portions? In the documentary film *Super Size Me* (2004), the narrator became critically ill by following such advice.

What if, as is often the case, there is insufficient evidence supporting the assertion? Suppose a manufacturer claims that a dietary supplement improves mood, facilitates bone joint movement, or dramatically increases metabolism for weight reduction. Suppose further that there exists no substantial scientific agreement in support of (or against) the claim. Should public health agencies be permitted to regulate in an environment of scientific uncertainty? Who should have the burden of proving the veracity of a health claim—the government or the commercial speaker? Does it matter if the product poses potential hazards to the consumer's health? For example, should the FDA be empowered to prevent a company from claiming that smokeless cigarettes are "less dangerous" in the absence of scientific agreement that they are?[82]

Inherently Deceptive or Misleading. The Supreme Court holds that even true advertisements that promote lawful activities merit no constitutional protection if they are inherently deceptive or misleading. Deceptive or misleading commercial speech is a form of fraud, undue influence, overreaching, or other vexatious conduct.[83] For example, states may prohibit optometrists from advertising and practicing under trade names[84] or attorneys from in-person solicitation of patients in hospital rooms.[85] The rationale is that these kinds of activities inherently risk deception. However, the constitutional position of "puffery" (exaggerated imagery) or "glamorous" advertising of hazardous products is less clear. Despite the intuitive sense that attractive, healthful images of smokers are inherently misleading,[86] the Court has not yet held that they stand outside the First Amendment.

STEP 2: IS THE ASSERTED GOVERNMENT INTEREST SUBSTANTIAL?

If commercial expression promotes a lawful activity and is not false, deceptive, or misleading, it warrants constitutional protection. The Court uses a balancing test that begins by asking whether the governmental interest is substantial. Public health regulation of commercial speech almost always fulfills this second *Central Hudson* criterion. The state has a significant, if not compelling, interest in protecting the health, safety, and welfare of its citizens. The Court recognizes the importance of injury or disease prevention and health promotion—for example, to enhance traffic safety,[87] promote temperance,[88] and reduce gambling.[89]

STEP 3: DOES THE REGULATION OF COMMERCIAL SPEECH DIRECTLY ADVANCE THE STATE INTEREST?

The third prong of the *Central Hudson* test requires that the regulation "directly and materially" advance the state interest. Nominally, this requires a "means/ends" inquiry (i.e., evaluating whether the advertising campaign adversely affects the public's health). In early cases, courts routinely deferred to the commonsense legislative judgment that advertising stimulates consumer demand.[90] In *Posadas de Puerto Rico Associates v. Tourism Company of Puerto Rico* (1986), the Supreme Court held that a law prohibiting gambling casinos from advertising to residents of

Puerto Rico was constitutional. Chief Justice Rehnquist noted: "[Puerto Rico] obviously believed [that] advertising of casino gambling aimed at [its residents] would serve to increase the demand for the product advertised. We think the legislature's belief is [reasonable]."[91]

This permissive approach to the third prong of the *Central Hudson* test has turned into "close scrutiny" in recent cases. These cases suggest that government must have a clear and consistent policy and evidence to demonstrate that its regulation is likely to achieve the asserted public health objective. (Empirical evidence, however, need not be systematic.)[92] In *Rubin v. Coors Brewing Company* (1995), the Court unanimously invalidated a federal statute that prohibited beer labels from displaying alcohol content. The government defended the act as necessary to prevent "strength wars" among brewers who would compete in the marketplace based on the potency of their beer. Although the governmental interest was substantial, the act did not directly advance that interest, "given the overall irrationality of the Government's regulatory scheme."[93]

In 44 *Liquormart, Inc. v. Rhode Island* (1996), the Court became even more insistent that government affirmatively demonstrate a relationship between means and ends. Rhode Island prohibited advertising the price of alcoholic beverages "in any manner whatsoever," except inside liquor stores, and asserted the goal of "temperance." Justice Stevens's plurality opinion declared,

> The State bears the burden of showing not merely that its regulation will advance its interest, but also that it will do so "to a material degree."... [T]he State has presented no evidence to suggest that its speech prohibition will significantly reduce market-wide consumption.... Thus, [any] connection between the ban and a significant change in alcohol consumption would be purely fortuitous. [Any] conclusion that elimination of the ban would significantly increase alcohol consumption would [rest on] "speculation or conjecture."[94]

While none of the opinions in 44 *Liquormart* garnered a majority, a strongly united Court in *Greater New Orleans Broadcasting Association v. United States* (1999) made clear its intention to use a more rigorous First Amendment standard.[95] The Court returned to the theme, introduced in *Coors Brewing*, that a lack of consistency and coherency in public health regulation is near fatal under the Court's evolving commercial speech doctrine. Congress's policy on gambling (which proscribed private casino advertising but promoted gambling on certain Native American land and in state-run lotteries) was "so pierced by exemptions and inconsistency that the Government cannot hope to exonerate it."[96]

Some of the language in *Greater New Orleans Broadcasting* has troubling implications from a public health perspective. Recall that in *Posadas,* the Court acceded to the commonsense legislative assumption that advertising restrictions decrease demand for socially harmful products. While accepting this assumption, the Court in *Greater New Orleans Broadcasting* said it was also reasonable to assume that advertising would merely channel consumers to a different venue or brand.[97] This argument is worrisome because it is exactly the claim made by tobacco and alcoholic beverage manufacturers, who insist that they are advertising only to achieve greater market share, not to stimulate demand.

In the aftermath of *Coors Brewing, 44 Liquormart,* and *Greater New Orleans Broadcasting,* government must demonstrate, most probably with credible evidence, that the regulation will, in fact, achieve the asserted public health goal[98] and not be an "ineffective" or "remote" method.[99]

STEP 4: IS THE REGULATION NO MORE EXTENSIVE THAN NECESSARY TO SERVE THE STATE'S INTEREST?

The government must show not merely that its regulation directly advances a public health objective but also that the means used are not more extensive than necessary to achieve that goal. Again, early cases readily accepted legislative judgments that commercial speech restrictions were no broader than necessary to pursue the public health goal.[100] In *Board of Trustees of the State University of New York v. Fox* (1989), the Court held that the fourth *Central Hudson* criterion did not require government to use the least restrictive alternative. "The ample scope of regulatory authority [in commercial speech cases] would be illusory if it were subject to a least-restrictive-means requirement, which imposes a heavy burden on the State":[101]

> [What] our decisions require is a "fit between the legislature's ends and the means chosen to accomplish those ends"—a fit that is not necessarily perfect, but reasonable; that represents not necessarily the single best disposition but one whose scope is "in proportion to the interest served"; that employs not necessarily the least restrictive means . . . but a means narrowly tailored to achieve the desired objective.[102]

While not explicitly questioning the rationale offered in *Fox,* the Court in *Coors Brewing, 44 Liquormart,* and *Greater New Orleans Broadcasting* conducted a more demanding inquiry. In these cases, the Court invalidated commercial regulations because less restrictive alternatives were, in fact, available to achieve the desired ends.[103]

The Supreme Court also used the fourth prong of the *Central Hud-*

son test to strike down comprehensive regulations governing the advertising and sale of cigarettes, smokeless tobacco, and cigars in *Lorillard Tobacco Co. v. Reilly* (2001).[104] (Because the Cigarette Labeling and Advertising Act preempted litigation related to cigarette advertising, the Court focused on smokeless tobacco and cigars in its First Amendment analysis.) Massachusetts placed a variety of restrictions on outdoor advertising, point-of-sale advertising, retail sales transactions, transactions by mail, promotions, sampling of products, and cigar labels. "The broad sweep of the regulations," said the Court, "indicates that the Attorney General did not 'carefully calculate the costs and benefits associated with the burden on speech imposed' by the regulations."[105] The Court was troubled by the outdoor advertising rule prohibiting product advertising within one thousand feet of a school, saying that it could include 87–91 percent of major cities. Similarly, it found that a point-of-sale rule requiring that products not be "placed lower than five feet from the floor of any retail establishment" within one thousand feet of a school violated both the third and fourth prongs of *Central Hudson*. The Court determined that the regulation did not advance the state's goal, nor was it narrowly tailored.

A year later, the Court continued to use the fourth prong of *Central Hudson* as the death knell of public health regulation. In *Thompson v. Western States Medical Center*, the Court found that a federal law which exempted "compounded drugs" (mixing of drugs to create a medication tailored to an individual patient's needs) from FDA approval, so long as providers did not advertise the product, amounted to an unconstitutional restriction on commercial speech.[106] The Court reasoned that the government failed to demonstrate that the speech restrictions were not more extensive than necessary to achieve state interests.

Theories for the Future of Commercial Speech

Earlier I asserted that the Supreme Court does not accord all commercial speech the same level of constitutional protection,[107] and that the Court's jurisprudence is in a state of transition. Here, I discuss several theories that help frame the key jurisprudential and policy issues.

THE FAIR BARGAINING THEORY: DISTINGUISHING TRUTHFUL FROM DECEPTIVE MESSAGES

The Supreme Court appears to subject two kinds of commercial speech—truthful and deceptive—to two different standards of review. The Court defers to regulation designed to assure a fair bargaining process between businesses and consumers. Thus, the Court characteristically approves government suppression of misleading, deceptive, or aggressive sales practices; or it approves government mandates to disclose truthful, beneficial consumer information. Regulation to assure fair market negotiations is consistent with the reasons for according a lower standard of constitutional review to commercial speech (i.e., to safeguard consumer health and safety). The Court vigorously reviews the suppression of truthful data, however, believing that consumers are rarely served by depriving them of information. The Court is suspicious of government policies designed to keep consumers ignorant.

THE INFORMATIONAL WORTH THEORY: THE ROLE OF IMAGE, CONTEXT, AND ASSOCIATION

Closely related to "fair bargaining" is the "informational worth" theory, by which the Court considers the informational value afforded to consumers by the advertisement. Commercial speech that informs consumers objectively about the product's price, quantity, ingredients, and quality deserves stronger constitutional protection. Most advertising does not convey objective information, but rather uses imagery, context, and association. The Supreme Court once said that "the use of illustrations or pictures in advertisements serves important communicative functions: It attracts the attention of the audience to the advertiser's message, and it may also serve to impart information directly."[108] The Court, however, could find that advertisements that depict hazardous products as rugged, athletic, adventuresome, or sexual have little informational worth.[109] Alluring images and associations do not inform consumers but may induce them to act against their self-interest in maintaining health and vitality.

THE ALTERNATIVE CHANNELS OF COMMUNICATION THEORY: DISTINGUISHING BLANKET PROHIBITIONS FROM "TIME, PLACE, AND MANNER" REGULATION

Since the Court does not desire to have consumers kept in the dark about relevant market information, it is particularly mistrustful of blanket prohibitions or content censorship. Justice Stevens's plurality opinion in *44 Liquormart* emphasizes the "special dangers that attend complete bans on truthful, nonmisleading commercial speech."[110] Accordingly, the Court rarely permits government to prevent completely the dissemination of truthful messages or to select the messages it will and will not allow.[111] The Court is more likely to cede to government the power to control the "time, place, and manner" of expression. This kind of regulation is "content neutral," meaning that government does not intend to censor a particular idea, but only to control its method of dissemination. Thus, regulation that leaves open alternative channels for consumers to hear messages is more likely to conform to the Constitution.[112]

THE UNLAWFUL PRACTICES THEORY: DISTINGUISHING CHILDREN FROM ADULTS

The judiciary gives greater deference to commercial speech regulation that is designed to effectuate a governmental interest to protect minors rather than adults[113]—although such deference was not evident in *Lorillard*. This is particularly true if the regulation filters out messages harmful to minors while, to the extent possible, leaving adults with alternative means of acquiring the information.[114] The Supreme Court has repeatedly recognized an independent governmental interest in protecting minors from harmful materials for several reasons.[115] If children and adolescents have legally restricted access to a hazardous product (e.g., cigarettes, alcoholic beverages, or handguns), advertisements that target this population arguably promote an unlawful activity. Additionally, minors are not yet fully able to assess and analyze independently the value of the message presented.[116] By the time they are capable of making a mature judgment, their health may be harmed irrevocably and their decisional capacity impaired by the product's addictive qualities.

THE UNDERLYING SOCIAL HARM THEORY: TAKING PUBLIC HEALTH INTERESTS SERIOUSLY

First Amendment theorists understandably urge that harmful messages, even those that are most unpopular, deserve protection in a vibrant democracy. The Supreme Court, moreover, has rejected the notion "that legislatures have broader latitude to regulate speech that promotes socially harmful activities."[117] However, justifications for commercial speech regulation must inevitably take account of the serious underlying harms caused by the products being sold.[118] The strength of the government's interests is classically relevant to constitutional analysis, even when the Court engages in close scrutiny. Thus, if the state's interest is compelling, such as a reduction in youth smoking, it should weigh heavily in the constitutional balance. Box 27, on cigarette advertising, illustrates these commercial speech theories.

BOX 27

REGULATION OF CIGARETTE ADVERTISING

Defendants ["Big Tobacco"] have marketed and sold their lethal product with zeal, with deception, with a single-minded focus on their financial success, and without regard for the human tragedy or social costs that success exacted.
Judge Gladys Kessler (2006)

Since the Surgeon General's first report was released in 1964,[1] government strategies to reduce cigarette smoking have focused on advertising restrictions and compelled disclosures.[2] Congress enacted the Cigarette Labeling and Advertising Act in 1965, requiring warning labels on all cigarette packages.[3] In 1971 Congress prohibited cigarette advertising on radio and television; the Supreme Court upheld the prohibition because, at that time, commercial speech did not receive constitutional protection.[4] A year later the Federal Trade Commission (FTC) required that all advertisements contain the same warning label used on cigarette packages.[5]

During the last decade, the government has explored more aggressive regulation to curb tobacco advertising and promotion. The FDA issued regulations on August 28, 1996, restricting the promotion and advertising of nicotine-containing cigarettes and smokeless tobacco to minors.[6] The FDA's theory was that it had the power to regulate cigarettes as a "nicotine delivery" device, but the Supreme Court disagreed and held that the agency lacked jurisdiction.[7] In *FDA v. Brown-Williamson* (2000), the Supreme Court was reluctant to allow the FDA's interpretation of its authority in the absence of clear congressional authorization. In the Court's view, if the FDA was entitled to regulate cigarettes, it would have to ban them entirely, and in examining almost a century of legislative history, the Court concluded that could not be the result Congress intended.[8]

The Master Tobacco Settlement Agreement (MTSA) negotiated in 1998 (see chapter 6) imposed tight controls on cigarette marketing, especially targeting youth, out-

Epigraph source: United States v. Philip Morris USA, Inc., 449 F. Supp. 2d 1 (D.C.C. 2006).

1 Department of Health, Education and Welfare, *Surgeon General's Report on Smoking and Health* (1964); see Department of Health and Human Services, *The Health Consequences of Involuntary Exposure to Tobacco Smoke: A Report of the Surgeon General* (Atlanta, GA: DHHS, 2006).

2 Lawrence O. Gostin, Peter S. Arno, and Allan M. Brandt, "FDA Regulation of Tobacco Advertising and Youth Smoking: Historical, Social, and Constitutional Perspectives," *JAMA*, 277 (1997): 410-18; Lawrence O. Gostin and Allan M. Brandt, "Criteria for Evaluating a Ban on the Advertisement of Cigarettes: Balancing Public Health Benefits with Constitutional Burdens," *JAMA*, 269 (1993): 904-9.

3 Pub. L. No. 89-92, §4, 79 Stat. 283 (1965). The original warning label read, "Caution: Cigarette Smoking May Be Hazardous to Your Health." The labeling act was substantially amended in 1970 to read, "The Surgeon General Has Determined that Cigarette Smoking Is Dangerous to Your Health." Pub. L. No. 21-222, §2, 84 Stat 88 (1970). It was amended again in 1984 by the Comprehensive Smoking Education Act to include four warnings on a rotational basis. 15 U.S.C. §1333 (1994).

4 *Capital Broadcasting Co. v. Acting Attorney Gen.*, 405 U.S. 1000 (1972) (mem) *aff'ing sub nom. Capital Broadcasting Co. v. Mitchell*, 333 F. Supp. 582 (D.D.C. 1971).

5 *In re Lorillard*, 80 F.T.C. 455 (1972). Congress imposed a similar requirement in 1984. 15 U.S.C. §1334 (1984).

6 FDA, Regulations Restricting the Sale and Distribution of Cigarettes and Smokeless Tobacco to Protect Children and Adolescents, Final Rule, 21§ CFR 897.2. See David A. Kessler et al., "The Food and Drug Administration's Rule on Tobacco: Blending Science and Law," *Pediatrics* (1997): 884-87; Leonard Glantz, "Controlling Tobacco Advertising: The FDA Regulations and the First Amendment," *American Journal of Public Health*, 87 (1997): 446-51; "Developments in Policy: The FDA's Tobacco Regulations," *Yale Law and Policy Review*, 15 (1996): 399-446.

7 *FDA v. Brown & Williamson Tobacco Corp.*, 529 U.S. 120 (2000).

8 In 2007, the Senate voted to expand the FDA's powers in response to recent food (*E. coli* in spinach) and drug (e.g., Vioxx) safety scandals. The bill (§ 1082) is awaiting House action and will allow the FDA to continually review drugs after they go to market. This implies there may be less deference in store for drugs such as nicotine to remain in the market when the FDA finds them unreasonably harmful.

door advertising, and product placement and sponsorship.[9] The settlement agreement transformed the country's visual landscape, removing ubiquitous images that had become cultural touchstones.[10] Nevertheless, annual revenues for tobacco advertising have risen dramatically. The FTC reported that in 2003 (the latest data available) cigarette manufacturers spent $15.15 billion, the most ever recorded.[11] Despite the MTSA, cigarette marketing now appeals to a younger audience, including multipurchase offers and giveaways such as hats and lighters.[12]

Throughout this extensive national debate, the public health community proposed systematic regulations:[13] imposing a "tombstone" format (e.g., black and white text only, no human or animal images or cartoon characters), limiting location (e.g., banning outdoor displays near schools or playgrounds), regulating promotions (e.g., banning nontobacco products such as T-shirts, hats, or posters), eliminating sponsorship (e.g., banning support for sporting and other events), and compelling disclosure of health information (e.g., intended use and age restrictions). These kinds of advertising restrictions raise important, and controversial, First Amendment issues.[14]

Misleading Imagery and Messages

Cigarette advertisements are replete with imagery that associates tobacco use with healthy, adventuresome, glamorous lifestyles. The government has strong justifications for curtailing images that do not convey truthful information useful to consumers. Images also can be misleading, suggesting that health warnings are exaggerated and that smoking is consistent with a robust and active existence. The Newport "Alive with Pleasure!" campaign, for example, used scenes of healthy outdoor activities, implying that tobacco use is safe and the choice of energetic people. Similarly, advertisements for "low-tar" cigarettes, such as Vantage and True, imply that they are a safe alternative to quitting. In both cases the FTC expressed concern about the "misimpressions" and "implied representations."[15] In a civil racketeering case against the tobacco industry in 2006, U.S. District judge Gladys Kessler ordered tobacco companies not to use terms such as *low tar, light,* and *mild,* and to undertake a massive media campaign to correct years of misrepresentations.[16]

Alternative Channels of Communication

Narrowly crafted regulations would not curtail essential messages or close off vital channels of information. First, regulations could be content neutral and avoid select-

[9] Master Settlement Agreement, http://www.naag.org/backpages/naag/tobacco/msa/msa-pdf/1109185724_1032468605_cigmsa.pdf.

[10] Barry Meier, "Lost Horizons: The Billboard Prepares to Give Up Smoking," *New York Times,* A1, A20, April 19, 1999. (For a discussion of tobacco litigation, see chapter 9.)

[11] *Federal Trade Commission Cigarette Report for 2003* (Washington, DC: FTC, 2005) (stating that $15 billion represents an increase of 21.5 percent from 2002, and 35 percent from 2001).

[12] *People ex rel. Lockyer v. R. J. Reynolds,* 124 P.3d 408 (Cal. 2005) (finding a violation of a statute regulating nonsale distribution of cigarettes, after a tobacco company distributed free cigarettes at a street fair and other events).

[13] For an excellent review, see Ken Cummins, *Selling Smoke: Cigarette Advertising and Public Health* (Washington, DC: American Public Health Association, 1986): 85–96.

[14] Martin H. Redish, "Tobacco Advertising and the First Amendment," *Iowa Law Review,* 81 (1996): 589–639; Howard Jeruchimowitz, "Tobacco Advertisements and Commercial Speech Balancing: A Potential Cancer to Truthful, Nonmisleading Advertisements of Lawful Products," *Cornell Law Review,* 82 (1997): 432–78; David C. Vladeck and John Cary Sims, "Why the Supreme Court Will Uphold Strict Controls on Tobacco Advertising," *Southern Illinois University Law Journal,* 22 (1998): 651–76.

[15] Matthew L. Meyers, Carol Jennings, William Lenox, et al., *Federal Trade Commission, Staff Report on the Cigarette Advertising Investigation* (Washington, DC: Federal Trade Commision, 1981); Federal Trade Commission, *Report to Congress Pursuant to the Public Health Cigarette Smoking Act* (Washington, DC: Federal Trade Commission, 1979).

[16] National Association of Attorney Generals, "Master Settlement Agreement," *National Association of Attorney Generals,* Oct. 13, 2006, http://www.naag.org/backpages/naag/tobacco/msa/msa-pdf/1109185724_1032468605_cigmsa.pdf.

ing particular facts for suppression. Manufacturers could still inform consumers about who is producing and selling what tobacco product, for what purpose, and at what price. For example, a requirement to use only black and white text would not dilute the factual quality of consumer messages. Second, regulations could impose reasonable "time, place, and manner" restrictions by limiting the placement, location, and visual presentation of tobacco advertising, provided the limitations were not ubiquitous, as in *Lorillard*.

Finally, regulations would leave open alternative channels of communication. The government would not foreclose the plethora of newspaper, magazine, direct mail, Internet, point-of-sale, and other media available to tobacco advertisers.[17]

Targeting Youth

Advertising continues to appeal to a youth audience despite the fact that promotion and sale of cigarettes and smokeless tobacco to people under eighteen years old is unlawful in every state. Tobacco company documents revealed strategies to capture the youth market. One internal R. J. Reynolds memo from the mid-1970s stated, "Evidence is now available to indicate that the 14- to 18-year-old group is an increasing segment of the smoking population. RJR-T must soon establish a successful new brand in this market if our position in the industry is to be maintained over the long term."[18] Canadian court documents also uncovered tobacco industry research on children, underscoring its strategic interest in the youth market.[19] Tobacco advertising, notably the "Joe Camel" campaign,[20] captured the attention of young people.[21] Similarly, promotional activities, including specialty items (e.g., free tobacco samples, lighters, and apparel), still reach large numbers of underage smokers.[22] Even the industry's antismoking ads perversely seem to be correlated with increased smoking among youth.[23] Youth are especially vulnerable—not only are they more susceptible to advertising, but young smokers are more likely to smoke heavily as adults.[24]

[17] Despite the ban on tobacco television advertising, brand names of tobacco products often appear in commercials for other brands, such as Viagra, Chevrolet, and Wendy's. Lara Zwarun, "Ten Years and One Master Settlement Agreement Later: The Nature and Frequency of Alcohol and Tobacco Promotion in Televised Sports, 2000 through 2002," *American Journal of Public Health,* 96 (2006): 1492–97.

[18] John Schwartz, "1973 Cigarette Company Memo Proposed New Brand for Teens," *Washington Post,* A2, Oct. 4, 1995.

[19] Kwechansky Marketing Research, *Project Plus/Minus-3 or Cry 11* (Montreal, QC: Imperial Tobacco, 1982).

[20] John P. Pierce, Elizabeth A. Gilpin, David M. Burns, et al., "Does Tobacco Advertising Target Young People to Start Smoking?" *JAMA,* 266 (1991): 3154–58; Joseph R. DiFranza and B.F. Aisquith, "Does the Joe Camel Campaign Preferentially Reach Eighteen to Twenty-four Year Old Adults?" *Tobacco Control,* 4 (1995): 367–71.

[21] David G. Altman, Douglas W. Levine, Remy Coeytaux, et al., "Tobacco Promotion and Susceptibility to Tobacco Use among Adolescents Aged Twelve through Seventeen Years in a Nationally Representative Sample," *American Journal of Public Health,* 86 (1996): 1590–93; Paul M. Fischer, John W. Richards, Jr., Earl J. Berman, et al., "Recall and Eye Tracking Study of Adolescents Viewing Tobacco Advertisements," *JAMA,* 261 (1989): 84–89, 84.

[22] George H. Gallup International Institute, *Teenage Attitudes and Behavior concerning Tobacco: Report of the Findings* (Princeton, NJ: George H. Gallup International Institute, 1992); William H. Redmond, "Effects of Sales Promotion on Smoking among U.S. Ninth Graders," *Preventative Medicine,* 28 (1999): 243–50.

[23] Melanie Wakefield, Yvonne Terry-McElrath, Sherry Emery, et al., "Effect of Televised, Tobacco-Company-Funded Smoking Prevention Advertising on Youth Smoking-Related Beliefs, Intentions, and Behavior," *American Journal of Public Health,* 96 (2006): 2154–60; Editorial, "When Don't Smoke Means Do," *New York Times,* November 27, 2006.

[24] Emanuela Taioli and Ernst L. Wynder, "Effect of the Age at Which Smoking Begins on Frequency of Smoking in Adulthood," *New Eng. J. Med.,* 325 (1991): 968–69; Scott L. Tomar and Gary A. Giovino, "Incidence and Predictors of Smokeless Tobacco Use among U.S. Youth," *American Journal of Public Health,* 88 (1998): 20–26; Department of Health and Human Services, *Reducing the Health Consequences of Smoking, Twenty-five Years of Progress: A Report of the Surgeon General, 1989 Executive Summary* (Center for Chronic Disease Prevention and Health Promotion, Office of Smoking and Health, 1989).

The Underlying Public Harms

The public harms attributable to cigarette smoking are unprecedented. Tobacco use is the single leading cause of preventable mortality, resulting in 438,000 premature deaths in the United States between 1997 and 2001.[25] This mortality is greater than that caused by AIDS, automobile crashes, alcohol, homicides, illegal drugs, suicides, and fires combined.[26] Moreover, since approximately 21 percent (45 million) of Americans smoke,[27] even relatively small changes in behavior could benefit the public's health. Reducing tobacco-related illnesses would also decrease economic burdens. Direct medical care expenditures attributable to smoking are estimated at $96.7 billion per year.[28] Sterile economic estimates, however, do not begin to measure the value to individuals, families, and society if tobacco-related disease were diminished. Decreased personal pain and suffering, enjoyment of more energetic lifestyles, and healthier parents and children are among the profound social benefits.

The constitutional debate over cigarette advertising is contentious, and its outcome surely is in doubt. Nevertheless, the public health case for regulation is powerful: Cigarette advertisements have low informational value, are misleading, appeal to children and adolescents, and result in profound social and economic harms. Narrowly tailored regulations would comport with prevailing constitutional doctrine if they remained content-neutral, regulated "time, place, and manner," and left open alternative channels of communication.

[25] Centers for Disease Control and Prevention, "Annual Smoking–Attributable Mortality, Years of Potential Life Lost, and Productivity Losses," *Morbidity and Mortality Weekly Report*, 54 (2005): 625-28.

[26] Ellen J. Hahn, Mary K. Rayens, Frank J. Chaloupka, et. al, "Projected Smoking Related Deaths among Youth: A 2000 Update," *University of California Scholarship Repository*, May 2002, http://repositories.cdlib.org/context/tc/article/1063/type/pdf/viewcontent/.

[27] Centers for Disease Control and Prevention, "Tobacco Use among Adults—United States 2005," *Morbidity and Mortality Weekly Report*, 55 (2006): 1145-48.

[28] Eric Lindblom and Katie McMahon, "Toll of Tobacco in the United States of America," *Campaign for Tobacco-Free Kids*, Oct. 30, 2006, http://www.tobaccofreekids.org/research/factsheets/pdf/0072.pdf.

COMPELLED COMMERCIAL SPEECH: HEALTH AND SAFETY DISCLOSURE REQUIREMENTS

> There is certainly some difference between compelled speech and compelled silence, but in the context of protected speech, the difference is without constitutional significance, for the First Amendment guarantees "freedom of speech," a term necessarily comprising the decision of what to say and what not to say.
>
> William J. Brennan (1988)

Federal and state regulations compel a great deal of speech for public health or consumer protection purposes. First, government requires businesses to label their products by specifying the content or ingredients (e.g., foods and cosmetics),[119] the potential adverse effects (e.g., pharmaceuticals and vaccines), and the hazards (e.g., warnings on packages of cigarettes, alcoholic beverages, or pesticides).[120] Second, government provides a "right to know" for consumers (e.g., performance of managed care organizations),[121] workers (e.g., health and safety risks), and the public (e.g., hazardous chemicals in drinking water).[122] Third, government mandates counteradvertising whereby industry or the media must provide health education as a counterbalance to advertisements of hazardous products (e.g., forced dissemination of antidrinking[123] or antismoking[124] messages). (For an interesting historical perspective on counteradvertising, see the "fairness doctrine"[125] and its application to cigarette advertisements.)[126]

Commercial disclosure requirements simply require businesses to provide more consumer information. The First Amendment, however, bestows not only a right to speak freely, but also a right to refrain from speaking.[127] The Court offers two complementary rationales for affording First Amendment protection to compelled speech. First, to compel a person to enunciate a view that she does not believe violates freedom of conscience or belief. This reasoning was used to invalidate state laws making flag salute and pledge compulsory[128] or requiring automobile owners to display license plates carrying the New Hampshire motto, "Live Free or Die."[129] Second, government-compelled speech may deter the speaker from expressing his own views. The Court struck down state laws prohibiting anonymous handbills[130] and campaign literature[131] because they discouraged the person's underlying right to publish and disseminate his work.[132]

The Court's compelled speech cases are not limited to requiring individuals to enunciate government messages. The Court has also limited the government's ability to force individuals to host or accommodate another speaker's message, such as requiring a St. Patrick's Day[133] parade organizer or the Boy Scouts to allow gay men to participate.[134]

The Supreme Court's compelled speech jurisprudence is concerned principally with political and social discourse, as opposed to product health and safety. However, in *United States v. United Foods Inc.* (2001), the Court made clear that its compelled speech doctrine applies to commercial speech.[135] In that case, the Court held that a federal statute requiring mushroom producers and importers to pay for generic advertising promoting the mushroom industry is coerced speech: "First Amendment values are at serious risk if the government can compel . . . [citizens to subsidize speech] on the side that it favors."[136] The Court said that, where the principal object is speech itself, compelled subsidies for commercial speech were impermissible. The Court's "compelled-subsidy" cases, however, are confusing and apparently inconsistent. Before *United Foods,* the Court had upheld mandatory contributions by fruit producers for generic advertising,[137] and in 2005, it upheld mandatory contributions by beef producers.[138]

The Court is likely to draw upon its case law in the commercial speech area when making decisions about compelled commercial speech. In its commercial speech cases, the Court has stressed that businesses have a fully protected First Amendment right to express truthful, nonmisleading commercial messages about lawful products.[139] The Court should support a corollary principle: that government has constitutional power to compel businesses to make accurate, nondeceptive disclosures for health, safety, or consumer protection purposes. Consequently, government labeling and product liability rules mandating content or ingredients, approved uses, potential adverse effects, or hazard warnings appear to be constitutionally permissible, and the Court is unlikely to subject these rules to exacting First Amendment scrutiny.[140] For example, the Second Circuit Court of Appeals upheld a Vermont law requiring labeling of mercury-containing lightbulbs, stressing that "mandated disclosure of accurate, factual, commercial information does not offend the core First Amendment values, . . . but furthers the goal of the discovery of truth."[141] If the judiciary engaged in close scrutiny of labeling requirements, an unelected branch could upset innumerable federal and state regulatory programs.

When commercial speech first attained constitutional legitimacy in *Virginia Pharmacy,* the Court stated that government had the power to assure that "the stream of commercial information flows cleanly as well as freely"[142] This includes the authority to compel businesses to issue disclaimers or additional information to render commercial messages nondeceptive.[143] The following year, the Court approved a state requirement that attorney advertisements include "some limited supplementation, by way of warning or disclaimer, . . . to assure that the consumer is not misled."[144] Later, it upheld a disclosure rule mandating attorneys who advertised contingent rates to state that clients would be responsible for litigation costs:[145] "Disclosure requirements trench much more narrowly on an advertiser's interest than do flat prohibitions on speech."[146]

Whereas government can require truthful disclosures relevant to health, safety, or consumer protection, interesting issues arise when the state mandates disclosures purely to satisfy consumer demands for information. In *International Dairy Foods Association v. Amestoy* (1996),[147] dairy manufacturers challenged a Vermont law requiring labeling of products from cows treated with recombinant bovine somatotropin (rBST) (a synthetic growth hormone that increases milk production). Vermont defended the regulation, not on the basis of health or safety but rather "strong consumer interest and the public's right to know."[148] The dairy products derived from herds treated with rBST are indistinguishable from products derived from untreated herds, and the FDA concluded that there are "no safety or health concerns." The Second Circuit Court of Appeals held that "consumer curiosity alone was not a strong enough state interest to sustain the compulsion of even an accurate, factual statement."[149]

The court in *Amestoy* seems to suggest that science-based risk assessments should be the gold standard. However, if scientific risk were the only factor in regulatory decision making, then labeling to satisfy consumer demands would not be justified. Consider the labeling of halal and kosher foods to inform religious communities about food content and preparation. The risk of consuming these foods is near zero. Yet labeling foods in this fashion is permitted because risk is a multifaceted concept that is embedded with values. What if government were to compel disclosure of genetically modified foods, as is already the case in Europe and under active consideration in America?[150] Consumers are keenly interested in knowing this information, even though science cannot identify meaningful health risks.[151]

In summary, the Supreme Court is likely to view two different kinds of commercial compelled speech quite differently. On the one hand, the Court is likely to permit government to compel disclosures of accurate, nondeceptive information—particularly if state justifications rely on a cognizable harm to health, safety, or a fair consumer/business bargaining process. On the other hand, the Court will more carefully scrutinize compelled commercial speech that fits within the rationale already articulated for political and ideological speech (i.e., regulation that undermines freedom of belief and chills the speaker's own desire and capacity to speak). The Court has already clarified that the right not to speak inheres in political and commercial speech alike,[152] and extends to statements of fact as well as opinions.[153] Thus, constitutional problems arise where government compels businesses to enunciate an objectionable message out of their own mouths, forces them to respond to a hostile message when they would prefer to remain silent, or requires them to be publicly identified or associated with another's message.[154] Under this rationale, compulsory counteradvertising may be harder to sustain if the manufacturer is forced to convey detailed educational content with which it disagrees. In some ways, that poses a real problem for public health, as counteradvertising can be an effective tool to reduce demand for dangerous products.

Two modern health threats illustrate poignantly the importance of sound regulation of commercial speech: obesity and smoking. Food and tobacco have been aggressively marketed to children and teenagers. Although they present different problems (underage smoking is unlawful but high-caloric diets are not), they both pose a major challenge to public health in an age of chronic disease.

FOOD MARKETING TO CHILDREN: A CASE STUDY

All these people understand something that is very basic and logical, that if you own this child at an early age, you can own this child for years to come. . . . Companies are saying, "Hey, I want to own the kid younger and younger and younger."

Mike Searles (1989)

Childhood obesity is so pervasive that some view it as an epidemic. In the United States, the rate of childhood obesity was about 4 percent in 1960, but rose to 16 percent by 2002, leaving 9 million children obese, with 15 percent more at risk for becoming obese. Type 2 diabetes, previously referred to as "adult onset" diabetes, has increased by over 100 percent in the childhood population.[155] Many factors contribute to this alarming increase in childhood obesity: sedentary lifestyles, greater frequency of eating out, both parents working outside the home, and consumption of higher calorie food with fewer nutrients.[156] But one of the major contributors to child obesity may be the ubiquitous marketing of food products to children.[157]

In 2004, the food industry spent $11 billion on marketing their products to children. Less than half was spent on traditional television advertising, with the rest devoted to innovative ways to influence children's diets.[158] The industry now promotes food through Web sites, cell phones, school events and materials, product placement, stealth marketing, character licensing, and even classic games such as chess.[159] Food marketing is integrated into every aspect of children's lives, and children are being targeted at younger and younger ages.

The Institute of Medicine's report *Food Marketing to Children and Youth: Threat or Opportunity* found that advertising has a significant impact on the preferences, purchase requests, and beliefs of children two to eleven years of age.[160] The purposeful targeting of young children in marketing is clearly illustrated in the epigraph by Mike Searles, former president of *Kids 'R Us*.

Innovative Ways to Influence Children

The food industry is adopting innovative ways of influencing children's eating habits. The Internet plays an important role in children's lives. Companies constantly barrage children with messages. Many companies have their own Web sites, where they have created games, known as advergames. After registering on these Web sites and enabling the receipt of promotional e-mails, children can play a multitude of alluring games. At Kraft.com, children "build" name-brand cookies with chocolate chips, cream fillings, and so on; the M&Ms Web site takes a classic game, Othello, and reformulates it using red M&Ms versus green M&Ms, with the colorful red and green characters from TV commercials and packaging cheering the player on.[161] On many of these Web sites, children compete with millions of others for high scores, all the time being bombarded by the food product the Web site is promoting. Nickelodeon, perhaps the most frequently accessed Web site for children, offers over 375 games, many of which are linked to sponsored games on other Web sites. When children reach the new page, the Nick.com insignia is still present, as advertisements for sugary foods, such as Cinnamon Toast Crunch, flash across the top of the page and promotional games for movies pop up below.

Web sites and advergames are only part of the larger advertising schemes. Character licensing also has become rampant. SpongeBob SquarePants sells Kraft Macaroni and Cheese. Movie releases, such as *Shrek 3* (2007), are linked directly to soda brands, kids' meals at fast-food restaurants, various candy brands, and other junk foods. Brand licensing and characters used in this fashion help children to transfer the warm, fuzzy feelings that they feel for a special character to the food product.

Stealth marketing is particularly insidious. A program called "Tremors" employs 250,000 teenagers to promote food brands to their friends without disclosing the promoter's financial ties. Although it is illegal to use product placement (e.g., actors drinking name-brand sodas) on shows designed for children, youth-oriented programs such as *American Idol* use product placement frequently.[162]

The combination of targeting children two to eleven years of age and the findings of the IOM report that advertising does influence children's purchase requests, preferences, and beliefs is powerful.[163] In addition, companies have invested in researching what is known as the "nag factor." In essence, companies teach children how to nag, knowing that parents tend to capitulate to their children's nagging.[164]

Public schools have become a battleground for food marketers. Schools in need of money and resources look to corporate sponsors. Preschools use papers and exercises provided by Froot Loops. Companies place vending machines selling their products throughout schools, provide new scoreboards with their brand centrally placed, provide convenience stands, and alter the nature of school lunches by making junk food more readily available in the schools.[165] (In 2006, major beverage companies, however, agreed to sharply limit the sale of soft drinks in schools—see chapter 5.) The "competitive foods" that are available in school stores, vending machines, and often in cafeterias enable children to select less nutritional alternatives to the regular school lunches.

Regulation of Food Marketing to Children

The obesity epidemic and the marketing to children of foods with low nutritional value and high calorie content have encouraged legislators to develop a variety of marketing regulations.[166] The regulations address concerns regarding the availability of such foods in schools, advertising to children, and use of the Internet. The government also has designed and implemented various social marketing programs to promote healthy eating habits and behaviors, in an attempt to combat obesity and our nation's obsession with fast food and junk food.

Limiting Availability of Junk Foods at Schools. In 2007, the Institute of Medicine released a report recognizing that children's easy access to soft drinks, sugary snacks, and other junk food contributes to the obesity epidemic.[167] The IOM report proposed a ban on the sale of these products in schools. However, there is currently no comprehensive federal regulation of food in schools. Nevertheless, the National School Lunch Program (NSLP) and the School Breakfast Program (SBP) require participating school districts to establish local school wellness policies.[168] Although participating school districts must adhere to certain dietary guidelines (e.g., no more than 30 percent of calories from fat), the GAO found that fat still accounted for a much greater proportion of school lunches.[169] The promotion of "competitive foods" in à la carte lines, school snack shops, and vending machines poses a major problem, with no comprehensive federal guidelines or regulations.[170] However, state and local governments have intervened. California passed legislation that raises the nutritional standards of competitive foods in schools and will ban all soft drinks by 2009.[171] Similarly, state and local governments regulate foods of minimal nutritional value (FMNV) in cafeterias, food service areas, and vending machines. Some schools have eliminated contracts with branded fast foods entirely.[172] Other schools have created guidelines for portion sizes and price.[173]

Regulating Advertising to Children. The legal regulation of food advertising is weak and fragmented. The tort system often seeks redress for harms caused by the fraudulent sale of food, such as misbranded meat,[174] misleading or deceptive advertising,[175] and failure to warn consumers of unreasonable risks (box 12, p. 213). The Federal Trade Commission (FTC) is authorized to regulate unfair and deceptive advertisements of food.[176] Current FTC guidelines are merely concerned with misleading consumers;[177] however, advertisements that are acceptable if addressed to an adult might be deceptive, unfair, or misleading when directed to a child.[178] Since young children's cognitive functions make them less capable of making distinctions than are adults, advertising to children may be inherently misleading, and therefore susceptible to regulation under the First Amendment.[179] At present, however, government barely regulates paid food advertisements to children—except for limiting commercial airtime per hour during children's programming on broadcast media and banning paid product placement in children's programming.[180] On a positive note, public pressure is beginning to affect industry behavior;[181] the Disney Company, for example, has pledged to stop using its characters to promote junk food.[182]

Regulating the Internet: Advergames. Marketing food to children via the Internet is a highly unregulated business. The only serious regulation is the FTC's limits on the amount of personal information that can be collected from children by a Web site.[183] In fact, some courts have ruled that games which are "sufficiently artistic and complex"[184] are protected under the First Amendment.[185] However, government may be permitted to regulate advergames that are not artistic and complex, where the primary goal is to sell products.[186]

Marketing food to children involves a complex web of divergent interests. The food industry is highly motivated to sell its products to children who will become lifelong consumers. Industry's economic interests lead to ever more sophisticated ways to influence the eating habits of youth. Government in turn seeks to regulate food marketing but has done so sporadically.[187] Legislators are influenced by special interests and large campaign contributions. At the same time, the judiciary is creating a protected sphere for commercial speech, which chills aggressive regulation of marketing. Children and their parents are caught in the middle, as parents seek to guide young people into a lifetime of more healthy eating and physical activity.

The field of public health is, in many ways, a battleground of ideas. The government's strategy is to capture the public's attention and, ultimately, to change behavior. Its methods are to deliver health messages to inform and influence the public, to suppress deceptive commercial messages, and to mandate private disclosures of health and safety risks. Government has good reason for seeking tighter control of the informational environment: An unfettered marketplace of ideas can result in grave public health consequences. But the government can go only so far in a constitutional democracy. When government acts as an educator or a censor, it intrudes on freedom of expression, one of the most powerful and persistent ideas in Western thought. These antithetical social visions—a free market of ideas and a regulated market to defend health and safety—cannot be easily reconciled. In the end, society must grapple with a values question: Which goal, freedom or health, matters most, and why?

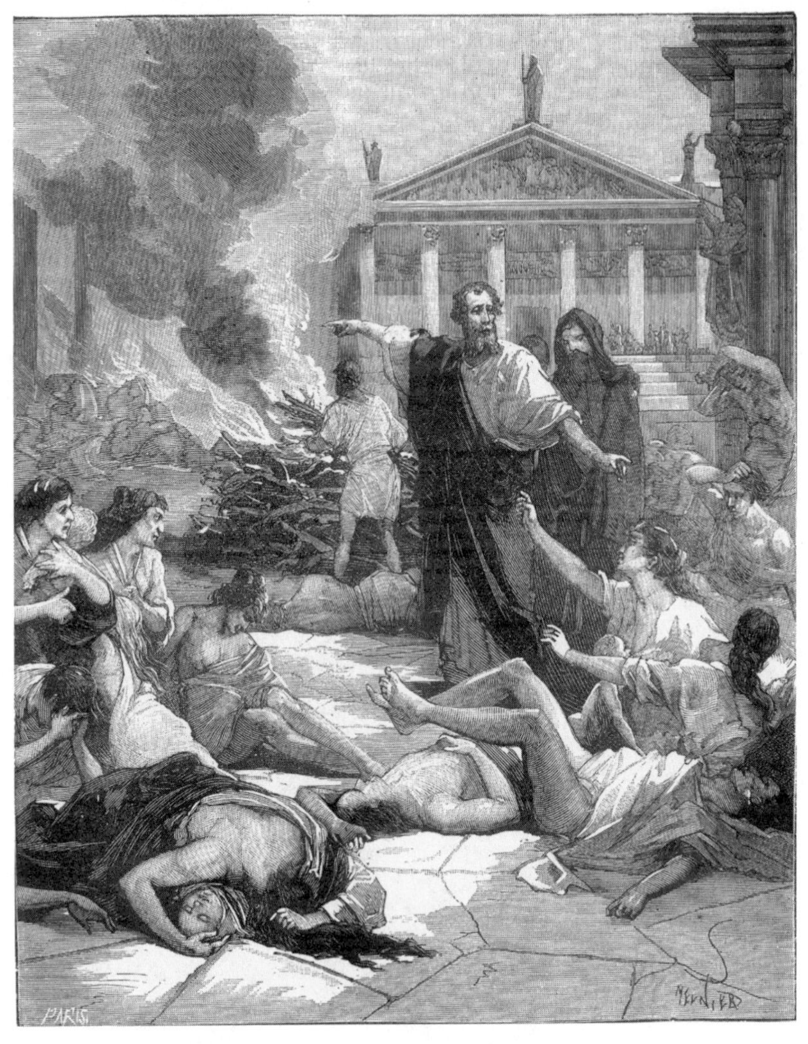

Photo 19. Hippocrates explaining the importance of contagion in a plague epidemic. This image depicts Hippocrates explaining the importance of contagion in an early plague epidemic. Long before the contagion theories of disease emerged, the ancient Greek physician understood the root causes of the spread of disease. Courtesy of The Image Works.

CHAPTER 10

Medical Countermeasures for Epidemic Disease

Bodily Integrity

Now I know these rods are alive, breathed Koch. Now I see the way they grow into millions in my poor little mice, in the sheep, in the cows even. One of these rods, these bacilli, he is a billion times smaller than an ox . . . but he grows, this bacillus, into millions, everywhere through the big animal, swarming in his lungs and brain, choking his blood-vessels, it is terrible.

Paul De Kruif (1926)

This chapter and the next are devoted to epidemics of infectious disease caused by bacteria, viruses, protozoa, fungi, or prions that can replicate in humans.[1] Microbial threats of public health significance cause serious or lethal human disease. Pathogens can be transmitted in many ways, including from person to person, from animals or insects to people, and from food or water to people. Microbial threats may occur naturally or be introduced intentionally through bioterrorism or biological warfare. Many of the same public health strategies used for epidemic disease are relevant for preventing or containing other hazards (e.g., release of chemicals, toxins, or radiological materials), but the primary concern here will be microbial threats.

Infectious diseases preceded the development of humans on earth.[2] Throughout civilization, organized society has struggled—often without hope or success—to contain microbial threats.[3] For most of history, society did not understand the etiology of infectious disease or how to prevent it. The social response was largely confined to crude separation of the ill from the rest of society through isolation or quarantine (see chapter 11).

Despite the dearth of knowledge, European physicians were already devising methods to prevent infectious disease a century before scientists discovered that germs were the etiologic agent. Although the basic principles underlying vaccination date back to the second century, vaccination as a public health practice emanated from the work of, among others, Dr. Edward Jenner, who developed a vaccine for the dreaded smallpox.[4] In 1796, Jenner observed that people who had cowpox rarely contracted smallpox. He induced cowpox in a young boy and later tried to infect the boy with smallpox, but the immunity provoked by the cowpox virus was effective against smallpox.[5] It was not until 1879 that Louis Pasteur advanced the theory of immunization. He discovered that neglected cultures of the bacteria that cause chicken cholera lost much of their ability to cause the disease, while fresh cultures failed to infect chickens previously inoculated with the old cultures.[6] Later, Pasteur established prophylactic inoculations for anthrax, swine erysipelas, and rabies; afterward, other researchers found vaccines for the bubonic plague and typhoid. Jenner called his cowpox inoculation a "vaccine," derived from the Latin *vaccinus,* pertaining to cows. Pasteur, in honor of Jenner's work, extended the meaning to include all prophylactic inoculations. By the close of the century, scientists demonstrated that inoculation with organisms in attenuated live or dead form afforded resistance to communicable diseases, a practice known as active immunization.[7]

It was also in the late nineteenth century that microbiologists such as Louis Pasteur, Robert Koch, and Gerhard Hansen discovered that microorganisms caused infectious diseases like anthrax, cholera, consumption, leprosy, and rabies.[8] They observed, moreover, that microbial disease could be spread from person to person. This meant that it would be possible to test persons for the presence of infection even before the onset of symptoms. Based on this discovery, in 1890 Robert Koch developed the tuberculin skin test, which diagnosed tuberculosis infection. Tuberculin testing, as well as other forms of infectious disease testing (such as for syphilis and gonorrhea), would soon be administered to larger populations as part of public health screening programs.

In a speech on bacterial research the same year he discovered a test for tuberculosis, Koch recalled, "Shortly after discovery of the tubercle bacillus, [I sought] substances that would be therapeutically useful against tuberculosis."[9] Though a treatment for tuberculosis had to await Selman Waksman's discovery of streptomycin in 1944, Alexander Fleming had noticed in 1928 that growth of the pus-producing bacterium

BOX 28

CONCEPTUALIZING THE DETERMINANTS OF HEALTH AND DISEASE

There are at least three ways of conceptualizing the determinants of health and disease: the microbial model, the behavioral model, and the ecological model. Despite considerable overlap, these three theories help explain the underlying rationales for the exercise of personal control measures and the political problems that result.

The microbial model, or germ theory, of public health probably conforms best to the lay perception of disease, together with its causes and methods of control.[1] Disease, in this view, is seen as a product of microbial infection, and the job of public health agencies is to identify the pathogen and to eliminate or contain it. This work can be done in a variety of ways. Vaccination controls microbes by denying them susceptible hosts. Mosquito abatement kills the vectors of insectborne diseases, such as yellow fever and encephalitis. Water purification and meat inspection help prevent harmful bacteria from entering the food chain. Case finding, medical treatment, and isolation curb transmission by people who are already infected. In each case, the intervention targets the pathogen. Under this conception of pathogen control, identifying cases and then intervening to break the cycle of infection safeguard the public's health.

The description of disease as being caused by contact with germs has a great deal of social acceptance. Nevertheless, restrictions placed on a person based on the microbial theory can be controversial. Resistance to traditional disease-control measures arises from a combination of social vulnerability and mistrust of government. Germ-based interventions encounter the stiffest public opposition when identifying or controlling the microbe means identifying or controlling the person who has it and the disease itself exposes its carriers to discrimination, ostracism, and other social risks.[2]

While the germ theory continues to undergird a great deal of public health work, the field has come to recognize another important determinant of health—human behavior. While this notion of disease is reflected in modern discourse about the roles of smoking, diet, and sedentary lifestyle in the development of chronic disease, the influence of behavior in transmitting infection (e.g., sexual or needle-sharing behavior) is also well recognized. Under the behavioral theory of disease control, public health assessment and interventions occur at the point of human conduct, whether at the individual, group, or organizational level. The behavioral model measures successful interventions in reductions of risk behavior. Modern surveillance, therefore, does not merely "count" cases of disease but monitors activities that give rise to morbidity and premature mortality.[3] From this perspective, the germ is less important than the behavior that moves it from one person to another or that makes people more susceptible to becoming ill when they encounter a pathogen.

Seeing public health predominately as the control of risky behavior can quickly become, for cultural and political reasons, a warrant for treating disease entirely as a matter of personal responsibility.[4] Ill health can be viewed, at least in part, as a just

Source: Box 28 is derived from Lawrence Gostin, Scott Burris, and Zita Lazzarini, "The Law and the Public's Health: A Study of Infectious Disease Law in the United States," *Columbia Law Review*, 99 (1999): 59-128.

[1] J.N. Hays, *The Burdens of Disease: Epidemics and Human Response in Western History* (New Brunswick, NJ: Rutgers University Press, 1998).

[2] Scott Burris, "Surveillance, Social Risk, and Symbolism: Framing the Analysis for Research and Policy," *Journal of Acquired Immune Deficiency Syndromes*, 25 (2000): S120-27.

[3] Danice K. Eaton, Laura Kann, Steve Kinchon, et al., "Youth Risk Behavior Surveillance: United States, 2005," *Morbidity and Mortality Weekly Report*, 55 (2006): 1-108.

[4] Robert Steinbrook, "Imposing Personal Responsibility for Health," *New Eng. J. Med.*, 355 (2006): 753-56 (discussing a West Virginia program providing "enhanced" benefits for recipients who sign a "Medicaid Member Agreement" to keep medical appointments, take medications, receive screenings, and follow health improvement plans).

dessert for wrongful behavior. Blame can feed the stigma of disease, adding to the social and psychological burdens.

A third account of disease control focuses on ecological understandings of health: the sources of disease in the social and physical environment. The ecological model conceives of illness not as an external threat, such as a discrete pathogen, nor as a function of personal choices, but rather as a product of society's interaction with its environment.[5] This understanding of public health does not see diseases that are listed on death certificates as "causes" of death at all, but merely as "pathways" along which more fundamental causes have exerted their effect. Ecological theorists emphasize social institutions, environmental conditions, and human inequality as the major health risks in a population.[6] The poor are more susceptible to illness not simply because they encounter more microbes or engage in less healthy behavior, but also because their access to health care and information on healthy living is blocked due to economic and social limitations. Ecological approaches have gained favor in explaining infectious diseases. These threats come from microbes, to be sure, and individual behavior also plays a role in their transmission. However, the ecological perspective offers a far broader view of the root causes, ranging from population growth, urban migration, and international travel to changes in the ecosystem, such as deforestation, flood, drought, and climatic warming.

[5] Mervyn Susser and Ezra Susser, "Choosing a Future for Epidemiology: From Black Box to Chinese Boxes and Eco-epidemiology," *American Journal of Public Health*, 86 (1996): 675-77.

[6] Bruce G. Link and Jo Phelan, "Social Conditions as Fundamental Causes of Disease," *Journal of Health and Social Behavior* (1995): 80-95 (stating that fundamental social causes of disease include money, knowledge, power, prestige, and interpersonal resources embodied in concepts of social support and social networks).

Staphylococcus aureus had stopped around an area in which an airborne mold contaminant, *Penicillium notatum*, had begun to grow. Fleming determined that a chemical substance had diffused from the mold, and named it penicillin.[10] It was not until 1939 that a team of Oxford University scientists led by Howard Florey identified and isolated substances from molds that could kill bacteria. That observation led to the mass production of penicillin for treating wounds during World War II.[11] By the mid-1940s, however, microbiologists were already aware that antibiotics had an Achilles' heel. Fleming observed in 1946 that "the administration of too small doses . . . leads to the production of resistant strains of bacteria."[12] Antibiotic-resistant strains of bacteria pose a problem that vexes public health to this day.

The realization that it was scientifically feasible to immunize persons against infection, test for the presence of infection, and treat the infection (thereby reducing contagion) led to the ascendancy of biological strategies against infectious diseases (see box 28). Public health law was closely modeled on the biological approach, and to this day, the law maintains a strong biological orientation. Indeed, it is relatively easy to sum-

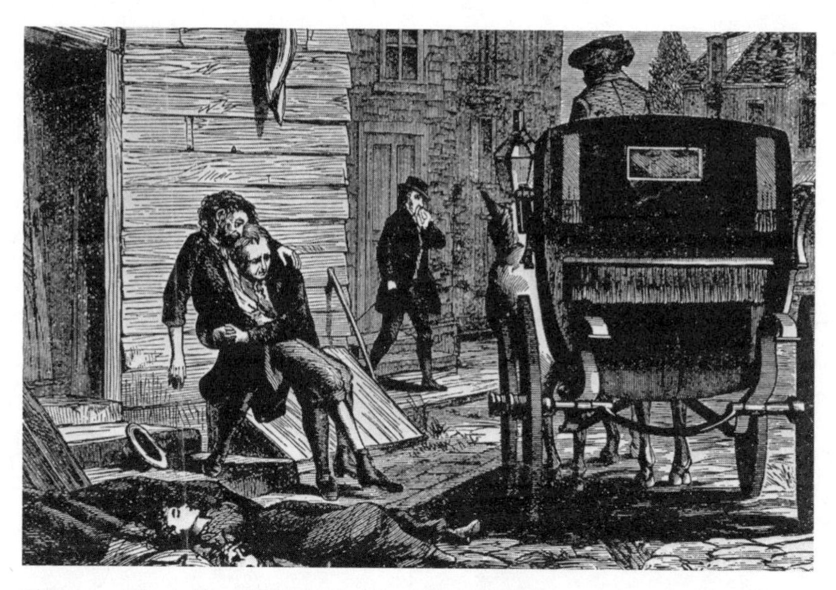

Photo 20. The yellow fever epidemic of 1793. During the 1793 yellow fever epidemic in Philadelphia, carriages rumbled through the streets to pick up the dying and the dead. This image, originally a woodcut, shows Stephen Girard, an American philanthropist and banker, on an errand of mercy. The epidemic was the largest yellow fever epidemic in American history and killed as many as five thousand people. © Bettmann/CORBIS.

marize biological strategies that have, to a greater or lesser extent, been codified in infectious disease laws. These statutes authorize public health officials to compel vaccination against specified infectious diseases. For diseases that cannot be prevented by immunization, public health authorities are empowered to identify cases of infection through testing, physical examination, and population screening. (Positive cases are reported to state health agencies, which also engage in partner notification to identify new cases: see chapter 8.) Physicians can treat persons with disease, voluntarily or sometimes compulsorily.

This chapter examines medical countermeasures for containing epidemic disease: immunization, screening, and medical treatment. The next chapter discusses traditional public health strategies of isolation, quarantine, and community containment (community hygiene, decreased social mixing, and international travel). A case study on pandemic influenza at the end of chapter 11 illustrates the legal and ethical dilemmas of both therapeutic and nonpharmacologic interventions.

COMPULSORY VACCINATION: IMMUNIZING THE POPULATION AGAINST DISEASE

> The first experiment (14 May 1796) was made upon a lad of the name of Phipps, in whose arm a little Vaccine Virus was inserted taken from the hand of a young woman who had been accidentally infected by a cow. Notwithstanding the resemblance which the pustule, thus excited on the boy's arm, bore to variolous inoculation, yet as the indisposition attending it was barely perceptible, I could scarcely persuade myself the patient was secure from the Small Pox. However, on his being inoculated some months afterwards, it proved that he was secure. This case inspired me with confidence; and as soon as I could again furnish myself with Virus from the Cow, I made an arrangement for a series of inoculations.
>
> Edward Jenner (1801)

Vaccinations are among the most cost-effective and widely used public health interventions—one of the ten great public health achievements of the twentieth century.[13] Vaccination programs have eradicated smallpox, virtually eliminated poliomyelitis,[14] and reduced vaccine-preventable diseases in many developed countries by 98–99 percent.[15] (And the need for affordable vaccines against the most deeply rooted diseases in developing countries is palpable.)[16] State vaccination laws, moreover, have been a great success. The rate of complete immunization of school-age children in the United States (more than 95 percent) is as high or higher than most other developed countries. More important, common childhood illnesses, such as measles, pertussis, and polio, which once accounted for a substantial proportion of child morbidity and mortality, have dramatically decreased.[17]

The Politics of Compulsory Vaccination

Despite its role in preventing infectious diseases, vaccination has provoked popular resistance throughout history.[18] Although vaccination was generally accepted in early America (actively supported, among others, by Thomas Jefferson), opposition arose in many quarters.[19] Some opponents expressed scientific objections about efficacy; some worried that vaccination transmitted disease or caused harmful effects; still others objected on grounds of religion or principle. Often, compulsory vaccination was seen as an unwarranted governmental interference with autonomy and liberty.[20]

The political, philosophical, and social struggles surrounding vaccination persist to this day. They are vividly reflected in legislative and judicial debates on the powers and limits of the state to compel vaccination, evoking strong beliefs in individual freedom. Vaccinations are performed on healthy people, most commonly children, and they are mandated for school entry. Consequently, vaccination poses unique ethical concerns.[21] Organized groups of parents, in particular, have struggled against mandatory vaccination and actively lobbied for liberal exemptions.[22] The Internet fuels their opposition, with Web sites openly hostile to immunization policies.[23] For example, some parents have vigorously resisted vaccinations, based on a deep-seated belief that thimerosal (a mercury preservative in some vaccines) causes autism, even though the Institute of Medicine found no evidence to support the claim.[24] As a result, several U.S. states ban thimerosal-containing vaccines,[25] and vaccine coverage for measles, mumps, and rubella (MMR) precipitously dropped in the United Kingdom.[26] The controversy over the human papillomavirus (HPV) vaccine to reduce cervical cancer, approved by the FDA in 2006, offers another illustration. Conservative religious groups publicly opposed the concept of making HPV vaccination mandatory for preadolescent girls, citing fears that vaccination against a sexually transmitted infection (STI) might send a subtle message condoning premarital sex.[27]

Public discourse about vaccination is often tense, with scientists and laypersons frequently talking at cross-purposes.[28] Scientists dispassionately measure the population benefits against economic costs, concluding that vaccines are among the most cost-effective prevention strategies.[29] The lay public, however, often mistrusts expert claims, despite the safety and efficacy of vaccination.[30] Parents, in particular, may be concerned with the health of *their* child and may feel strongly that the risk of a catastrophic vaccine-induced injury should not be imposed by governmental fiat.

Perceptions differ sharply depending on whether the risk of vaccination is viewed from an individualistic or societal perspective. From the perspective of a single child, there may be a slightly greater risk if she is vaccinated than if she were to remain unvaccinated.[31] For example, oral poliovirus vaccines (OPV, a now-discontinued vaccine that contained a

BOX 29

VACCINES AND THE COLLECTIVE ACTION PROBLEM

"Bandwagoning" and "free riding"

Broad exemptions from vaccination requirements create "collective action" problems—what may be in individuals' interests may not be in the public's interests. The most noticeable concern is clustering of refusals ("bandwagoning") in communities.[1] Vaccination behavior is affected by the decisions of others in the community. Clustering may occur because people who share religious beliefs live in close proximity to each other. Or individuals may refuse vaccinations in response to highly visible adverse events among their neighbors. Clustering behavior can lead to precipitous declines in vaccination rates.[2] For example, in Japan in the 1970s, the percentage of infants vaccinated against pertussis plummeted following media reports of neurological injuries to two infants caused by the DPT vaccine. The government eliminated the vaccine coverage requirement, and a major outbreak of pertussis ensued.[3]

Similarly, individuals perceive that they can "free ride" by relying on herd immunity for protection against disease. So long as the majority of the community agrees to be vaccinated, there is protection for the few who refuse. But if too many people opt out, everyone becomes vulnerable to disease. The traditional answer to the free rider problem is enforced compliance, because voluntary cooperation cannot be assured.

Collective action problems place two ethical values in conflict: autonomy and equity. Individuals claim the right to bodily integrity by refusing vaccination. However, by exercising a right to autonomy, individuals place others at risk. Enforced compliance is perceived as fairer because everyone in the community equitably shares the burdens and benefits of vaccination. This still leaves room for exemptions for medical reasons or genuine religious beliefs. So long as exemptions are limited, everyone receives the protection of herd immunity.

1 John C. Hershey, David A. Asch, Thi Thumasathit, et al., "The Roles of Altruism, Free Riding, and Bandwagoning in Vaccination Decisions," *Organizational Behavior and Human Decision Processes,* 59 (1994): 177–87.

2 Thomas May and Ross D. Silverman, "Clustering of Exemptions as a Collective Action Threat to Herd Immunity," *Vaccine,* 21 (2003): 1048–51.

3 Eugene J. Gangarosa, A.M. Galazka, C.R. Wolfe, et al., "Impact of Anti-vaccine Movements on Pertussis Control: The Untold Story," *Lancet,* 351 (1998): 356–61.

live attenuated virus) caused the only cases of poliomyelitis in the United States in the late twentieth century; an unvaccinated child's risk of contracting wild poliovirus was negligible.[32] Government-imposed vaccination should be understood in this light. The state is explicitly asking parents to forgo their right to decide the welfare of their children, not necessarily for the child's benefit but for the wider public good.[33] From a societal perspective, the choice not to immunize may be optimal to the individual if there is herd immunity; but in the aggregate, this choice could lead to failure of that herd immunity.[34] Affording individuals the right to refuse vaccination, then, is not for the greatest good of the community. Rather, as Hardin suggests, the right of refusal can contribute to a "tragedy of the commons" if too many people make the decision not to immunize (box 29).[35]

School and Day Care Vaccination Laws

> Beginning in the 1830s [smallpox] attacks gradually intensified, and by the time of the Civil War the disorder was once again a serious problem. By chance, the rise of smallpox coincided with the enactment of compulsory school attendance laws and the subsequent rapid growth in the number of public schools. Since the bringing together of large numbers of children clearly facilitated the spread of smallpox, and since vaccination provided a relatively safe preventive, it was natural that compulsory school attendance laws should lead to a movement for compulsory vaccination.
>
> John Duffy (1978)

The driving force behind compulsory vaccination laws was a series of outbreaks of smallpox.[36] Laws mandating immunization first appeared in the early nineteenth century, with Massachusetts enacting the first law in 1809.[37] In 1827, Boston became the first city to require all children entering public schools to give evidence of vaccination.[38] By the time of the 1905 landmark decision in *Jacobson v. Massachusetts,* many states required citizens to submit to smallpox vaccination, and almost half required compulsory child vaccination as a condition of school attendance.[39] Antivaccinationists, however, attempted to repeal or thwart such laws through political routes, judicial challenges, and refusals to comply.[40]

Modern immunization statutes were enacted in response to the transmission of measles in schools in the 1960s and 1970s. Legislatures were influenced by the significantly lower incidence rates of measles among schoolchildren in states with immunization laws.[41] They were also influenced by the experience of states that strictly enforced vaccination requirements and school exclusions in outbreak situations without significant community opposition.[42] Rather than having health departments mandate immunization, legislatures required immunization as a condition of attendance in schools or licensed day care.[43] A nationwide Childhood Immunization Initiative was launched in 1977, which stressed the importance of strict enforcement of school immunization laws. Within the next few years, thirty states reformed their laws or regulations, and vaccination levels among children rose to 90 percent.[44]

Currently, all fifty states have school immunization laws.[45] Although the CDC makes recommendations based on guidance by the Advisory Committee on Immunization Practices (ACIP),[46] states have ultimate responsibility for determining which vaccines should be required.[47] From an ethical perspective, states should mandate vaccines primarily for diseases that are highly contagious, cause significant morbidity and mortality, and pose a major health threat to students, teachers, or the community.[48] States require, as a condition of school entry, proof of vaccination against a number of diseases on the immunization schedule, such as diphtheria, pertussis (whooping cough), tetanus (lockjaw), measles, mumps, rubella, polio, and hepatitis B.[49] State laws often require schools to maintain immunization records and report data to public health agencies.[50]

While the exact provisions differ by state, all immunization laws grant exemptions for children with medical contraindications to immunization.[51] Thus, if a physician certifies that the child is susceptible to adverse effects from the vaccine, the child is exempt. This may occur when a child is allergic to vaccine components or has an immune deficiency, such as occurs when being treated for cancer. All states (except West Virginia and Mississippi) also grant religious exemptions for persons who have sincere religious objections to immunization.[52] Some statutes require parents to disclose their religion, while others are more liberally worded.[53] Twenty states also grant exemptions for parents who profess philosophical objections to immunization.[54] These statutes allow parents to refuse vaccination because of their "personal," "moral," or "other" beliefs. The process for obtaining a nonmedical exemption varies depending on the specific state law, and the complexity in the application process is inversely related to the proportion of exemptions filed.[55] In practice, exemptions for all reasons constitute only a small percentage of total school entrants.[56] However, children with exemptions and their surrounding communities have had considerably higher rates of vaccine-preventable disease,[57] with major outbreaks of measles, polio, pertussis, and rubella.[58] For example, research suggests that states permitting personal belief exemptions and those with easily obtained exemptions had higher nonmedical exemption rates and increased incidence of pertussis.[59]

Adult Immunization Laws

The federal and state governments do not mandate vaccinations for adults, except for persons entering military service. The Department of Defense can compel service members to receive vaccinations. However, Congress, in response to the Gulf War, proscribed the administration of investigatory new drugs, or drugs unapproved for their intended use, to service members without their informed consent, unless a presidential waiver is issued.[60] The military discontinued mandatory anthrax vaccinations in 2004 after a federal court issued a preliminary injunction.[61]

The National Immunization Program recommends certain immunizations for adults, but the law does not require it.[62] However, some employers require certain immunizations as a condition of working with people who are sick or vulnerable to infection, or for those who handle or are exposed to dangerous pathogens.[63] Health officials may also recommend immunizations in the aftermath of natural disasters, such as earthquakes or hurricanes, because of, for example, contaminated water and unsanitary conditions (e.g., tetanus and typhoid).[64]

Travel and Immigration Immunization Laws

Whereas immunizations were once required for persons traveling oversees, none is currently required. Depending on the travel destination, health officials may recommend immunizations such as typhoid, hepatitis A and B, meningococcal disease, yellow fever, and Japanese encephalitis.[65]

As of July 1, 1997, all individuals seeking permanent residence in the United States must submit documentation that they have been inoculated against all vaccine-preventable diseases. This includes infants and children brought into the country for international adoption. [66]

The Constitutionality of Compulsory Vaccination

The judiciary has firmly supported compulsory vaccination because of the overriding importance of communal well-being.[67] The vaccine program, of course, must be scientifically warranted and not arbitrary or discriminatory, as detailed in *Wong Wai v. Williamson* (1900), when health officials required inoculation of Chinese residents in San Francisco based purely on race.[68] In the seminal case *Jacobson v. Massachusetts* (1905), the Supreme Court held that vaccination was squarely within the state's police powers (see chapter 4).[69] The state's power to require children to be vaccinated as a condition of school entrance has been widely accepted and judicially sanctioned.[70] In *Zucht v. King* (1922), the Supreme Court upheld a local government mandate for vaccination as a prerequisite for attendance in public school.[71] Enforcement mechanisms may include denying unvaccinated children admission to schools (which is commonly employed), criminally punishing the parents of unvaccinated children (which is seldom used in modern days), or ordering a school to be closed (an extreme measure that is rarely undertaken).

Public Health and Religion in Conflict: Challenges under the First Amendment. Antagonists of vaccination often frame their objections in terms of the First Amendment: "Congress shall make no law respecting an establishment of religion [the Establishment Clause], or prohibiting the free exercise thereof [the Free Exercise Clause]." Does a law that requires people to submit to vaccination against their religious beliefs violate the Free Exercise Clause? Though almost all states currently grant religious exemptions, compelling a person to submit to vaccination against his religious beliefs would be constitutional.[72] The Supreme Court's jurisprudence makes clear that the right of free exercise does not relieve an individual of the obligation to comply with a "valid and neutral law of general applicability."[73] In *Prince v. Massachusetts*, for example, the Court held that a mother could be prosecuted under child labor laws for using her children to distribute religious literature.[74] The Supreme Court of Arkansas in 1965 explicitly upheld a compulsory vaccination law that did not exempt persons with religious beliefs: The "freedom to act according to religious beliefs is subject to a reasonable regulation for the benefit of society as a whole."[75]

While states are not constitutionally obliged to grant religious exemptions, they are permitted to do so. As mentioned, forty-eight states offer some form of religious exemption from school immunization laws. State supreme courts (with the exception of Mississippi)[76] have permitted legislatures to create exemptions for religious beliefs.[77] Even so, courts sometimes strictly construe religious exemptions, insisting that the belief against compulsory vaccination must be "genuine," "sincere," and an integral part of the religious doctrine.[78] In other cases, however, courts readily accept parents' claims for religious exemptions without searching inquiry into their legitimacy.[79] Public health advocates have decried the liberal use of religious exemptions, believing that they have resulted and will continue to result in outbreaks of vaccine-preventable diseases among children and their communities.[80]

Legislatures often limit the scope of religious exemptions by applying them only to "recognized" and "established" churches or religious denominations.[81] The intention is to limit the number of people who can opt out of vaccination requirements. Individuals with sincerely held religious convictions that are not recognized or established, however, have challenged these statutory provisions on two grounds. First, they argue that because these statutes provide preferential treatment to particular religious doctrines, they violate the Establishment Clause.[82] Second, they argue that because these provisions discriminate against persons with nonestablished religious beliefs, they violate equal protection of the law.[83] Although the case law is still in flux, there exists judicial precedent to support each of these claims.[84]

Philosophical Exemptions. As stated above, twenty states allow philosophical or conscientious exemptions, which carry an even lower burden of proof than religious exemptions.[85] Philosophical exemptions vary by state and may recognize objections based on "personal," "philosophical," or "moral convictions." Where available, parents claim the exemption with increasing regularity. In states offering both religious and philosophical exemptions, the latter far exceeds the former.[86] As is the case with religious exemptions, states are constitutionally permitted to exempt conscientious objectors from vaccine requirements, but they are not obliged to do so under the Constitution.

Other Constitutional Claims: Education and Liberty. Objections that school vaccination laws interfere with a child's "right to education" have been raised with little success.[87] For example, the Arizona Court of Appeals rejected the argument that "an individual's right to education would trump the state's need to protect against the spread of infectious disease."[88] Similarly, courts are unlikely to find that a person's constitutionally protected liberty interests override the state's police power to mandate vaccination. In *Cruzan v. Director, Missouri Department of Health,* for example, the Supreme Court, referencing *Jacobson v. Massachusetts,* noted that medical privacy is not absolute and must be weighed against the public good.[89] As a result, the judiciary is unlikely to recognize a right that includes refusal of state-mandated vaccination.[90] (For a summary of constitutional law and vaccination, see box 30.)

BOX 30

A SUMMARY OF CONSTITUTIONAL LAW AND VACCINATION

Constitutional adjudication regarding vaccines is hardly a picture of clarity. Certainly, states have inherent authority under the police power to mandate vaccinations directly or as a condition of school entry. The police power allows states to override individual claims to autonomy or bodily integrity, and the power is not limited to periods of outbreaks, epidemics, or emergencies. Courts uphold mandatory vaccination, so long as it is scientifically justified and not exercised arbitrarily or as a pretext for discrimination. The Supreme Court in *Jacobson* also implied that states must exempt those who would be medically harmed by vaccination.[1]

Although the states must offer medical exemptions, they are not constitutionally obliged to offer religious or philosophical exemptions.[2] The First Amendment Free Exercise Clause probably allows states to require universal vaccinations—even if vaccination is against an individual's religious beliefs—because such laws are "neutral" and apply to everyone.[3] Most states, however, do offer such exemptions—forty-eight states have religious exemptions and twenty states have philosophical exemptions. (Individuals seeking a waiver on religious grounds may have to demonstrate that their objection is actually based on religion rather than secular values.)[4] States that choose to exempt individuals for religious reasons must not fall afoul of the First Amendment Establishment Clause, which forbids government from making any law "respecting an establishment of religion." For some courts, this means that the state may not limit religious exemptions to "recognized" or "established" churches or religious denominations.[5] This kind of claim also has been framed as a violation of the Fourteenth Amendment's Equal Protection Clause, because it favors those with established religious beliefs over nonestablished religious beliefs.[6]

Arguments based on the Establishment or Equal Protection Clauses can be troubling to public health advocates, who fear that it would open the floodgates for religious exemptions. Perhaps the best way to meet public health objectives, while still respecting the Constitution, is to require individuals to demonstrate that their beliefs are internally consistent, based on coherent (although not necessarily "established" or recognized") religious doctrine, and sincerely held. Researchers have demonstrated that a deliberative process for religious exemptions limits the number of those exempt from vaccination and is consistent with a sound public health approach.[7]

[1] *Jacobson v. Massachusetts,* 197 U.S. 11 (1905).

[2] *Brown v. Stone,* 378 So.2d 218 (Miss. 1979).

[3] *Employment Div. v. Smith,* 494 U.S. 872 (1990).

[4] *Mason v. General Brown Cent. Sch. Dist.,* 851 F.2d 47 (2d Cir. 1988) (holding that parents' sincerely held belief that immunization was contrary to "genetic blueprint" was a secular, not a religious, belief); *Hanzel v. Arter,* 625 F. Supp. 1259 (S.D. Ohio, 1985) (holding that parents with objections to vaccination based on "chiropractic ethics" were not exempt); see *Wisconsin v. Yoder,* 406 U.S. 205, 215 (1972) ("To have the protection of the Religion Clauses, the claims must be rooted in religious belief").

[5] *Sherr v. Northport-East Northport Union Free Sch. Dist.,* 672 F. Supp. 81 (E.D.N.Y. 1987).

[6] *Dalli v. Board of Educ.,* 267 N.E.2d 219 (S. Jud. Ct. Mass. 1971).

[7] Jennifer S. Rota, Daniel A. Salmon, Lance E. Rodewald, et al., "Process for Obtaining Nonmedical Exemptions to State Immunization Laws," *American Journal of Public Health,* 91 (2000): 645–48.

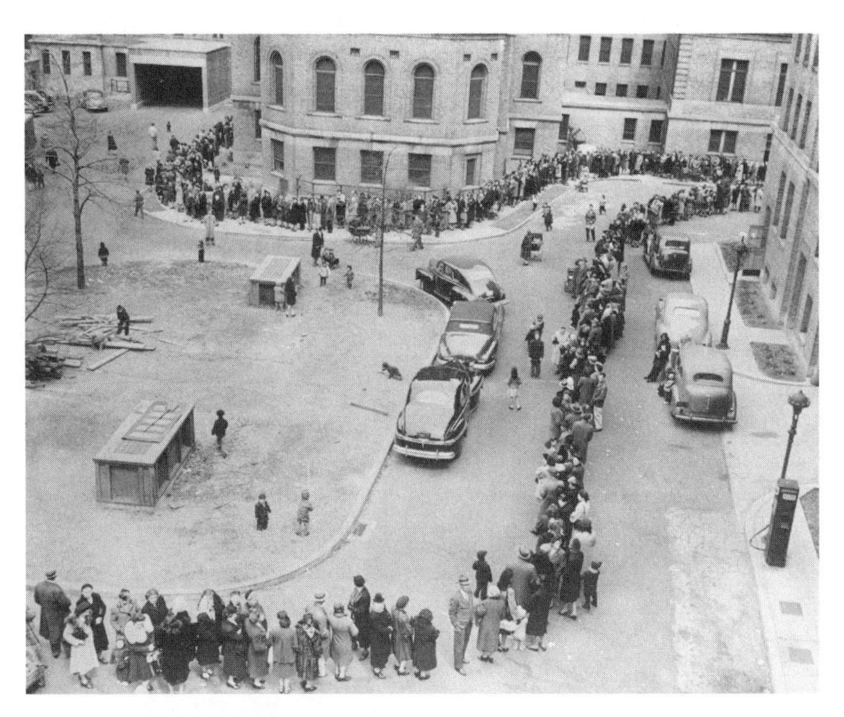

Photo 21. The long queue for smallpox vaccinations. This 1947 photograph displays thousands of New Yorkers flocking to the Morrisania Hospital in the Bronx for vaccination against smallpox after New York officials asked all residents to get vaccinated. Vaccination remains an important public health intervention today, particularly given the potential threat posed by emerging infectious diseases such as pandemic influenza. © Bettmann/CORBIS.

Ensuring Stable Vaccine Supplies

Despite the promise of vaccines, the United States has struggled to ensure a stable vaccine supply, at reasonable cost and delivered efficiently to consumers.[91] Vaccine manufacturers are leaving the industry, creating the risk of severe shortages. In 1967, twenty-six companies were licensed to produce vaccines for the U.S. market, but less than half are licensed today.[92] Presently, only a handful of companies produce all routine vaccines and, for many, there is only one supplier.[93] Vaccine production has been unreliable even for seasonal influenza, which is the leading cause of vaccine-preventable mortality; only a fraction of the recommended population is vaccinated each year.[94] For example, the United States lost half its supply of influenza vaccine in 2004–5, when the United Kingdom withdrew Chiron Corporation's license due to bacterial contamination.[95] The best way to ensure preparedness for current and emerging infectious diseases is to increase capacity for the manufacture and delivery of childhood and seasonal vaccines. This requires planning, market incentives, and sound regulation.

Planning and Market Incentives. Public/private strategies, rather than private markets, are most likely to succeed in ensuring a stable vaccine supply, as a result of the "unique risks and constraints" associated with this endeavor.[96] Market forces create disincentives that inhibit vaccine development: high investment costs,[97] limited or variable markets,[98] and regulatory compliance.[99] The Institute of Medicine recommends a National Vaccine Authority (NVA) to advance the development, production, and procurement of vaccines.[100] With or without an NVA, government can create incentives by boosting demand through seasonal vaccine awareness programs, issuing purchasing contracts, and providing price guarantees or subsidies.[101]

Liability and Compensation. In the 1980s, a liability crisis brought on by concerns about the safety of diphtheria and tetanus toxoids and pertussis vaccine led to supply shortages and calls for rationing. Vaccine prices skyrocketed, and research on new vaccines was threatened. [102] In response, Congress created the National Vaccine Injury Compensation Program (NVICP)—tort reform legislation designed to compensate individuals quickly, easily, and fairly.[103] Though tort liability for industry and fair compensation for patients offer a sound dual approach to vaccine policy, the current NVICP needs reform (see box 31).[104]

The NVICP created a no-fault system that pays for injuries caused by specific immunizations;[105] Congress added influenza to NVICP in 2004. Special masters at the Federal Claims Court adjudicate compensation, based on a Vaccine Injury Table. To recover, claimants must show that a listed vaccine caused their injury. Compensation comes from a Compensation Trust Fund financed by a tax on each administered dose. As of June 2006, 11,830 claims had been filed, of which 1,985 were compensated; over $6.8 billion has been paid in awards since the NVICP began in 1988.[106]

Patients can opt out of NVICP, which has led to a sustained critique that legal liability represents a major disincentive for the industry. President Bush's influenza plan in 2005, for example, would have virtually banned lawsuits (except for willful misconduct) and assigned liability determinations to a political figure (the HHS Secretary). However, the

BOX 31

GOVERNMENT VACCINE INITIATIVES

A series of events during the 1980s and 1990s threatened the viability of vaccine policy and stimulated legislative initiatives.

National Childhood Vaccine Injury Act of 1986

In the early 1980s, manufacturers expressed concern that substantial tort costs would discourage research and innovation. At the same time, consumer groups believed it was morally wrong to make parents prove that manufacturers were at fault before obtaining compensation for vaccine-induced injuries. As a result, Congress enacted the National Childhood Vaccine Injury Act of 1986.[1] The act established four programs: (1) the National Vaccine Program in the Department of Health and Human Services is responsible for most aspects of vaccination policy (e.g., research, development, safety and efficacy testing, licensing, distribution, and use); (2) the Vaccine Injury Compensation Program compensates persons who suffer from certain vaccine-induced injuries according to values set in a Vaccine Injury Table; (3) the Vaccine Adverse Events Reporting System requires health care providers and manufacturers to report certain adverse events from vaccines;[2] and (4) a vaccine information system requires all health care providers to give parents standardized written information before administering certain vaccines.

Comprehensive Childhood Immunization Act of 1993

A second important event took place between 1989 and 1991 that refocused federal attention on immunization policy. Several major outbreaks of measles produced some 50,000 cases of disease, 11,000 hospitalizations, and 130 deaths, mostly among unvaccinated children.[3] These outbreaks led Congress to enact the Comprehensive Childhood Immunization Act of 1993. The Children's Immunization Initiative created an entitlement to free vaccines for eligible children, supported state efforts to deliver vaccines, increased community participation and provider education, enhanced measurement of immunization status, and developed combined vaccines to simplify the immunization schedule.[4]

State Immunization Registries

Despite the Children's Immunization Initiative, vaccination rates among preschool-age children stayed below the levels in many developed, and even some developing, countries.[5] As recently as the mid-1990s, approximately one-third of infants born annually in the United States had not received all of their recommended immunizations by age two.[6] Policymakers concluded that efforts to vaccinate children were being hindered by incomplete and inaccurate information. Immunization information that parents im-

[1] 42 U.S.C.A. § 300aa(1); see Derry Ridgway, "No-Fault Vaccine Insurance: Lessons from the National Vaccine Injury Compensation Program," *Journal of Health Politics, Policy and Law*, 24 (1999): 59–90.

[2] Institute of Medicine, *Vaccine Safety Forum* (Washington, DC: National Academies Press, 1997).

[3] Centers for Disease Control and Prevention, "Measles—United States, 1992," *Morbidity and Mortality Weekly Report*, 42 (1993): 378–81; National Vaccine Advisory Committee, "The Measles Epidemic: The Problems, Barriers, and Recommendations," *JAMA*, 266 (1991): 1547–52.

[4] Centers for Disease Control and Prevention, "Reported Vaccine-Preventable Diseases—United States, 1993, and the Childhood Immunization Initiative," *Morbidity and Mortality Weekly Report*, 43 (1994): 57–60; General Accounting Office, PEMD-94-28.

[5] General Accounting Office, *Preventive Health Care for Children: Experience from Selected Foreign Countries*, HRD-93-62 (Aug. 1993), http://archive.gao.gov/t2pbat5/149648.pdf.

[6] Centers for Disease Control and Prevention, "Vaccination Coverage of Two-Year Old Children—United States, 1991–92," *JAMA*, 271 (1994): 260–61.

parted to health care providers was frequently incorrect or insufficient.[7] States began to develop immunization data systems to track children, identify those who needed to be vaccinated, and generate notices when a child's vaccinations were due or past due.[8] As a result of this and other initiatives, vaccination rates among preschool-age children have improved significantly.[9]

[7] Centers for Disease Control and Prevention, "Impact of Missed Opportunities to Vaccinate Preschool-Aged Children on Vaccination Coverage Levels—Selected U.S. Sites, 1991-1992," *Morbidity and Mortality Weekly Report*, 38 (1994): 709-18, 717-18.

[8] National Vaccine Advisory Committee, *Developing a National Childhood Immunization System: Registries, Reminders, and Recall* (Washington, DC: U.S. Department of Health and Human Services, 1994); Lawrence O. Gostin and Zita Lazzarini, "Childhood Immunization Registries: A National Review of Public Health Information Systems and the Protection of Privacy," *JAMA*, 274 (1995): 1793-99.

[9] Centers for Disease Control and Prevention, "Immunization Information System Progress—United States, 2004," *Morbidity and Mortality Weekly Report*, 54 (2005): 1156-57.

political critique may overstate the negative influence of liability on vaccine production. Vaccine litigation, although a serious concern, has been relatively rare, with few reported cases and most with small penalties for companies that comply with FDA standards.[107]

Mass use of untested vaccines, particularly during a public health emergency, could result in numerous adverse events. Health care workers and patients would be less likely to volunteer without a fair compensation system, as the failed smallpox vaccination campaign demonstrated in 2003 (see box 32). A no-fault system like NVICP could provide relief for injured patients and greater certainty for industry. New vaccines, such as experimental influenza A (H5N1) vaccines, may not be covered under NVICP, so vaccines would need to be added early in development. Moreover, NVICP has become adversarial, burdensome on claimants, and time consuming. A reformed system would have to take account of important issues: an overwhelmed program, resulting in delays; insufficient money in the compensation trust fund; and injustices caused by excessive burdens placed on injured patients. In return, policymakers would have to consider tort reform, which could spare the industry lawsuits based on strict liability but perhaps not those for recklessness or gross negligence.

To encourage rapid development of vaccines in a public health emergency, Congress enacted the Public Readiness and Emergency Preparedness (PREP) Act in December 2005.[108] The PREP Act provides immunity from liability (except for "willful misconduct") for all claims resulting from the use of medical countermeasures during a public health emergency. The Secretary for Health and Human Services has primary responsibility for declaring an emergency that would justify removing financial risk barriers.[109] Civil libertarians vigorously opposed PREPA

BOX 32

THE NATIONAL SMALLPOX VACCINATION CAMPAIGN

A case study at the intersection of public health and national security

Even though the World Health Organization certified the global eradication of smallpox on May 8, 1980, and the last vaccinations in the United States were given in the 1970s,[1] laboratories in Atlanta, Georgia, and Koltsovo, Russia, maintain stocks of live virus.[2] The WHO, having vociferously debated their destruction,[3] resolved in 2006 to temporarily retain the two existing stocks of virus for the purpose of international research.[4]

The terrorist attacks of September 2001 and the anthrax deaths that occurred soon afterward changed the course of smallpox policy.[5] Questions about the security of Russian laboratories after the fall of the Soviet Union, combined with concerns that all countries may not have destroyed their smallpox virus stocks, led to the fear that smallpox virus might have fallen into the hands of rogue nations or terrorist organizations. With a heightened sense of its own vulnerabilities, the United States launched a program to prepare for a potential smallpox attack.

The national smallpox vaccination plan announced on December 13, 2002, represented an extraordinary policy decision: mass vaccination against a disease that did not exist with a vaccine that had well-documented risks.[6] Based on the belief that the risk of serious adverse events in a general-population campaign outweighed the risk of a smallpox outbreak, the administration opted for a prerelease vaccination of selected groups.[7] The plan had several phases: immediate and mandatory vaccination of half a million military personnel who were or might be deployed in high-threat areas;[8] voluntary vaccination of up to 500,000 health care workers and smallpox response

[1] Brendon Kohrs, "Bioterrorism Defense: Are State Mandated Compulsory Vaccination Programs an Infringement upon a Citizen's Constitutional Rights?" *Journal of Law and Health*, 17 (2002-3): 241-69.

[2] Research stocks of the virus are being kept frozen in laboratories at the CDC in Atlanta and the Russian State Research Center for Virology and Biotechnology in Koltsovo. George W. Conk, "Reactions and Overreactions: Smallpox Vaccination, Complications, and Compensation," *Fordham Environmental Law Journal*, 14 (2002-3): 439-97. Destruction of the known research stocks of the virus has been intensely debated. WHO campaigned for the destruction of the known stocks of the virus, but the Clinton administration decided against destruction of the U.S. supply. Lawrence K. Altman, "Health Group Votes to Kill Last Virus of Smallpox," *New York Times*, May 26, 1996; Judith Miller and William J. Broad, "Clinton to Announce that U.S. Will Keep Sample of Lethal Smallpox Virus, Aides Say," *New York Times*, April 22, 1999.

[3] Lawrence K. Altman, "Destruction of Smallpox Virus Backed in WHO Committee," *New York Times*, September 10, 1994 (reporting that WHO recommended unanimously that the smallpox virus be destroyed on June 30, 1995).

[4] World Health Organization, Executive Board, EB117/33, 117th Session, Jan. 16, 2006. Provisional agenda item 4.7.

[5] David A. Koplow, *Smallpox: The Fight to Eradicate a Global Scourge* (Berkeley: University of California Press, 2003).

[6] Department of Health and Human Services, *Declaration Regarding Administration of Smallpox Countermeasures*, 60 Fed. Reg. 4,212 (Jan. 28, 2003) (declaring vaccinia [smallpox] a covered countermeasure).

[7] The public health and national defense communities within the Bush administration actively debated whether to vaccinate a core group of health care workers and other critical personnel—a control and containment strategy—or to initiate a program to vaccinate the general population. In 2002, the ACIP finally decided that a focused immunization campaign would be more beneficial. Advisory Committee on Immunization Practices, "Recommendations for Using Smallpox Vaccine in a Pre-Event Vaccination Program," *Morbidity and Mortality Weekly Report*, 52 (2003): 1-16.

[8] White House, "Protecting Americans: Smallpox Vaccination Program," press release, Dec. 13, 2002, http://www.whitehouse.gov/news/releases/2002/12/20021213-1.html.

teams within thirty days;[9] vaccination of up to 10 million health care personnel and other first responders, such as firefighters and police; and vaccination with a new, not yet approved vaccine for members of the public who insisted on access.[10]

The military smallpox vaccination program went essentially as planned; in less than six months the Department of Defense administered 450,293 smallpox vaccinations.[11] The plan to vaccinate up to 500,000 civilian health care workers who would be responsible for vaccinating the public in the event of a smallpox attack faltered badly, however, and was officially "paused" in June 2003, with a response rate of less than 10 percent of eligible physicians and nurses.[12]

The campaign, if successfully implemented, would have subjected healthy volunteers to the risk of adverse effects ranging from mild and self-limited to severe and life-threatening. Vaccinated individuals also could transmit vaccinia to close contacts.[13] The program's justification was the risk of intentional release of smallpox virus, but the White House did not disclose evidence that the virus existed outside the two known repositories.[14] The ACIP and the CDC both said the risk was "low" and "indeterminate."[15] Never before had a vaccination program been undertaken where there was no natural hazard, but only a hypothetical threat posed by the possibility of a terrorist attack.

The national smallpox vaccination campaign was the subject of intense criticism.[16] The Institute of Medicine's principal findings were that the White House failed to communicate the policy's rationale and curtailed the CDC from communicating with key constituencies.[17] The American Public Health Association stated that the CDC's implementation plan did not provide adequate resources, "including costs derived from monitoring adverse events, treating complications, and training personnel."[18] The vaccine industry and hospitals that administered vaccinations sought and received tort immunity in 2002.[19] Health care workers requested compensation for injuries result-

[9] Edward P. Richards, Katharine C. Rathbun, and Jay Gold, "The Smallpox Vaccination Campaign of 2003: Why Did It Fail and What Are the Lessons for Bioterrorism Preparedness?" *Louisiana Law Review*, 64 (2003-4): 851-904.

[10] The vaccine was unlicensed until 2004. Vincent A. Fulginiti, Arthur Papier, J. Michael Lane, et al., "Smallpox Vaccination: A Review, Part I. Background, Vaccination Technique, Normal Vaccination and Revaccination, and Expected Normal Reactions," *Clinical Infectious Diseases*, 37 (2003): 241-43.

[11] John D. Grabenstein and William Winkenwerder, "US Military Smallpox Vaccination Program Experience," *JAMA*, 289 (2003): 3278-82; Richard Stevenson and Sheryl Gay Stolberg, "Bush Lays Out Plan on Smallpox Shots: Military Is First," *New York Times*, Dec. 14, 2002.

[12] Donald G. McNeil, "Two Programs to Vaccinate for Smallpox are 'Paused,'" *New York Times*, June 19, 2003; Donald G. McNeil, "Threats and Responses: Bioterror Threat; Many Balking at Vaccination," *New York Times*, Feb. 7, 2003.

[13] Christine Casey, Claudia Vellozzi, Gina T. Mootrey, et al., "Surveillance Guidelines for Smallpox Vaccine (Vaccinia) Adverse Reactions," *Morbidity and Mortality Weekly Report*, 55 (2006): 1-16; Joanne Cono, Christine G. Casey, and David M. Bell, "Smallpox Vaccination and Adverse Reactions: Guidance for Clinicians," *Morbidity and Mortality Weekly Report*, 52 (2003): 1-28.

[14] Grabenstein and Winkenwerder, "US Military Smallpox Vaccination Program Experience"; Stevenson and Stolberg, "Bush Lays Out Plan on Smallpox Shots."

[15] Advisory Committee on Immunization Practices, "Recommendations for Using Smallpox Vaccine in a Pre-Event Vaccination Program."

[16] Thomas May, Mark P. Aulisio, and Ross D. Silverman, "The Smallpox Vaccination of Health Care Workers: Professional Obligations and Defense against Bioterrorism," *Hastings Center Report*, 33 (2003): 26-33 (arguing that there is no professional moral obligation to receive smallpox vaccination as a matter of either public health or national security).

[17] Institute of Medicine, *The Smallpox Vaccination Program: Public Health in an Age of Terrorism* (Washington, DC: National Academies Press, 2005); see Thomas May and Ross D. Silverman, "Should Smallpox Vaccine Be Made Available to the General Public?" *Kennedy Institute of Ethics Journal*, 13 (2003): 67-82.

[18] American Public Health Association, "Policy Statement on Smallpox Vaccination," *American Public Health Association*, http://www.apha.org/legislative/policy/smallpox.htm.

[19] *Homeland Security Act of 2002*, Pub. L. No. 107-296, 116 Stat. 2135, §304 (stating that if the Secretary of HHS declares smallpox vaccination to be a "countermeasure . . . to the chemical, biological, radiological, nuclear, and other emerging terrorist threats," there shall be immunity from tort liability for "any person who is . . . a manufacturer, or distributor," or is a "health care entity under whose auspices any qualified person administers the smallpox vaccine").

ing from smallpox vaccination,[20] but Congress did not enact a plan until April 2003, after highly publicized cases of serious adverse events. In the end, the government could not secure the needed participation of public health and health care professionals. The unifying theme was a lack of planning and collaboration with major stakeholders that resulted in a loss of trust in government, and ultimately led to the plan's failure.

The national smallpox vaccination program offers a poignant case study at the intersection of public health and national security. The order for vaccinations came from the highest level—the president of the United States. It began with intense media coverage of smallpox in the aftermath of the trauma of September 11, and continued with the build-up to the war in Iraq. Public health and health care professionals remained deeply skeptical and prevaricated in the face of a president's call to action. In many ways, the breakdown in trust between national security and public health was sad and remarkable—a lesson that, if not learned well, could harm America's national interests in a time of crisis.

[20] Naomi Seiler, Holly Taylor, and Ruth Faden, "Legal and Ethical Considerations in Government Compensation Plans: A Case Study of Smallpox Immunization," *Indiana Health Law Review*, 1 (2004): 3-27.

for delegating broad power to the executive branch and undermining state vaccine laws.[110]

Biodefense Vaccine Development—Project Bioshield. Many of the issues discussed above are also relevant to biodefense vaccine development. The biotechnology industry has not systematically developed countermeasures for potential agents of biological warfare and terrorism because the market is speculative; research and development historically have focused on products of commercial value.[111] The Department of Defense sought to increase economic incentives in the mid-1990s by creating the Joint Vaccine Acquisition Program, which contracts out promising biodefense vaccines to the private sector.[112] However, the Institute of Medicine concluded that the vaccine acquisition program is poorly organized and underfunded, and even puts military readiness at risk.[113] Effective countermeasures are not available for many of the biological terrorism agents deemed most dangerous by the CDC; for example, botulinum toxin, plague, tularemia, and viral hemorrhagic fevers lack licensed vaccines.[114]

To encourage companies to develop new biodefense countermeasures, Congress enacted the Project Bioshield Act in 2004.[115] Project Bioshield encourages the development of vaccine countermeasures by: (1) relaxing procedures for procurement of property or services for biomedical research and development; (2) authorizing the FDA to permit rapid distribution of promising yet unapproved and unlicensed new drugs and antidotes in emergencies; and (3) establishing a Special Reserve Fund of $5.6 billion over ten years to purchase medical countermeasures against a broad array of chemical, biological, radiological, and nuclear agents.[116] The Department of Homeland Security[117] has thus far authorized special reserve funds for countermeasures against anthrax, smallpox, botulinum toxin, and radiological or nuclear devices.[118]

When President Bush proposed Project Bioshield in his 2003 State of the Union address, he reasoned that the promise of lucrative sales to the government would generate strong interest in the private sector.[119] Companies, however, often need more than funding. The industry has expressed concerns about liability associated with developing untested countermeasures. Critics also expressed concerns that the project was restricted to intentional acts of terror and not naturally occurring infectious diseases such as pandemic influenza. In the end, delays and bureaucracy, together with lack of coordination with the private sector, have stalled Bioshield.[120] Even the development of a safer, more effective anthrax vaccine—the government's highest priority—has been mired in disputes.[121] Congress has been debating enacting Bioshield II to overcome several of these problems: reducing safety testing requirements, reducing tort liability, and creating a new federal agency for developing countermeasures for biodefense and natural disease outbreaks.[122] Government watchdog groups, however, have criticized the bill for pandering to the pharmaceutical industry while providing insufficient protection for patients.

Vaccines for Poor Countries—The Role of the International Community. As intractable as the problems seem for ensuring a stable vaccine supply in developed countries, the difficulties are compounded for poorer nations. Millions of people die each year from diseases such as pneumococcal disease, malaria, and HIV/AIDS, mostly in developing countries.[123] Vaccines arguably offer the best hope for tackling these and other "neglected" diseases concentrated in poor countries.[124] Moreover, vaccination is generally cost-effective.[125] Economists estimate, for example, that a malaria, HIV, or TB vaccine would cost approximately $15, $17, or $30 per life-year saved, respectively. Yet there is a dearth of research and development relative to the social need.[126] The private sector is unlikely to pay the high costs of vaccine development for diseases endemic in poor countries, where governments cannot afford the high prices required for offsetting development costs.[127]

International organizations have proposed advance market commitments (AMC) as an innovative way to provide investment incentives for vaccine manufacturers.[128] Under an AMC, sponsors commit to fully or partially "subsidize the purchase of an as yet unavailable vaccine against a specific disease causing high morbidity and mortality in developing countries."[129] The Group of Eight industrialized nations (G8) agreed on a pilot AMC proposal in 2006. The G8 nations would offer from $800 million to $6 billion to subsidize the purchase of a vaccine for one disease, probably pneumococcal infection.[130] The routine use of vaccines to prevent deadly pneumococcal infections in developing countries could substantially reduce infant and child mortality and contribute to the United Nations' ambitious goal of reducing child mortality by two-thirds by 2015.[131] (See chapter 7.)

Incentives for vaccine development are necessary but insufficient. It is also important to link incentives with access to vaccines once they are developed. The divide in access to vaccines between developed and developing countries has widened over the past two decades.[132] In poor and isolated areas of developing countries, for example, vaccines for common diseases such as TB, measles, tetanus, and whooping cough reach less than one in twenty children.[133] The disparities are not caused simply by the high cost of vaccines. Many developing countries also have poorly managed and equipped health service delivery systems, which in turn is often the result of decades of underinvestment and neglect.[134]

The Swine Influenza Immunization Program: A Case Study

> Just about everybody in public health knows something about 1976. . . . The swine flu program has become part of public health lore, with the moral of the tale depending on who is telling it and why it is being told. But the swine flu program is not the stuff of folklore. It is far too complex. There are no villains. It does not lend itself to easy analysis.
>
> Walter R. Dowdle (1997)

After outbreaks of influenza among army recruits in 1976, the CDC identified the causative strain as swine flu, a virus transmitted easily through human-to-human contact.[135] The CDC feared the population would not have resistance to the disease. The media was already speculating that this epidemic would become as catastrophic as the 1918 swine flu pandemic, which caused 20 million deaths worldwide, including 500,000 in the United States.[136] David Sencer, the CDC director, advised President Ford to initiate mass immunization, reasoning that it was safer to gamble with money than lives. The president announced an ambitious public health program designed to immunize the American population at a cost of $134 million, and Congress followed with the requested appropriation.

As would be expected, there were massive logistical problems in manufacturing and distributing the vaccine, and political quarrels ensued. Liability risks posed perhaps the greatest challenge. The insurance industry, fearing massive liability exposure, informed pharmaceutical companies that it would not provide liability insurance for the swine flu vaccine, which posed a serious threat to the vaccine supply. Congress again acted quickly with a modified version of the Tort Claims Act that would underwrite liability costs. Despite waning support among top health officials, the program lurched forward. On October 1, the first vaccinations were given, and ten days later, three elderly people in Pittsburgh died shortly after receiving the vaccine. Despite health officials' claims that the deaths were not causally related to the vaccine, the media developed a "body count" mentality. On October 14, the president and his family received immunizations on prime-time television to reassure the public.

In November, a physician in Minnesota reported a case of ascending paralysis, called Guillain-Barre syndrome. After surveillance activities revealed an increased incidence of the syndrome, the swine flu immunization program was brought to an end on December 16, with the president's reluctant agreement; 45 million people had been vaccinated. The federal government changed hands in January 1977. President Carter's Secretary of Health, Education and Welfare, Joseph Califano, fired David Sencer and reimplemented the Victoria flu program (a component of the larger swine flu program) for high-risk individuals only.

The swine flu immunization program provides an intriguing illustration of policymaking in circumstances of uncertainty. Many commentators held government scientists primarily responsible.[137] For example, in a controversial report commissioned by Secretary Califano, Richard Neustadt and Harvey Fineberg found that health officials assumed an air of arrogance, manipulating their constitutional superiors to comply with "expert" recommendations. The report described overconfidence among scientific experts based on meager evidence, conviction fueled by personal agendas, and zeal by scientists to make their lay superiors do right.[138]

In retrospect, health officials did err in recommending a massive immunization campaign with substantial economic cost and potential harmful effects in circumstances of scientific uncertainty. The available data were inadequate to predict whether swine flu would be contained within narrow outbreaks or become a more serious epidemic.[139] Nevertheless, the roles played by the media, industry, and politicians are also instructive. The media made swine flu salient in the public mind, exaggerating both the health effects of the disease and the risk of vaccine-induced injury and death. The pharmaceutical industry convinced political leaders to hold it harmless against lawsuits while it profited from a massive vaccination program actively promoted by government. Politicians in both the executive and legislative branches wanted to position themselves to gain credit for a successful public health program (e.g., President Ford hoped to pin his reelection prospects on mobilizing the immunization program). At the same time, politicians wanted to avoid the blame for failure to respond to an emergent public health risk (e.g., Congress capitulated to demands for large expenditures first to fund the vaccination campaign and then to assume the liability costs).

The swine flu epidemic is instructive in many ways, but it still fails to answer the critical question: whether, in the face of scientific uncertainty, it is better to err on the side of excess caution or aggressive intervention. Consider the appropriate response to suspected bioterrorism with a microbial agent such as anthrax or smallpox. In an emergency, to whom should vaccines be made available, and under what circumstances would the government be justified in mandating vaccination? There are evident costs both of action and inaction: The costs of inaction, if the risk materializes, are lost lives, but the costs of overreaction, if the risk is exaggerated, are wasted public funds and unnecessary burdens of vaccine-induced injury and diminished autonomy.

TESTING AND SCREENING

Disease screening is one of the most basic tools of modern public health and preventive medicine. Screening programs have a long and distinguished history in efforts to control epidemics of infectious diseases and targeting treatment for chronic diseases. . . . In practice when screening is conducted in contexts of gender inequality, racial discrimination, sexual taboos, and poverty, these conditions shape the attitudes and beliefs of health system and public health decision-makers as well as patients, including those who have lost confidence that the health care system will treat them fairly. Thus, if screening programs are poorly conceived, organized, or implemented, they may lead to interventions of questionable merit and enhance the vulnerability of groups and individuals.

Institute of Medicine (1999)

Although the terms are often used interchangeably, there is a distinction between testing and screening. *Testing* refers to a medical procedure that determines the presence or absence of disease, or its precursor, in an individual patient.[140] Individuals are often selected for testing because of a history of risk or clinical symptoms. In contrast, *screening* refers to the systematic application of a medical test to a defined population.[141] Typically, medical testing is administered for diagnostic or clinical purposes, whereas screening is undertaken for broader public health purposes, such as case finding: identifying previously unknown or unrecognized conditions in apparently healthy or asymptomatic persons.[142]

Screening is often fraught with political controversy. Legislatures may wish to appear to be "doing something" about an urgent health problem.[143] Screening, however, reveals the identity of individuals and subjects them to potential stigma and discrimination. Because it can be costly and impose burdens, public health agencies should evaluate screening programs under two broad criteria: Does screening have adequate predictive value? Will screening achieve an important public health objective?[144] Equally important, screening programs must be socially just, avoiding stigma and fairly distributing benefits and burdens.

Scientific Measures of Accuracy: Positive Predictive Value

Careful policy assessments begin with understanding a screening test's vital characteristics: its validity, determined by measures of sensitivity and specificity, its reliability (i.e., repeatability), and its yield, or the amount of disease detected in the population.[145] Validity is a screening test's ability to determine which individuals within a population actually have a disease and which do not. Validity has two components: sensitivity and specificity. Sensitivity is a test's ability to identify accurately those who have a particular disease; specificity is a test's ability to identify accurately those who do not have that disease. Sensitivity and specificity are often inversely related; high sensitivity is generally achieved at the expense of low specificity, and vice versa. From a policy perspective, sensitivity and specificity pose difficult trade-offs. If a test has low sensitivity, a significant number of persons actually infected will escape detection (false negatives).[146] Conversely, a test with low specificity will misclassify and mislabel many healthy people as having the infection (false positives).

Reliability is the consistency of a screening test's results when the test is performed more than once on the same individual under similar conditions. Two major factors affect consistency: methodological variation (e.g., inadequate quality control) and observational variation (e.g., insufficient operator training). Obviously, unreliable tests are of little value, since clinicians and patients cannot depend on the results.

A screening program's yield is the amount of previously unrecognized disease identified by the test. The most cost-effective screening programs achieve a high yield.[147] However, programs that detect a nominal number of persons with disease can sometimes be justified if early detection and intervention can avert transmission (e.g., TB in congregate settings) or serious consequences (e.g., hyperthyroidism).

In summary, screening programs have value only if they are scientifically sound, showing high sensitivity and specificity, reliability, and yield. Thus, screening programs, in order to be effective, must use technically superior tests, trained test operators, and quality laboratories, and they must detect a significant number of cases that would not otherwise be identified. But even if a test is accurate in all these ways, it may still have low positive predictive value (PPV). PPV measures the proportion of people with positive test results who actually have the disease.[148] PPV is determined mostly by a test's specificity and the disease's prevalence.[149] Even highly valid tests have poor PPV in a low-prevalence population. (See table 18 for a worksheet explaining how to calculate PPV.)

The State of Illinois powerfully illustrated the problems with screening in a low-prevalence population by mandating premarital HIV screening in the late 1980s.[150] The legislature assumed that screening marriage applicants, who would then be counseled on the risks of unprotected sex, could prevent HIV. However, during the first six months of the program, screening identified only eight HIV-positive persons, at a cost of $2.5 million ($312,000 per infected individual). The annual cost was nearly 1.5 times the state appropriation for all other AIDS surveillance and prevention programs combined. At the same time, the marriage rate dropped in Illinois and rose in adjacent states.[151] This analysis suggests that policymakers need to think carefully about the likely costs and benefits of screening in low-prevalence populations.

TABLE 18. Positive predictive value and prevalence

The PPV of a particular test is the number of persons who test true positive divided by the total number of persons who test true positive and false positive. Even highly valid tests have a poor PPV in a low-prevalence population. Consider the following two-by-two table, which shows the possible results of testing on a person infected or not infected with a disease.

Test Results:	Infected	Not Infected
Positive	True positives	False positives
Negative	False negatives	True negatives

Positive predictive value (PPV) = true positives/(true positives + false positives)

Consider the screening for HIV of 10,000 previously undiagnosed people from the general population in the United States—where about one person out of 1,000 has undiagnosed HIV[a]—and a sub-Saharan African country with an undiagnosed HIV prevalence of 20 percent. The tests used for preliminary HIV screening have sensitivities and specificities in the range of 99.9 percent.[b] This means that one out of each 1,000 infected people will test false negative (and the rest true positive), and one person out of each 1,000 noninfected people will test false positive (and the rest true negative).

In our group of 10,000 screened Americans, one would expect 10 true cases of HIV and 9,990 people without the disease. With a sensitivity of 99.9 percent, one would expect that all 10 cases would be caught, so there would be no false negatives. With a specificity of 99.9 percent, one would expect 9,980 true negatives and 10 false positives. Dividing the true positives by the total number of people who test positive on the test yields a PPV of 50 percent. This means that a person who tests positive is equally likely to have HIV as not.

Test Results:	Infected	Not Infected	*Total*
Positive	10	10	20
Negative	0	9,980	9,980
Total	10	9,990	10,000

PPV = 10 / 20 or 50 percent

Now consider the use of the same test in our sub-Saharan African population of 10,000 with a 20 percent HIV prevalence. One would expect 2,000 HIV infections in this group of people. The test would be expected to register 1,998 true positives and two false negatives. It would also be expected to register 7,992 true negatives and eight false positives. This yields a PPV of 99.6 percent, meaning that the vast majority of people who test positive really are. Thus, the value of a screening test is strongly dependent on the actual level of disease in populations being screened.

TABLE 18. *(continued)*

Test Results:	Infected	Not Infected	*Total*
Positive	1,998	8	2,006
Negative	2	7,992	7,994
Total	2,000	8,000	10,000

PPV = 1,998 / 2,006 or 99.6 percent

[a] Centers for Disease Control and Prevention, "Rapid HIV Test Distribution—United States, 2003–2005," *Morbidity and Mortality Weekly Report,* 55 (2006): 673–76.

[b] Roger Chou, Laurie Hoyt Huffman, Rongwei Fu, et al., "Screening for HIV: A Review of the Evidence for the U.S. Preventive Services Task Force," *Annals of Internal Medicine,* 143 (2005): 55–73. Note that, in the United States, a preliminary positive test is confirmed using a Western blot test, which looks for HIV proteins and is extremely accurate. When the confirmatory test is done, the chance of a false positive drops to around one in 250,000.

Public Health Purposes

Policymakers sometimes assume that acquisition of knowledge about a population's health status must promote the public's welfare. For example, legislators proposed screening as an immediate response to publicized cases of HIV transmission from health care workers to patients and rapists to victims.[152] These legislative initiatives, on their face, may appear to be appropriate responses to a health emergency, but screening should not be regarded as an inherent good. Policymakers should have an important public health purpose and demonstrate that the screening program actually will achieve the stated purpose. What is the marginal usefulness of the test? Given what is known about the person, does the test yield new information, and are effective responses available?

One of the most important measures of a successful screening program is whether it is acceptable to the population.[153] Public acceptance is important because behavior change is most likely if persons at risk participate in public health programs. Public acceptance is also important for political reasons, since democratic support is crucial to the legitimacy of public health activities. Public acceptance is, of course, far from simple; in urgent situations the public may clamor for strong measures, while persons at risk resist compulsion. Community acceptance of screening depends in part on the target population and the voluntariness of the screening.

The "Targeting" Problem

From a scientific and public health perspective, screening in higher prevalence populations is preferable (table 18). High-prevalence screening finds more cases, at less cost per case, and generates fewer false positive results. High-prevalence screening, then, is more cost-effective and less burdensome. Given its clear advantages, one would expect that public health authorities would almost always target populations at high risk of infection. However, this is not always the case, and there may be good reason. If the risk group is vulnerable, narrowly targeted screening may expose the population to social risk. Think about a disease that disproportionately affects minorities (e.g., TB among homeless persons, or HIV among gays, African Americans, or Latinos).[154] Or, in the analogous field of genetics, think about the stigma associated with screening African Americans for sickle cell anemia or Ashkenazi Jews for Tay-Sachs disease or breast cancer.[155]

Public health officials face a dilemma. If they target the narrow high-risk population, they reinforce existing bigotry, thereby creating harms to individuals and to the group itself.[156] Alternatively, public health officials may choose to screen a much broader population that includes but is not limited to risk groups. This broad population-based approach, however, unnecessarily screens many individuals who are unlikely to be infected. There is no simple answer to this dilemma because it involves a values choice: Which is more important, the most efficient screening program or the program that is least burdensome to vulnerable communities? In the end, policymakers need to make a hard choice and will have to weigh efficiency against social justice.[157]

Problems of Compulsion and Consent: A Taxonomy

Policymakers not only have to make difficult choices about how to target screening; they also have to decide politically volatile issues of compulsion and informed consent.[158] Politicians sometimes are drawn to compulsory screening as a way to protect the public. However, groups that bear the burden of compulsion vigorously insist on maintaining personal autonomy—a claim that civil liberties organizations strongly support. This section explores the problem of compulsion by offering a taxonomy of screening, while the next section examines screening from a constitutional perspective.

The terms *voluntary* and *compulsory* appear simple enough: The former connotes unfettered freedom to choose and the latter the absence of freedom. Between these two extremes, however, is a gradation of different kinds of screening that warrants exploration. It is possible to identify at least five forms of screening: compulsory, conditional, routine with advance agreement (opt-in), routine without advance agreement (opt-out), and voluntary.[159] Some of the most controversial public health debates turn on the structure of the screening program, because this determines whether vulnerable individuals can provide fully informed consent, as the HIV screening case study later in this chapter reveals.

Compulsory Screening. Pursuant to their police powers, states may compel citizens to submit to medical screening without informed consent. (The screening program, however, must have a legitimate public health purpose and be administered fairly.)[160] Various states require screening for specific diseases, such as TB in schools and workplaces,[161] syphilis among newborns,[162] and HIV and TB among prison inmates.[163] This body of law contains a morass of confusing, sometimes contradictory, provisions. First, statutes define a class of persons to which the compulsory power applies. The class may be generic, such as persons who are "reasonably suspected" of having an infection.[164] Alternatively, the class may single out certain groups, such as sex offenders,[165] migrant laborers,[166] prostitutes,[167] pregnant women,[168] newborns,[169] or inmates.[170] Second, statutes define a set of circumstances that triggers a screening requirement, such as when a person is "exposed" to bloodborne infection.[171] Finally, statutes specify procedures that public health officials must follow, ranging from unfettered discretion to procurement of a judicial order prior to screening.[172]

Conditional Screening. The government can make access to certain privileges or services contingent upon undergoing medical screening. Some states, for example, mandate STI screening to obtain a marriage license or PPD tuberculin skin screening to work in a school or nursing home.[173] The federal government requires TB, HIV, and other health testing for immigrants to the United States.[174] (Screening of travelers and immigrants for TB, HIV, and STIs is prevalent around the globe.[175] The International Health Regulations permit countries to screen applicants for long-term residence, but limit screening of short-term visitors to those who pose an immediate risk of spreading disease.[176]) Conditional screening is not mandatory in the strict sense of the term because persons can avoid the test by forgoing the privilege or service sought. However, if the privilege or service has great importance to the individual, the screening requirement may be perceived as highly coercive.[177]

Routine Screening with Advance Agreement (Opt-In). There are few concepts used with less care and precision than "routine screening." Routine screening is sometimes used to refer simply to "universal screening":

Each member of a defined population is routinely tested to ensure widespread identification of infected persons. However, this definition fails to explain the essential characteristics of the screening: whether individuals are informed they are being tested, how they are informed (e.g., individually or by public notice), when they are informed (before testing or after the fact), and whether they can withhold consent.

There are at least two forms of "routine" screening: with advance agreement (opt-in) and without advance agreement (opt-out). In opt-in screening, all individuals in the defined population are routinely "offered" testing (e.g., they are notified that a certain test is a standard part of the treatment they are about to receive). As part of the informational process, individuals are told that they have the right to give or withhold consent; they are not actually tested until they have consented. A clearer term for this kind of program would be "routine offering" with informed consent.

Routine Screening without Advance Agreement (Opt-Out). In opt-out screening, all individuals in the defined population are routinely and automatically screened unless they expressly ask that the test not be performed. A critical question is how they are informed that testing will take place: Does the physician or nurse orally explain the procedure face-to-face? Is it signposted in the hospital ward? Or is it explained in pamphlets distributed to patients? This kind of "routine screening" does not necessarily ensure informed consent. Individuals may not be aware they are being screened, and even if they are aware, they may not fully understand the purposes of the test or their right to withhold consent. Yet opt-out screening does not expressly coerce because it theoretically respects a person's express desire not to be tested.

There are important policy implications of choosing between these two forms of routine screening. Opt-in screening is more respectful of personal autonomy and the importance of informed consent. Opt-out screening, however, reaches a larger population and is less expensive. In opt-out screening, health professionals do not have to provide pretest counseling, rendering the program less time consuming and costly. Consequently, policymakers face hard trade-offs between screening programs that capture a larger population and programs that are more respectful of individual rights.

Voluntary Screening. Voluntary screening is the norm in medicine and public health, and any deviation from the norm requires careful justification. Voluntary screening requires advance provision of information about the nature of the test, full understanding by a competent person, and the freedom to choose to be tested or to decline. Nondirective counseling is thought to be "best-practice" where individuals are informed of the options and the choice is left to them.

Compulsory Screening from a Constitutional Perspective: Unreasonable Search and Seizure

Since the guarantees of the U.S. Constitution constrain principally actions by the state, the legal battleground over screening has centered on government, as well as private entities acting in accordance with federal or state rules that require or authorize testing.[178] The primary constitutional impediment to testing is the Fourth Amendment's right of people to be "secure in their persons" and not subjected to "unreasonable searches and seizures." Though the Fourth Amendment is popularly perceived as applying solely to personal or residential searches (see chapter 12), the Supreme Court has long recognized that searches also include the collection and subsequent analysis of biological samples.[179] Privacy and security are threatened by the invasion of bodily integrity involved in collecting the sample and performing the chemical analysis, which extracts personal information.

The constitutional issue is whether the analysis of blood, urine, or other tissue is "reasonable." Reasonableness is the point at which the government's interest in a particular search or seizure outweighs the loss of individual privacy or freedom that attends the government's action.[180] In most criminal cases, a search is unreasonable unless it is accomplished pursuant to a judicial warrant issued upon probable cause; if the warrant requirement is impracticable, the courts require, minimally, "reasonable suspicion" based upon an individualized assessment.[181]

The Supreme Court, in drug screening cases, held that when the state has "special needs beyond the normal need for law enforcement," the warrant and probable or reasonable cause requirements may not be applicable.[182] Many screening programs are not conducted for law enforcement purposes, thus falling under the special needs doctrine.[183] For example, courts have upheld compulsory STI screening for persons accused or convicted of sexual assaults,[184] arguing that they are justified by the "special need" to inform rape victims of potential exposure.[185]

If screening is for public health rather than criminal justice purposes, the courts balance governmental and privacy interests to determine the reasonableness of the search. On one side of the balance is the government's interest in public health and, on the other, the individual's expectation of privacy.[186] The courts weigh the state's interests in public health and safety quite heavily, but sometimes perceive individual interests as nominal: "Society's judgment [is] that blood tests do not constitute an unduly extensive imposition on an individual's privacy and bodily integrity."[187] As a result, most courts have assumed a permissive posture when reviewing government screening programs.[188] Even for highly stigmatized diseases such as HIV, the courts have upheld screening of firefighters and paramedics,[189] military personnel,[190] overseas employees in the State Department,[191] immigrants,[192] and sex offenders.[193]

In *Ferguson v. City of Charleston* (2001), the Supreme Court considered the special needs doctrine in an intriguing case involving drug testing of pregnant women.[194] In *Ferguson,* the Medical University of South Carolina (MUSC), together with law enforcement, developed a policy to test pregnant patients suspected of drug use without their consent, and to arrest those who tested positive. Although the intent was benevolent (protecting the health of the mother and child), the Court found that the policy did not fit within the "special needs" doctrine; the purpose served by the MUSC searches was "ultimately indistinguishable from the general interest in crime control."[195]

Screening that is scientifically accurate and achieves an important public health purpose is often justified, even if it imposes a burden on vulnerable groups. Nevertheless, apart from *Ferguson,* the Supreme Court's Fourth Amendment jurisprudence tends to accept state public health interests without carefully considering whether the screening will in fact achieve those objectives. Compulsory screening, rather than furthering the state's interests, may dissuade individuals at risk from accessing the health care system. At the same time, by focusing on the physical intrusion of the blood test, the courts do not sufficiently weigh the informational privacy concerns entailed in compelled disclosure of sensitive information.[196]

A CASE STUDY ON HIV SCREENING: PUBLIC HEALTH AND CIVIL LIBERTIES IN CONFLICT?

On September 22, 2006, the CDC issued a sweeping revision of its guidelines for HIV screening in health care settings that reversed decades of thinking on AIDS policy. Previous guidelines recommended HIV testing only for persons at high risk or in health care settings with high HIV prevalence.[197] This reflected a civil liberties approach that constrained testing with costly, time-consuming procedures for pretest counseling and written informed consent. Health care professionals often did not implement HIV screening due to the financial and administrative burdens, or because conducting risk assessments or discovering HIV prevalence in their facilities was impractical.[198] For example, relaxing certain procedural requirements, such as written informed consent, has been shown to be associated with increased testing rates.[199]

The new guidelines represent a radical departure by encouraging HIV screening for all individuals ages thirteen to sixty-four as a part of routine medical care, irrespective of lifestyle, perceived risk, or HIV prevalence.[200] The recommendations incorporate opt-out testing, which notifies all patients that testing will be performed unless an individual specifically declines. Separate written informed consent would no longer be required; instead, general consent for medical care would be sufficient. Similarly, pretest counseling would not be required. (See box 33 for a discussion of HIV screening in a global context.)

The Social and Historical Context: HIV Testing from the 1980s to the Present

HIV screening policy originated in the 1980s, when the scientific and social context was markedly different than it is today. At that time, individuals were unlikely to benefit from HIV testing: Treatments were rudimentary, offering prophylaxis against some opportunistic infections but holding out little hope of a longer, healthier life. More striking were the social risks.[201] Family and friends ostracized persons living with HIV/AIDS; employers, landlords, and insurers discriminated against them; and partners or even members of the community threatened them with violence. Policymakers criminalized HIV transmission and spoke about tattooing or quarantining persons with HIV infection, leading to fears of reprisal. Exclusion from school and other ordinary aspects of life symbolized the struggle for equality, as AIDS joined race, sex, and disability as part of the civil rights movement of the 1980s and 1990s. It was fully understandable, given the negligible therapeutic benefits and the pronounced stigma, that the law would safeguard personal autonomy and privacy, and proscribe discrimination.

Scholars have wrestled with the question of whether the civil rights paradigm still is justified, given the transformative scientific and social developments over the last decade. Rapid testing now enables HIV test results to be provided in twenty minutes, as compared with one to two

BOX 33

HIV SCREENING: A GLOBAL PERSPECTIVE

AIDS is no longer just a disease. It is a human rights issue.
Nelson Mandela (2003)

HIV screening from a global perspective is, if anything, more complex and controversial, than in the United States. While the CDC recommends universal HIV screening of the population, UNAIDS and WHO advise routine screening only in high-risk/high-yield health care settings: patients assessed for STIs, pregnant women, and patients in community-based health services where HIV is prevalent and antiretroviral treatment is available. The UNAIDS/WHO guidelines give considerably greater attention to ameliorating social risks, advocating the "three Cs" of voluntary counseling and testing (VCT): confidentiality, counseling, and consent. The guidelines adopt a human rights approach: individual informed consent, linkages to treatment and psychosocial support, privacy, and antidiscrimination.[1]

International organizations have come under increasing pressure to expand the scope of HIV screening.[2] Despite a historic UN General Assembly Declaration of Commitment to effective HIV prevention and treatment in 2001, the pandemic is intensifying.[3] As of 2006, nearly 40 million people worldwide were living with HIV, with 4 million newly infected and 3 million losing their lives each year. Sub-Saharan Africa is the global epicenter of the pandemic.[4] Countries such as Lesotho and Swaziland, with nearly one in three adults infected, are characterized as countries "dying of AIDS." And life expectancy in countries such as Botswana has dropped from seventy-four years to twenty-seven.[5]

Despite the extreme burden of HIV/AIDS, prevention efforts are failing.[6] Fewer than one in five people at risk of HIV infection have any access to HIV prevention information, and most HIV-infected individuals in the world do not know their status.[7] Consequently, the vast majority of the twelve thousand people around the world who become infected every day will not become aware of their status until they develop symptoms. During that period, they will unknowingly spread HIV to their sexual and needle-sharing partners, and will not receive treatment. Botswana, Malawi, and Lesotho have dramatically increased testing and awareness with routine HIV screening. Lesotho's "know your status" campaign has brought testing out of medical settings into communities, with a village-to-village prevention strategy.

Epigraph source: Nelson Mandela, "Remarks at the First 46664 Concert at Greenpoint Stadium," Cape Town, South Africa, November 29, 2003.

[1] UNAIDS/WHO, *Policy Statement on HIV Testing* (Geneva: UNAIDS, 2004).

[2] Richard Holbrooke, "AIDS: The Strategy Is Wrong," *Washington Post,* Nov. 29, 2005 (arguing that the world health community has been shamefully quiet on the need for testing and detection); Richard Holbrooke, "Sorry, but AIDS Testing Is Critical," *Washington Post,* Jan. 4, 2006 (arguing that the human rights mindset for testing was locked in twenty years ago); *Clinton Supports Wider AIDS Testing* (CNN television broadcast, March 28, 2006) (regarding former president supporting rapid testing even in remote areas of the globe).

[3] UN General Assembly, *Declaration of Commitment on HIV/AIDS,* RES/S-26/2, June 27, 2001. See also UN General Assembly, *Scaling Up HIV Prevention, Treatment, Care and Support,* A/60/737, March 24, 2006.

[4] UNAIDS, *2006 Report on the Global AIDS Epidemic,* UNAIDS/06.20E (May 2006).

[5] Lawrence O. Gostin, *The AIDS Pandemic: Complacency, Injustice, and Unfulfilled Expectations* (Chapel Hill: University of North Carolina Press, 2004).

[6] Jim Yong Kim and Paul Farmer, "AIDS in 2006: Moving toward One World, One Hope?" *New Engl. J. Med.,* 355 (2006): 645-49 (describing five lessons of the AIDS pandemic: charging for services poses an insurmountable barrier, health care system improvement is needed, more trained health care personnel are needed, extreme poverty makes it difficult to comply with therapy, and international aid must be increased).

[7] UNAIDS, *2006 Report on the Global AIDS Epidemic.*

The fault lines between the public health and human rights approaches to HIV screening are increasingly clear.[8] In many poor countries, HIV testing still evokes feelings of fear and shame. In this social environment, concerns about coercion abound. Individuals may submit to testing due to authoritarian or hierarchical structures in their communities.[9] Problems of illiteracy, custom, social exclusion, or retribution may make it hard to refuse the offer of testing. Women and girls, for example, may suffer physically, socially, or economically when they feel compelled to accept testing. At the same time, medical treatment is extremely limited in many poor countries, so that the value of screening is undermined. HIV screening is, therefore, one of the great conundrums of AIDS policy: Should international health organizations promote routine HIV screening linked, where possible, to prevention and treatment? Or, should they persevere with a policy of pre- and post-test counseling, informed consent, and programs targeted to high-risk populations? Perhaps there is a way to adopt both the public health and human rights perspectives, but currently there is a large divide between the two communities.

[8] Joanne Csete, "Scaling Up HIV Testing: Human Rights and Hidden Costs," *HIV/AIDS Policy and Law Review*, 11 (2006): 1-10 (arguing that routine HIV testing violates human dignity, exposes people to abuse, and does not reduce stigma).

[9] *C v. Minister of Correctional Services* 1996(4) SA 292 (holding that a prisoner given an HIV test after being informed of the right to refuse, but not given pretest counseling, had not given informed consent).

weeks previously. Highly active antiretroviral therapy (HAART) can extend the healthy life of people living with HIV/AIDS from less than one year to decades. And treatment and counseling significantly reduce the spread of HIV in the population. HAART reduces infectiousness, and knowledge of HIV infection reduces risk behavior.[202] Health economists conclude that HIV screening is cost-effective.[203]

Public health organizations recommend screening to foster earlier detection, identify and counsel persons with unrecognized infection, and link them to clinical and prevention services.[204] Researchers estimate that a quarter of the more than 1 million Americans living with HIV are unaware of their status.[205] Moreover, nearly 40 percent of individuals who test positive receive an AIDS diagnosis within one year after the test. The large number of cases that are undiagnosed, or diagnosed late in the course of HIV disease, represent lost opportunities for prevention and treatment.[206] Universal, as opposed to risk-based, screening also has the advantage of being less stigmatizing, because it does not single out vulnerable populations and applies equally to all socioeconomic classes and racial groups.

Pregnant Women and Infants: A Successful Illustration of Routine Screening

In the absence of effective treatment, 15 to 30 percent of HIV-infected mothers transmit the infection to their newborns in utero, during birth, or through breast-feeding.[207] Yet in 1994, the AIDS Clinical Trials Group (ACTG) 076 made the dramatic discovery that a regimen of antiretroviral medication given to mother and infant could reduce perinatal transmission by two-thirds.[208] As a result of routine screening and treatment, the estimated number of infants born with HIV declined from a peak of approximately 1,650 in 1991 to current rates of fewer than 240 a year. Perinatal transmission rates could be reduced further, to less than 2 percent, through universal screening of pregnant women in combination with HAART, cesarean delivery, and avoidance of breast-feeding.[209]

The CDC responded to ACTG 076 by issuing guidelines for treatment of pregnant women that year[210] and for counseling and screening in 1995.[211] However, the political response to the deaths of babies from HIV disease was as predictable as it was unscientific. In 1996, Congress enacted a law implicitly supporting mandatory newborn screening,[212] and New York adopted such a proposal.[213] The sponsor of the New York statute, Assemblywoman Nettie Mayersohn, reasoned that it was "criminal" to allow the suffering of "innocent and helpless victims." However, knowing the HIV status of infants would not reduce perinatal transmission, and at the time, the benefit of early treatment of newborns was yet to be proven. It became apparent that only screening pregnant women and treating those who were HIV-infected could reduce perinatal transmission. In 1999, the Institute of Medicine made a bold proposal for routine universal screening of pregnant women,[214] which led to revision of the CDC prenatal testing guidelines in 2001.[215] Whereas the IOM panel recommended opt-out voluntary testing, the CDC required written informed consent.

The CDC's 2006 guidelines fully embrace the IOM proposal. Screening should now become part of a routine panel of prenatal tests unless the woman declines. No additional process or written consent is required for testing. Abandoning the normal approach of nondirective counseling, the CDC recommends that health care professionals address a woman's reasons for declining the test and inform her about the importance of testing.

Barriers to Implementation: Legislation and Liability

HIV-specific legislation has been enacted in every state.[216] State law, although highly disparate, could be a barrier to implementation of CDC guidelines.[217] First, state law stipulates who can perform testing, counseling, and partner notification services. Rigorous training and certification requirements could limit the capacity of hospitals and physicians or dental offices to offer these services. Second, state laws explicitly require pretest counseling with prescribed content areas, including the uses and limits of the test, confidentiality assurances, transmission routes, symptoms of HIV disease, treatment options, and test result recipients. Third, connected to pretest counseling, state law requires informed consent, often in writing and also conforming to the content areas just discussed. Finally, states regulate post-test activities, such as by requiring confirmatory tests in licensed laboratories and face-to-face counseling. A few states even require counseling whether the test is positive or negative.

Existing state law is inconsistent with CDC guidelines, raising a problem of federalism. Given the states' primacy in infectious disease control, state legislation would likely prevail over federal guidelines, but states may fear loss of CDC funding if they do not comply with national guidelines. If states do not reform their laws, they may pose insuperable obstacles to routine screening. State law reform, therefore, is important if the CDC is to fully achieve its objectives. Federal/state partnerships in crafting model legislation to harmonize AIDS policy would benefit all stakeholders, particularly if government initiated a process of civic engagement with affected communities.

Enduring Conflicts

AIDS policy has been mired in controversy since the earliest moments of the epidemic.[218] Should the health system treat HIV differently than other diseases, given the history of animus and discrimination? Alternatively, should HIV be incorporated into a standard public health model? "AIDS exceptionalism" can be seen in policies ranging from HIV testing and named reporting to partner notification—all of which have been viewed with suspicion for undermining privacy and autonomy.[219] AIDS advocates stress the value of individual rights, while health professionals stress the communal interest in prevention and treatment. The CDC, which for decades adopted a "rights" approach, is moving demonstrably toward public health. This can be seen in its support of named HIV reporting, universal screening of pregnant women and infants, and now routine screening of the population. (See the case study in chapter 8 on named reporting.)

Certainly, AIDS advocates have muted their objections to routine testing as the benefits to their community have become more apparent. Nevertheless, the differences between the civil liberties and public health models endure.[220] Although the CDC emphasizes the importance of respecting patient wishes, the guidelines leave open the possibility that individuals will be tested without prior informed consent. Whether due to vulnerability, lack of initiative, lax hospital procedures, or cultural differences, some patients unknowingly will receive HIV tests. Though the CDC properly recognizes the value of early diagnosis as a bridge to treatment, the guidelines do not provide a mechanism for referral to treatment. Patients may be diagnosed with HIV, but there is no guarantee that they will get into care.

The AIDS policy debates have in many ways framed the discourse in modern society. The American polity has searched, often in vain, to reconcile the difficult trade-offs between personal freedom and the common good. Perhaps we are witnessing a counterbalance to the civil rights approach of the late twentieth century. When we think about vulnerable communities, it may not be enough to focus absolutely on their rights; we must also consider their health and collective well-being. That may be the message of the evolution toward a new public health model for combating HIV/AIDS.

HIV screening demonstrates that case finding is far from a neutral scientific pursuit. Rather, screening is political: Elected officials perceive some groups as blameworthy and some as innocent. Screening is also rich in symbolism: The public health response helps to construct diseases socially on dimensions of race, gender, nationality, and socioeconomic status. Finally, screening is fraught with complex choices and weighing of values: cost, efficiency, autonomy, and justice. Perhaps the lesson is that tidy evaluative criteria are only part of a textured understanding of screening. Politics, symbolism, and values appear to be just as important as science in understanding the complexities of case finding.

COMPULSORY PHYSICAL EXAMINATION AND MEDICAL TREATMENT

> No right is held more sacred, or is more carefully guarded, by the common law, than the right of every individual to the possession and control of his own person, free from all restraint or interference of others, unless by clear and unquestionable authority of law.
>
> Horace Gray (1891)

Clinical testing and public health screening identify individuals who are infected with a contagious pathogen. Public health laws similarly authorize physical examination to determine the presence of disease; these powers often are contained in STI or TB statutes. Legal powers also exist for the medical treatment of persons diagnosed with an infectious disease. Treatment affords both individual and collective goods: It benefits individuals by ameliorating symptoms and sometimes providing a cure, and it benefits society by reducing or eliminating infectiousness. But these dual advantages of treatment are placed at risk if individuals do not take the full course of their medication. Inconsistent treatment can result in drug resistance, so that modern therapies become less effective. Because of the benefits to individuals and the community, and the problem of drug resistance, public health officials have an abiding interest in compulsory treatment. However, mandatory treatment represents a serious intrusion into a person's bodily integrity, which requires careful justification.[221] This section discusses the primary justifications for mandatory treatment, together with the common law, statutory, and constitutional rights of individuals to refuse.

The Common Law Right to Refuse Treatment: Informed Consent

As the epigraph by Justice Horace Gray suggests, patients have a deeply rooted common law right to refuse treatment that is embodied in the concept of informed consent.[222] Bioethicists ground the right to refuse treatment on personal autonomy and self-determination. Absent a statutory power to impose treatment, physicians are bound to respect the wishes of competent patients. The doctrine of informed consent traditionally includes the following components:[223] *information*—doctors must disclose the material benefits, risks, and alternatives;[224] *competency*—individuals must be capable of understanding;[225] *voluntariness*—patients must make a free choice, without undue influence, fraud, or duress;[226] and *specificity*—patients must consent to the actual treatment provided.

Mandatory Treatment under Public Health Statutes

Public health statutes frequently authorize mandatory treatment, which has the effect of overriding common law. Most STI[227] and TB[228] laws, for example, grant the power to compel physical examination and medical treatment.[229] Statutes often impose conditions for mandatory treatment, such as being a danger to the public; others may require a violation of some rule or order, such as noncompliance with a health directive; still others limit treatment to active, or contagious, cases of infection.

New York City, for example, in response to a resurgence of multidrug-resistant TB in the 1990s, revised its health code to permit detention of nonadherent individuals. In *City of New York v. Antoinette R.* (1995), a court upheld an order of hospitalization based on clear and convincing evidence of a patient's inability to comply with a prescribed course of medication.[230]

The Constitutional Right to Refuse Treatment

The right to refuse treatment, most importantly, has been grounded in federal and state constitutions.[231] In a series of cases over the last two decades, the Supreme Court has recognized that a competent person has a constitutionally protected "liberty interest" in refusing unwanted medical treatment. The Court embraced the principle of bodily integrity in cases involving abortion[232] and the rights of persons with terminal illness[233] and mental illness.[234] The Court's jurisprudence provides ample reason to believe the Constitution safeguards treatment decisions, which are among "the most intimate and personal choices a person may make in a lifetime, choices central to personal dignity and autonomy."[235]

The Supreme Court's recognition of a right to bodily integrity does not mean that the right is absolute.[236] The Court uses a balancing test that weighs personal liberty against state interests (see figure 34). The judiciary usually supports public health decisions to compel treatment, provided that the treatment is reasonably necessary to safeguard the population.[237] A series of cases concerning forced administration of antipsychotic medication, although not directly analogous to infectious disease treatment, provides insight into the Court's view of mandatory treatment.

In *Washington v. Harper* (1990), the Supreme Court recognized a "significant" constitutionally protected liberty interest in avoiding unwanted medication but found an overriding state interest in treating a prisoner who was seriously mentally ill.[238] The *Harper* Court defined the constitutional standard for compelled treatment to include: danger to self or others, treatment in the person's medical interest, and administration of medication by a licensed physician acting in accordance with the standards in the profession. According to the Court, this amounts to a constitutionally permissible "accommodation" between the individual's liberty interest and the state's authority to reduce risks to self or others.

In *Riggins v. Nevada* (1992), the Court reiterated that an individual

STATE INTERESTS	INDIVIDUAL INTERESTS
Preserving Health State interest is weak with competent adults but is strong when safeguarding the welfare of children and incompetent adults.	**Personal Autonomy** Interest in making personal decisions and determining own actions without interference.
Harm Prevention State interest strengthens as probability of transmission and severity of harm increase.	**Bodily Integrity** Interest becomes stronger as invasiveness and duration of treatment increase.
Preservation of Effective Therapies State interest in avoiding drug-resistant strains of disease increases as evidence of nonadherence in individuals and groups increases.	**Liberty** Interest in personal freedom if treatment is under conditions of civil confinement or supervision.

Constitutional Standard: For mandatory treatment of competent adults, the state must demonstrate dangerousness (significant risk of transmission) and medical appropriateness of treatment.

Figure 34. Mandatory treatment: Balancing individual and state interests.

has a constitutionally protected liberty interest—an interest that only an "essential" or "overriding" state interest might overcome. The Court, citing *Harper,* noted that the state had to show that the treatment was "medically appropriate and, considering less intrusive alternatives, essential for the sake of Riggins' own safety or the safety of others."[239]

Finally, in *Sell v. United States* (2003), the Court held, under the framework of *Harper* and *Riggins,* that the Constitution permits the government to administer antipsychotic drugs involuntarily to render a mentally ill defendant competent to stand trial if the treatment is medically appropriate, substantially unlikely to have side effects that may undermine the trial's fairness, and taking account of less intrusive alternatives, is necessary to further significantly important governmental interests.[240] Civil libertarians hailed *Sell* for the strict conditions under which treatment may be imposed.[241] However, Justice Breyer, writing for the Court, cautioned that if compulsory treatment is imposed for a "different purpose," such as dangerousness, then the ostensibly narrow *Sell* test need not be applied—and of course, in most cases the driving force behind the desire to compel medication is danger to self or others.

In the Supreme Court trilogy of *Harper, Riggins,* and *Sell,* the conflict between free will and state power comes up against age-old problems—the nature of personal autonomy, the sanctity of bodily integrity, and the police power to protect individuals and society. The lines dividing therapeutic benefit, self-determination, and societal protection are fine, and there is no field that illustrates the conundrums better than mandatory treatment.

Justifications for Mandatory Treatment

The state has three interrelated interests in compulsory treatment: health preservation (harm to the individual), prevention (harm to others), and preservation of effective therapies (continued usefulness of key medications).[242]

Preservation of Health or Life. The state has an interest in preserving a person's health or life, although paternalism usually provides insufficient justification for compelled treatment of a competent adult (see chapter 2).[243] Courts have recognized a right to refuse consent in cases of terminal illness,[244] mental illness,[245] and infectious disease.[246] The judiciary also has upheld the right to refuse treatment based on religious conviction.[247] Courts do, however, permit beneficial treatment for children and incompetent persons. Parents, for example, may not withhold medical treatment from their children if it poses a serious health threat.[248] Similarly, courts often empower surrogate decision makers to authorize treatment in the best interests of incompetent adults.[249]

Harm Prevention. The most telling justification for imposing infectious disease treatment is to prevent harm to others. Since persons with infectious disease can transmit the infection through casual contact (e.g., measles) or behavior (e.g., herpes simplex or hepatitis B), the state has a substantial interest in treatment that reduces contagiousness. The Supreme Court has held that health authorities may impose serious forms of treatment, such as antipsychotic medication, if the person poses a danger to himself or others, given the treatment is medically appropriate and beneficial to the person.[250] Lower courts, using a similar harm prevention theory, have upheld compulsory physical examination[251] and treatment[252] of persons with infectious disease. Conversely, courts have found compulsory treatment unconstitutional where the person was not dangerous[253] or the treatment was not medically appropriate.[254] Consequently, public health officials (if authorized by statute) can require individuals to submit to medical treatment if they pose a significant risk of transmission and the treatment is beneficial.

Preservation of Effective Therapies. The state has an interest, connected to harm prevention, in preserving the effectiveness of antiviral or antibacterial medications. Drug resistance has been a major concern ever since the discovery of penicillin. Today, resistance to antibiotics[255] (e.g., staphylococcus infections[256] or TB[257]) and antiviral medications (e.g., HIV or influenza)[258] is a serious problem in the health system. As the incidence of multidrug resistance increases, society faces the specter of revisiting a pretherapeutic era when infectious disease was a scourge.

Patients develop drug-resistant disease in two ways. First, transmitted, or primary, drug resistance occurs when a person becomes infected with organisms that are already resistant to one or more drugs. Second, acquired, or secondary, drug resistance occurs when pathogens genetically change and multiply as a result of ineffective therapy. If persons with disease take their medication in an incomplete or sporadic fashion, or if they receive a suboptimal dosage, then organisms can acquire drug resistance.[259]

Drug resistance has many causes, including prescribing patterns of physicians (e.g., overuse of antibiotics) and patient dislocation (e.g., homelessness and inadequate access to health care).[260] The government's interest in reducing drug-resistant disease therefore can be accomplished, in part, by modifying physician prescribing patterns through incentives or regulations and by providing compliance-enhancing services for vulnerable patients (e.g., support and economic incentives). These services are often seen as costly and sometimes as ineffective, however, so public health officials may resort to compulsion to ensure that "nonadherent" patients take the full course of their medication. One method of accomplishing that goal, widely used in TB and now discussed for HIV, is directly observed therapy (see box 34).

Directly Observed Therapy for Tuberculosis

The state's interest in ensuring the completion of treatment may not always require compulsory hospitalization. Treatment in the community can often be assured through directly observed therapy, commonly used in the management of TB.[261] Directly observed therapy (DOT) is a compliance-enhancing strategy in which each dose of medication is observed by a family member, peer advocate, community worker, or health care

BOX 34

MANDATORY HIV TREATMENT

Balancing individual and collective interests

In constitutional litigation, the courts weigh collective interests in societal health and safety against individual interests in bodily integrity. However, it is not always easy to balance these interests, particularly when the person is a competent adult. On one side is the state's interest in preventing harm: What is the probability of the risk and the severity of the harm? On the other side is the individual's interest in bodily integrity: How intrusive is the treatment, both in terms of its invasive quality and its duration? This analysis may help explain why a single injection of an antibiotic to eliminate a syphilis infection is constitutional, as is a short course of antituberculosis medication. But would compulsory HIV treatment or directly observed therapy pass constitutional muster?

Compulsory HIV treatment that is highly effective and time-limited might be constitutionally acceptable, even if it does not necessarily represent good public policy. For example, mandatory treatment of an HIV-infected pregnant woman who was refusing medication might pass constitutional muster. The courts could give great weight to protecting the baby, particularly if a single dose of antiretroviral medication could substantially reduce the risk.

Compulsory HIV treatment that is highly burdensome, however, probably would not be constitutional. Treatment of gay men to reduce sexual transmission, for example, would be deeply intrusive. Antiretroviral treatment would have to be administered indefinitely, throughout the lifespan, in order to maintain a reduction in infectiousness. Courts would be unlikely to endorse such a sweeping interference with bodily integrity. Therefore, when commentators talk about the prospect of mandatory HIV treatment or DOT, it is important to consider the impracticality and extensive personal burdens entailed in such proposals.[1]

[1] Gregory M. Lucas, "Directly Observed Therapy for the Treatment of HIV: Promises and Pitfalls," *Hopkins HIV Report*, 13 (2001): 12–15 (arguing that the frequent dosing requirements of HAART makes DOT impractical, but the introduction of drugs with prolonged serum half-lives has rekindled interest); Jennifer Adelson Mitty, Grace Macalino, Lynn Taylor, et al., "Directly Observed Therapy (DOT) for Individuals with HIV: Successes and Challenges," *Medscape General Medicine*, 5 (2003); Office of ADS Research Advisory Council (OARAC), *Guidelines for the Use of Antiretroviral Agents in HIV-1-Infected Adults and Adolescents* (Bethesda, MD: National Institutes of Health, 2006).

professional.[262] Supervised therapy can take place in a variety of locations, ranging from a personal residence or place of employment to a clinic, physician's office, or even a street corner. Supervised therapy can be either voluntary, which requires informed consent, or mandatory. Contemporary understandings of DOT go beyond supervised swallowing of drugs to include multiple enablers and enhancers: patient incentives (e.g., free food, transport, and medicines), social support (e.g., assistance with housing, health insurance, and psychosocial problems), intensive staff supervision, and tracing of defaulters.[263]

Legal and policy analysis of compulsory DOT requires careful balancing of public health and individual interests. Directly observed therapy is frequently thought to be relatively unintrusive because it does not involve confinement. However, its imposition does affect an individual's liberty, dignity, and privacy. Individuals may have to show up for treatment at specific places and times, interfering with freedom of movement. Moreover, treatment may take place in public places known for infectious disease management, resulting in stigma or discrimination, or treatment may occur at the individual's home, interfering with privacy.

Public health benefits must be sufficiently strong to override these personal interests. A significant proportion of individuals who self-administer antituberculosis medication do not complete the full course of treatment.[264] DOT appears to be effective in securing higher rates of completion of treatment; although the empirical evidence is mixed,[265] many DOT programs achieve treatment completion rates of over 90 percent.[266] Moreover, DOT substantially reduces the rates of primary and acquired drug resistance and relapse, supporting the state's interests in harm prevention and preservation of effective medications.[267] For this reason, the World Health Organization supports DOT and its wide use around the world.[268]

If individuals with infectious disease have a history of nonadherence to treatment regimens and they pose a significant risk, DOT may be justified. The more difficult question is whether public health officials should apply DOT to a large population, absent individualized risk assessments (universal DOT). International[269] and U.S.[270] public health agencies, as well as expert committees,[271] recommend universal supervised therapy for TB. Their reasoning is that it is difficult to predict who will or will not take the full course of their medication, so that a population-based approach is fairer and more effective. If DOT were to be applied only to groups assumed less likely to cooperate (e.g., the mentally ill, drug-dependent, homeless, or uninsured), it would be prejudicial and stigmatizing.[272]

The best public health policies often require a nuanced approach. Universal DOT may well be preferable in locales with low treatment completion rates but may be unnecessarily burdensome where rates are already high.[273] More importantly, DOT may be most effective when used in combination with compliance-enhancing services—surveillance, access to health care (e.g., drug dependency and mental health treatment), support services (e.g., transportation and child care), and monetary incentives.[274]

Expedited Partner Therapies for STIs

Prevention and control strategies for containing STIs are based on case finding, education, counseling, and treatment of individuals and their partners.[275] Health professionals can offer, or even compel, STI treatment to patients; however, it is not easy to reach their sex partners. The CDC is therefore exploring an innovative, albeit controversial, practice known as expedited partner therapy (EPT).[276] EPT involves treating the sex partners of persons with STIs without an intervening medical evaluation. Rather, clinicians provide medications or prescriptions directly to patients for use by their partners. While limited, data indicate that not only can EPT reduce the incidence of chlamydial and other sexually transmitted infections,[277] but it can also reduce reinfection rates.[278]

EPT is fraught, however, with medical and legal risk. Without an individual clinical evaluation, partners may use the medications inappropriately, causing adverse effects and contributing to drug resistance. In addition, health professionals face potential liability in tort or for licensing violations that may be viewed as contrary to standard clinical practice or medical ethics. A systematic review of the legal environment suggests, however, that EPT may be permissible or possible in most jurisdictions but proscribed in others.[279] STIs are a "hidden epidemic" with a worryingly high prevalence among America's youth.[280] Any strategy that reaches people and offers treatment may be worth pursuing, perhaps even if it is not possible to provide individualized counseling and clinical assessment.

Medical interventions (vaccination, testing, and treatment) can be powerful levers in preventing or containing disease epidemics. But for many endemic and emerging diseases where there are no clear scientific answers, the only strategy may be crude forms of containment. The next chapter examines the long-standing public health powers of isolation, quarantine, and community containment strategies. These are perhaps the most divisive powers used in public health, as they deprive individuals of the most basic human right: the freedom of movement.

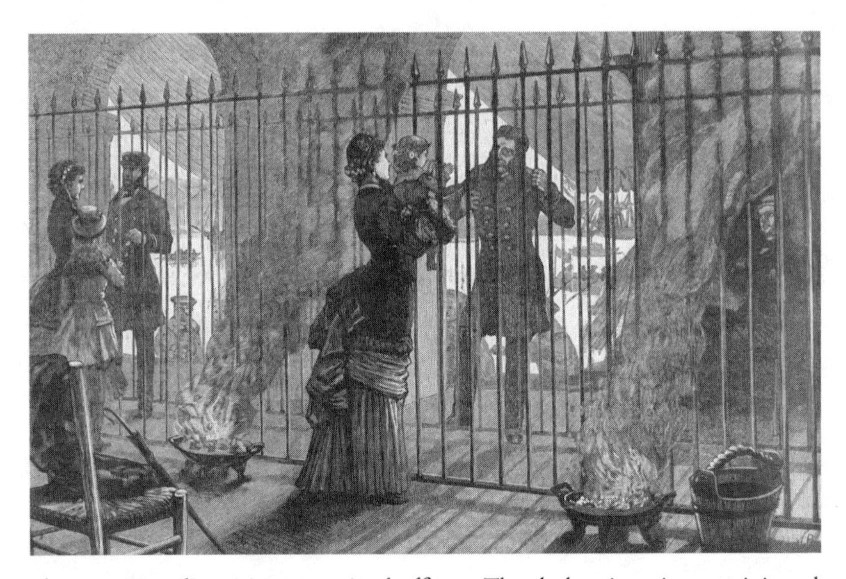

Photo 22. Families visit quarantined officers. The cholera invasion precipitated the necessity for quarantine. Here, the artist depicts wives and children visiting quarantined merchant ship officers after a cholera outbreak in Toulon and Marseille. The vapors from burning "sulfate of nitrostyle" were believed to disinfect and kill cholera germs.

CHAPTER 11

Public Health Strategies for Epidemic Disease

Association, Travel, and Liberty

Everybody knows that pestilences have a way of recurring in the world, yet somehow we find it hard to believe in ones that crash down on our heads from a blue sky. There have been as many plagues as wars in history; yet always plagues and wars take people equally by surprise.

Albert Camus (1948)

The previous chapter examined vaccination, screening, and treatment, and their effects on bodily integrity. Considerable resources are devoted to developing therapeutic countermeasures, which undoubtedly can be highly successful. Yet medical interventions may fail to impede the epidemic spread of disease: Vaccines may be unavailable or ineffective against a novel infection, pharmaceuticals can become resistant, and medical supplies may be extremely scarce, particularly in a public health emergency. This chapter explores traditional public health strategies, which raise vital social, political, and constitutional questions because they interfere with the most basic human rights—association, travel, and liberty. But nonpharmaceutical interventions may be the only option available, so it is important to take a hard look at their impact on individuals, political systems, and the economy.

The social response of excluding those with epidemic disease from society has remained essentially the same throughout history. The obvious explanation is that people with disease are seen as vessels of transmission, hence justifying restraint, but this does not seem entirely consistent with the fact that civilizations had vastly different understandings of the causes of diseases and their methods of transmission. In fact, many societies actively rejected theories of contagion.[1] Although the persistence of personal control measures has no simple explanation, it may be related to how communities organize themselves to ward off threats to health and safety, and how they view those who are perceived as public menaces. Government measures to separate the ill from society are deeply complex, imbued with the social meaning of "community" and "the other," as well as competing economic interests and political controversy.

The social divisiveness may be even greater when those who seek to harm the populace or destabilize the political system deliberately release dangerous pathogens. Bioterrorism can be terrifying, evoking the most basic human instinct to protect self and society from external threats. Even when the hazard causes minimal loss of life, such as the 2001 anthrax attacks, bioterrorism evokes trepidation and fear. Whereas there is often little political interest in naturally occurring infectious diseases, bioterrorism captures the attention of the most senior government officials; bioterrorism, as a national security problem, is a matter of "high politics."[2]

This chapter first discusses the most controversial and enduring public health powers: isolation and quarantine. Isolation of infected persons and quarantine of asymptomatic persons can take place in a variety of settings (e.g., home, work, hospital) and with different levels of coercion or enforcement. Next, the chapter examines a range of disease mitigation strategies in the community, including personal hygiene, decreased social mixing, and international travel and border controls. Community containment strategies were widely used in previous epidemics, and policymakers are considering their use in case of a future influenza pandemic.[3] Isolation, quarantine, and community containment are civil measures designed to prevent harm to the public and are not intended to punish individuals for morally culpable behavior. (Civil measures should be contrasted with criminal penalties, which are backward-looking and aim to sanction wrongdoers.)[4] Finally, the chapter presents a case study on pandemic influenza to illustrate the challenging legal and ethical problems associated with medical countermeasures and public health strategies.

A BRIEF HISTORY OF THE ANCIENT POWER OF QUARANTINE

> If the bright spot be white in the skin of his flesh, and
> in sight be not deeper than the skin . . . then the priest
> shall shut up him that hath the plague seven days. . . .
> And the priest shall look on him again the seventh day

and, behold, if the plague be somewhat dark, and
the plague spread not in the skin, the priest shall
pronounce him clean. . . . But if the scab spread
much abroad in the skin . . . and if the priest see
that, behold, the scab spreadeth in the skin, then the
priest shall pronounce him unclean: it is a leprosy.

Leviticus 14:4–8

Command the children of Israel, that they put out of
the camp every leper, and every one that hath an issue,
and whosoever is defiled by the dead.

Numbers 5:2

The story of the legal regulation of the person is interwoven with the great contagious maladies of leprosy, syphilis, and pest.[5] The Old Testament describes the inspection and sequestration of lepers.[6] The crusaders found "lazarettos," places of isolation, still in existence outside the walls of Jerusalem and incorporated the word into their language to mean a house for the reception of diseased persons.[7] Lazarettos were built outside the gates of principal European cities, often under the religious order of St. Lazarus. These places of asylum confined not only persons with infectious diseases but also the insane and others whose separation from society was deemed beneficial to the populace.[8]

Governmental edicts separated those with disease from the community during the early Middle Ages: Emperor Justinian's order in 532 that persons arriving from plague-contaminated localities should be "cleansed" in places set aside for that purpose, the Council of Lyons's policy in 583 restricting the association of lepers with healthy persons, and the Lombard king Rothari's 644 edict isolating lepers.[9]

Multiple methods existed to exclude the contagious from society. The ill were confined in their homes for the duration of their illness, and upon death, they were passed through the windows and removed from the city. Lepers had to forbear communicating with the healthy; they wore special costumes, sounded a clapper, and could not appear in markets, inns, or taverns. Sanitary cordons were established along borders, whereby countries isolated themselves from their neighbors during periods of epidemic, leaving only special passages of egress.[10]

These were all variations of land sanitary laws, but much of the history of personal control was exercised through maritime laws. Overseers of public health were thought to regulate seafaring vessels as far back as the year 1000. Certainly by the fourteenth century, Venetian overseers were authorized to spend public funds to quarantine ships, goods, and persons on an island in the lagoon. Soon after, Venice appointed a public bureau of sanitation, and neighboring city-states, which were engaged in Mediterranean commerce, established sea lazarets.[11]

From these beginnings, the quarantine system began. The first compendium of Venetian legislative acts on the plague, around 1127, required merchants and travelers to remain for a period of forty days in the House of St. Lazarus before entering the city.[12] Sanitary bulletins were incident to quarantines and cordons. When persons and ships were proclaimed free of disease, they were given official bills of health indicating they were free to enter or leave a geographic area. Health officials had considerable powers and duties, including inspection, disinfection (e.g., by fire or lime), and isolation of people, animals, and goods (e.g., garments, food, and merchandise) thought capable of carrying disease. Offenses against quarantine, both land and maritime, were severely punished—with whipping, forced service on sick galleys or hospitals, even exile or death.[13]

Early Quarantine Laws in the United States

Quarantine has been practiced in the United States, mostly at a local level, since the early colonial period.[14] The earliest municipal ordinances were enacted in Boston in 1647; East Hampton, Long Island, in 1662; and New York in 1663.[15] During the next century, states such as Massachusetts[16] and New York[17] enacted quarantine statutes. By the time the Constitution was drafted, quarantine was well established.[18] Persons with infectious diseases have been detained for prevention or treatment from the framing era up until the present day. The last "leper home" closed as recently as 1998,[19] and many states still maintain places for the treatment of tuberculosis.

Although quarantine is principally a state and local power, the federal government also has a long history of quarantine regulation. The Fourth Congress, in response to a yellow fever epidemic in 1796, enacted the first federal quarantine law, which authorized federal officials to assist in state quarantines.[20] Several years later, Congress replaced the act with a federal inspection system for maritime quarantines.[21] Then, on April 29, 1878, Congress passed a federal quarantine act "to prevent the introduction of contagious or infectious diseases into the United States."[22] Congress assigned responsibilities for quarantine to the Marine Hospital

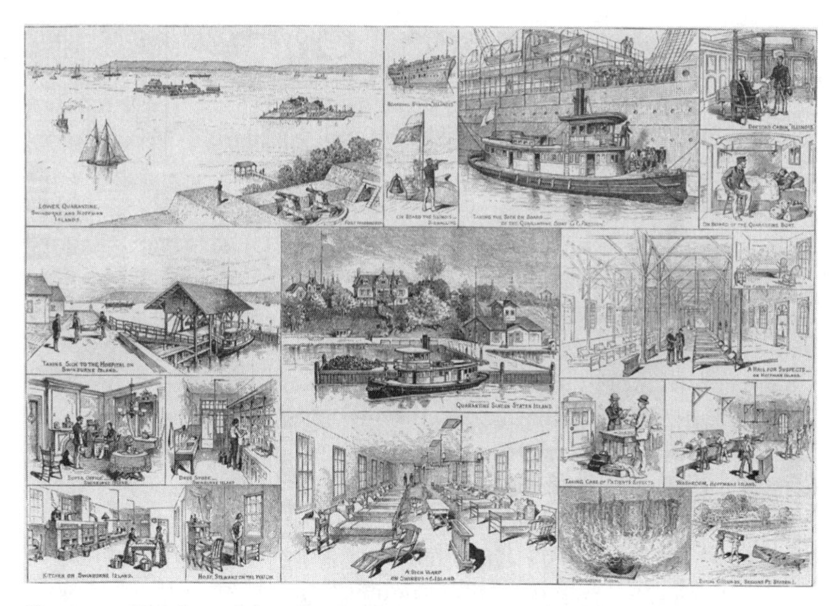

Photo 23. Sketches of the New York quarantine establishment. These sketches show the range of quarantine measures taken to prevent the spread of communicable disease in New York. © A. Berghaus/CORBIS.

Service (MHS), which had been established in 1798. The 1878 Quarantine Act, however, was extremely limited, stating merely that federal quarantine regulations could not conflict with state or municipal quarantine. In 1893, Congress expanded the role of the MHS, granting the federal government the power to enact and enforce quarantine rules to prevent the introduction of diseases, both foreign and interstate.[23] This was a time when the conflict between federal and state quarantine regulations sparked a federalism debate in the courts.[24] The courts ruled that, though states have quarantine authority,[25] federal law could preempt state power to control disease at the nation's borders or in interstate commerce[26] (see box 8, p. 156).

Society and Politics

It is difficult to exaggerate the dread caused by disease epidemics and the destabilizing effects on people and their communities.[27] A pestilence was a scourge, decimating the population and presenting a threat to the common security as momentous as war.[28] Thus society, through its institutions, felt justified in taking whatever measures necessary to defend itself. The prevailing social response was to exclude sufferers from the community to safeguard healthy members. The measures taken were harsh and punitive, subjecting individuals to indefinite periods of restraint, unbearable isolation from human companionship, and total deprivation of liberty.

Persons suffering from or exposed to disease came to be viewed as more than public menaces. They were loathed and reviled, often blamed for their own condition. Sufferers were shut out from normal social intercourse, and boundaries were created between them and the wider community. It was not simply a matter of expelling, isolating, or separating sufferers. They were outcasts, socially dead. The awful finality of exclusion from the human community was symbolized by a funeral service for lepers: "He was clad in a shroud, the solemn mass for the dead was read, earth was thrown upon him, and he was then conducted by the priests . . . outside the confines of the community."[29] Thus, disease bred fear and provoked punitive actions. The community justified this harsh treatment in part by blaming sufferers and branding them as "the other," deserving of ostracism.

Even in relatively more enlightened times, personal control measures have been applied in ways that may be better explained by animus than by science. Several campaigns of restraint in nineteenth- and twentieth-century America demonstrate the influence of prejudice:[30] isolation of persons with yellow fever, despite its mode of transmission by mosquitoes;[31] arrest of alcoholics, especially poor Irishmen, in the false belief that cholera arose in part from intemperance;[32] mass confinement of prostitutes "suspected" of having syphilis in state-run "reformatories";[33] house-to-house searches and forced removal of children thought to have poliomyelitis;[34] and quarantine of people of Chinese descent during a plague epidemic in San Francisco.[35]

Tuberculosis during the postbacteriologic era and AIDS in the modern era offer interesting illustrations of social intolerance. "Lungers" (the diseased organ representing their persona) were exiled to "Bugsville." Health officials exercised their authority almost exclusively against vagrants, immigrants, and the poor, who were thought to be careless in their hygiene and "fractious and intractable" in their behavior.[36] Public health campaigners, such as Hermann Biggs and Charles Chapin, insisted that "autocratic," "radical," and "arbitrary" powers encroaching on liberty were necessary for the commonweal.[37] In retrospect, the reduced incidence of TB probably resulted from medical treatment and vastly improved sanitary conditions rather than the segregation of the ill.[38]

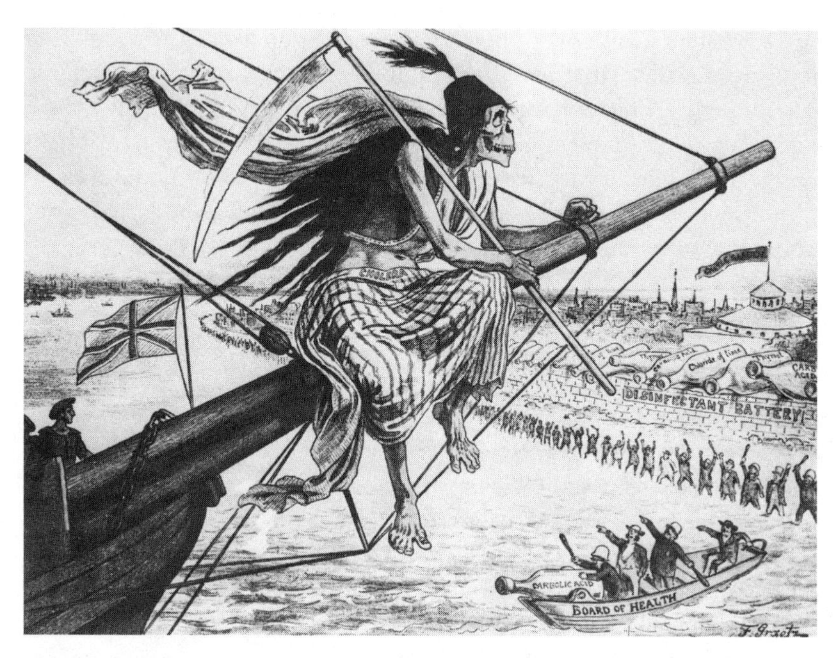

Photo 24. The threat of cholera at Ellis Island. "The kind of 'assisted emigrant' we can not afford to admit." So reads the caption to this 1883 *Puck* drawing, which shows members of the New York Board of Health wielding a bottle of carbolic acid, a disinfectant, in their attempts to keep cholera at bay. © Bettmann/CORBIS.

Though persons with HIV were spared systematic sanctions,[39] the community showed exaggerated fears of contagion and segregationist instincts during the first decade of the epidemic (e.g., burning the home of Ryan White because his mother insisted he attend school).[40] Persons with HIV, particularly those associated with disfavored subgroups, such as gays and injecting drug users, were blamed for their disease and contrasted with "innocent" "AIDS babies" and hemophiliacs.[41] (This is reminiscent of *venereal insontium,* or venereal disease of the innocent, in the early twentieth century.)[42] Popular indignation was evident in proposals for punitive measures, such as branding victims with a tattoo,[43] isolating them,[44] and establishing special institutions.[45] Both tuberculosis and AIDS earned their respective sobriquets: *phthisiophobia*[46] and AIDS phobia (often associated with homophobia).[47]

Throughout history, communicable disease has created vexing problems of fear and misapprehension, blame and ostracism of marginalized groups, and social controversy. As recently as 2003, SARS fueled negative stereotypes, with overtones that those of Asian descent were unclean and irresponsible. In Toronto, the public stopped patronizing Chinese restaurants; in Singapore, the names of superspreaders were made public; and in parts of Asia, service industry workers wore "fever-free" stickers.[48] The connection between disease, societal protection, and nationalism is evident, as ideas of "racial contagion" permeate modern debates about international travel and immigration.[49]

ISOLATION AND QUARANTINE: LAW, ETHICS, AND PUBLIC POLICY

> Investigations by the Department of Human Services have revealed that you have been engaged in activities which are potentially harmful to the public health. You have been counseled as to the nature and risk of these activities. Nevertheless, there is evidence to suggest that you have continued to participate in these activities. Now, therefore, I, Commissioner of the Department of Human Services, order you, [name], to cease and desist from activities which are deemed to constitute a threat to public health, effective immediately. If you fail to honor this order, a court injunction may be sought to compel your compliance.
>
> State of Maine, Department of Human Services (1993)

Public health authorities possess a variety of powers to restrict the autonomy or liberty of persons who pose a danger to the public.[50] They can direct individuals to discontinue risk behaviors ("cease and desist" orders),[51] compel them to submit to physical examination or treatment, or detain them temporarily or indefinitely. This section discusses two different, but overlapping, powers of detention—*isolation* of known infectious persons and *quarantine* of asymptomatic persons exposed to disease.

Definitions

Although the terms *isolation* and *quarantine* often are used interchangeably, both in public health statutes and in common parlance, there is a technical distinction between them.

Quarantine. Historically, quarantine was the detention and separation of persons suspected of carrying a contagious disease, especially travelers or voyagers before they were permitted to enter a country or town and mix with inhabitants.[52] As suggested by the word *quarantine* (derived from the Italian *quaranta* and the Latin *quadragina*), the period of observation was forty days, which was assumed to be the maximum duration of acute, as opposed to chronic, forms of disease.[53] The forty-day period was also symbolic (e.g., Christ fasted for forty days in the desert [*Quarentena*] and Noah's flood lasted forty days and nights).[54] The modern definition of quarantine is the restriction of the movement of persons who have been exposed, or potentially exposed, to infectious disease, during its period of communicability, to prevent transmission of infection during the incubation period.[55] Quarantine of exposed persons is designed to prevent the spread of dangerous, highly contagious biologic agents, such as smallpox, plague, and Ebola virus, particularly if medical countermeasures are ineffective or unavailable.

Isolation. In contrast, isolation is the separation, for the period of communicability, of *known* infected persons in such places and under such conditions as to prevent or limit the transmission of the infectious agent.[56] Modern science usually can detect, through testing and physical examination, whether a person actually has an infectious condition. Accordingly, *isolation* often is the appropriate term. Two kinds of isolation statutes exist: those that authorize confinement of infected persons on the basis of disease status alone ("status-based" isolation) and those that authorize confinement of infected persons who engage in dangerous behavior ("behavior-based" isolation). The distinction between status-based and behavior-based isolation is pivotal; the first concerns an immutable health status, whereas the second directly targets those who engage in risk behavior. In either case, isolation is frequently linked to treatment, which is offered to, or even imposed on, detained persons.[57]

The Many Faces of Isolation and Quarantine: Lessons from SARS

The terms *isolation* and *quarantine* appear straightforward but have acquired many different meanings. Governments in Asia and North America, for example, used multiple forms of civil confinement during the SARS epidemic (see box 35): medical isolation, institutional quarantine, home

BOX 35

SEVERE ACUTE RESPIRATORY SYNDROME

During 2002-3, Severe Acute Respiratory Syndrome (SARS) affected twenty-nine countries within a matter of months, infecting 8,098 people and killing 774 worldwide.[1] After China, Hong Kong, and Taiwan, Canada was hit the hardest.[2] SARS sent massive shock waves around the world, causing widespread fear and confusion among health care officials and citizens who had to cope with uncertainty regarding the cause, source, modes of spread, and appropriate interventions for the disease.[3]

The WHO has favored maximum control measures when new, poorly understood, and highly pathogenic diseases, such as SARS, emerge. Invasive measures such as quarantine and isolation are justified "when, in the view of national health authorities, they can be expected to protect populations against infection, keep the disease from spreading into the general population, and help prevent international spread to other countries, particularly through air travel."[4] Consequently, quarantine and isolation were widely used in Asia and Canada to reduce SARS transmission. In Toronto, between 13,000 and 30,000 people were quarantined. In Beijing and Taiwan, those numbers were even higher: 30,000 people in Beijing and 131,000 people in Taiwan.[5]

Isolation was used for persons who posed the greatest risk of transmission, persons who met the medical criteria for probable SARS cases, with symptoms such as high fever, coughing, and breathing difficulty. Isolation generally took place in inpatient acute care hospitals.[6] Persons in quarantine who developed symptoms of infection were subsequently placed in isolation.

Though quarantine was accomplished by a variety of means, home quarantine was predominant for asymptomatic contacts of infected persons. Contact cases were instructed to remain at home for a ten- to fourteen-day period after the last exposure, with follow-up, usually by telephone, from a local public health worker. The instructions for quarantine included sleeping separately from others, using personal

[1] World Health Organization, "Summary of Probable SARS Cases with Onset of Illness from 1 November 2002 to 31 July 2003," *World Health Organization*, Sept. 26, 2003; Jane Speakman, "Quarantine in Severe Acute Respiratory Syndrome (SARS) and other Emerging Infectious Diseases," *Journal of Law. Medicine and Ethics*, 31 (2003): 61-74.

[2] Public Health Agency of Canada, "Learning From SARS—Renewal of Public Health in Canada: A Report of the National Advisory Committee on SARS and Public Health," *Public Health Agency of Canada*, Oct. 2003, http://www.phac-aspc.gc.ca/publicat/sars-sras/naylor/index.html; Ontario Ministry of Health and Long-Term Care, "For the Public's Health: Initial Report of the Ontario Expert Panel on SARS and Infectious Disease Control," *Ontario Ministry of Health and Long-Term Care*, Dec. 2003, http://www.health.gov.on.ca/english/public/pub/ministry_reports/walker_panel_2003/walker_panel.html; Archie Campbell, "Spring of Fear," *SARS Commission*, December 2006, http://www.sarscommission.ca/report/index.html.

[3] Natalie Pawlenko, "Public Health Response to Terrorism: A Regional Approach. Isolation and Quarantine: A SARS Perspective" (2004), http://biodefense.umdnj.edu/documents/PH%20Response%20to%20Terrorism_Quarantine.pdf.

[4] World Health Organization, *Severe Acute Respiratory Syndrome (SARS) Multi-Country Outbreak* (Geneva: World Health Organization, 2003) (measures are justified when, in the view of national health authorities, they can be expected to protect populations against infection, keep the disease from spreading into the general population, and help prevent international spread to other countries, particularly through air travel).

[5] Speakman, "Quarantine in Severe Acute Respiratory Syndrome"; Pawlenko, "Public Health Response to Terrorism."

[6] Mark A. Rothstein, M. Gabriela Alcalde, Nanette R. Elster, et al., *Quarantine and Isolation: Lessons Learned from SARS* (Louisville, KY: Institute for Bioethics, Health Policy and Law, 2003); Sheela V. Basrur, *Toronto Public Health's Response to the Severe Acute Respiratory Syndrome (SARS) Outbreak 2003* (Ontario: Ministry of Health Staff Report, 2003); Health Canada, *Interim Guidelines: Public Health Management of SARS Cases and Contacts* (Ontario: Health Canada, 2003) (providing that all "people meeting the 'probable' case definition should be isolated in hospital").

items, such as utensils and towels, exclusively, and wearing a mask when near household members.[7]

The quarantine of contact cases was also used for health care workers.[8] Since it was difficult to identify all possible exposures in hospitals, all persons who had been in hospitals in which SARS was transmitted were considered contacts and were quarantined immediately. To prevent a shortage of essential health care staff, health care workers were subject to work quarantines, "which required them to travel directly from home to work without using public transportation and without stopping at any other destination."[9] During the time they were not at work, they had to follow home quarantine rules.

Less restrictive measures, including closure of public places, schools, and work sites, and cancellation of public events were also widely used.[10] At the other extreme, highly restrictive measures were used in China, including cordoning off certain neighborhoods and closure of public transit.[11]

While Canadians generally adopted voluntary approaches, public health officials in countries such as China, Hong Kong, and Singapore utilized more coercive measures. In Hong Kong, for example, barricades and tape were used in an attempt to confine residents in a large housing complex where over three hundred people were known to be infected with SARS. Singapore took drastic measures to enforce quarantine orders. For example, three telephone calls were made per day to the home of each individual in quarantine to confirm that the individual was there. Surveillance cameras were placed in homes where people were quarantined and, to avoid fraud, the inhabitants were required to take their temperature on camera. Electronic wrist- or anklebands were also used as enforcement measures. Singaporeans, moreover, faced a fine of over $5,000 for breaching home quarantine orders. Chinese citizens faced even harsher penalties, such as a jail sentence of up to life imprisonment and execution for anyone violating quarantine.[12]

A lack of alternatives made the use of quarantine and isolation an important element in controlling SARS. Nevertheless, the efficiency of the quarantine is still in doubt. Reports indicate that SARS was diagnosed in 0.22 percent of quarantined contacts in Taiwan, 2.7 percent in Hong Kong, and 3.8 percent in Beijing.[13] Also, in Toronto only a small

[7] Tomislav Svoboda, Bonnie Henry, Leslie Shulman, et al., "Public Health Measures to Control the Spread of the Severe Acute Respiratory Syndrome during the Outbreak in Toronto," *New Engl. J. Med.,* 350 (2004): 2352–61; Government of Hong Kong Special Administrative Region, Department of Health, "Health Advice for People Who Have Been in Contact with SARS Patients," Jan. 2004, http://www.chp.gov.hk/files/pdf/grp-contact-en-2004052100.pdf (health officials asked four thousand residents to go home and stay there indefinitely as the capital clambered to contain the deadly SARS virus); Singapore Ministry of Health, "Information for Home Quarantine," http://www.moh.gov.sg/corp/sars/information/quarantined.html.

[8] For example, more than half of Toronto's 850 paramedics ended up under ten-day quarantine during the outbreak.

[9] Nola M. Ries, "Public Health Law and Ethics: Lessons from SARS and Quarantine," *Health Law Review,* 13 (2004): 3–6.

[10] Basrur, *Toronto Public Health's Response* (addressing the closure of a work site, public schools, public health programs unrelated to the SARS outbreak, conferences, meetings, and businesses); David M. Bell, "Public Health Interventions and SARS Spread, 2003," *Morbidity and Mortality Weekly Report,* 10 (2004): 1–14. For a description of events and procedures related to quarantine of schools, hospitals (including visitors), and foreign workers, see Singapore Ministry of Education, "Procedure If a SARS Case Arises in a School, PSEI or Hostel," http://www.moe.gov.sg/sars/procedures.htm; Singapore Ministry of Health, "Chronology of SARS Events in Singapore," http://www.gov.sg/moh/sars/news/chronology.html.

[11] Joseph Kahn, "The SARS Epidemic, Beijing: Quarantine Set in Beijing Areas to Fight SARS," *New York Times,* April 25, 2003.

[12] "China Warns SARS Spreaders Could Face Execution," *CBC News,* May 15, 2003.

[13] Bell, "Public Health Interventions and SARS"; Kow-Tong, Chien-Jen Chen, Yi-Chun Wu, et al., "Use of Quarantine to Prevent Transmission of Severe Acute Respiratory Syndrome—Taiwan, 2003," *Morbidity and Mortality Weekly Report,* 52 (2003): 680–83; Centers for Disease Control and Preven-

percentage of quarantined persons had a suspect or probable SARS diagnosis, and even a smaller percentage of quarantined persons had a laboratory-confirmed case of SARS.[14] In hindsight, over-recognition of contacts resulted in overestimating the number of persons requiring quarantine. The public feared SARS because of its novelty, communicability, and rapid spread. Some trepidation proved rational, but in the end the 9.6 percent case fatality rate was less than first feared, and the total number of deaths was a small fraction of the estimated 35,000 seasonal influenza deaths in the United States alone.[15]

---

tion, "Efficiency of Quarantine during an Epidemic of Severe Acute Respiratory Syndrome—Beijing, China, 2003," *Morbidity and Mortality Weekly Report,* 52 (2003): 1037–40 (studies indicate that focusing only on persons who had contact with an actively ill SARS patient would have reduced the number of persons in quarantine by approximately 66 percent, without compromising its effectiveness).

[14] Svoboda et al., "Public Health Measures to Control SARS" (public health officials in Toronto identified 23,103 contacts of SARS patients as requiring quarantine, while only 225 residents met the case definition of SARS).

[15] Richard P. Wenzel and Michael B. Edmond, "Managing SARS amidst Uncertainty," *New Engl. J. Med.,* 348 (2003): 1947–48. There was, however, significant variability in the SARS death rate depending on age, with an over 50 percent mortality rate among those age sixty-five or older. Public Health Agency of Canada, "Learning from SARS."

quarantine, quarantine of travelers, and geographic quarantine (see table 19). Because isolation and quarantine deprive individuals of liberty and disrupt society, they must be carefully evaluated. Critical evaluative criteria include: What is the place of confinement and how onerous are the restrictions on movement? What are the levels of compulsion and intrusiveness of enforcement? How large a population is confined? What are the logistical, social, political, and economic impacts? How can health officials monitor the health status of quarantined populations and ensure that their basic needs are met? Are the benefits and burdens fairly distributed, particularly for the poor and for ethnic minorities?

Medical Isolation. Isolation of an infectious individual is widely accepted as a prudent and effective health measure. Medical isolation offers personal benefits by facilitating close monitoring of the patient's health and provision of treatment. It also provides societal benefits, because segregation from the public, coupled with treatment, prevents transmission. Medical isolation usually takes place in a hospital or other health care setting with trained personnel. However, this intervention can be costly and difficult; in a public health emergency, hospitals would have to cope with a large and sustained surge in demand for medical care, requiring increased capacity for staff, beds, and equipment.

Home Quarantine. During the SARS outbreaks and in current pandemic planning, policymakers stressed "home" or "self" quarantine, sometimes called "sheltering in place," or euphemistically, "snow days."

TABLE 19. Isolation and quarantine: Application, benefits, and challenges

	Definition	Application	Benefits	Challenges
Medical Isolation	Segregation in a hospital or other health care setting of an infectious individual	Infected individuals who require medical care	Availability of medical services, supplies, and support Ease of monitoring	High-risk work environment Hospital setting can facilitate disease spread Limited capacity
Home Quarantine ("Shelter in Place")	Home-based segregation of exposed or potentially exposed persons for the period of communicability of the disease	Persons who (1) meet the criteria for confirmed or probable exposure, (2) do not require hospitalization, and (3) have a home environment in which basic needs can be met and protection of household members is feasible	Socially and politically acceptable Minimal utilization of community resources Most logistically feasible Easy to solicit cooperation	Availability of support services Requires mechanisms for monitoring and enforcement Need to minimize contact with household members
Institutional Quarantine	Segregation in an alternate facility, such as school, hotel, or dormitory, of exposed individuals or groups	Exposed individuals who do not have an appropriate home setting, such as travelers, homeless populations, or people whose residence is in a congregate institution, such as a prison or mental hospital	Ease of monitoring Takes advantage of existing infrastructure	Congregate setting can facilitate disease spread Limited capacity Resource intensive
Work Quarantine	Persons permitted to work but must observe rules of home or insti-	Persons for whom home or institutional quarantine is indicated but who provide	Reduces risk of disease transmission while minimizing social and eco-	Need for careful and consistent preshift monitoring at work site to prevent

TABLE 19. *(continued)*

	Definition	Application	Benefits	Challenges
	tutional quarantine while off duty. Monitoring for symptoms and social distancing while at work	essential services (e.g., health care workers)	nomic impact of disruption of essential services Clinical monitoring at work reduces the staff required for active monitoring at quarantine site	inadvertent exposures May require transportation to and from work site to minimize interactions Must maintain close cooperation and communication between work-site and local health authorities
Quarantine of Travelers	Isolation on an airplane or ship of passengers until the threat level has been established or the period of communicability has passed	Passengers who are suspected of being exposed or have symptoms of a quarantinable disease	Ease of monitoring Prevent introduction of disease into a new area	Availability of support services Resource intensive Disrupts travel industry
Geographic Quarantine ("Cordon Sanitaire")	Legally enforceable order that restricts movement into or out of the quarantined community or neighborhood. Designed to reduce likelihood of transmission to persons outside affected area	All members of a community in which extensive transmission is occurring and where restrictions placed on exposed individuals are insufficient to prevent further spread	Reduces need for urgent evaluation of large numbers of potential contacts to determine indications for activity restrictions Reduces or eliminates spread of disease outside the quarantined area	Difficult to gain public trust and acceptance Requires good communication mechanisms with affected population Requires cooperation with neighboring jurisdictions that may not be using a similar intervention Care must be taken to avoid unjust distribution of harms and benefits

Key Evaluative Criteria: How onerous are the restrictions on movement? What are the levels of compulsion and intrusiveness of enforcement? How large a population is confined? What are the logistical, social, political, and economic impacts? How can health officials monitor the health status of quarantined populations and ensure that their basic needs are met? Are the benefits and burdens fairly distributed?

Home quarantine has multiple advantages: It is less onerous, more socially and politically acceptable, and logistically simpler. Most people do not mind staying at home for a period of time to safeguard themselves and their family. However, home quarantine can be difficult to monitor and enforce, as individuals may feel impelled to go to work, shop for necessities, or meet close family members, such as a child at day care or school. Home quarantines are ostensibly voluntary, but the state could resort to compulsion if symptomatic individuals chose to leave home. During the SARS outbreaks, enforcement ranged from no monitoring to placards, phone calls, and intrusive forms of surveillance (thermal scanners, web cameras, and electronic bracelets).[58] Home quarantine also can place household or family members at risk because they are living in close proximity.[59] Finally, government may have to ensure that vulnerable people (e.g., the elderly, disabled, children) receive health care, clothing, heating, food, and water.

Work Quarantine. Health officials during SARS similarly employed "work" quarantines, which restricted the movement of asymptomatic health care workers to their homes and workplaces.[60] When individuals under work quarantine were not at their workplace, they were required to follow the rules of home quarantine. The justification for work quarantine is to keep essential employees at their jobs while monitoring them closely. This strategy, of course, entails risk, as health care workers may transmit infection to patients who are congregated together and susceptible to infection.

Quarantine of Travelers. Travelers can pose special risks of disease transmission: They may originate from areas with endemic disease or outbreaks of novel infection, they often travel together in closed conditions, and they disperse to multiple locations, interacting with the populace. During the SARS outbreaks, North American officials quarantined airplanes and cruise ships if passengers had suspicious symptoms, until specialists could determine the threat level.

Institutional Quarantine. Though medical isolation and limited forms of quarantine are primarily directed to individuals or small groups, health officials have discussed mass quarantines in institutions or geographic areas. In China, Hong Kong, and Singapore, apartment complexes were quarantined, and public officials proposed designating special infectious disease hospitals to contain SARS patients. Other potential institutional venues include military bases, gymnasiums, stadiums, hotels, and dormitories. Historically, residents of congregate institutions such as prisons, mental hospitals, and nursing homes were not permitted to leave during epidemics. They suffered badly, as infection spread rapidly in closed, overcrowded conditions.[61]

Geographic Quarantine. Cordon sanitaire is a historic form of quarantine—literally a guarded line between infected and uninfected districts, to prevent intercommunication and spread of a disease or pestilence.[62] Sometimes also called "perimeter" or "geographic" quarantine, a sanitary cordon restricts travel into or out of an area circumscribed by a real or virtual sanitary barrier.

Mass quarantines in large institutions or geographic areas are unlikely to be effective or politically acceptable because they are so personally intrusive and socially disruptive. They deprive a large population of liberty even though many individuals may not be a risk to the public. Congregating healthy and infected individuals together can rapidly spread epidemic disease. Mass quarantines can also operate unfairly, disproportionately burdening ethnic minorities and the poor, as the quarantine of Chinese Americans in San Francisco at the turn of the twentieth century illustrated.[63] Beyond liberty and justice concerns are the sheer logistics of a mass quarantine. During federal bioterrorism "tabletop" exercises, officials predicted numerous deaths in the event of a smallpox or plague epidemic, as a result of congregating large numbers of people together. The logistics of a mass quarantine, moreover, would be daunting: There is no plausible way to determine who should be quarantined; substantial resources are required for monitoring and enforcement; and it is infeasible to ensure sanitary conditions in the quarantined area, which would require medical care, clothing, food, and water for large confined populations.[64] The constitutional problems of ensuring due process for a large confined population would also be overwhelming.

Above all, quarantine of all kinds is politically charged. It is frequently associated with overbearing government, and the socioeconomic repercussions loom large. A sizable proportion of the public opposes compulsory quarantine, expressing concern about overcrowding, transmission of infection, and inability to communicate with family members.[65] Compliance with public health advice requires public acceptability and trust in government. Perhaps quarantine would be worth the sociopolitical costs if the intervention impeded the spread of infection, but the evidence, particularly for mass quarantines, is limited.[66]

Legal Authority for Isolation and Quarantine

Legal authority for the exercise of public health powers can be found at every level of governance—international, federal, state, and local. This leads to inevitable problems of federalism: Which government may act, which set of legal rules applies, and in what circumstances? In theory, the WHO's International Health Regulations (IHR) cover regional or global health hazards; federal law applies to controlling disease arriving from foreign countries and interstate transmission of infection; and state or local law is concerned with health threats confined to a single state, city, or county. Beyond this relatively simplistic explanation lies a highly complex problem regarding the "lead" government official in any given situation. Public health preparedness, above all, requires clear lines of authority in an emergency. This section explains state and federal public health powers, and chapter 7 discusses the IHR.

State authority to compel isolation and quarantine within its borders is derived from the police power.[67] Even though all jurisdictions have authorized quarantine, state laws vary significantly. Typically, powers of detention are found in three kinds of infectious disease law: STIs,[68] TB,[69] and communicable diseases (a residual class of conditions ranging from measles to malaria).[70] When a novel infectious disease emerges, states sometimes find that they lack the power to act, as occurred with SARS.[71]

Ordinarily, different state approaches are not a problem, but variation could prevent or delay an efficient response in a multistate public health emergency. Cooperation among state and national authorities is necessary but is undermined by disparate legal structures. In addition, state quarantine laws are often old and do not reflect contemporary scientific understanding of disease.[72] In the light of the recent threats, however, many states have begun to reconsider their emergency response systems. The president's 2002 National Strategy for Homeland Security precipitated this action, urging states to review their quarantine authority as a priority.[73]

The Center for Law and the Public's Health at Georgetown and Johns Hopkins universities drafted two model acts to modernize and codify public health law, including quarantine authorities—the Model State Emergency Health Powers Act (MSEHPA) (2001) and the Turning Point (TP) Model Public Health Act (2003). These model laws were designed to ensure that states have ample power to respond to health threats, and to introduce constitutionally required due process protections for isolation and quarantine. Thirty-seven states have adopted provisions from the MSEHPA,

BOX 36

TWO MODEL PUBLIC HEALTH LAWS

A response to the anthrax attacks

A week after the terrorist attacks of September 11, 2001, letters containing anthrax were mailed from Trenton, New Jersey, to the three major network news stations in New York City and two tabloid newspapers. Nine people were infected, but most cases were not immediately identified as anthrax infections. Within a month, one victim was dead. Soon after, letters were sent to the offices of Senators Tom Daschle and Patrick Leahy, causing the closure of the Hart Senate Office Building and, briefly, the House of Representatives. Congressional staffers were offered prophylactic treatment for inhalation anthrax (ciprofloxacin hydrochloride), but public health officials failed to recognize the risk that spores would leak from the letters and contaminate other mail. Several postal workers and recipients of mail that had been in contact with the original letters were infected, leading to accusations of unfairness. In all, this series of as yet unsolved attacks sickened twenty-two people, killing five.[1]

In the midst of these events, the CDC asked the Center for Law and the Public's Health at Georgetown and Johns Hopkins universities to draft what became known as the Model State Emergency Health Powers Act (MSEHPA). The act addresses five key public health functions: preparedness and planning, surveillance, management of property, protection of persons, and communication and public information. The MSEHPA is designed to standardize and clearly delineate the powers states have when responding to public health emergencies. Drafted in recognition of the fact that most public health statutes predated modern judicial conceptions of individual rights, the act provides clearer standards and stronger guarantees of due process.[2]

Under the act, coercive public health powers can be exercised in response to an outbreak only after the governor has declared a state of emergency.[3] A declaration gives public health officials the power to carry out examinations necessary for diagnosis and treatment. Authorities have the power to conduct isolation and quarantine when warranted to prevent a substantial risk of transmission of infection, but they must adhere to human rights principles: the least restrictive alternative, safe and habitable environments, and fulfilling individual needs for medical treatment and necessities of life. Although the act was created with recognition that exigencies may prevent a predetention hearing, the government is required to petition for a court order within ten days of issuing a quarantine or isolation directive, and detainees have the right to counsel.

Nonetheless, some scholars criticized the act for providing insufficient protection of civil liberties, particularly those concerning due process safeguards for isolation or quarantine.[4] Other scholars argued that coercive powers are often ineffective and may cause health workers to underrely on medical countermeasures;[5] while still others ex-

[1] Centers for Disease Control and Prevention, "Update: Investigation of Bioterrorism-Related Anthrax and Adverse Events from Antimicrobial Prophylaxis," *Morbidity and Mortality Weekly Report*, 50 (2001): 973-76.

[2] Lawrence O. Gostin, "The Model State Emergency Health Powers Act: Public Health and Civil Liberties in a Time of Terrorism," *Health Matrix*, 13 (2003): 3-32; Lawrence O. Gostin, "Public Health Law in an Age of Terrorism: Rethinking Individual Rights and Common Goods," *Health Affairs*, 21 (2002): 79-93.

[3] *Model State Emergency Health Powers Act* §§ 401-5 (2001) ("During a state of public health emergency, the public health authority shall use every available means to prevent the transmission of infectious disease").

[4] George J. Annas, "Blinded by Bioterrorism: Public Health and Liberty in the Twenty-first Century," *Health Matrix*, 13 (2003): 33-70.

[5] Wendy E. Parmet, "Quarantine Redux: Bioterrorism, AIDS, and the Curtailment of Individual Liberty in the Name of Public Health," *Health Matrix*, 13 (2003): 85-116.

pressed concerns that extraordinary powers might be used in response to routine public health events.[6] The MSEHPA, in an era of deep concern about terrorism and civil liberties, became a lightning rod for debates about public health preparedness and conformance with the rule of law.[7]

During discussions on the MSEHPA, legislators asked for model laws that could be used for everyday problems in public health. They recognized that the law is a critical tool for public health but the existing framework is insufficient.[8] Responding to this need, the Robert Wood Johnson Foundation funded the multidisciplinary Public Health Statute Modernization National Collaborative.[9] In September 2003, the Turning Point Model State Public Health Act was published.[10]

The Turning Point Act is the most comprehensive model state public health law ever introduced in the United States (see further chapter 1). Acknowledging that traditional public health powers, such as surveillance, quarantine, and isolation, are among the most outdated provisions in existing state law, the collaborative intended to modernize powers within a framework that balances protection of the public's health with respect for individual rights. The act establishes a public health agency's mission and essential services, provides a full range of powers to control infectious and chronic disease, and provides safeguards for individuals. The act applies to all "conditions of public health importance." This non-disease-specific framework allows practitioners considerable flexibility in responding to new and emerging threats without resorting to last-minute legal updates as problems emerge. With respect to compulsory powers, such as quarantine and isolation, the act stresses the need to seek voluntary compliance. When compulsory powers are exercised, the act provides due process of law.

The Turning Point Model Act, together with the MSEHPA, represents a new approach to state public health law reform in the twenty-first century: legislators, with key professionals in the public health system, making their own choices based on model provisions developed by and for public health practitioners.

6 Wendy E. Parmet and Wendy K. Mariner, "A Health Act That Jeopardizes Public Health," *Boston Globe,* Dec. 1, 2001.

7 Lawrence O. Gostin, "When Terrorism Threatens Health: How Far Are Limitations on Personal and Economic Liberties Justified?" *Florida Law Review,* 52 (2003): 1-65 (Dunwody Distinguished Lecture in Law, with commentaries by four leading scholars).

8 Lawrence O. Gostin, "Public Health Law Reform," *American Journal of Public Health,* 91 (2001): 1365-68.

9 Susan Hassmiller, "Turning Point: The Robert Wood Johnson Foundation's Effort to Revitalize Public Health at State Level," *Journal of Public Health Management and Practice,* 8 (2002): 1-5; James G. Hodge, Lawrence O. Gostin, Kristine Gebbie, et al., "Transforming Public Health Law: The Turning Point Model State Public Health Act," *Journal of Law, Medicine, and Ethics,* 34 (2006): 77-84.

10 Turning Point Public Health Statute Modernization National Collaborative, "Turning Point Model State Public Health Act," Sept. 16, 2003, http://www.publichealthlaw.net/Resources/Modellaws.htm. Legislators, however, have not given the same attention to the Turning Point Model Act as they gave to the MSEHPA. Dan M. Fox, "The Politics of Policy Development in Public Health: Notes on Three Stories," *Journal of Public Health Management Practice,* 8 (2002): 65-67.

and other states are now considering adoption of the TP Model Act.[74] The two model laws are similar in many respects, but the MSEHPA is designed for a large-scale health event and its powers are triggered by a governor's declaration of a public health emergency.[75] The TP Model Act reflects the modern mission and essential functions of health departments, providing a set of powers and safeguards for day-to-day use (see box 36).[76]

BOX 37

CDC COMMUNICABLE DISEASE REGULATIONS

The CDC promulgated proposed communicable disease control regulations in late 2005.[1] The proposed regulations empower the federal government to exercise public health powers to prevent the introduction, transmission, and spread of communicable diseases from foreign countries into the United States (e.g., at international ports of arrival), and from one state or possession into another. The federal government has a major interest in preventing the spread of communicable diseases entering the United States or crossing state lines. But to what extent do these powers conform to the rule of law?

Scope of Federal Power

The Public Health Service Act authorizes the "apprehension, detention, or conditional release" of individuals for only a small number of diseases listed by executive order.[2] The proposed rules would significantly expand the scope of federal power by defining "ill person" to include the signs or symptoms commonly associated with quarantinable diseases—e.g., fever, rash, persistent cough, or diarrhea. This inclusive approach embodies an important conceptual shift, affording the CDC greater flexibility and adaptability. The proposed rules, however, capture a wide and undifferentiated range of signs and symptoms.

Federal Quarantine Power: Personal Liberty

The proposed regulations empower CDC quarantine officers to provisionally quarantine ill passengers for up to three business days. Thereafter, officers can order full quarantine on grounds of a reasonable belief that a person or group is in the qualifying stage of a quarantinable disease. The length of quarantine may not exceed the period of incubation and communicability of the disease, which can range from weeks to several months. During periods of quarantine, officers can "offer" individuals vaccination, prophylaxis, or treatment, but a refusal may result in continued deprivation of liberty. HHS is authorized to pay for necessary medical and other services, but it is not bound to do so.

The CDC does not intend to provide individuals with hearings during provisional quarantine, but individuals can request an administrative hearing to contest a full quarantine order. The administrative hearing comports with some basic elements of due process: notice, a hearing officer, and communication with counsel. Still, there are notable deficiencies that may violate principles of natural justice: (1) individuals must affirmatively request a hearing, which may delay or prevent independent review for those who do not understand or take the initiative; (2) the proceedings can be informal, with the regulations even permitting hearings exclusively based on written documents; and (3) the hearing officer may be a CDC employee who makes a recommendation to the CDC director. The European Court found a similar scheme in the United Kingdom to violate Article 5 of the European Convention on Human Rights, which requires a hearing by a "court."[3]

Surveillance and Contact Investigations: Cost and Privacy

The proposed rules impose obligations to screen passengers at borders (e.g., visual inspection, electronic temperature monitors); report cases of illness or death to the CDC; distribute Health Alert Notices to crew and passengers; collect and transmit personal passengers; order physical examination of exposed persons; and require pas-

[1] *Public Health Service Act* §§361-68 (42 U.S.C. 264-71) (authorizing the Secretary to make and enforce regulations to prevent the introduction or transmission of communicable diseases from foreign countries and from one state into another); Department of Health and Human Services, Control of Communicable Diseases (Proposed Rule), 42 CFR Parts 70 and 71 (Nov. 30, 2005).

[2] Exec. Order 13295, of April 4, 2003. Also see 68 F.R. 17255.

[3] *X v. United Kingdom*, judgment of Nov. 27, 1981, 46 Eur. Ct. H.R. (ser. A).

sengers to disclose information on their contacts, travel itinerary, and medical history. The travel industry critiqued the requirement to collect passenger data because of annualized costs of $118–$425 million.[4] Further, privacy advocates expressed concern about the disclosure of sensitive personal data.

Sanitary Measures: Economic Interests

The PHSA empowers the CDC to provide for inspection, fumigation, disinfection, sanitation, pest extermination, and destruction of contaminated animals or goods.[5] The rules specify that the CDC shall not bear the expense of sanitary measures, hence property owners incur the costs. The government's power to inspect and abate hazardous conditions has historical precedent, but the political Right vociferously contested destruction of property without compensation. However, requiring agencies to compensate property owners would chill health regulation and pass the cost of private health hazards to the public. This is particularly true for screenings at ports and borders, where individuals may be transporting infected or contaminated animals or goods that pose a risk to the public's health.

The CDC had not promulgated a final rule governing communicable diseases as of early 2007. As indicated, the proposed rules were controversial—applauded by many in the public health community but criticized by those concerned with the invasion of liberty, privacy, and property.

[4] Centers for Disease Control, Division of Global Migration and Quarantine, *Regulatory Impact Analysis of Proposed 42 CFR Part 70 and 42 CRF Part 71* (Sept. 26, 2005) (noting that the health benefits of the database could exceed $1.2 billion on an annualized basis).

[5] 42 C.F.R. 70.2

The federal government's current quarantine authority is contained in the Public Health Service Act of 1944 (PHSA).[77] The act grants the Secretary of Health and Human Services (formerly the Surgeon General) the power to make and enforce regulations to prevent the introduction, transmission, or spread of communicable diseases into or within the United States; to authorize the inspection, fumigation, disinfection, sanitation, pest extermination, and destruction of animals and articles that are sources of dangerous infection to humans; and to apprehend, detain, or conditionally release individuals for "quarantinable diseases" specified by the president in executive orders.[78] (As of 2006, the president had specified cholera, diphtheria, infectious TB, plague, smallpox, yellow fever, viral hemorrhagic fevers [Lassa, Marburg, Ebola, Crimean-Congo, and South American], SARS, and pandemic influenza.) The federal government can enforce quarantine regulations through criminal sanctions or judicial injunction.[79]

The CDC gave notice in late 2005 of proposed communicable disease control regulations, promulgated by authority of the PHSA.[80] The Secretary justified the use of federal powers based on the human and economic costs of dangerous biologic agents such as smallpox, plague, West Nile virus, and monkeypox. The regulations, if adopted, would expand the scope of federal authority to include powers of quarantine, surveillance, and sanitary measures. The proposed regulations empower the CDC to provisionally quarantine ill passengers for up to three business days, with the authority to order full quarantine thereafter. No hearings would be provided for provisional quarantine, but individuals could request an administrative hearing to contest a full quarantine (see box 37).

Constitutional Review of Isolation and Quarantine: Pre–Civil Rights Era

The Constitution does not explicitly mention quarantine. However, in discussing imports and exports, it does recognize the right of states to execute inspection laws, which are incident to quarantines.[81] Chief Justice Marshall suggested, as early as 1824, that states have the inherent authority to quarantine under their police powers.[82] Since Marshall's time, numerous courts have upheld detention powers,[83] mostly in the late nineteenth[84] and early twentieth[85] centuries. Their hallmark was the deference shown by the courts, with regulation regarded as presumptively valid.[86] Indeed, litigation during this period usually did not challenge states' constitutional authority to detain, but merely inquired whether statutes delegated too much discretion to executive branch health officials, or alternatively, whether health officials acted *ultra vires* (i.e, outside of the scope of their statutory authority).[87] In other litigation, plaintiffs sought damages against state or municipal government not for deprivation of personal liberty but for deprivation of property. For example, if health officials confiscated a hotel,[88] apartment,[89] or vehicle[90] for purposes of quarantine, litigants pressed for economic damages.

The major impetus for judicial activity in the public health field was the sporadic occurrence of epidemics[91] of venereal disease,[92] tuberculosis,[93] smallpox,[94] scarlet fever,[95] leprosy,[96] cholera,[97] and bubonic plague.[98] In this context, private rights were subordinated to the public interest, and individuals were seen as bound to conform their conduct for society's good.[99] As one court put it, quarantine does not frustrate constitutional rights because there is no liberty to harm others.[100] Even when courts recognized that personal containment cuts deeply into private rights, they would not allow the assertion of those rights to thwart public policy.[101] This preference for social control over individual autonomy emerged as a major characteristic of judicial rulings of the period.[102]

The judiciary, even during this early period, did assert some control over isolation and quarantine. Following a "rule of reasonableness" established in *Jacobson,* courts insisted that powers are justified by "public necessity"[103] and that states may not act "arbitrarily" or "unreasonably."[104] In practice, however, this standard left basic questions unanswered: How was "rationality" or "necessity" to be judged? For example, a New York court left the question of necessity to "the people."[105] The courts during this period set three limits on civil confinement, even though their decisions were not always clear or consistent (see chapter 4).

The Subject Must Be Infectious. Health authorities had to demonstrate that individuals had, in fact, been exposed to disease and posed a public risk.[106] The courts appeared hesitant to stigmatize citizens in the absence of reasonable proof.[107] Even here, however, social prejudice often provided the principal basis for action. The Ohio Supreme Court upheld a quarantine regulation that "all known prostitutes and people associated with them shall be considered as reasonably suspected of having a venereal disease." "Suspect conduct and association" were deemed sufficient to justify imposition of control measures, and the court did not appear unduly concerned with whether the woman actually had venereal disease.[108] An Illinois court accepted similarly unfounded assumptions: "Suspected" prostitutes were considered "natural subjects and carriers of venereal disease," making it "logical and natural that suspicion be cast upon them."[109]

Safe and Habitable Conditions Must Be Provided. The courts periodically insisted on safe and healthful environments for quarantine because public health powers are designed to promote well-being and not to punish.[110] On this theory, the quid pro quo for loss of autonomy or liberty on grounds of public health is that the state must take reasonable steps to avert harm by providing sanitary conditions, as well as safe and adequate treatment.[111] The Supreme Court in *Youngberg v. Romeo,* for example, held that civilly committed mental patients have a right to "conditions of reasonable care and safety," "freedom from bodily restraint," and "adequate food, shelter, clothing and medical care."[112]

Confinement Must Be Fair and Just. One of the most invidious measures in public health history was struck down in *Jew Ho v. Williamson.*[113] Public health officials had quarantined an entire district of San Francisco containing a population of more than fifteen thousand persons, ostensibly to contain an epidemic of bubonic plague. The quarantine was made to operate exclusively against the Chinese community. The court held the quarantine unconstitutional on grounds that it was unfair: Health authorities acted with an "evil eye and an unequal hand."[114] *Jew Ho* serves as a reminder that quarantine can be used as an instrument of prejudice and subjugation of vulnerable individuals or populations.[115]

Constitutional Review of Isolation and Quarantine in the Modern Era

Although these early cases still have influence, constitutional doctrine has changed markedly since the civil rights era of the 1960s. As explained in chapter 4, the Supreme Court has devised a "tiered" approach to constitutional adjudication, which requires "heightened scrutiny" of state powers that invade an important sphere of liberty, such as "the right to travel."[116] The Court has described civil commitment as a uniquely serious form of restraint because it constitutes a "massive curtailment of liberty."[117] Although modern cases often concern civil commitment of the mentally ill, they also should apply to isolation and quarantine. As one court explained, "Involuntary commitment for having communicable tuberculosis impinges on the right to liberty, full and complete liberty, no less than involuntary commitment for being mentally ill."[118]

Compelling State Interest. Under the Supreme Court's "strict scrutiny" analysis, the state must have a compelling interest that is substantially furthered by the detention.[119] Consequently, only persons who pose a significant risk of transmission can be confined.[120] In *O'Connor v. Donaldson,* the Supreme Court held that, without providing treatment, the state could not detain a nondangerous mentally ill person who is capable of surviving in the community.[121] Lower courts have gone further by requiring actual danger as a condition of civil confinement in both mental health[122] and infectious disease[123] contexts. For example, in the case of *In re City of New York v. Doe,* the court required clear and convincing evidence of the person's inability to complete a course of TB medication before permitting restraint.[124]

"Well-Targeted" Intervention. Mass confinement of a large group of people (e.g., everyone in a geographic area) raises constitutional questions. If some members of the group could not, in fact, transmit infection, the state action is overbroad. The Supreme Court finds overinclusive restraints constitutionally problematic because they deprive some individuals of liberty without justification. Consequently, public health officials should, to the extent feasible, target quarantine orders to those who demonstrably pose a risk to the public.

Least Restrictive Alternative. Given the strict standard of review, the courts could require the state to demonstrate that there are no alternatives that are less restrictive and would achieve the public health objective.[125] The state, for example, might have to offer directly observed therapy as a less restrictive alternative to confinement. However, the state probably does not have to go to extreme or unduly expensive means to avoid confinement.[126] The judiciary, for example, is not likely to require the state to provide economic incentives and benefits as an inducement to compliance. In the context of TB, New York City health officials aptly argued that they could not be required "to exhaust a pre-set, rigid hierarchy of alternatives that would ostensibly encourage voluntary compliance . . . regardless of the potentially adverse consequences to the public health."[127]

Procedural Due Process. Persons subject to detention are entitled to procedural due process. As the Supreme Court recognized, "There can be no doubt that involuntary commitment to a mental hospital, like involuntary confinement of an individual for any reason, is a deprivation of liberty which the State cannot accomplish without due process of law."[128] The procedures required depend on the nature and duration of the restraint.[129] Certainly, the state must provide elaborate due process for long-term nonemergency detention.[130] Noting that "civil commitment for any purpose constitutes a significant deprivation of liberty,"[131] and that commitment "can engender adverse social consequences," the Court has held that, in a civil commitment hearing, the government has the burden of proof by "clear and convincing evidence."[132]

In *Greene v. Edwards*, the West Virginia Supreme Court held that persons with infectious disease are entitled to procedural protections similar to those of persons with mental illness facing civil commitment.[133] These procedural safeguards include the right to counsel, a hearing, and an appeal. Such rigorous procedural protections are justified by the fundamental invasion of liberty occasioned by long-term detention,[134] the serious implications of erroneously finding a person dangerous, and the value of procedures in accurately determining complex facts, which are important to predicting future dangerous behavior.

COMMUNITY CONTAINMENT STRATEGIES

Isolation and quarantine are the most discussed and controversial public health strategies. Health officials, however, have a variety of additional nonpharmacological tools to stem infectious diseases. Disease mitigation measures in the community include personal hygiene, social distancing, and international border controls. Although these strategies are not as intrusive as isolation and quarantine, they still raise critical social, political, economic, and logistical considerations. Several empirical and policy evaluations of community containment have been published as part of strategic planning for highly pathogenic influenza.[135]

One historical study of the 1918 influenza pandemic concluded that there was insufficient evidence of effectiveness for community containment strategies. The single exception was "protective sequestration," defined as measures to protect a discrete, healthy population from infection prior to the disease reaching the population. This intervention is executed through restrictions on community members leaving the site, restrictions on visitors entering a circumscribed perimeter, and quarantine of visitors for a period of time prior to their admission into the community. Shielding a healthy population, however, worked only in island communities or other remote locations. In most other contexts, influenza spread inexorably.[136]

Community Hygiene

Hygienic measures to prevent the spread of respiratory infections are broadly accepted and have been widely used in previous epidemics, such as influenza[137] and SARS.[138] Infection control includes hand washing, disinfection, respiratory hygiene (etiquette for coughing, sneezing, and spitting), and personal protective equipment (PPE—masks, gloves, gowns, eye protection). Evidence of effectiveness varies and depends on the setting—hospital, community, or congregate facility (school, nursing home, prison). Strong evidence supports hand hygiene in all settings,[139] while PPE, disinfection, and aerosol-generating procedures should be standard hospital practices.[140] However, the effectiveness of community hygiene is unclear, and further research is important to understand its appropriate role in a future pandemic. For example, mask use was common, even legally required, in the 1918 influenza pandemic and SARS outbreaks. However, masks that are not well fitted or that become blocked by moisture from breathing may be ineffective.[141]

Even if hygienic measures are effective, professionals and the public must use them properly and sustainably. Infection control (e.g., tight-fitting N95 respirators) is challenging and must be used reliably until the risk subsides. Studies demonstrate inconsistent infection control in hospitals, and the general public has not uniformly adopted even basic hygiene practices such as hand washing.[142] Consequently, it is vital to train professionals and monitor their infection control practices. Public education campaigns grounded in risk communication science are equally important, as the acceptability of health measures is vital to community adherence.

Decreased Social Mixing / Increased Social Distance

Past experience shows that social separation and community restrictions form a significant response to pandemics.[143] It is assumed but not proven that decreased social mixing slows the spread of respiratory disease. Thus, in the face of pandemics, governments have closed public places (child care facilities, malls, workplaces, mass transit) and canceled public events (sports, arts, conferences). During the SARS outbreak, for example, health officials ordered widespread closures of schools, hospitals, factories, and hotels. As fear rises, the public itself may shun social gatherings. Predicting the effect of policies to increase social distance, however, is difficult, as infected persons and their contacts may be displaced into other settings.

Policymakers are particularly interested in school closures as a disease mitigation strategy.[144] Modeling studies suggest that, because children are efficient transmitters of infection, school closures would impede the spread of epidemics.[145] The key question, of course, is whether students would stay at home or disperse to malls, cinemas, and other crowded spaces. Closing schools for short periods of days or weeks would not have major social ramifications, but pandemics can endure for many months or longer. During this time, children and adolescents would miss the support structure of the school system—e.g., learning, social development, in-school meals. In addition, parents would have to stay home to care for young children, which would affect public services and productivity, because essential workers would be absent from their jobs for prolonged periods.

All forms of decreased mixing entail social separation from family, friends, and neighbors. Social isolation, particularly for long durations, can cause loneliness, emotional detachment, and depression; disrupt social and economic life; and infringe on individual rights. Community restrictions raise profound questions of faith and family. Coming together with fellow human beings in civic or spiritual settings affords comfort in a time of crisis. When people lose loved ones to a dreaded disease, there is a yearning to express grief in churches, social groups, and funeral services. But even these assemblies would be discouraged or disallowed.

As with other disease mitigation strategies, the vulnerable would suffer most, particularly those who cannot stock up on food, water, and clothing, or those who need assistance to function, such as physically and mentally disabled persons. Assuring the necessities of life is primarily a governmental function, but there is also a vital role for the community. The First Nation Māori call this *whānaungatanga* (neighborliness). Supported by the ethical values of unity and reciprocity, it means helping and caring for neighbors, family, and friends—being committed to getting through together, working cooperatively where there are needs to be met.[146]

The effects of social distancing on the economy also could be catastrophic, because the engine of production and wealth (workers and consumers) would not be participating fully in the economy. Travel, trade, and business would be severely compromised, with serious economic disruptions. The constitutional questions are equally complex, because the Supreme Court finds travel and free association to be fundamental rights.[147] Undoubtedly, the courts would uphold reasonable community restrictions, but legal and logistical questions loom: Who has the power and under what criteria to order closure, and for what period of time? Enforcement and assurance of population safety remain critical but unanswered questions.

International Travel and Border Controls

> Whether naturally occurring or intentionally inflicted, microbial agents can cause illness, disability, and death in individuals while disrupting entire populations, economies, and governments. In the highly interconnected and readily traversed "global village" of our time, one nation's problem soon becomes every nation's problem.
>
> Institute of Medicine (2003)

The forces of globalization render disease control a matter for national and international public health agencies. Nearly forty newly emergent infectious diseases have been identified during the last thirty years, caused by rapid, high-volume international travel, commerce, and human migration; mass relocation of rural populations to overcrowded cities; widespread changes in climate, ecology, and land use; and intense interchange between people and domesticated or wild animals (see chapter 7). In 2004, for example, a man with fever and chills arrived from Sierra Leone in Newark, New Jersey, and by the time he died of Lassa fever less than a week later, he had exposed 188 people.[148] A year earlier, infected rodents imported from Africa caused a multistate outbreak of human monkeypox.[149]

It is for these reasons that the United States and the global community have an abiding interest in the health of immigrants, refugees, travelers, expatriates, and other globally mobile populations. As mentioned, the PHSA grants the HHS Secretary the power to prevent the introduction, transmission, and spread of communicable diseases from foreign countries into the United States and from one state to another.[150] The CDC's Division of Global Migration and Quarantine (DGMQ) has delegated authority to operate quarantine stations at ports of entry, medically examine travelers to the United States, and govern the international and interstate movement of persons, animals, and cargo.

During the 1960s, fifty-five federal quarantine stations were active at U.S. seaports, airports, land border crossings, consulates, and territories. Yet overconfidence in the ability of science to overcome infectious disease led to the dismantling of most stations, so that by the early twenty-first century only eight stations remained. Spurred by the SARS outbreaks in 2002–3 and heightened biosecurity concerns, Congress allocated funds for significant expansion of quarantine stations.[151]

In fact, the term *quarantine stations* is deceptive. Although they have the power to quarantine travelers, their main function is to inspect people and cargo (e.g., review shipping manifests, screen immigrants, and visually examine travelers). The Institute of Medicine (IOM), however, suggests a more active, anticipatory role that would involve leadership in biosurveillance and disease control. The IOM recommends a "quarantine network" with a strong infrastructure, surge capacity for emergencies, research, and performance evaluation.[152]

Border controls, which were used during the SARS outbreaks,[153] can be far-reaching: entry or exit screening, reporting, health alert notices, collection and dissemination of passenger information, travel advisories or restrictions, and physical examination or management of sick or exposed individuals. Border controls, authorized under the IHR and regulations proposed by the CDC, also include sanitary measures at frontiers or on conveyances: inspection, fumigation, disinfection, pest extermination, and destruction of infected or contaminated animals or goods.

WHO and Canadian officials, however, found that screening of and restrictions on travelers were not highly effective during the SARS outbreaks.[154] The economic impact of restrictions on travelers and trade was enormous. The SARS epidemic, which killed fewer than one thousand people, was responsible for an estimated 2 percent fall in GDP across East Asia. Similarly, an influenza pandemic could cost $900 billion globally in a single year.[155]

Sovereign nations seek to safeguard their citizens' health from external threats, even in a global world where people, animals, and goods diffuse across state boundaries. Although border protection is legitimate, it can severely disrupt travel, trade, and tourism, as well as infringe civil liberties. Freedom of movement is a basic right protected by the U.S. Constitution and international treaties, but it is subject to limits when necessary for the public's health.[156] The World Trade Organization similarly defends free commerce but permits science-based trade restrictions to protect the public's health.[157] Consequently, international law requires a careful balance between the free flow of trade and travel, and respect for the rights to privacy, association, and liberty.

PANDEMIC INFLUENZA: A CASE STUDY ON MEDICAL COUNTERMEASURES AND PUBLIC HEALTH INTERVENTIONS

Highly pathogenic influenza A (H5N1) has captured the close attention of policymakers, who regard pandemic influenza as a national security threat. The virus is endemic in avian populations in Southeast Asia, with serious outbreaks now in Africa, Europe, and the Middle East. International trade, travel, and migratory birds will likely bring the infection to other continents. The economic consequences are severe, with millions of birds culled or dead from infection and bans placed on poultry imports.

Although the H5N1 virus is highly contagious among birds, it is rare in humans because of a significant species barrier.[158] A few cases of human-to-human transmission have occurred, principally involving intimate contact, but transmission has not continued beyond one person. The virus appears highly pathogenic, with a reported death rate exceeding 50 percent.

Although the prevalence is currently very low (and pales in comparison to pandemics of HIV, malaria, and tuberculosis), health officials express concern about the potential for pandemic spread. Historically, the world has experienced three to four influenza pandemics per century. The twentieth century witnessed the Spanish flu (1918, H1N1, 20–50 million deaths), Asian flu (1957, H2N2, 1–2 million deaths), Hong Kong

TABLE 20. Brief definitions of public health interventions for an infectious disease outbreak

Community hygiene is the community's use of basic hygienic measures (e.g., hand washing, cough etiquette) to reduce the risk of transmission of infection.
Hospital infection control involves the use of technical strategies in hospitals (e.g., particulate respirators, surgical face masks, hand sanitizers, disinfectants, and vaccines) to prevent medical personnel from becoming exposed to or transmitting infection in the health care setting.
Social distancing is used to decrease contact between people, thus minimizing opportunities for the disease to spread. Social distancing measures can include closing public places, cancelling public events, and encouraging people to remain in their homes.
International travel and border control measures are designed to check the global spread of infected individuals and goods. Techniques can include: entry or exit screening, reporting, health alert notices, collection and dissemination of passenger information, travel advisories or restrictions, and physical examination or management of sick or exposed individuals.
Quarantine is the restriction, during a period of communicability, of the activities of *healthy* persons who have been exposed to a case of communicable disease, to prevent disease transmission during the incubation period if infection should occur.
Isolation is the separation, for the period of communicability, of *known* infected persons in such places and under such conditions as to prevent or limit the transmission of the infectious agent.

flu (1968, H3N2, 700,000 deaths), and Swine flu (1976, H1N1, no pandemic). Through adaptive mutation or viral reassortment, the virus could become highly transmissible among humans. Recent evidence that the 1918 pandemic was caused by an avian influenza virus lends credence to the theory that current outbreaks could have pandemic potential.[159] Extrapolating from the 1918 pandemic, modeling studies indicate that, in the absence of intervention, 500,000 to 1 million Americans could die, with tens of millions of deaths globally.[160] In response, the United States[161] and the WHO[162] issued strategic plans in 2005–6. Therapeutic countermeasures and public health interventions are the two principal strategies. Table 20 defines the public health interventions, and table 21 depicts the communal benefits of these interventions, the rights infringed, and recommendations for improved preparedness.

Medical Countermeasures: Vaccines and Antivirals

Vaccination and, to a lesser extent, antiviral medication (oseltamivir [Tamiflu®] or zanamivir [Relenza®]) are the most important interventions for

TABLE 21. Public health strategies: Public benefits and private rights

Intervention	Public Benefits	Private Rights	Recommendations
Isolation and Quarantine: Hospital, home, work, institution, cordon sanitaire	Separate the infected or exposed from the healthy	Free movement, personal health and livelihood, nondiscrimination	Safe/humane settings, necessities of life, logistics, due process, social justice
Community Hygiene: Hand washing, disinfection, respiratory etiquette, masks	Reduce transmission in families and the community	Minimal, but requires behavior change	Public education grounded in risk communication science
Hospital Infection Control: Disinfection, hand hygiene, PPE, HCW vaccination	Reduce transmission among patients, HCWs, and their families/communities	HCW autonomy, freedom of religion and conscience	Training/monitoring in infection control, greater acceptance of vaccination
Decreased Social Mixing: Close public places, cancel public events, restrict mass transit	Slow spread of infection in public settings	Free association, mental and social destabilization, economic disruption	Target closures to high-risk settings based on evidence
Border Controls: Screening (entry/exit), reporting, health alerts, passenger data, travel advisories, inspection, disinfection, pest extermination	Prevent cross-border spread of infectious disease	Disruption of travel, tourism, business, trade	Adequate resources for surveillance, treatment, and response in affected areas and at U.S. borders
Medical Countermeasures: Vaccines, antivirals	Prophylaxis, reduced infectiousness, treatment	Bodily integrity, fairness to disadvantaged, intellectual property, business and trade	Stable, economically viable supplies: incentives, public/private partnerships, tort reform, compensation

reducing morbidity and mortality associated with influenza.[163] Indeed, most of the $6.7 billion federal influenza plan is devoted to medical countermeasures: $4.7 billion for cell-based vaccine technology and stockpiling of experimental vaccines, and $1.4 billion for antiviral medicines. The FDA has already approved one pandemic influenza vaccine for use by humans, but significant concerns remain about the vaccine's future efficacy and the ability of manufacturers to quickly produce adequate quantities.[164]

Despite the promise of medical countermeasures, there is a chronic mismatch between public health needs and private control of production. Vaccine production has been unreliable even for seasonal influenza, which is the leading cause of vaccine-preventable mortality; only a fraction of the recommended population is vaccinated each year.[165] For example, America lost half its supply in 2004–5, when the United Kingdom withdrew Chiron Corporation's license due to bacterial contamination. The best way to ensure pandemic preparedness is to increase the baseline for seasonal countermeasures.

PLANNING AND MARKET INCENTIVES

Public/private strategies, rather than private markets, are most likely to ensure a supply of stable, economically viable vaccines to meet a potentially massive public need.[166] Market forces create disincentives that inhibit vaccine development: high investment costs, limited or variable markets, and regulatory compliance. Vaccine manufacturers are leaving the industry, creating a risk of severe shortages. In 1967, twenty-six companies were licensed to produce vaccines for the U.S. market, but today there are less than half that number; only four companies supply influenza vaccine, with only two manufacturing domestically—MedImmune (FluMist only) and Sanofi Pasteur.[167]

The Institute of Medicine recommends a National Vaccine Authority to advance the development, production, and procurement of vaccines.[168] With or without such an institution, government can create incentives by boosting demand through seasonal vaccine awareness programs, issuing purchasing contracts, and providing price guarantees or subsidies. Recognizing the need, the G7 finance ministers announced a pilot advance market commitment for vaccines of public health importance.[169]

SOUND REGULATION

The vaccine industry must undergo rigorous regulatory hurdles, which are necessary for safety and efficacy but result in increased costs and delays. The Food and Drug Administration licenses vaccines, conducts regular Current Good Manufacturing Practice inspections, and requires that each lot of vaccine be tested for contaminants before public release. The industry therefore faces multiple, overlapping regulatory requirements. Since manufacturers must be licensed and begin commercial production in advance of or soon after the start of a pandemic, regulatory requirements should be timely, efficient, and well coordinated.[170]

INTELLECTUAL PROPERTY

Potential patent disputes must be anticipated because they have significant cost implications for commercial vaccines. The H5N1 virus cannot be grown in fertilized chicken eggs without modification through reverse genetics, which is a patented technology. Similarly, newer cell-based technologies, which promise more efficient mass production, are subject to intellectual property (IP) protection. Although IP affords incentives for innovation, it can also impede rapid and large-scale vaccine production in a public health emergency.

The federal government plans to stockpile 81 million courses of Tamiflu, costing more than $1.4 billion, sufficient to treat a quarter of the population. Hoffmann-LaRoche, the patent-holder until 2016, originally stated that the global demand was well in excess of its production capacity; yet the company adamantly resisted world pressure to allow the compulsory licensing of Tamiflu under the Trade-Related Aspects of Intellectual Property Rights Agreement (TRIPS, Art. 31), which allows countries to produce a product without the patent-holder's authorization (see chapter 7). Instead, Roche increased its manufacturing capacity and in April 2007 announced that demand for Tamiflu had slowed down to a degree that actually required cutting back production.[171]

LIABILITY AND COMPENSATION

Tort liability protection for industry and fair compensation for patients offer a sound dual approach to vaccine policy. Such a system already exists in the national Vaccine Injury Compensation Program (VICP), but it needs reform (see chapter 10). Patients can opt out of VICP, which has led to a sustained critique that legal liability represents a major disincentive for the industry. The president's influenza plan virtually bans lawsuits (except for willful misconduct) and assigns liability determinations to a political figure (the HHS Secretary).[172] The political critique, however, overstates the negative influence of liability on vaccine production.

Influenza vaccine litigation has been rare, with ten reported cases during the past twenty years, most with small verdicts.[173]

ETHICAL ALLOCATION OF SCARCE RESOURCES

The most challenging question facing bioethics is how to ration scarce life-saving resources: "Who shall live when not all can live?"[174] Given the devastating social, economic, and political ramifications of a serious pandemic, the following rationing criteria are worth consideration.[175]

(1) *Prevention / Public Health.* The historic mission of public health is prevention, so countermeasures to impede transmission should be a high priority. Rapid deployment of vaccines or prophylaxis to groups at risk of acquiring infection could contain localized outbreaks. For example, ring vaccination of direct contacts in a family, congregate setting, or local community could be an effective intervention to maximize lives saved.

(2) *Scientific/Medical Functioning.* If the first political priority is public health, then it is vital to protect individuals who innovate and produce vaccines or antivirals, provide treatment, and protect the public's health. These are critical social missions necessary to save lives and provide care for the sick. Priority, for example, could be given to key personnel in developing countermeasures (scientists and laboratory workers), delivering health care (nurses, physicians, and hospital staff), and devising public health strategies (epidemiologists and health officials).

(3) *Social Functioning / Critical Infrastructure.* A large-scale pandemic could result in key sectors of society not being able to function. Many public and private actors are necessary for the public's health and safety: first-responders (ambulance, fire, and humanitarian assistance), security (police, national guard, and military), essential products and services (water, food, and pharmacies), critical infrastructure (transportation, utilities, and telecommunications), and sanitation (undertakers, garbage, and infectious waste). Continued functioning of governance structures would also be important, such as the executive, legislative, and judicial systems.

(4) *Medical Need / Vulnerability.* Medical need, which is a widely accepted rationing principle, targets those who most require

medical intervention. It requires a scientific or epidemiologic judgment about at-risk groups that may vary. Seasonal influenza disproportionately burdens infants and the elderly, but highly pathogenic strains may affect young adults, as occurred with Spanish flu.

(5) *Intergenerational Equity.* The "medical need" criterion often favors the elderly because they are most vulnerable to influenza complications. However, there may be reasons not to routinely favor this age group.[176] Interventions may be less beneficial to the elderly than to younger, healthier populations, because vaccines produce fewer antibodies in older people. All human lives have equal worth, but interventions targeted toward the young may save more years of life. Would a "fair innings" principle militate in favor of children, young adults, and pregnant women?[177]

(6) *Social Justice / Equitable Access.* The allocation of benefits should not favor the rich, powerful, or politically connected. The Gulf Coast hurricanes seared into the American consciousness the inequities that could ensue in a public health emergency, as evacuation and relief services disfavored the poor and minorities. Special efforts, therefore, should be made to ensure fair distribution of life-saving countermeasures to traditionally underserved populations.

Public Health Strategies for Pandemic Influenza

Public health strategies are difficult to evaluate. First, evidence of effectiveness is often historical or anecdotal, with few systematic studies. Second, an intervention's effectiveness depends on the transmission pattern, which cannot be fully understood in advance. Key issues include viral shedding (infectivity during pre- and postsymptomatic stages), mode and efficiency of transmission (large droplet, aerosol, or contaminated hands and surfaces), incubation period, and serial interval between cases.[178] Third, an intervention's usefulness depends on the pandemic phase. In the pandemic alert period, surveillance, medical prophylaxis, and isolation are important tools; during a pandemic, the focus shifts to delaying the spread through population-based measures.[179] Thus, the key question is: Which measure, or combination of measures, works best at each stage of the pandemic? Multiple targeted approaches are likely to be most effective but can have deep adverse consequences for the economy and civil liberties.

Community Hygiene. If community hygiene (e.g., hand washing, disinfection, respiratory etiquette, and PPE) is to play a significant role in a future pandemic, the public must be clearly informed of measures they can take. In past epidemics, misinformation has been rampant, causing public anxiety, reliance on word of mouth, and purchase of ineffective or expensive products.[180] People have an interest in being provided adequate information to make informed decisions about their own health. Strategic plans should take account of geographic and cultural differences, which can be accomplished by civic engagement and consultation with affected communities.

Increased Social Distance. Government policies to restrict social gatherings raise problems of individual rights, social connectedness, economic prosperity, and survival of the disadvantaged. People have a right to association and assembly, which should be restricted only when necessary to reduce a significant health risk. Social separation, moreover, can cause isolation and loneliness, which can make individuals anxious or depressed and affect the social fabric of a community. The closure of schools, workplaces, and conferences can affect personal livelihoods, trade, and tourism. Additionally, lost profits due to closures may cause companies to go out of business, leading to job loss and other economic hardships. Finally, if people are instructed to avoid public places, such as markets, stores, and pharmacies, or if those places are required to close, there will be a need for people to procure food, medicine, and other necessities. These problems will affect everyone in society, but mostly will impose a hardship on the poor, who have no other means of survival.[181]

International Travel and Border Controls. Restriction of international travel, as discussed in many national influenza plans, would have an enormous global economic impact. World travel and tourism account for about 10 percent of global GDP and 8 percent of global jobs, generating more than $4 trillion in economic activity in 2005.[182] During the SARS outbreaks, tourist arrivals in Asia dropped 30–80 percent for various countries in the region. After travel bans were put in place, almost half the planned international flights to Southeast Asia were cancelled. Even Australia, which was largely unaffected by the disease, saw a 20 percent decline in international arrivals. Even if countries do not officially close their borders during an influenza pandemic, voluntary travel advisories would disrupt trade, transport, and tourism.

Isolation and Quarantine. Modeling studies predict that voluntary household-based quarantine and medical isolation can be partially effective in limiting the morbidity and mortality of an influenza pandemic, even if compliance is not uniform.[183] Isolation and quarantine therefore are likely to play a limited role in the early stages of pandemic influenza, but they are not considered effective or practical for later stages. Unlike SARS, influenza's transmission characteristics allow little time for isolation and quarantine: Influenza has a short serial interval (the mean interval between the onset of illness in two successive patients is two to four days), and infectivity is maximal early in the illness.

The exercise of compulsory public health powers requires rigorous safeguards: scientific risk assessments, safe and habitable environments, procedural due process, the least restrictive alternative, and attention to the principles of social justice. Pandemics are deeply divisive. To be successful, the government must gain the public's trust by acting transparently. The way we respond to a health crisis—whether we choose to exercise authoritarian powers, whether or not we protect the vulnerable—reflects profoundly on the kind of society we aspire to be.

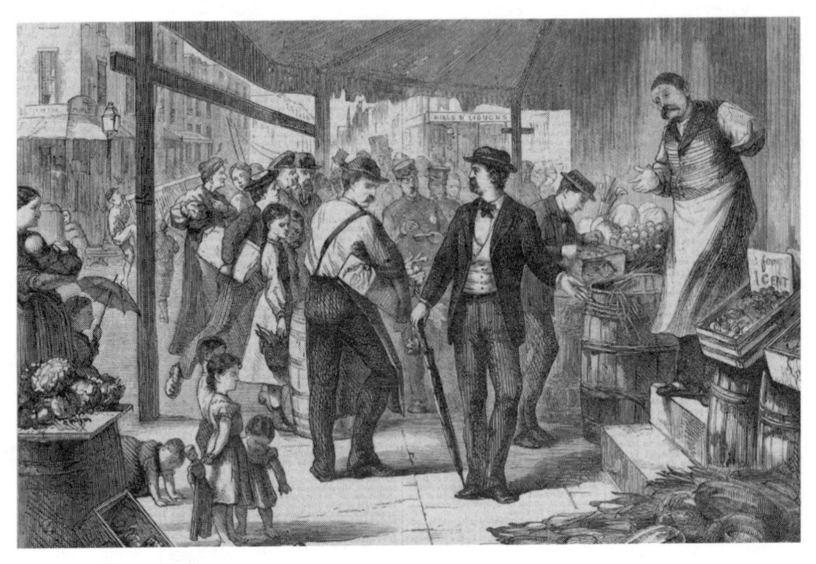

Photo 25. Inspections of fruit in New York markets. This image depicts early public health efforts to ensure the sale of healthy food. Picture Collection, The Branch Libraries, New York Public Library. Aster, Lenox, and Tilden Foundations.

CHAPTER 12

Economic Liberty and the Pursuit of Public Health

We think it is a settled principle, growing out of the nature of well ordered civil society, that every holder of property, however absolute and unqualified may be his title, holds it under the implied liability that his use of it may be so regulated, that it shall not be injurious to the equal enjoyment of others having an equal right to the enjoyment of their property, nor injurious to the rights of the community. All property in this commonwealth, as well that in the interior as that bordering on tide waters, is derived directly or indirectly from the government, and held subject to those general regulations, which are necessary to the common good and general welfare.

Chief Justice Lemuel Shaw (1851)

The sovereign power in a community may and ought to prescribe the manner of exercising individual rights over property. . . . The powers rest on the implied rights and duty of the supreme power to protect all by statutory regulations, so that, on the whole, the benefit of all is promoted. . . . Such a power is incident to every well regulated society.

John Woodworth (1827)

I have discussed a series of conflicts between public interests in health and well-being and private interests in freedom from governmental interference. Thus far, the private interests examined involve personal freedoms: autonomy, privacy, bodily integrity, and liberty. A great deal of the history and regulatory content of public health, however, involves private economic interests: freedom to enter legally binding agreements, own and use property, and engage in businesses and professions without undue government interference.

Commercial regulation creates a tension between individual and collective goods. In a well-regulated society, public health officials set clear, enforceable rules to protect the health and safety of workers, consumers, and the population at large. Yet regulation impedes economic freedoms and business interests. It is not surprising, therefore, that public health regulation of commercial activity, like the regulation of personal behavior, is highly contested terrain.

Industry and commerce are widely and legitimately thought to be essential to social progress and economic prosperity. Business and trade create greater productivity, more employment, and higher living standards. These benefits are highly relevant to healthy populations because of the positive correlation between health and socioeconomic status (see chapter 1). Community well-being is determined to a large extent by improved standards of living and increased general wealth.

Important and influential economic theories (e.g., laissez-faire and, more recently, a market economy or free enterprise) support private enterprise as a means of economic growth. These theories favor free markets and open competition; regulation that hampers private initiative is often seen as detrimental to social progress.[1] Commercial regulation, if it is desirable at all, should redress market failures (e.g., monopolistic and other anticompetitive practices) rather than restrain free enterprise. Modern proponents of market economy stress the importance to economic growth of the profit incentive and the undeterred entrepreneur.[2]

Public health advocates are opposed to unfettered private enterprise and suspicious of free-market solutions to social problems.[3] They are concerned more with the manifest harms to the community posed by an industrial economy and the resulting urbanization. It is not difficult to identify the public health risks of unbridled commercialism. Manufacturers can pose significant risks to the health and safety of employees, who may be exposed to toxic substances or unsafe work environments. Businesses may produce noxious by-products, such as waste or pollution, or sell contaminated foods, beverages, drugs, or cosmetics. Property owners may create public nuisances, such as unsafe buildings, accumulations of garbage, or dangerous animals. Persons engaged in trades, occupations, or professions may pose harms to consumers due to lack of qualifications or expertise. At the same time, migration to the cities for jobs brings the manifest health risks of overcrowding, substandard housing, rodents, infestations, and squalor.

This chapter explores the complex trade-offs between the benefits of regulation to advance the common good and the resulting retardation of economic growth. It first examines the law relating to three of the most common forms of commercial regulation: licenses, inspections, and nuisance abatements. These regulatory techniques protect the public's health and safety but undoubtedly interfere with economic liberty. Next, the chapter reviews the major claims of economic liberty: economic due process, freedom of contract, limits on eminent domain, and compensation for regulatory takings. Throughout this chapter, the key normative issue concerns the appropriate weight to be afforded to economic freedom. How important are contract and property rights compared with political and civil liberties? When government acts for the public's health, how concerned should we be about impeding commercial opportunities?

THE REGULATORY TOOLS OF PUBLIC HEALTH AGENCIES

Chapter 5 examined the structure, functions, and powers of public health agencies. It is important also to consider the specific methods of regulation. Public health officials possess a number of regulatory tools: licensing trades, professions, and institutions; inspecting for violations of health and safety standards; and abating public nuisances (see figure 35).

Licenses and Permits

Licenses and permits are an integral part of civil society[4] and a staple of public health practice.[5] (A related but different requirement is registration, which involves recording data such as names, dates, and events for identification and informational purposes.)[6] A license is authoritative permission to hold a certain status or to perform certain activities that would otherwise be unlawful (e.g., practice a trade or profession, keep a dog, or carry a firearm).[7] Consequently, legislative language is phrased in terms of a prohibition and then permission: "No person shall engage in the [specified] activities unless she has obtained a license from the [specified] agency."[8]

Licenses are administered principally by state public health agencies or by a body authorized by the legislature or agency.[9] (Because licenses are historically state functions, they pose especially complex problems

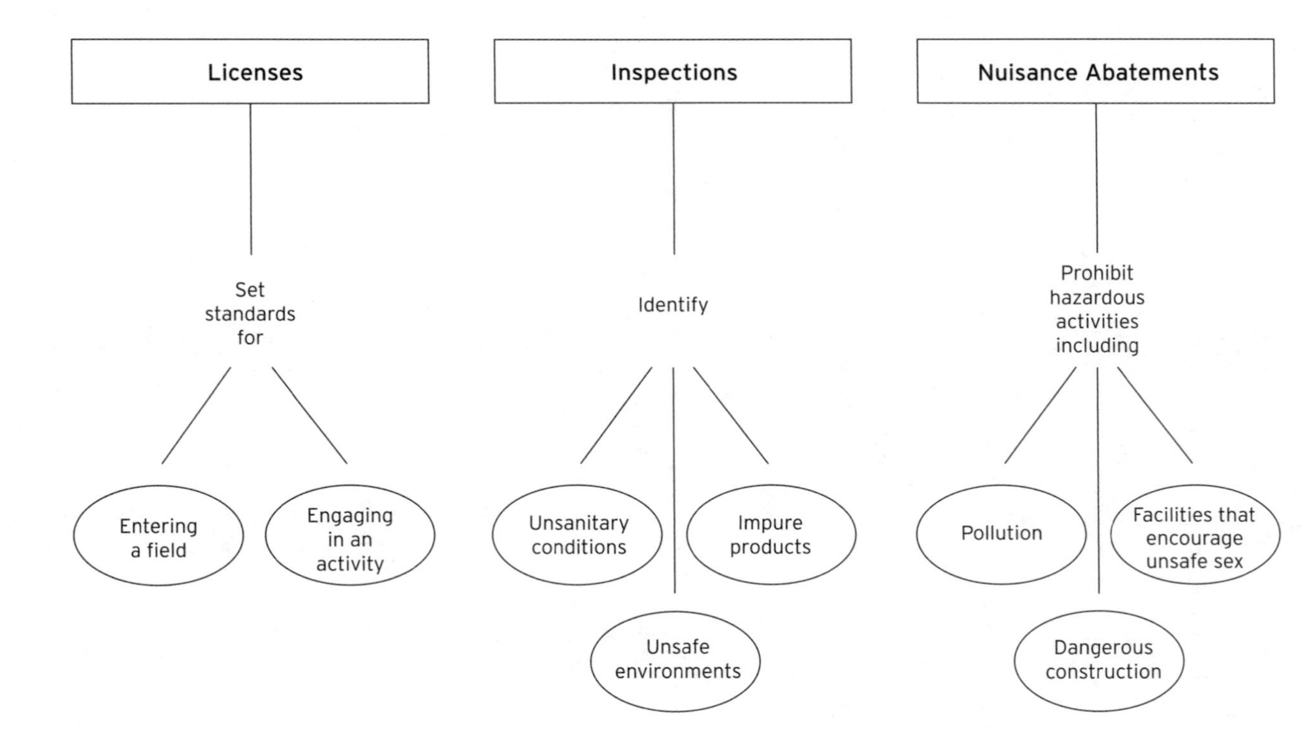

Figure 35. Regulatory tools of public health agencies.

BOX 38

MULTISTATE PRACTICE: TELEMEDICINE AND DISASTER RELIEF

Health care and emergency response professionals historically are regulated by states, but professional practice increasingly has multijurisdictional dimensions. Telemedicine and cybermedicine, for example, entail rapid access to shared and remote medical expertise by means of telecommunications, the Internet, and other information technologies, no matter where the patient or relevant information is located. Health care professionals may view medical records and images, correspond with patients, and make clinical judgments (e.g., diagnosis, prognosis, treatment) in multiple states. Complex questions arise about the right of individuals to practice in states where they are not licensed. Professionals also fear legal liability for their actions if patients are harmed by the negligent exercise of clinical judgment.

Legal issues related to licensure similarly arise during natural disasters or other public health emergencies, such as the Gulf Coast hurricanes Katrina and Rita in 2005. During times of crisis, volunteers typically travel to affected states to render assistance.[1] In these and other contexts, it is important to ensure that individuals have a valid license or permission to practice, at least temporarily, in the state. Absent such permission, the professional may be liable under state statute or tort law. To address this problem, the National Conference of Commissioners on Uniform State Laws has approved a Uniform Emergency Volunteer Healthcare Practitioners Act. If adopted by the states, the act will standardize states' licensure practices for out-of-state professionals during emergencies and make clear the legality of volunteers working outside their jurisdiction. However, the conference deferred adopting portions of the act applying to workers' compensation coverage and civil liability of volunteers until 2007.[2] Federal intervention may be required to reduce liability risks—for instance, by setting a national standard or facilitating cooperative arrangements among the states. The Emergency Management Assistance Compact (EMAC), for example, is a congressionally ratified organization for interstate mutual aid. Through EMAC, a state impacted by disaster can request and receive assistance from other member states, resolving upfront liability concerns.[3] Forty-seven states—all but Alaska, California, and Wyoming—have joined this compact through enactments of their legislatures.

[1] Center for Law and the Public's Health, "Hurricanes Katrina and Rita—Legal Issues concerning Volunteer Health Personnel," *Center for Law and the Public's Health at Georgetown and Johns Hopkins Universities,* http://www.publichealthlaw.net/Research/Katrina.htm ("In response to Hurricanes in the Gulf Coast region, volunteer medical personnel have been utilized to provide medical assistance to a large number of impacted persons. . . . Utilizing these volunteers in times of an emergency, however, presents challenges for hospital, public health, and emergency authorities, and raises a host of legal issues").

[2] *Uniform Emergency Volunteer Healthcare Practitioners Act* §§ 4–6 (2006).

[3] James G. Hodge, Jr., Lance A. Gable, and Stephanie H. Calves, "The Legal Framework for Meeting Surge Capacity through the Use of Volunteer Health Professionals during Public Health Emergencies and Other Disasters," *Journal of Contemporary Health Law and Policy,* 22 (2005): 32–39.

when professionals practice in multiple jurisdictions, particularly during a public health emergency such as a natural disaster—see box 38.) Licensing authorities may include the health department, a board of regents, a special licensing agency, or a professional or occupational board. Members of licensing boards, of course, should not have a direct or pecuniary interest in the license.[10] The courts readily allow public health officials to administer licensing systems, provided the legislature has adequately stated the facts, conditions, or qualifications for issuing the license.[11]

Licenses are part of a regulatory system that sets standards for entering a field or engaging in an activity. Agencies can set any licensing conditions reasonably necessary to protect the public's health, safety, morality, or general welfare.[12] Agencies license a broad range of professions, trades, and occupations in such areas as health care (e.g., physicians, nurses, pharmacists, and dentists)[13] and public safety (e.g., barbers, plumbers, and electricians).[14] (Note that many private professional or occupational specialties, such as medical specialties, nursing specialties, and dietitians, also operate credentialing systems designed to obtain recognition for their members' special qualifications.)[15] Licensing authorities set standards relating to qualifications, experience, and safe practice. In addition, agencies license public health institutions (e.g., hospitals, nursing homes, and laboratories).[16] Here, they can set standards relating to the security and health of patients or residents. Finally, agencies license businesses (e.g., alcohol beverage retailers, food services, and tattoo parlors).[17] The agency can set standards relating to the safety of workers, the purity of goods, or protection of consumers from fraud, deception, or unreasonable risks.

A licensing system does not merely sift out the unqualified or unsafe; it also offers continuous supervision by inspecting, monitoring, and punishing violators (e.g., withdrawal of licenses, as well as civil or criminal penalties). Consequently, licensing systems regulate both prospectively, by limiting entry into the field and imposing operational requirements, and retrospectively, by punishing transgression of standards.

State and local governments have the power to impose reasonable license fees.[18] However, fees must be proportionate to the government's regulatory costs.[19] Thus, if the license has a revenue-raising purpose (the fee is considerably higher than the administrative and policing costs), it may be invalidated as an impermissible tax.[20]

Social and Economic Fairness. Although licensing is important for health, safety, and prevention of fraud, it raises questions of social and economic justice. Licensing can be unfair because it parcels out a privilege based upon officials' discretion, which can be exercised in a discriminatory fashion against racial[21] or religious[22] minorities, women,[23] or other disenfranchised groups.[24] For example, in striking down a licensing system that was hostile to Chinese Americans, the Supreme Court said, "Though the law be fair on its face and impartial in appearance, yet, if it is applied and administered by public authority with an evil eye and unequal hand . . . [it is] a denial of equal justice."[25] Similarly, licenses can operate to exclude disadvantaged individuals because they cannot meet educational and qualification standards that may be set artificially high.[26] For example, the American Medical Association forced the closure of many existing black medical schools when it co-opted medical licensing in the early twentieth century, resulting in marked declines in the number of African American physicians.[27]

Members of the regulated profession may dominate or influence licensing authorities, creating the appearance or reality of exclusionary practices.[28] Licensing grants monopoly power to the profession or occupation,[29] which can enable private actors to exclude people for anticompetitive reasons.[30] Seen in this way, a licensing system, even if it originated in the public interest, can be used by the regulated group to limit new entrants, thus ensuring those already in the field higher incomes and professional status.[31]

Procedural Fairness. A license can be a valuable property interest that triggers a constitutional right to procedural due process (see chapter 4).[32] Licensing authorities may proceed informally, but they must comport with fundamental fairness when determining whether to grant or deny applications. Citizens who face official denial or revocation of a professional license may be entitled to legal representation, an adequate opportunity to present their case and cross-examine witnesses, a reasonable record of the proceedings, and reasons for the decision.[33]

Constitutionally Troublesome Conditions. Regulations requiring a license for the exercise of a right or freedom raise important constitutional concerns. For example, licenses may burden the free exercise of religion (e.g., religious processions),[34] expression (e.g., adult cinemas),[35] or assembly (e.g., bathhouses).[36] Courts will not necessarily overturn licensing decisions that burden the exercise of constitutional interests, but they will require neutral health and safety standards as well as the absence of unbridled discretion and arbitrary decision making.[37]

Inspections (Administrative Searches)

An inspection, or administrative search, of public or commercial premises is perhaps the most important and commonplace method of monitoring and enforcing compliance with health and safety standards. It also is among the oldest state powers, mentioned expressly in the Constitution.[38] An inspection is an official investigation or oversight—a formal and careful examination of a product, business, or premises to ascertain its authenticity (e.g., possession of a valid license), quality (e.g., purity and fitness for use), or condition (e.g., safe and sanitary). Inspection laws authorize and direct public health officials to conduct administrative searches to ensure private conformance with health and safety regulations. Inspection systems operate in many different public health contexts, ensuring the safe construction and maintenance of buildings or residences,[39] purity of food and drugs,[40] sanitary condition of farms[41] or restaurants,[42] safe workplace environments,[43] and control of pesticides[44] and toxic emissions.[45]

Search and Seizure under the Fourth Amendment. Although administrative searches are conducted in the public interest, they invade a sphere of privacy protected explicitly in the Constitution.[46] The Fourth Amendment guarantees the "right of people to be secure in their persons, houses, papers, and effects, against unreasonable searches and seizures." For most of the nation's history, public health inspections were rarely challenged and presumed to be constitutional.[47] However, in 1967, in the companion cases *Camara v. Municipal Court*[48] and *See v. City of Seattle*,[49] the Supreme Court held that public health inspections are governed by the Fourth Amendment and are presumptively unreasonable if conducted without a warrant.[50]

Administrative search warrants, therefore, are generally required for health or safety inspections of both residential[51] and private commercial property.[52] However, the judiciary permits searches without a warrant in at least three circumstances. First, a legally valid consent justifies an administrative search,[53] and in practice, most health and safety inspections are conducted with the permission of an authorized person (e.g., the owner or occupier of the property).[54] Second, public health officials may inspect premises in an emergency to avert an immediate threat to health or safety.[55] Third, under the so-called open-fields doctrine, inspectors may search a public place[56] (e.g., an eating area of a restaurant)[57] or test pollutants emitted into the open air.[58]

Generally speaking, courts issue warrants in criminal investigations only on evidence of probable cause to believe that a person has committed an offense.[59] However, courts issue warrants for health and safety inspections on grounds that are far less stringent than in criminal investigations.[60] To obtain a warrant for an administrative search, public health agencies need only demonstrate specific evidence of an existing violation of a health and safety standard,[61] or a reasonable plan supported by a valid public interest.[62]

Public health officials may not use an inspection to investigate a crime.[63] If the primary purpose is to discover evidence of criminal activity, they must obtain a search warrant based on probable cause.[64] Agencies often have both a public health and criminal investigative purpose, of course; after all, violation of health and safety standards can itself result in criminal penalties. Provided that the public health purpose is dominant, courts will not invalidate an otherwise lawful inspection that combines criminal law and administrative objectives.[65] Similarly, public health officials may seize criminal evidence if it is discovered during a lawful inspection.[66]

The courts have carved out a major exception to the general rule that agencies must obtain a warrant for inspection. Courts permit reasonable inspections of pervasively regulated businesses without a warrant.[67] In *New York v. Burger* (1987), the Supreme Court held that an inspection without a warrant of a pervasively regulated industry is reasonable if (1) there is a substantial public interest for the regulatory scheme, (2) the search is necessary to achieve the objective, and (3) the enabling statute gives notice to owners and limits the discretion of inspectors.[68] The courts permit inspections without warrants for a wide range of heavily regulated (and often hazardous) businesses, such as mining,[69] firearms,[70] alcoholic beverages,[71] propane,[72] and transport.[73] They also permit inspections without warrants for licensed businesses with substantial public health significance, such as nursing homes[74] and health care facilities.[75] Finally, the courts allow health inspectors to conduct routine audits of data (e.g., medical or pharmacy records) that, by statute, they have a legal right to search.[76] The judiciary permits administrative searches of pervasively regulated businesses without a warrant because of the importance of routine inspections in enforcing health and safety standards (warrants may afford owners time to conceal hazards)[77] and the reduced expectation of privacy in highly regulated commercial activities.[78]

The courts place certain limits on the time, place, and scope of searches without a warrant.[79] Further, if public health officials violate the Fourth Amendment (e.g., by not obtaining a warrant when it is required or exceeding the proper scope of the search), the exclusionary rule may apply (i.e., health officials are prohibited from using illegally collected evidence).[80] However, the judiciary often does not apply the exclusionary rule to administrative proceedings if the regulatory subject is facing civil penalties or minimal burdens.[81]

Nuisance Abatement

> [A public nuisance encompasses] that class of wrongs that arise from the unreasonable, unwarrantable or unlawful use by a person of his own property, real or personal, or from his own improper, indecent or unlawful personal conduct, working an obstruction of, or injury to, a right of another or of the public. . . . It is a part of the great social compact to which every person is a party, a fundamental and essential principle in every civilized community, that every person yields a portion of his right of absolute dominion.
>
> H. Wood (1893)

> Many wrongs are indifferently termed nuisance or something else, at the convenience or whim of the writer. Thus, injuries to ways, to private lands, various injuries through negligence, wrongs harmful to the physical health, disturbances of the peace . . . are commonly spoken of as nuisances.
>
> Joel Bishop (1889)

In law, a nuisance is a condition or situation (e.g., a loud noise, foul odor, or environmental contamination) that is harmful or offensive to the public or to a member of it, for which there is a legal remedy—an unlawful interference in the enjoyment of a person's or community's legally protected interests. The linguistic origins of the term illustrate its basic character: a hurt, injury, or annoyance.[82]

Private and public nuisances have common origins[83] but are distinct doctrines. A private nuisance, discussed in chapter 6, is an unreasonable interference with the possessor's use and enjoyment of property (e.g., flooding or contaminating adjoining land). Private nuisances principally are part of the common law and are redressed through the tort system.

A public nuisance, also known as a common nuisance, is an unreasonable interference with the community's use and enjoyment of a public place or harm to common interests in health, safety, and welfare.[84]

Public nuisances need not involve interference with interests in property but include all activities that harm common pool resources, such as silence, clean air and water, or species diversity.[85] The interest claimed must be common to the public as a class, and not applicable merely to one person or even a small group.[86] Public nuisances were originally part of the common law but are now principally legislative and enforced by public health agencies.

Public nuisance suits can be brought either by government (e.g., cities, counties, and states) or by private citizens. In private actions for public nuisance, however, individuals must show that they suffer an interference with their enjoyment of property distinct from the general public interest.[87] That is, private plaintiffs must demonstrate injury different in kind from the harm suffered by the public in general. Contemporary firearms litigation illustrates the role of public versus private actions for common nuisance. Municipalities have brought suit against the firearm industry under various tort theories, including public nuisance for conduct that poses a threat to the public's health and safety.[88] At the same time, private actions for public nuisance have been brought by civic organizations suing on behalf of harmed members and by victims, or their descendants, who have been personally harmed by gun violence.[89] Most courts, however, have not been sympathetic to public or private actions for common nuisance related to firearm violence, believing it is an unreasonable expansion of the theory of a "public right." [90] In fact, in 2005, Congress precluded most public nuisance suits against gun manufacturers or sellers[91] (see chapter 6).

A public nuisance is exceptionally difficult to define[92]—a point (as we will see) of significance, since the Supreme Court resurrected the doctrine in a famous "regulatory takings" case in 1992. In common law, a public nuisance is an act or omission "which obstructs or causes inconvenience or damage to the public in the exercise of rights common to all."[93] Early American illustrations of public nuisances included explosives,[94] garbage and offal,[95] decaying animals,[96] improper sewage,[97] and hogs kept in a filthy condition.[98]

Today, public nuisances are usually defined by the legislature. Alternatively, the legislature delegates to state and local public health agencies the power and duty "to define, prevent, and abate nuisances."[99] The legislative or administrative definition is often broad and virtually coterminous with the police power (e.g., "anything which is injurious to health, or indecent or offensive to the senses, or to an obstruction to the free use of property, so as to interfere with the comfortable enjoyment of life or property").[100] Legislatures or agencies also specify as public nuisances particular conditions such as "a breeding place for flies, rodents, mosquitoes,"[101] a place that is conducive to "high risk sexual activity,"[102] or keeping pigeons in a residential area.[103]

As mentioned above pertaining to federal firearms legislation, legislatures sometimes act to immunize certain industries from nuisance actions, believing that their activities are necessary to the economy or another public interest. Granting immunity, however, can interfere with private economic interests. For example, in *Gacke v. Pork Xtra, L.L.C* (2004), the Supreme Court of Iowa held that Iowa law granting nuisance immunity to animal feeding operations violated the state constitution because it deprived property owners of a remedy for the "taking" of their property resulting from the noxious odors that emanated from animal feeding.[104]

Legislative or administrative definitions of nuisances are presumed constitutional, but courts reserve the right to determine the presence of a nuisance. The standard for judicial review (unless the regulatory action affects a constitutionally protected interest, such as free expression)[105] is whether the nuisance abatement is reasonably necessary to avert a health threat,[106] even if it represents "a derogation of pre-existing private rights of property."[107] Consequently, the courts have sustained a wide spectrum of traditional nuisance abatements, including noxious odors,[108] diseased crops,[109] hazardous waste,[110] pollution,[111] unsanitary or dangerous buildings,[112] fire hazards,[113] and lead paint in homes.[114]

Courts have also sustained nuisance abatements in response to public health problems of more recent origin, such as unsafe health care practitioners,[115] public meeting places that increase risks of STIs (e.g., adult entertainment),[116] and violence by abortion protesters.[117] For example, in several cities public health agencies have successfully used nuisance laws to close down bathhouses in response to the HIV epidemic, believing that they create opportunities for anonymous sex.[118]

Courts possess broad equitable powers to alleviate nuisances. These powers include issuing injunctions to abate nuisances (e.g., ordering cleanup, repair, discontinuance of hazardous activity, or closure), awarding damages to the injured parties, or destruction of property. If abatement is the remedy, public policy suggests that, where there is no emergency, the person should be given reasonable time and opportunity to rectify the hazardous condition.[119] If the public health agency has to intervene, it should avoid unnecessary property damage.[120]

In summary, public health agencies have ample methods to regulate commercial activities, including licenses, inspections, and nuisance abatements. At the same time, these regulatory techniques, if applied in an arbitrary or discriminatory manner, can be unjust and may trample the constitutional protection of liberty and property interests. One question that has long troubled scholars is the relative importance of economic freedoms. I now turn to the discussion of economic rights, which have taken on increased importance in contemporary political discourse.

ECONOMIC LIBERTY: CONTRACTS, PROPERTY USES, AND "TAKINGS"

The regulatory techniques used by public health officials safeguard the public's health and safety but interfere with economic liberties. The Framers intended to defend economic freedoms, as evidenced by several constitutional provisions. Notably, the Constitution prevents the state from depriving persons of property (or life or liberty) without due process of law (economic due process),[121] from impairing the obligations of contracts (freedom of contract),[122] and from taking private property for public use without just compensation ("takings") (see figure 36).[123] Here, I examine the normative and constitutional justifications for economic liberties.

Economic Due Process

Conservative scholars argue that economic liberties are important in the constitutional design and deserve protection from commercial regulation.[124] Their claim is that individuals have a right to possess, use, and transfer private property, engage in a business, or pursue the profession of their choosing.[125]

In support of their claim, these scholars cite the Fifth and Fourteenth Amendments of the Constitution, which prohibit the federal government and the states from depriving any "person" (including corporations)[126] of "life, liberty, or property, without due process of law." Known as economic substantive due process, this constitutional theory holds that government must act fairly and nonarbitrarily. Courts applying this theory typically use a means-ends analysis to inquire into the extent to which the regulation furthers a reasonable or important public interest. Substantive due process theory would allow the courts to invalidate public health regulation if it unreasonably infringed on personal economic freedoms.

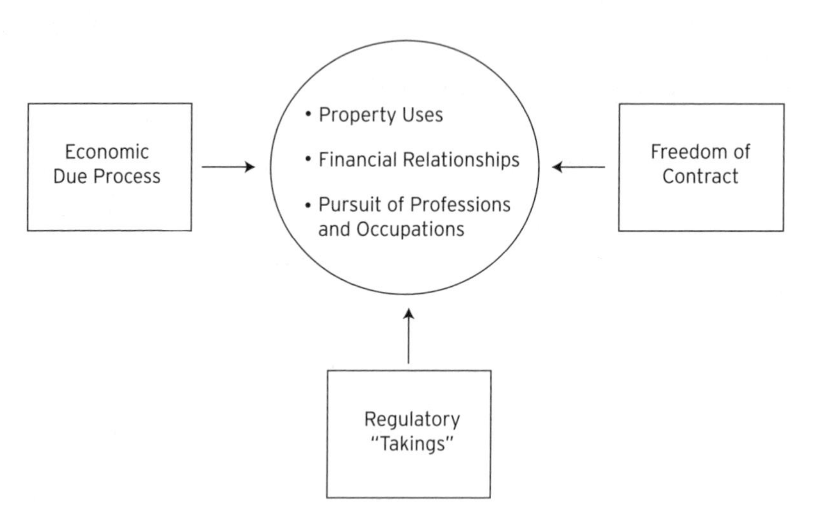

Figure 36. Economic liberties protected under the U.S. Constitution.

Despite the claim for constitutional protection of economic rights, the Supreme Court has rarely overturned state regulation, seeing public health as a sufficient justification for government infringement of economic liberty. Not long after the Constitution was ratified, the Supreme Court explored the idea that private property deserved protection as part of the natural law.[127] However, none of these early cases involved public health regulation. Indeed, when the Supreme Court examined a challenge to sanitary regulation of slaughterhouses in 1873, it said that government had the undoubted power to restrict occupational freedoms for the common good.[128]

During the nineteenth century, the Supreme Court began to find that business regulation could violate due process but still affirmed the state's power when it came to public health.[129] The Court ushered in a new era in constitutional protection of economic rights in *Lochner v. New York* (1905), when it struck down a state law regulating the hours that bakers could work. (In the same term, Justice Harlan wrote the Court's famous opinion in *Jacobson v. Massachusetts,* upholding state compulsory vaccination laws.)[130] Justice Holmes wrote a prescient dissent in *Lochner,* arguing that economic due process would erode government's ability to protect the public's health and safety:

> The liberty of the citizen to do as he likes so long as he does not interfere with the liberty of others to do the same, which has been a shibboleth for some well- known writers, is interfered with by school laws, by the Post Office, by every state or municipal institution. . . . But a constitution is

> not intended to embody a particular economic theory, whether paternalism and the organic relation of the citizen to the State or of *laissez faire*.[131]

The *Lochner* era, from 1905 to 1937, was a time when the Court most prized economic freedoms and aggressively invalidated numerous attempts at social and economic regulation. The Court struck down a great deal of legislation designed to protect the public's health and security, such as the minimum wage, consumer protection, and licensing. In 1937, the Supreme Court repudiated the *Lochner* doctrine, and scholars almost universally condemned it. The major flaw of economic due process was that it permitted courts to substitute their view for that of the legislature as to what is in the best interests of society and the economy. Since Franklin Delano Roosevelt's New Deal, the Court has granted police power regulation a strong presumption of validity, even if it interferes with economic and commercial life (see chapter 3).

Modern conservative scholars have sought to resurrect the *Lochner* doctrine.[132] As Judge Richard Posner remarked, "There is a movement afoot (among scholars, not as yet among judges) to make the majority opinion in *Lochner* the centerpiece of a new activist jurisprudence."[133] This "movement" empathizes with the promarket, antiregulation philosophy underlying *Lochner*, and it has regained influence in political and academic circles.[134] The judiciary, however, has not endorsed the political theory or constitutional interpretation of *Lochner*, and for good reason. It is for democratically elected assemblies to strike a balance between a well-ordered, safe society and the property rights of individuals.

Freedom of Contract

Conservative commentators have urged stronger protection of a number of interrelated economic rights against health regulation. Perhaps the most important of these is freedom of contract. The right of contract is often favored because it epitomizes free economic relationships and the ability to plan and conduct business in a predictable, orderly fashion. Unlike economic due process, which must be inferred from the Due Process Clause, the Constitution expressly provides for the right of contract: No state shall pass any "Law impairing the Obligation of Contracts."[135]

Despite the express constitutional language, the Contract Clause has become a relatively unimportant limitation on public health powers. The clause applies only to the states; most challenges to federal restrictions on contractual freedom must be brought under the Due Process Clause of the Fifth Amendment, which, as we have just seen, is quite limited.[136] More importantly, the clause applies only to existing contracts; states are free to limit the terms of future contracts.[137] Most public health regulation, of course, is intended to govern future economic relationships. In rare cases, however, public health regulation affects existing contracts. In such cases, the Supreme Court has emphasized that the police power "is an exercise of the sovereign right of the Government to protect the lives, health, morals, comfort, and general welfare of the people, and is paramount to any rights under contracts between individuals."[138] Consequently, public health regulation, even if it interferes with existing economic relationships, is presumed to be constitutionally legitimate.

The modern Court uses a three-part test to assess government regulation that interferes with private contracts:[139] (1) Is there a substantial impairment of a contractual relationship? (2) If so, does it serve a significant and legitimate public purpose? (3) Is it reasonably related to achieving the goal?[140] Like substantive due process, this is a highly permissive standard that generally affirms governmental power to regulate contractual relationships reasonably in the public interest. Public health regulation ordinarily meets this deferential test because it usually prescribes health and safety practices that have incidental effects on commercial transactions; it is intended for important public purposes; and if it is based on science or established practice, it is reasonably likely to achieve a public health objective. For example, in *RUI v. One Corp. v. City of Berkeley* (2004), the Ninth Circuit Court of Appeals upheld a living wage law designed to alleviate poverty. The Court found no infringement of contracts, noting that "the power to regulate wages and employment conditions lies clearly within a state's or municipality's police power," and that legislative bodies are given broad authority to exercise such power.[141]

Aggressive use of the Contract Clause is another means by which some conservative activists try to block health and safety regulation. Adopting a philosophy of natural rights or libertarianism, these scholars sometimes propose revolutionary changes to judicial interpretation of the Contract Clause. Richard Epstein, for example, asserts that the freedom of contract should apply to both public and private contracts; to both rights and duties of contracts, so that government could not relieve existing contractual obligations or impose new ones; and to prospective, as well as retroactive, modification of contracts. This position threatens forward-looking health and safety regulation. Of particular concern is the claim that the Contract Clause could restrain the police power: "Even health or safety measures may be attacked, notwithstanding the soundness of their ends."[142]

It may be that individuals in a state of nature would seek freedom to do what they wish with their wealth and property. But individuals are not in a state of nature; they are embedded in a society where their interactions may be regulated for the sake of the collective. Limits on sound regulation sometimes benefit the economic interests of discrete individuals, but society as a whole would suffer from deteriorated health and safety standards. Contract rights, therefore, should give way when they come in conflict with the public interest, and decisions about when a public purpose justifies impairment of economic relationships should be a policy determination.[143]

Eminent Domain: "Taking" Property for Public Use with Just Compensation

The federal government and the states have the power of eminent domain, which is the authority to confiscate private property for government purposes. However, the Fifth Amendment imposes a significant constraint on this power: ". . . nor shall private property be taken for public use, without just compensation."[144] Thus, government may take property only (1) for a "public use" and (2) with "just compensation."[145]

Theories supporting the Takings Clause relate to basic fairness and justice. The "public use" constraint is intended to reserve government's power to confiscate private property only for legitimate public purposes. Under this theory, government may not use the power of eminent domain to confer a private benefit, taking one person's property solely to enrich another private party.[146] The "just compensation" constraint is intended to ensure that individuals do not have to bear public burdens, which should be borne by the community as a whole. Consequently, the Takings Clause is about government spreading loss when pursuing the public interest.[147]

No one would quarrel with the idea of justice in the ownership and allocation of private property, but this seemingly innocuous constitutional provision has been intensely divisive. It has created deep fault lines between those who view the state as a vehicle for the common good and others who see protection of private property as the natural right of citizens. Modern controversy has swirled around two defining questions in the law of eminent domain: What is a "taking" and what is a "public use"? Both of these constitutional questions have important public health dimensions, because they help determine when and how the state can interfere with economic rights to promote the common good. Powers of eminent domain can be exercised for many public health purposes—e.g., to renovate unsanitary or unsafe buildings,[148] to convert private animal shelters to serve the public need of controlling dangerous animals,[149] and to confiscate hospitals for care or even quarantine during a public health emergency.[150]

WHAT IS A "TAKING"? COMPENSATION FOR REGULATORY TAKINGS

> Attorney General Meese . . . had a specific, aggressive, and it seemed to me, quite radical project in mind: to use the takings clause of the Fifth Amendment as a severe brake on federal and state regulation of business and property.
>
> Charles Fried (1991)

> Many of the changes in takings law . . . correspond quite closely to a blueprint for the takings doctrine proposed by Professor Richard Epstein. . . . This observation [is] both remarkable and troubling. After all, Epstein's work was almost universally criticized . . . [and its] proposed end result—the overturning of a century's worth of health, safety, and economic regulation—would sink this country in a constitutional crisis. . . . What we have found is a large and increasingly successful campaign by conservatives and libertarians to use the federal judiciary to achieve an anti-regulatory, anti-environmental agenda.
>
> Douglas T. Kendall and Charles P. Lord (1998)

Government confiscation or physical occupation of property is a "possessory" taking that certainly requires compensation. But does government regulation that only diminishes the value of private property also require just compensation? An expansive interpretation of takings would shackle public health agencies by requiring them to provide compensation whenever regulation significantly reduced the value of private property. Since public health regulation, by definition, restricts commercial uses of property, it has become a focal point for a sustained conservative critique of social action itself.[151] As Justice Holmes warned as early as 1922, "Government hardly could go on if to some extent values incident to property could not be diminished without paying for every such change in the general law."[152] The law of regulatory takings is complex and muddled and, therefore, beyond the scope of a book on public health law. (See box 39 for a brief explanation.)

During the early twentieth century, the Supreme Court held that government regulation that "reaches a certain magnitude" also is a taking requiring compensation.[153] The question, of course, is when does a regulation go so far that it becomes a taking? Initially, this idea of "regulatory" takings was not highly problematic for public health agencies because the Court indicated that government need not compensate property owners when regulating within the police power.[154] However, regulatory takings took on public health significance in the 1992 case of *Lucas v. South Carolina Coastal Council*.[155] In *Lucas*, Justice Antonin Scalia, the most intellectually powerful conservative voice on the Court, said that a person suffers a per se, or categorical, taking if regulation denies all economically beneficial or productive use of real property[156] and there were no similar restrictions "that background principles of the State's law of property and nuisance already place upon land ownership."[157] (Temporary restrictions on land use do not rise to the level of a per se taking.)[158] Justice Scalia suggested that common law nuisance was the key to resolving the question of when regulation amounted to an uncompensated taking; an owner who lost the value of her land would suffer a taking if the public health regulation was not considered a nuisance under the common law.[159]

Lucas focused on the reasonable expectations of the buyer at the time the property was purchased. In that case, the buyer knew there were government restrictions on the use of the property at the time of the purchase, so she couldn't then complain that there had been a taking. However, the Court now appears to draw a distinction between common law rules that existed prior to purchase and other regulations. In *Palazzolo v. Rhode Island* (2005), the Court held that a property owner could bring a takings claim for statutes and regulations (as opposed to common law nuisance) that were in place at the time the property was acquired.[160]

The Court's reasoning in *Lucas* is problematic because it forces public health agencies to define and abate public hazards according to vague and outdated common law understandings of nuisance. Even the most astute legal scholars perceive common law nuisance as confusing and indecipherable.[161] The complexity was compounded in *Palazzolo*, which drew an even more unfathomable distinction: challenges to common law

BOX 39

REGULATORY TAKINGS DOCTRINE: HARDLY A MODEL OF CLARITY

The Supreme Court's regulatory takings jurisprudence is "hardly a model of clarity."[1] Regulatory takings cases are commonly divided between "per se" takings, where there are categorical rules, and other regulatory takings, where there is a balancing test.[2] The Court has established two categories of regulatory action that are deemed per se takings, which give rise to an unqualified constitutional obligation to compensate the property owner. First, if the regulation results in a permanent physical invasion of the owner's property, however minor, the state must provide just compensation.[3] This per se regulatory takings rule makes sense because a permanent physical invasion is a serious incursion on property rights similar to the government taking ownership.

A second categorical rule applies to all regulations that completely deprive an owner of "all economically beneficial use" of property.[4] Under *Lucas v. South Carolina Coastal Council* (1992), the government must pay just compensation for such "total regulatory takings," except to the extent that "background principles of nuisance and property law" independently restrict the owner's intended use of the property.[5]

Two subsequent Supreme Court cases explain further the *Lucas* doctrine. In *Palazzolo v. Rhode Island* (2005), the Court held that a property owner could bring a per se takings claim for statutes and regulations (as opposed to common law nuisance) that were in place at the time the property was acquired.[6] Palazzolo was repeatedly denied planning permission for development of his coastal property. Even though he knew about the restrictive rules prior to buying the land, the Court permitted a regulatory takings claim for the loss of all economic value in his property. Property rights advocates hailed the decision in *Palazzolo*,[7] although on remand he lost his regulatory takings claim.[8] In *Tahoe-Sierra Preservation Council, Inc. v. Tahoe Regional Planning Agency* (2002), the Supreme Court made clear that when government enacts *temporary* regulation denying a property owner all viable economic use of property, there is no per se taking. Rather, temporary moratoria on land use are to be decided by applying the balancing factors discussed below.[9]

Outside of these two relatively narrow categories of per se takings—physical invasion of property and total loss of economic value—regulatory takings are governed by a balancing test established in *Penn Central Transportation Co. v. New York City* (1978) that takes into account: (1) the economic impact of the regulation on the property

[1] "Leading Cases," *Harvard Law Review*, 119 (2005): 169-414, 297.

[2] It is important to emphasize that zoning laws are not considered regulatory takings. The Supreme Court considers land use restrictions to be within the states' broad police powers. *Village of Euclid v. Ambler Realty Co.*, 272 U.S. 365 (1926) (upholding a zoning regulation even though it reduced the value of land because the regulation bore a rational relationship to public health and safety).

[3] *Loretto v. Teleprompter Manhattan CATV Corp.*, 458 U.S. 419 (1982) (holding that a state law requiring landlords to permit cable companies to install cable facilities in apartment buildings effected a taking).

[4] *Lucas v. South Carolina Coastal Council*, 505 U.S. 1003, 1029 (1992).

[5] Under *Lucas*, "background principles" can bar any type of per se claim, whether based on physical occupation or denial of all economic value.

[6] *Palazzolo v. Rhode Island*, 533 U.S. 606 (2001). The Court, however, determined there was no per se taking because the land still had economically valuable use. The Court remanded for a balancing analysis under *Penn Central*.

[7] Harold Johnson, "Supreme Court Strikes a Blow for Property Rights," *Wall Street Journal*, July 3, 2001.

[8] *Palazzolo v. Rhode Island*, 2005 WL 1645974, *14 (holding that "Palazzolo could have had little or no reasonable expectation to develop the parcel as he has now proposed. Constitutional law does not require the state to guarantee a bad investment").

[9] *Tahoe-Sierra Preservation Council, Inc. v. Tahoe Regional Planning Agency*, 535 U.S. 302 (2002).

owner; (2) the extent to which the regulation has interfered with investment-backed expectations; and (3) the character of the governmental action.[10]

The Court has noted that these three inquiries—permanent physical invasion, loss of all economically beneficial use, and the *Penn Central* balancing test—share a common touchstone: "Each aims to identify regulatory actions that are functionally equivalent to the classic taking in which government directly appropriates private property or ousts the owner from his domain."[11] Accordingly, each criterion focuses directly on the severity of the burden imposed by the government upon private property rights.

In *Agins v. City of Tiburon* (1980), a case involving municipal zoning, the Supreme Court said that there is a taking if the ordinance does not "substantially advance legitimate state interests."[12] This test was highly solicitous of property rights, as it finds a taking even in cases where the intrusion on the owner is slight. But in *Lingle v. Chevron U.S.A.* (2005), the Supreme Court ruled unanimously that *Agins* is not a valid method of identifying compensable regulatory takings. It prescribes an inquiry in the nature of a due process test, which has no proper place in the Court's takings jurisprudence.[13]

Lingle represents a victory for public health regulation. It abandons the "heightened scrutiny" of the "directly advances" formula, which would have given judges the power to interfere with a multitude of government actions on land use, zoning, rent control, and the environment. The Court indicated that regulatory takings could be found only in those situations that are so dire as to be "functionally equivalent to the classic [physical] taking." The case appropriately limits the potential use of the Takings Clause and may return the Court to a path of restraint in the creation of economic rights.[14] However, much still depends on the Roberts Court, which could resurrect the regulatory takings doctrine by using either *Lucas* or a *Penn Central* balancing test with a bite.

[10] *Penn Central Transportation Co. v. New York City*, 438 U.S. 104, 124 (1978).
[11] *Lingle v. Chevron USA, Inc.*, 544 U.S. 528, 539 (2005).
[12] *Agins v. City of Tiburon*, 447 U.S. 255, 260 (1980).
[13] *Lingle*, 544 U.S. at 545.
[14] "Judicial Takings and Givings," *Washington Post*, May 29, 2005.

rules, which cannot be brought if they were in place at the time of purchase, and challenges to statutes and regulations, which can be made even if they were in place at the time of purchase. Consequently, when democratically elected government, according to modern standards, regulates to avert a public harm or promote a public good, it cannot be certain whether it will be compelled to compensate property owners. This narrowing of what may be considered a nuisance and expansion of property interests effectively constrains police power regulation. The Court, in effect, has simultaneously frozen the understanding of public health that existed in earlier times, while allowing the normative value of property to expand to meet modern libertarian expectations.

Lucas poses a threat to public health regulation because it adopts a rule imposing a categorical duty to compensate property owners. As the Supreme Court itself recognized, "Land-use regulations are ubiquitous and most of them impact property values in some tangential way—often in completely unanticipated ways. Treating them all as *per se* takings would transform government regulation into a luxury few governments could afford."[162] Public health regulation, however, rarely obliterates the value of property, and the future of *Lucas,* therefore, is uncertain. Although lower courts have been highly reluctant to apply this rule and find a per se taking,[163] the conservative wing of the Supreme Court and property rights advocates outside the Court still have ambitions to revitalize a categorical rule of regulatory takings.[164] For example, the Supreme Court of Ohio found a per se taking when state regulations designed to protect public drinking water prevented coal mining operations.[165] And strong property rights protections have been enacted by the states to constrain environmental regulation.[166]

Most regulatory takings cases do not involve a complete loss of property value. These cases are governed by a balancing formula established in *Penn Central Transportation Co. v. New York City* (1978) that takes into account:[167] (1) the economic impact of the regulation on the property owner; (2) the extent to which the regulation has interfered with investment-backed expectations; and (3) the character of the governmental action.[168] Balancing tests of this kind often suggest a permissive standard of review, but this does not mean that the Supreme Court will not use *Penn Central* as a strong vehicle for protection of property rights in the future. For example, federal courts have ruled that steps taken to protect the public's food supply[169] or even to protect trade secrets (e.g., compelled disclosure of the ingredients in cigarettes)[170] can constitute a taking under the more flexible *Penn Central* test.

If Charles Fried in the epigraph was correct in describing a conservative plan to use the Takings Clause as a severe constraint on public health regulation, then the outcome remains uncertain. Much depends on the direction of the Supreme Court, which, at present, has several members apparently committed to expansion of the regulatory takings doctrine.[171] This split among the Justices is likely to be manifested in many property rights cases to come. It is too soon to tell whether the Roberts Court will elevate economic justice to a new level in our constitutional democracy.

WHAT IS A "PUBLIC USE"? *KELO V. NEW LONDON*

The concept of the public welfare is broad and inclusive. . . . The values it represents are spiritual as well as physical, aesthetic as well as monetary. It is within the power of the legislature to determine that the community should be beautiful as well as healthy, spacious as well as clean, well-balanced as well as carefully patrolled . . . . If those who govern the District of Columbia decide that the Nation's Capital should be beautiful as well as sanitary, there is nothing in the Fifth Amendment that stands in the way.

Justice William O. Douglas (1954)

That alone is a just government, which impartially secures to every man, whatever is his own.

James Madison (1792)

The Fifth Amendment authorizes the state to take private property only for a justifying "public use." If the government took property to confer a private benefit, the taking would be unconstitutional, even if the owner were fully compensated.[172] Classically, the state may not take the property of one person for the sole purpose of transferring it to another private person.[173] It would obviously be unjust to use the power of eminent domain purely to transfer wealth from one private party to another. However, what if the state's purpose were to advance the public interest in health, welfare, prosperity, or another public good, but nevertheless conferred an economic advantage on private parties?

The term *public use* is susceptible to a narrow or broad interpretation. In its narrow sense, public use literally is "use by the public," where the government takes ownership (e.g., a public utility) or grants access to the public (e.g., a park, road, or railway). In its broader sense, public use is when the taking benefits the public. The Supreme Court historically has preferred an expansive understanding of public use, defining it more as a "public purpose." Court decisions have conceived of public use as virtually coterminous with the police powers.[174] Like the "rational basis" test discussed in chapter 4, the Court has upheld the power of eminent domain provided it is "rationally related to a conceivable public purpose."[175] The Court has afforded elected bodies due deference, moreover, in deciding what forms of development benefit the public. The Supreme Court, for example, was highly permissive in upholding the District of Columbia's use of eminent domain to acquire slum properties and transfer them to private developers to remove blight in the city, as expressed in Justice Douglas's epigraph.[176]

The Supreme Court's expansive understanding of public use was affirmed in a bitterly contested 5–4 decision in *Kelo v. New London* (2005), where the Court ruled that government could use its eminent domain power to take property for the purpose of spurring private economic development. In *Kelo,* homeowners in an economically distressed city challenged the condemnation of their property under a comprehensive urban renewal plan designed to increase jobs and augment tax revenue. The Court found that economic development is a "long accepted function of government," and refused to limit the use of eminent domain to properties that are "blighted" or to require government to show a "reasonable certainty" that the expected public benefits actually would ensue.[177]

The decision was widely criticized within the Court and by American politicians, and was commonly seen as benefiting large corporations at the expense of homeowners and small businesses. Four dissenting Justices fervently appealed to the Founders' vision of the "security," "sanctity," and "inviolability" of private property and the "natural rights" of property owners, declaring, "The specter of condemnation hangs over all property."[178] And Justice Thomas said, "Losses will fall disproportionately on poor communities. Those communities are not only systematically less likely to put their lands to the highest and best social use, but are also the least politically powerful."[179] Public opinion polls showed overwhelming disapproval of the ruling;[180] the House passed the Private Property Protection Act by a vote of 376 to 38, denying federal funds to cities and states that use eminent domain for private commercial development;[181] and states rushed to proscribe such uses of eminent domain.[182] Local town boards in New Hampshire even threatened to seize the property of Justices Breyer and Souter for joining the majority in *Kelo.*[183]

Was the almost universal denunciation of *Kelo* justified, or was it part of an overly romantic American ideal of the private home and the small business owner fighting big government?[184] Certainly private owners can endure hardship when their property is taken by eminent domain: They may have a sentimental attachment, the compensation may not be enough to make them feel "whole," and private developers may gain economic windfalls.[185] Undoubtedly, eminent domain is used more often in poor, minority neighborhoods than in well-heeled communities.[186]

Despite the hardship for the few, eminent domain can bring significant benefit to the many. The exercise of police powers entails trade-offs, almost by definition, so that individual interests are diminished while collective interests are enhanced. And eminent domain, even for economic development, *does* confer substantial benefits for the public's health, safety, and welfare. Land-use policy goes to the heart of local government planning for healthy and prosperous societies, which would be

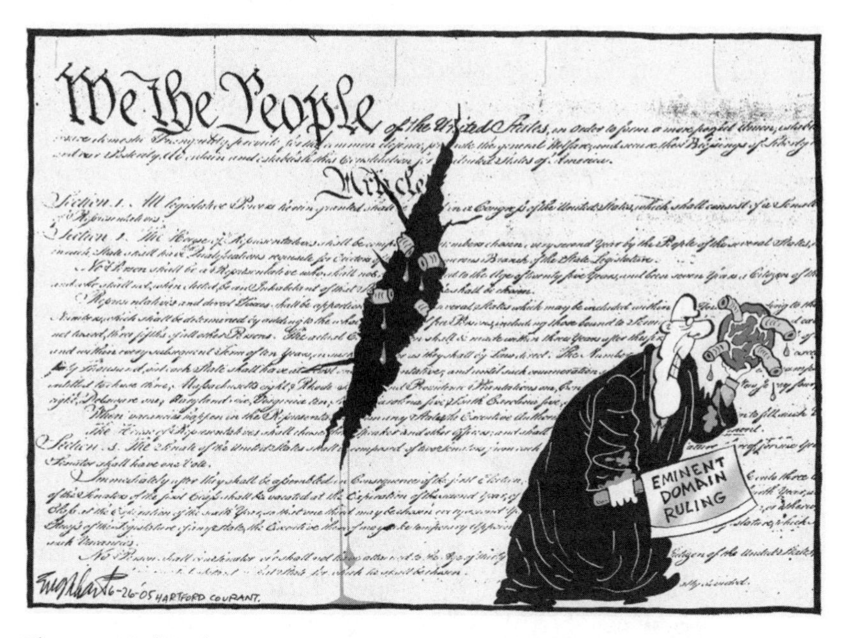

Photo 26. Political cartoon criticizing the *Kelo* ruling. The depicted cartoon represents the rampant public hostility in response to the *Kelo* ruling. *Kelo* was attacked by critics as expanding the scope of the government's eminent domain power and stripping individuals, especially the poor and vulnerable, of their property rights. © 2005 Bob Englehart.

thwarted without the power of eminent domain.[187] For example, improving run-down urban areas can diminish some of the more intractable problems of slum living: alcohol and drug abuse, firearm and other violence, lead exposure in children, contamination of drinking water, asthma from cockroaches or mold, exposure to pests and toxins, and a dearth of facilities for nutritious food, recreation, and exercise that can increase risks of obesity and chronic diseases.

When desperately poor urban communities are revitalized through a comprehensive plan of improvement, the vast majority of people in those neighborhoods benefit: The area is more beautiful and livable, jobs are more plentiful, and problems of the inner city discussed above are curtailed. In *Kelo,* the city of New London was suffering from deep economic and social disadvantage and had been designated as a "distressed municipality"—showing steep economic decline, high unemployment, and fewer residents in 2005 than in 1920. The city council's comprehensive development plan promised parks, a river walk, jobs, an environmental cleanup, and a "small urban village" with restaurants and shopping.

When Justice Thomas and other economic conservatives contend that the poor and vulnerable are exploited, what do they mean? In New London, and in most comparable cities, the overwhelming majority of residents voluntarily sell their homes, and the whole community benefits from the improvements. Poor people usually do not choose to live in derelict neighborhoods with no prospect of hope or change, and most want the government to pursue well-designed plans for social and economic improvement. It is too easy to champion the few "holdouts" who, by refusing to sell their property, can spoil plans to rejuvenate public spaces and improve the well-being of residents.

It is well to consider that the most vocal critics of *Kelo* were not the people of New London or their elected representatives, but rather those who routinely defend private entrepreneurs and free markets.[188] The conservative wing of the Supreme Court has long sought to limit government control over private property.[189] And the Institute of Justice, which brought *Kelo* and has since waged a tenacious public campaign against eminent domain, describes itself as an activist libertarian organization for individual economic liberty.[190] Libertarian groups make emotive claims regarding state exploitation of the downtrodden and the vulnerability of "a family's home or church."[191] Yet, in other important ways, *Kelo* was a highly conservative decision, upholding a federalist vision of local democratic decision making, judicial restraint, and due deference to elected officials.[192] Granting city leaders latitude to seek innovative solutions for struggling urban communities is better than having federal judges sit in judgment of whether land-use plans are sufficiently "public."[193]

Government must make hard choices when faced with desperately poor and dilapidated inner cities. It is not possible to act boldly for the common good while privileging a small handful of property owners. Nor is it possible to revitalize communities without conferring some economic advantage on private developers. The essence of public health is that it seeks to benefit most of the population while acting deliberatively, transparently, and fairly.

The constitutional interpretation of the Takings Clause for which I have advocated—both for regulatory takings and urban redevelopment—is not intended to show disrespect for private property. Instead, as articulated by the Georgetown University Environmental Law and Policy Institute, it suggests that individual property rights must be defined in relation to the rights and needs of all other citizens to health, safety, and environmental protection. And it reflects the conclusion that resolution of the conflict between private rights and public goods is primarily for democratically elected representatives of the people rather than the judiciary. Philosophical opponents of state regulation drive the property rights movement in the United States. If the public had to pay every time government regulated, it would chill state action for the common good. And if cities could not exercise powers of eminent domain, it would seriously impede rejuvenation of long-neglected communities. At the same time, other property owners and other citizens would suffer harm to their health, well-being, and the environment in which they live.[194]

Certainly, the courts should curtail powers of eminent domain intended to provide special favors for private developers. But government should be empowered to exercise these powers to clean up environmental hazards, ameliorate unsanitary or unsafe conditions, and reinvigorate communities stricken by violence, drug abuse, or other detriments to the public's health.

THE NORMATIVE VALUE OF ECONOMIC LIBERTY

When health is absent
Wisdom cannot reveal itself,
Art cannot become manifest
Strength cannot fight,
Wealth becomes useless
And intelligence cannot be applied.

Herophilus (325 B.C.)

As we have seen throughout this book, government regulation for the public's health inevitably interferes with personal or economic liberties. The Supreme Court usually grants the legislature deference in the exercise of police powers. A permissive approach to government regulation is justified, in part, by democratic values; citizens elect representatives to make complex policy choices.[195] A legislative choice to prefer collective health and well-being over individual interests deserves respect and insulation from aggressive judicial scrutiny. This is broadly the judicial approach to public health regulation that affects personal autonomy. Heightened scrutiny is reserved for those rare instances where public health interventions intrude on fundamental rights and interests, such as total deprivation of liberty.

The normative issue is whether there is something in the nature of economic liberty that warrants a departure from the normal deference to public health regulation. Put another way, how important is unbridled freedom in property uses, financial relationships, and the pursuit of occupations? I see no reason why the diminution of economic liberties should be taken more seriously than the many deprivations of personal autonomy and privacy that routinely occur with public health regulation (e.g., vaccination, reporting, and contact tracing). Courts generally understand that some loss of individual freedom is necessary for the common welfare. Regulation that interferes with civil liberties does not cause conservative thinkers undue concern; nor is there any discussion of compensation to those who must forgo liberty for the collective good.

The same logic ought to apply to economic regulation for the common welfare. The reason for the governmental intervention usually is to prevent owners from using their private property in ways that are harmful to the public interest. Thus, the state's aim is not to deny economic opportunity per se, but only to foreclose commercial activities that are detrimental to the public's health and safety. The creation of private wealth, moreover, hardly can be regarded as a fundamental interest akin to loss of personal freedom, for private wealth creation is not essential to the achievement of a healthy and fulfilling life. Rarely does economic regulation affect an individual's basic ability to obtain the necessities of life, such as food, shelter, and medical care. Indeed, the purpose of such regulation is to meet the needs of the many.

The conservative claim, of course, is not only that economic liberties have intrinsic value, but that they have instrumental value as well. They claim that preserving economic liberty will help create wealth for the community at large. Even assuming that economic freedom reliably leads to greater overall prosperity, it is still reasonable for a legislature to make a social choice that favors immediate health and safety benefits over future wealth creation. A community cannot benefit from increased prosperity if it experiences excess morbidity and mortality from hazardous commercial activity.

Government, to be sure, ought not carelessly or gratuitously interfere with economic freedoms. If government has a reason, however, based on averting a risk to the public's health, then there is nothing in the nature of economic liberty that should prevent the state from intervening, nor is there any reason why the state should provide compensation for regulating private commercial activities deemed detrimental to the communal good.

PART FOUR

The Future of the Public's Health

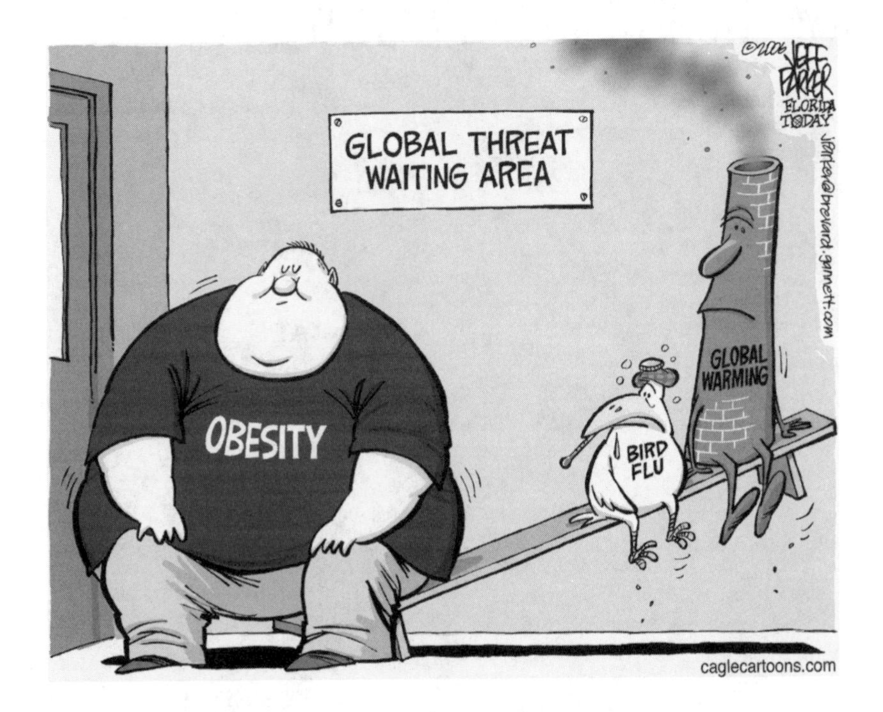

Photo 27. Increased attention to obesity. This cartoon is one example of the significant attention that the obesity epidemic has garnered in the popular press. It depicts obesity as a threat to the United States on a par with pandemics and climate change. © 2006 Parker.

CHAPTER 13

Concluding Reflections on the Field

> Public health is the science and the art of preventing disease, prolonging life, and promoting physical health and efficiency through organized community efforts for the sanitation of the environment, the control of community infections, the education of the individual in principles of personal hygiene, the organization of medical and nursing service for the early diagnosis and preventive treatment of disease, and the development of the social machinery which will ensure to every individual a standard of living adequate for the maintenance of health; organizing these benefits in such fashion as to enable every citizen to realize his birthright of health and longevity.
>
> Charles-Edward Winslow (1920)

Public health typically is regarded as a positivistic pursuit, and undoubtedly, our understanding of the etiology and response to disease is heavily influenced by scientific inquiry. Nonetheless, this book has been devoted to the core idea that law is essential for creating the conditions for people to lead healthier and safer lives. Law creates a mission for public health agencies, assigns their functions, and specifies the manner in which they may exercise their authority. The law is a tool in public health work, used to influence norms for healthy behavior, identify and respond to health threats, and set and enforce health and safety standards.[1]

The essential job of public health agencies is to identify what makes people healthy and what makes them sick, and then to take the steps necessary to make sure that the population encounters a maximum of the former and a minimum of the latter. At first glance, this would seem to be uncontroversial, but the pursuit of public health creates fundamental social and political disputes almost by definition. Public health is rooted in the biomedical and social sciences, but from the moment of asserting some collective responsibility for the population's health, officials have to manage a complex political process and operate with finite resources. Public health agencies, in particular, confront inherent problems concerning politics and money, leadership and jurisdiction, and legitimacy and trust.[2] These are not barriers to good public health that somehow can be overcome by law. They are, rather, unavoidable conditions of public health, conditions with which agencies must find ways to cope to achieve the gains in health that are possible in an imperfect political, social, and economic environment.

This chapter offers brief concluding reflections on the public health field and its inescapable connection to politics and government in a constitutional democracy. The chapter ends with a case study on perhaps the most controversial modern problem facing public health: the prevention of chronic diseases caused by overweight and obesity. America, and most of the rest of the world, is experiencing an epidemiological transition from infectious to chronic disease. The challenge for the field is how far it can legitimately go in influencing or controlling individual behaviors that pose little risk to others. If public health officials are proactive they risk losing political support, but if they remain passive they ignore the most common causes of illness, disability, and premature death in the population.

PUBLIC HEALTH, POLITICS, AND MONEY

> From my perspective, as a White House official watching the budgetary process, and subsequently as head first of a health care financing agency and then of a public health agency, I was continually amazed to watch as billions of dollars were allocated to financing medical care with little discussion, whereas endless arguments ensued over a few millions for community prevention programs. The sums that were the basis for prolonged, and often futile, budget fights in public health were treated as rounding errors in the Medicare budget.
>
> William Roper (1994)

The ability of public health authorities to attract support is essential to their success, for, as its daily practice reminds us, public health operates in a world of choices in the allocation of limited resources. The great sanitarian Hermann Biggs famously remarked that "public health is purchasable,"[3] but because there will always be limits on how much we are willing to buy, public health will always turn on allocational decisions. Thus, the field of public health is as inherently political (i.e., concerned with the distribution of resources in society) as it is technological (i.e., concerned with the deployment of scientific knowledge).[4]

If the field of public health is essentially political, one might assume that attracting public and financial support would not be difficult, given the undoubted communal benefits of health. But, as the epigraph from William Roper illustrates, the condition of public health is one of paradox. Most people support a high level of public health, fewer are eager to pay for it, and many are positively opposed to changing their own activities to promote it. Public health officials have enormous legal power, yet they often cannot exercise it for political, cultural, or resource reasons. The public cares passionately about health threats, but often in inverse relation to the quantitative magnitude of the risk (see chapter 2). The measures that provide the most societal benefit often provide little or no discernible benefit to any one person, and vice versa.[5] Although there is a virtually bottomless purse for treating illness, it appears there is little in the budget to prevent it or, more generally, to ensure the conditions in which people can be healthy.[6]

Even within the relatively modest budgets devoted to public health, there remain hard choices. Public health officials are inevitably faced with the need to divide a small pie among many worthy competitors for resources. Injuries, HIV, emerging infectious diseases, bioterrorism, chronic disease, and many other health threats are, in some sense, in competition for prevention resources. Difficult decisions must be made about the most effective allocation of funds. Thus, rationing—a controversial notion in medicine—is, in public health, a "moral imperative . . . in the face of scarce resources."[7]

LEADERSHIP AND JURISDICTION

Public health agencies face the challenge of explaining why injury and disease prevention and health promotion are important and deserve the support of policymakers and the public. Effective public health work requires leaders who can win battles in the halls of government. Programs have to be approved by executives and funded by legislators in an environment of scarcity, and often political polarization. Effective leaders understand the value of the political process and seize it as an opportunity to define important health issues and take the lead in solving them.

Public health scholars and practitioners perceive a crisis in leadership, despite its importance.[8] Although some health department leaders are astute politically and have established their credibility in government and the community, many others view politicians and legislators as unwelcome impediments to effective public health action.

Public health leadership requires planning, collaboration with each of the branches of government, building popular support, and the capacity to exercise political skill. Public health policy development requires prioritizing health problems, identifying solutions, and determining who can best implement them. Ideally, public health policy should include long-range planning that forecasts resource needs, maintains the public health infrastructure, and anticipates new health threats. Without long-range planning, health departments may find crises—such as an environmental accident, a disease outbreak, bioterrorism, or a natural disaster—driving their priority setting and policymaking. Arguably, this has already occurred, as public health leaders have been tugged and pulled from one crisis to another, ranging from anthrax, smallpox, and SARS to avian influenza. From the leadership point of view, a planning process that includes communities in identifying priorities and fashioning responses is an excellent way to create political support for health programs, quite apart from its benefits in building better programs in the first place.

Even the most powerful and best-led public health agency could not exercise direct authority over the full range of activities that affect health. Occupational safety, environmental protection, and the purity of food and drinking water are often the province of other agencies, and much of the behavior that public health officials try to change (e.g., diet, exercise, and smoking) is not subject to direct legal regulation at all. And in other spheres, such as reduction of socioeconomic disparities, public health agencies play only a marginal role. Since many determinants of health are outside the jurisdiction of health agencies, in developing policy, public health officials must collaborate with other federal and state agencies (e.g., environment, agriculture, highway safety, housing, welfare, social services, and law enforcement), community-based organizations (e.g., nongovernmental organizations, activists, and consumers), the private sector (e.g., business, labor, and health care), philanthropic organizations (e.g., the Gates, Clinton, and Ford foundations), and academic institutions (e.g., schools of public health, nursing, dentistry, medicine, and law).

Public health agencies often can accomplish their goals only by instigating and coordinating health-enhancing activities in these spheres. Thus, every health agency faces the challenge of using its expertise and persuasive power to encourage and facilitate others to take actions that are consistent with the goals of public health. The jurisdictional problem, therefore, casts the health agency in the roles of educator and persuader. It also requires the health department to act as an expert for other agencies and to coordinate government policy affecting the population's health.

LEGITIMACY AND TRUST

Public health agencies rely on voluntary cooperation by those at risk and the support of the population at large. Consequently, they must appear credible in the advice they render and trustworthy in their practices. Despite its importance, agencies face considerable challenges in maintaining public confidence both because they are organs of government and because, by necessity, they are engaged in a highly political process.

Public health agencies are fixtures of public administration, part of the structure of government since the earliest times of the republic (see chapter 5). As such, they possess the trappings of government: generalized mistrust, doubts about efficiency, and fear of oppression. If the public perceives health officials simply as the tool of an overreaching government captured by special interests, their ability to win compliance and support is compromised. Likewise, public health measures become subject to general legal limitations on governmental activity and to prevailing attitudes about the sorts of things government ought to do. This dynamic can be seen in multiple public health activities characterized as the "Nanny State"—e.g., seat belts, motorcycle helmets, water fluoridation, smoking bans in public places, and obesity prevention. Many disputes in public health turn less on its goal, which everyone professes to support, and more on the proper scope of government intervention to achieve it.

To maintain legitimacy and trust, public health authorities rely on expert knowledge derived from the sciences of public health. Scientific decisions are thought to be more objective and systematic, and less captive to political ideology. Health officials know that this expertise gives them the authority and the ability to convince. Yet health officials, to be effective, must be willing to embrace and excel in the political process. It is precisely this political involvement that risks weakening the impression of professional neutrality and expertise from which public health officials draw their public credibility.

Winning and maintaining the trust of those at risk of disease and of the general public are preconditions for effective public health programs. This helps explain the importance of finding a way to maintain scientific rigor while still engaging effectively in the political process.

There is perhaps no better illustration of the challenges faced by the field than the raging contemporary debates about the legitimate role of public health in preventing overweight and obesity. This book concludes by exploring this problem, which provides a way to summarize the various legal tools available to prevent or ameliorate disease, together with the formidable political problems of accomplishing public health goals in a way that is acceptable to society.

POWERS AND LIMITS IN PUBLIC HEALTH: A CASE STUDY ON OBESITY AND CHRONIC DISEASE

Government can give people the information, legislate and regulate to encourage sustainable living, help business to function in a more environmentally responsible way. . . . But it can't "do it" by itself. "Doing it" will depend on the decisions and choices of millions of individuals and companies. Our task is to empower them to make the right ones. . . . Government has to encourage, it has to inform, but, if necessary, in a tougher way than ever before. Our public health problems are not, strictly speaking, public health questions at all. They are questions of individual lifestyle—obesity, smoking, alcohol abuse, diabetes, sexually transmitted disease. These are not epidemics in the epidemiological sense. They are the result of millions of individual decisions, at millions of points in time. These individual actions lead to collective costs. . . . But the question still hangs in the air: whose responsibility is it? The individual? The state? The company? Should it be a proper area for Government intervention at all? . . . Now we have legislation on a host of matters pertaining to public health: food, air, water quality, drinking and driving, drug classification, seatbelts, childproof medicine bottles, speed restrictions. . . . I want the health debate to be about prevention as much as cure, about personal responsibility as much as collec-

> tive responsibility, about the quality of living as much as life expectancy. . . . It means changes in Government, business and people, but that is the way the modern state should work.
>
> Tony Blair (2006)

Previous chapters explored the traditional public health activities of communicable disease control and commercial regulation. These activities have deep historical roots and strong public support. The public intuitively understands the dangers of transmission of infectious disease within the population and accepts, even demands, state action. Since the dangers are hidden and individuals are powerless to protect themselves, the polity relies on the state to monitor and respond to epidemic disease. The citizenry may keenly debate the necessity of vaccination, treatment, or quarantine in particular cases, but it does not question the legitimacy of government efforts to control infectious diseases.

Commercial regulation also has a strong level of public acceptance. Businesses are vital to society, but they can pose risks to employees from unsafe workplaces, to communities from toxic exposures, and to consumers from hazardous products. The public expects government to regulate businesses to reduce these harms, understanding that the market cannot adequately protect those placed at risk. Critics may contest commercial regulation that is excessively burdensome or unnecessary, but everyone accepts the basic premise that the state has a responsibility in this sphere.

The same cannot be said about prevention of chronic diseases, such as cardiovascular disease, cancer, or diabetes. Here, the polity actively disputes the claim that government has a significant role to play. The reason is that a person's own behavior is often the root cause of the disease. Individuals make personal choices about their diet, exercise, and lifestyle, so disease is often thought of as a matter of personal, not governmental, responsibility. The state can inform, even persuade individuals to make the healthy choice, but it cannot limit that choice or, worse, coerce individuals. After all, a person's decision about what to eat or whether to exercise affects only him- or herself, so many do not see government intervention as justifiable.

There are, however, serious problems with this story of individualism and personal responsibility. As Tony Blair explains, "Millions of individual decisions, at millions of points in time" impose enormous collective costs. These personal choices result in substantial, and increasing, burdens of disease in society that adversely affect human well-being, the community, and the economy. Individual behaviors result in illness, pain, disability, and death, which profoundly affect the happiness of individuals, the functioning of social groups, and the prosperity of nations, with massive costs in medical care and lost productivity.[9]

There is another problem with the story that individuals must live with the consequences of their own choices. People certainly have a degree of freedom in making choices about their lifestyle, but individuals are embedded in societies, and their environments profoundly affect the decisions that they can and do make. Government can help structure the physical and social environment to help people make healthier choices. But should public health agencies intervene, given the prevailing culture of individual liberty and free enterprise?

This case study explores a series of important questions at the intersection of law, health, and politics. What is the legitimate role of government in influencing or controlling personal behavior? What is the appropriate level at which the obesity epidemic should be tackled—the individual, corporations, or society as a whole? If government has a role to play, how far should it go—education, persuasion, and disclosure, or even taxation, zoning, regulation, and liability? It will be helpful first to examine the obesity epidemic and ask whether it is an epidemic at all in the traditional sense of the term.

The Obesity "Epidemic": The Burden of Illness and Death in the Population

> People must take responsibility for their own lives. They must recognize that the pose of helplessness is not just detrimental to their individual dignity, it also saps them and their communities of the spirit of enterprise that makes a healthy and vibrant society. The real epidemics threatening Britain today are not smoking or obesity; they are passivity, the culture of victimhood and stifling government paternalism.
>
> *London Times* (2004)

Obesity, one of the ten leading U.S. health indicators,[10] is associated with increased risk of death from type 2 diabetes, hypertension, coronary heart disease, stroke, and certain cancers.[11] Yet the proportion of overweight and obese children and adults is alarmingly high.[12] In 2005, 60.5 percent of adults in the United States were overweight, 23.9 percent were obese, and 3 percent were extremely obese. African Americans had the highest obesity prevalence at 33.9 percent.[13] The prevalence of adult obesity increased significantly in every state during the last decade, so that no state will meet the Department of Health and Human Services "Healthy People 2010" goals.[14] Similarly, 16 percent of children and adolescents were overweight, an increase of nearly 50 percent over a five-year period.[15] Obesity could shorten the average lifespan of an entire generation by two to five years, which would result in the first reversal in life expectancy since the government started tracking data in 1900. Already, average adult life expectancy in the United States may be four to nine months shorter than it would be if no Americans were obese.[16] The global dimensions of obesity are equally apparent, with more than one billion adults overweight, and at least 300 million of them clinically obese.[17]

Despite the magnitude of these data, public health researchers have been roundly criticized for exaggerating the health threat. Conservative commentators have accused the CDC of overly zealous and careless advocacy.[18] In 2005, the CDC acknowledged that, due to a statistical error, it had overestimated the number of deaths caused by poor diet and physical inactivity, and lowered its estimate from 400,000 to 320,000 deaths per year.[19] Later that year, CDC researchers reported 112,000 obesity-attributable deaths, far lower than the original estimate.[20] These variable estimates are probably the result of different assumptions about confounding variables, such as smoking, substance abuse, and socioeconomic status.[21]

However, even the lowest estimates of excess deaths are disturbing, vastly exceeding the mortality rates of well-recognized public health problems such as AIDS, vehicle crashes, and injuries.[22] At the highest estimates, the death rates from obesity approach those of smoking, a point emphasized by the Surgeon General.[23] And the CDC struck back at its detractors by stating that "our principal conclusions remain unchanged: Tobacco use and poor diet and physical inactivity contributed to the largest number of deaths, and the number of deaths related to poor diet and physical inactivity is increasing."[24]

Critics of the public health approach object to the way obesity is characterized as an "epidemic," saying it conveys an unwarranted sense of urgency. Critics argue that, by evoking the image of impending crisis, agencies can more easily justify public health regulation. In one sense, obesity is correctly described as an epidemic: "A disease affecting many people at the same time." But in another, it lacks some of the elements of disease epidemics, notably "spreading from person to person."[25] "Whatever the problems with obesity," writes Richard Epstein, "it is not a communicable disease, with the fear and pandemonium that real epidemics let loose in their wake."[26] The dangers posed by pathogens are concealed, and individuals are powerless to defend themselves. But the dangers of obesity are well known and controllable. People feel capable of making their own choices about diet and exercise, and many say they do not need government to protect them.

This is why obesity regulation is so troubling to segments of the political community. Unlike a "true" communicable disease epidemic, obesity does not appear to be a *public* health problem in the classical sense. A person's decision about what to eat or whether to exercise is purely self-regarding; the individual's choice affects no one but him- or herself. Each person's decision can have powerfully adverse consequences for his or her vitality and longevity, but it still leaves other individuals to make their own choice. Seen in this way, diet and exercise are matters of individual or parental responsibility, and do not fall within the appropriate sphere of government.

The public is uncomfortable with government telling or forcing people to behave in certain ways because it is overtly paternalistic, suggesting that officials know best about what is good for the individual and her family. Modern society is often antipaternalistic, prizing personal sovereignty and distrusting governmental interference in private matters. But there are other ways to view government's role in combating obesity that may justify limiting people's choices for their own good. Seeing obesity from a population and social justice perspective may provide insights into why government has an important role to play.

A Population-Based Approach to Obesity

Some support limited state action to curb obesity because individuals lack sufficient willpower to defer immediate gratification for long-term health benefits.[27] Although people often struggle with their immediate cravings and fail to safeguard their long-term interests, this is still a highly individualistic way to see the problem of obesity. Obesity regulation to protect people from their own temptations is explicitly paternalistic and does not overcome prevailing cultural and political concerns.

Public health paternalism is best understood from a population-based perspective, where the principal concern is overall societal welfare rather than individual preferences. Obesity regulation is intended to benefit the community as a whole. Its goal is not to affect the choices of any particular person but to build a healthier population. Even if decisions on what to eat are primarily self-regarding, the aggregate effects of people's choices are countless preventable disabilities and deaths. There is little doubt that if society could be structured in ways that make it even a little bit easier for individuals to make healthier choices, it would result in greater societal well-being and productivity. Government's responsibility is to the collective, as well as the individual, so it may be just as important to safeguard the population from chronic disease as it is from infectious disease.

There is also an economic argument that is frequently used in response to claims that government policy is paternalistic. Obesity-attributable medical expenditures reached $75 billion in 2003, with substantial additional indirect costs in lost productivity.[28] The costs of obesity are rapidly increasing, moreover.[29] Critics of state regulation argue that individuals absorb the cost of their own illness, so there is no "public" issue at play, but taxpayers finance about half of all medical costs through Medicare and Medicaid, and employers cover much of the rest. The government has a legitimate interest in controlling medical and social costs of individuals' unhealthy behaviors, which are borne by society at large.[30]

This still leaves the consequential question about whether government interventions would, in fact, reduce chronic disease and, if so, what interventions would work best. Many of the strongest critiques of state action suggest that it does not work and would provoke a popular backlash against heavy-handed governmental interference. Centralized solutions will fail, they argue, because they cannot take account of the wide variation in circumstances among individuals, ranging from differences in genetics to environmental factors.[31]

This claim, of course, misses the central understanding of epidemiology, which is captured in Geoffrey Rose's prevention paradox: A prevention measure that brings much benefit to the population will not benefit each participating individual.[32] For example, tiny changes in the eating and exercise habits of millions of people may have little effect on any given person but would have enormous benefits for overall population health precisely because excess weight is such a prevalent cause of chronic disease. The prevention paradox, in turn, creates a sociopolitical problem: Individuals are less likely to accept and support interventions that offer them little personal advantage. This is particularly true if individuals believe they have the right to make ill-advised or beneficial decisions on their own without the state meddling in their personal lives.

Perhaps there is no way to frame obesity regulation to overcome the objection that it is paternalistic, and all one can do is argue that there remains a role for benign paternalism in the modern state. If state measures are, in the words of Hermann Biggs, "plainly designed for the public good," then at least the polity should consider them.[33] If paternalistic measures significantly reduce illness and premature death with minimal burdens on individual freedom, should they be out-of-bounds simply because they fail to meet a philosophical standard of self-sovereignty? Should a caring society refuse to act when its members suffer such high burdens of preventable disease? If so, public health agencies would become powerless to effectively respond to one of the most common causes of disability and death.[34]

A Social Justice Approach to Obesity

There is another way to view the problem of obesity that offers a further justification for government intervention. Racial minorities and the poor suffer substantial and disproportionate burdens from obesity. Poor diet and sedentary lifestyles are undoubtedly a contributing cause of socioeconomic disparities in health.[35] Government passivity, leaving individuals free to make unfettered choices, will almost certainly perpetuate health disparities. A social justice perspective requires the state to identify and ameliorate the common causes of disease and premature death among the most deprived.[36] It supports systematic action to redress persistent patterns of disadvantage, even if ill health is attributable to personal lifestyles (see chapter 1).

The most disadvantaged do not have even remotely the same chances for living a healthy life that are afforded to more prosperous people. They are bombarded with commercial information about unhealthy foods; their communities are inundated with fast-food establishments; their neighborhoods lack playgrounds and fields for recreation; and they live in poorly lit, violent areas that discourage outside activity. The poor cannot afford the whole foods, health clubs, and leisure time that make it so much easier for the prosperous to eat well and exercise. A central tenet of social justice is the obligation to help give everyone a fair chance to live a healthier life.

Corporate Responsibility

Thus far, we have thought about individual responsibility and governmental obligation to control obesity. But what about corporate responsibility? Are businesses partly to blame for the increasing weight of the population and, if so, should they be held to account? Several companies have voluntarily changed their practices (e.g., removing trans fats from products or fattening foods from schools), but most have not self-regulated.[37] Many public health advocates place the blame squarely on the food industry.[38] "Big Food," pejoratively analogized to "Big Tobacco," offers energy-dense nutrient-poor foods with high levels of added sugar, salt, and saturated or trans fats. These foods are not only fattening but psychologically, perhaps physically, addictive.[39] The industry often serves this food in oversized portions. For example, a single "super-size" meal at McDonald's typically contains more than the recommended daily amount of calories, fat, sodium, and cholesterol (see chapter 6).[40]

Sugary cereals, sugary drinks, and high-fat foods are aggressively marketed to the public with alluring, well-funded advertising campaigns. These foods are, moreover, disproportionately marketed to children and adolescents (see chapter 9). Even adults, however, may find it difficult to make informed choices, as the nutritional content is often concealed or hard to find, particularly in restaurants.

But as those who prefer market-oriented solutions remind us, Big Food is on both sides of the fence. Along with high-fat foods, there are low-fat foods, with their own advertising campaigns, which create a real or mistaken impression that they are healthy. And then there is the ubiquitous diet and exercise industry, which occupies a desirable market niche extolling the benefits of good eating and an active lifestyle.[41] In truth, America is bombarded by messages and images of stick-thin beauty on the one hand and gluttonous self-indulgence on the other. Within the din, the question remains whether corporations should be held to account or whether the market will self-correct. Given the vast profits of getting consumers to buy more and more food, irrespective of its nutritional value, and the fact that the market currently is not stemming the tide of obesity, perhaps there is a legitimate role for regulation.

The rest of this chapter briefly explores the various alternatives open to the state to reduce chronic disease by influencing human behavior. My claim is not that politicians should simply adopt these measures, which still require careful examination of their effectiveness. Rather, it is that the polity should remain open to innovative ways of preventing obesity, given the devastating effects on population health, particularly for the most disadvantaged among us.

Obesity Regulation: Using the Law as a Tool to Facilitate Healthier Lifestyles

The public health community is actively discussing policies designed to influence personal behavior to reduce overweight and obesity, even though these are deeply controversial.[42] Using the models of legal intervention developed in chapter 1, table 22 describes the principal ideas for obesity prevention (see further chapters 5, 6, 8, and 9). (There are also medical interventions, such as bariatric surgery, facilitated by Medicare's classification of obesity as a disease.)[43]

Disclosure. Consumers often eat foods without understanding their nutritional content or harmful effects. Labels on packaged foods are often obfuscatory by design,[44] restaurants usually make no disclosures at all,[45] and many consumers are not even aware of the risks from added sodium, fat, and sugar. Government has the power to require companies to disclose the nutritional content of foods and provide health warnings. Canada and the United States, for example, mandate labeling of trans fatty acids on prepackaged foods.[46] Product labeling and health warnings help consumers make more informed choices about their diet. Disclosure requirements also can powerfully affect corporate behavior. For example, box 10 (p. 177) describes a decision by Kraft Foods to remove trans fat from the ultimate American comfort food—the Oreo cookie—in response to the FDA's disclosure rule. Even fast-food restaurants, which are not bound by the FDA rule, changed their products; for example, KFC decided to stop using trans fats in fried foods.[47] Disclosure rules can be beneficial to the public's health, as suggested by the FDA estimate that by 2009 trans fat labeling will have prevented from 600 to 1,200 cases of coronary heart disease and 250 to 500 deaths each year.[48]

Industry often resists disclosure rules, asserting that they can be confusing and inconsistent. Restaurants argue that disclosure is impracticable because they constantly change their menus. But it may be precisely because labeling influences consumer purchasing patterns that companies often oppose mandatory disclosure: "It is unrealistic for the manufacturers to remove all fat, sugar and salt," argues a food executive, "because nobody would buy the result."[49] Disclosure, as a government

TABLE 22. Legal interventions to control overweight and obesity

Interventions	Definition	Public Health Benefits	Arguments in Favor	Arguments Against
Disclosure (e.g., nutritional labeling)	Require food manufacturers and restaurants to disclose nutritional contents of food (e.g., fat, sugar, calories)	Inform consumers about the nutritional benefits and risks of food	Clear nutritional information allows consumers to make more informed choices. Consumers are unaware of the dangers of fast food	Too difficult to provide accurate information, particularly in restaurants that change their menus Food labels are often misleading and inconsistent
Tort Liability	Litigation against food companies and restaurants for deceptive practices, false claims, unreasonably hazardous products, etc.	Force fast-food restaurants to offer healthier alternatives and give consumers accurate information Prevent marketers of unhealthy food from targeting children	Discovery may uncover deception (e.g., reveal company manipulation of addictive ingredients) Change public opinion Alter business practices in favor of more healthy alternatives	Counter to public opinion, which sees food consumption as a personal choice Hard to prove that fast-food consumption caused disease, given confounding variables
Surveillance (e.g., diabetes surveillance)	Diabetes surveillance provides data for monitoring population health, feedback, action alerts, and recommendations sent to physicians and patients	Improve diabetes epidemiology Provide individual and aggregate feedback and support to providers and patients	Majority of patients do not know their glycosylated hemoglobin values and do not adequately manage the disease	Impinges on clinical autonomy Interferes with therapeutic relationship Increased reporting responsibilities are time-consuming Informed consent and confidentiality Opt-out system is complex

TABLE 22. *(continued)*

Interventions	Definition	Public Health Benefits	Arguments in Favor	Arguments Against
Regulation of Food Marketing to Children and Youth	Regulation of television and print advertising, Web sites and advergames, character licensing and stealth marketing (e.g., limiting air time during children's programs)	Advertising influences eating habits and purchasing patterns of children and their parents	Advertisements can be deceptive and misleading Children are less capable of making distinctions	Freedom of commercial speech Paternalistic
Taxation	Impose higher taxes on calorie-dense, nutrient-poor foods	Decrease consumption of unhealthy foods Generate revenue to subsidize healthful foods, physical activity programs, obesity prevention, nutrition education Focus on maximizing health benefits, not monitoring dietary choices per se	Many countries use fiscal measures to promote availability of and access to certain foods Effective: compare with taxes on alcohol and tobacco use	Paternalistic Could affect poor people disproportionately (regressive tax) Freedom of choice Tax revenues are often used to cover budget deficits May raise food prices without any impact on demand No consistency on which foods to tax Slippery slope with concerns that more and more foods will be taxed

School and Workplace Policies	Encourage school and workplace policies such as removing vending machines, providing healthier menus, more physical activity, and nutritional/physical education	Reduce high-calorie temptations at school and work Provide more opportunity for exercise Enhance learning and working	Influence nutrition and physical activity on a regular basis and help establish healthful eating habits Offer courses on health maintenance Prevent undue influences on young people	Difficult to implement Resource intensive Inefficient if dietary habits do not change at home Insufficient federal school meal funding
The "Built" Environment: Zoning	Use zoning laws to limit prevalence of fast-food outlets, expand recreational opportunities, and encourage the development of healthier lifestyles	Give people greater choice and opportunity to eat healthy, recreate, and exercise, especially in poor neighborhoods	Fast-food chains create traffic and pollution, contribute to truancy, tarnish aesthetics, and drive out stores that offer healthier alternatives Governments often use zoning powers to restrict business Access to healthier foods Easy to adapt to changing community needs	Paternalistic Access to healthier food alone will not prevent overeating Could affect poor people disproportionately Might only affect certain areas in a locality Slippery slope to an outright ban of fast food Restricts competition
Food Prohibitions (e.g., trans fat ban)	Require food manufacturers and restaurants to remove certain ingredients that pose particular health hazards	Reduce certain hazardous ingredients from the food supply	Improved diets as consumers avoid hazardous ingredients Consumers may not be able to discern any difference in taste or desirability of the product	Expensive for food industry to make the switch Restriction on trade Freedom of choice

intervention, is most consistent with prevailing cultural values of consumer autonomy. Thus, informing personal choices rather than restricting them is most likely to find political acceptance.

Tort Liability. Box 12 (p. 213) shows how advocates are adapting strategies in tobacco litigation for use in litigation against the food industry. Legal theories range from inadequate disclosure of health risks, misleading advertisements, targeting children, and deceptive practices under consumer protection laws[50] to serving foods that are dangerous beyond the extent ordinarily understood by consumers.[51] A key component of this litigation is the claim that the food industry has reasonable alternatives to reduce foreseeable risks, such as substituting unsaturated fats for trans fats or simply using less sugar and salt. The Second Circuit Court of Appeals in *Pelman v. McDonald's* (2005) gave some hope to public health advocates when it permitted plaintiffs' claims alleging deceptive representation of the nutritional benefits of McDonald's food to go to trial.[52] But beyond this case, food litigation has been largely unsuccessful.

Although litigation may be unsuccessful and deeply unpopular, it can result in modest short-term changes in corporate policy and perhaps longer-term changes in popular culture, as occurred with tobacco litigation. Still, politicians bristle at the idea that businesses should be subjected to liability for serving food that people willingly buy and eat. They believe food litigation is paternalistic, anticapitalistic, and an inefficient way to regulate. And this view has prevailed in state legislatures, which have enacted "commonsense consumption" or "personal responsibility" laws that sharply limit tort liability.[53]

Surveillance. Infectious disease surveillance is a well-accepted part of public health practice, but the idea that the state should monitor chronic diseases is much more controversial. New York City has adopted an aggressive diabetes surveillance program, including mandatory laboratory reporting of glycosylated hemoglobin, recommendations for doctors to manage patients with poor glycemic control, and advice to patients on diabetes management. The public health objectives are to improve monitoring of diabetes and provide feedback and support to physicians and patients.

The close involvement of public health officials in clinical practice and patient compliance represents a new way of thinking about surveillance and follow-up to track and manage chronic diseases. But civil libertarians and health providers vehemently oppose aggressive surveillance, believing it interferes with patient autonomy and privacy, as well as clinical freedom. A key question is whether surveillance and case management of a disease with a crippling effect on the public's health offer sufficient benefits to offset the limited invasion of patient privacy and clinical freedom (see further chapter 8).

Targeting Children and Adolescents. The food industry spends more than $11 billion annually on advertising to children and adolescents, and often employs highly innovative methods, such as Internet marketing, advertising games, and stealth marketing.[54] America's youth is exposed to approximately forty thousand food advertisements annually, the vast majority of which are for candy, cereal, and fast foods.[55] Studies suggest that advertising can significantly shape the eating habits of young people and the purchasing patterns of their parents.[56] Young children, especially, are unable to understand the persuasive intent of advertising or to view it critically.[57] Consequently, regulatory strategies include restricting food advertising during children's programs; counteradvertising to promote good nutrition and physical activity; limiting the use of cartoon or other characters; and restricting Web-based games and promotions.

Regulating the content of food advertising on television, the print media, and the Internet is deeply controversial, with constitutional overtones. Certainly, the public supports, and the Constitution permits, regulation of misleading messages directed toward young people. However, there is no consensus on which messages are misleading and which simply alluring—no clear line between deception and puffery. Moreover, adults as well as children watch most media outlets, so there is a concern about censorship. Consequently, the food industry aggressively asserts its First Amendment rights to creatively advertise its products, even in the face of a growing problem of childhood obesity. Still, regulation of advertising to children and adolescents may be politically acceptable given the potential for manipulation of vulnerable youth and the state's responsibility to protect children (see further chapter 9).

Taxation of Unhealthy Foods. Public health advocates believe that food costs are out of balance, with healthy foods costing more than unhealthy ones. They have proposed a "fat tax" as a proactive response to a food industry and consumer culture that increasingly promotes high-fat, low-nutrition products as the cheapest, tastiest, most convenient, and most available dietary options. Colloquially known as a "junk food," "snack," or "Twinkie" tax, the objective would be to provide a disincentive for purchasing calorie-dense, nutrient-poor foods. The revenue from the tax could also be used to promote healthy nutrition and antiobesity programs. For example, a national tax of one cent per twelve-ounce soft drink would generate $1.5 billion annually, and similar revenues could be generated with a tax on candy, chips, and other snack foods.[58] The WHO has lent support to the concept, noting that food-purchasing patterns could be influenced through taxes and subsidies, with potential benefits to the public's health.[59]

The public is often stridently opposed to taxation of food products, particularly those most desired by consumers.[60] A fat tax is paternalistic, because it penalizes consumers for behaviors that do not harm others. It is also regressive, because poor people are the primary consumers of high-fat foods, and the costs of the tax weigh more heavily on them. But most of all, people wonder how it is possible to decide which foods should be taxed and why. Would distinctions be made, for example, between a snack food made with canola oil and one made with palm oil? Or what about fruit juices, juice drinks, regular sodas, and diet soda? Finally, would a tax on, say, fast-food hamburgers be acceptable if the government did not tax steaks, French fries, or crème brulé in upscale restaurants? The public opposes a fat tax not only because government is levying a charge for eating their favorite foods, but also because they don't know what foods might be taxed next. Food, after all, is not like tobacco, which is never beneficial. People need food to survive, and any food may be acceptable when eaten in moderation.

"Junk" Food and Physical Education in Schools. The food industry has introduced its foods and brand images in public schools throughout America (see chapter 9). To obtain badly needed funds, schools allow food companies to sell their products in vending machines and cafeterias, and to advertise ubiquitously on school property. Even meals served under the National School Lunch Program contain fat and calories exceeding federal guidelines.[61] And only a minority of schools require daily physical education classes. But government can do a great deal to prevent companies from flooding schools with sugary beverages and high-fat foods.[62] It can require schools to adhere to dietary guidelines and portion size for snacks and school lunches, or even ban certain foods from vending machines, shops, and cafeterias.[63] Indeed, as explained in chapter 5, several companies have voluntarily removed unhealthy beverages and snack foods from schools.[64] At the same time, schools can increase opportunities for health education and physical activities.

School districts can make nutrition education a part of their curriculum, require more physical education, and create opportunities for active lifestyles for students.

Many of these policies should be uncontroversial because they involve the health of children and adolescents, who are forming lifetime habits and are not in a position to fully discern the dangers of high-calorie foods and sedentary lifestyles.[65] Yet many believe that diet and physical activity are the responsibility of parents, not schools. And, in any case, they argue that school policies are ineffective if children's dietary habits do not change at home.

The Built Environment: A "Zoning" Diet. The environment in many poor minority neighborhoods is not conducive to healthy living, providing limited access to healthy foods, recreational facilities, and safe places for walking and playing.[66] Consequently, governments could facilitate healthier eating and exercise patterns, particularly in poorer neighborhoods, by altering the "built environment"—a broad term that encompasses the man-made structures that constitute people's living spaces. Local officials could limit the number of fast-food restaurants, build recreational parks and bike paths, expand mass transportation, and provide lighting and playgrounds in housing developments.[67] Many communities have, for example, passed zoning restrictions on fast-food outlets, including wholesale prohibitions, limited bans on "formula" restaurants (fast-food chains with standardized menus, name, and appearance), bans in certain vicinities, quotas on the number of restaurants, and limits on the distance from residential areas.[68] By regulating how land and buildings are used, governments can encourage the development of alternative, more health-conscious food retailers.[69]

Land use for public health purposes used to be a well-accepted practice in local government, but it is much more controversial today.[70] Critics believe that government officials should not impose their values on the public—telling people what they should eat and how they should live: "It is coercive, moralistic, nostalgic, [and lacks honesty]."[71] They prefer free markets so that businesses are permitted to sell foods in places where consumers are willing and happy to buy their products. Critics also maintain that affording access to healthier food alone will not prevent overeating, as individuals will search out the foods that they prefer. But there are undoubted social, economic, and physical influences on eating habits, and government could strive to make healthier foods an easier choice for the public.[72]

Food Prohibitions. Perhaps the most coercive, and politically divisive, form of obesity regulation is an outright ban on foods or ingredients deemed to be particularly harmful. A growing body of scientific evidence links trans fatty acids to coronary heart disease. The Institute of Medicine concluded there is no safe level of trans fat consumption,[73] and they provide no known benefit to human health.[74] In 2003, Denmark became the first country to set an upper limit on the percentage of industrially produced trans fat in foods.[75] In May 2005, Tiburon, California, adopted a voluntary prohibition on cooking with trans fat oils.[76] More recently, New York City banned trans fatty acids from restaurants, and other cities and counties are adopting similar plans.[77] Supporters believe that eliminating a known health risk from foods will decrease morbidity and premature mortality in the population. Customers may not even be able to discern a difference in taste or desirability of the product.

The fierce debates about the propriety of a trans fat ban focus on scientific credibility, effectiveness, cost, and legitimacy. At one time, the government actively promoted refined oil products high in trans fat, encouraging low-income populations to choose margarine over butter. A key question today is whether there is sufficiently robust evidence that trans fat is more dangerous than saturated fat to justify new public policies.[78] In light of experience with apparently contradictory government health messages, the public may doubt the credibility of current pronouncements. Moreover, a trans fat ban could drive the market back toward saturated fats.[79] Consumers, believing their risks are reduced, may eat more fried foods, leading to even higher levels of obesity and chronic disease.

The food industry believes that government prohibitions violate the basic tenets of competitive markets and free trade. Removing trans fat from foods is expensive, and industry leaders believe it affects the food's taste and desirability, thus driving consumers to their competitors' products. Local bans can have a potentially far-reaching impact on states, the nation, and countries worldwide. Multinational corporations such as McDonald's and Burger King use similar food processing in restaurants throughout the globe, so a ban in one dense metropolitan area can affect operations everywhere.

Perhaps the strongest objection to a trans fat ban is that it is highly paternalistic: The state decides what people may eat because it is "better for them." People see government bans as heavy-handed, interfering with a person's right to order what he or she wants. The conventional wisdom is that people are capable of deciding what to eat, making the trade-offs between taste, current pleasures, and future health consequences. And, of course, banning saturated fats is a more logical problem to address because the public consumes much more of them. So critics worry that the state might ban popular foods high in saturated fat, such as pizza and cheesecake.[80]

Despite the undoubted political risks, should public health agencies push for strong measures to control obesity, perhaps even banning hazardous foods? The justification lies in the epidemic rates of overweight and obesity, the preventable morbidity and mortality, and the stark health disparities based on race and socioeconomic status. Major cities have sought voluntary bans on trans fats, which companies have largely ignored. If the problem involved pathogens, tobacco, or lead paint, most would support aggressive measures to protect innocent victims from hazards created by others. But comfort foods also have hidden hazards; it is nearly impossible to tell if they are laden with fat and, if so, what kind.[81] Nearly everyone agrees that some form of legal response is at least presumptively justifiable when a risk is imposed by one person on another. Although paternalism has a pariah status, it is at least worth considering whether it is ever justified to regulate harms that are apparently self-imposed but deeply embedded in society and pervasively harmful to the public.

THE FUTURE OF PUBLIC HEALTH LAW

In this book, I have sought to provide a fuller understanding of the varied roles of law in advancing the public's health. The field of public health is purposive and interventionist. It does not settle for existing conditions of health but actively seeks effective techniques for identifying and reducing health threats. Law is a very important but perennially neglected tool in furthering the public's health. Public health law should not be seen as an arcane, indecipherable set of technical rules buried deep within state health codes. Rather, public health law should be seen broadly as the authority and responsibility of government to ensure the conditions for the population's health. As such, public health law has transcending importance in how we think about government, politics, and policy.

Though government has a responsibility to ensure the conditions for health, it cannot overreach in a democratic society. This leads to one of the most complicated problems in the field: how to balance the collective good achieved by public health regulation with the resulting infringements of individual rights and freedoms. The difficult trade-offs between collective goods and individual rights form a major part of the study of public health law.

Finally, it is important to recall that public health, and the law itself, are highly political, influenced by strong social, cultural, and economic forces. As these forces shift over the years, as different political ideologies and economic conditions take hold, the field of public health will change and adapt. It has always been that way in public health, and it is likely to remain that way in the future, providing intellectually enticing and socially important terrain for scholars and practitioners to explore.

John Ruskin, the nineteenth-century British scholar whose work ranged from art history, literary criticism, and mythology to the pervasive health hazards of the industrial economy, captured better than most the essential message of this book:

> I desire, in closing the series of introductory papers, to have this one great fact clearly stated. There is no wealth but life. Life, including all its powers of love, of joy, and of admiration. That country is richest which nourishes the greatest number of noble and happy human beings; that man is richest, who, having perfected the functions of his own life to the utmost, has also the widest helpful influence, both personal and by possessions, over the lives of others.[82]

Notes

1. A THEORY AND DEFINITION OF PUBLIC HEALTH LAW

SOURCES FOR CHAPTER EPIGRAPHS: James A. Tobey, *Public Health Law: A Manual of Law for Sanitarians* (Baltimore, MD: Williams and Wilkins, 1926): 6–7; Charles V. Chapin, foreword to *Public Health Law,* by James A. Tobey, xv; Geoffrey Rose, *The Strategy of Preventive Medicine* (Oxford: Oxford University Press, 1992): 101; William Farr, "Vital Statistics or the Statistics of Health, Sickness, Disease and Death," in *McCulloch's Statistical Account of the British Empire* (1837), reprinted in *Mortality in Mid Nineteenth Century Britain,* ed. Richard Wall (Farnborough, England: Gregg International, 1974): 567 (see also Major Greenwood, *Medical Statistics from Graunt to Farr* [Cambridge: Cambridge University Press, 1948]: 71); Nassim Nicholas Taleb, "Scaring Us Senseless," *New York Times,* July 24, 2005; William Foege, "How to Effect Change in the Population," in *Implications of Genomics for Public Health: Workshop Summary, Institute of Medicine* (Washington, DC: National Academies Press, 2005): 27; Michael Marmot, "Life at the Top," *New York Times,* February 27, 2005; C. E. A. Winslow, *The Life of Hermann M. Biggs* (Philadelphia: Lea and Febiger, 1929): 120.

1. Organized groups of teachers, scholars, and practitioners in law and health are active and visible, including the American Society of Law, Medicine, and Ethics; the American Health Lawyers Association; and the American College of Legal Medicine. More recently, the Centers for Disease Control and Prevention established a public health law program (see Richard A. Goodman, Anthony Moulton, Gene Matthews, et al., "Law and Public Health of CDC," *Morbidity and Mortality Weekly Report,* 55 [2006]: 29–33), and a group of public health attorneys and academics formed the Public Health Law Association. Analogous organizations, such as the World Association for Medical Law, operate on a global scale.

2. Several recent volumes make important contributions to the field of public health law in the United States. See, e.g., Frank P. Grad, *The Public Health Law Manual,* 3d ed. (Washington, DC: American Public Health Association, 2005); Richard A. Goodman, Mark A. Rothstein, Richard E. Hoffman, et al., *Law in Public Health Practice,* 2d ed. (New York: Oxford University Press, 2007); Kenneth R. Wing, *The Law and the Public's Health,* 7th ed. (Chicago: Health Administration Press, 2006). For valuable texts in other countries, see Christopher Reynolds (with Genevieve Howse), *Public Health: Law and Regulation* (Sydney: Federation Press, 2004); Robyn Martin and Linda Johnson, eds., *Law and the Public Dimension of Health* (London: Cavendish Publishing, 2001); Tracey M. Bailey, Timothy Caulfield, and Nola M. Ries, eds., *Public Health Law and Policy in Canada* (Markham, ON: Butterworths, 2005).

3. Lu Ann Aday, *Reinventing Public Health: Policies and Practices for a Healthy Nation* (San Francisco: Jossey-Bass, 2005).

4. Dan E. Beauchamp, *The Health of the Republic: Epidemics, Medicine, and Moralism as Challenges to Democracy* (Philadelphia: Temple University Press, 1988): 4.

5. Severine Deneulin and Nicholas Townsend, "Public Goods, Global Public Goods, and the Common Good," *ESCR Research Group on Wellbeing in Developing Countries,* Sept. 2006, http://www.welldev.org.uk/research/workingpaperpdf/wed18.pdf (arguing that the concept of global public goods could be more effective if it were broadened beyond the individual level: "living well" or the "good life" does not dwell in individual lives only, but also in the lives of communities that human beings form).

6. Garrett Hardin, "The Tragedy of the Commons," *Science,* 162 (1968): 1243–48. The tragedy of the commons is based on the premise that rational actors will always seek to maximize their own self-interest. Hardin illustrates his point by supposing that the common pasture of a small hamlet becomes the grazing area for everyone's cows. Each farmer would increase his herd because the utility of adding one more cow to his own herd would be greater than the costs to the individual since the costs would be spread over everyone. All farmers would follow this train of thought as self-interested beings, and the commons would become a desolate wasteland.

7. Jo Ivey Boufford and Phillip R. Lee, *Health Policies for the Twenty-first Century: Challenges and Recommendations for the U.S. Department of Health and Human Services* (New York: Milbank Memorial Fund, 2001); Kay W. Eilbert, Mike Barry, Ron Bialek, et al., *Measuring Expenditures for Essential Public Health Services* (Washington, DC: Public Health Foundation, 1996); Trust for America's Health, *Public Health Leadership Initiative: An Action Plan for Healthy People in Healthy Communities in the Twenty-first Century* (Washington, DC: Trust for America's Health, 2006); Leslie M. Beitsch, Robert G. Brookes, Nir Menachemi, et al., "Public Health at Center Stage: New Roles, Old Props," *Health Affairs,* 25 (2006): 911–22.

8. Norman Daniels, *Just Health: A Population View* (New York: Cambridge University Press, 2007); Sudhir Anand, Fabienne Peter, and Amartya Sen, eds., *Public Health, Ethics, and Equity* (Oxford: Oxford University Press, 2004) (if health

is prerequisite to a person functioning, inequalities in health constitute inequalities in people's capability to function, hence a denial of equality of opportunity).

9. *General Comment 14: The Right to the Highest Attainable Standard of Health,* U.N. ESCOR, 22d Sess., Agenda Item 3, U.N. Doc. E/C.12/2000/4 (2000).

10. Michael Walzer, *Spheres of Justice: A Defense of Pluralism and Equality* (New York: Basic Books, 1983).

11. *Id.*

12. Jared Diamond, *Collapse: How Societies Choose to Fail or Succeed* (East Rutherford, NJ: Viking Adult, 2005).

13. Lisa F. Berkman and Ichiro Kawachi, eds., *Social Epidemiology* (New York: Oxford University Press, 2000).

14. Howard Markel, *When Germs Travel: Six Major Epidemics That Have Invaded America and the Fears They Have Unleashed* (New York: Vintage, 2005); Allan M. Brandt, *No Magic Bullet: A Social History of Venereal Disease since 1880* (New York: Oxford University Press, 1987); Wendy E. Parmet, "Health Care and the Constitution: Public Health and the Role of the State in the Framing Era," *Hastings Constitutional Law Quarterly,* 20 (Winter 1992): 267–334.

15. Jonathan Mann, Lawrence Gostin, Sofia Gruskin, et al., "Health and Human Rights," *Journal of Health and Human Rights: An International Journal,* 1 (1994): 6–22.

16. Institute of Medicine, *The Future of the Public's Health in the Twenty-first Century* (Washington, DC: National Academies Press, 2002).

17. "Regulatory capture" entails powerful interest groups improperly influencing regulatory decisions. See, e.g., George J. Stigler, "The Theory of Economic Regulation," *Bell Journal of Economics and Management Science,* 2 (1971): 3–21.

18. Lawrence O. Gostin and Peter D. Jacobson, *Law and the Health System* (New York: Foundation Press, 2005).

19. Carmen DeNavas-Walt, Bernadette D. Proctor, and Cheryl Hill Lee, U.S. Census Bureau, *Income, Poverty, and Health Insurance Coverage in the United States: 2004* (Washington, DC: U.S. Government Printing Office, 2005) (15.7 percent of the population was without health insurance coverage in 2004); Robin A. Cohen and Michael E. Martinez, *Health Insurance Coverage: Estimates from the National Health Interview Survey, 2005* (Atlanta: Centers for Disease Control, 2006); U.S. Census Bureau, "Census Bureau Revises 2004 and 2005 Health Insurance Coverage Estimates," March 23, 2007, http://www.census.gov/Press~Release/www/releases/archives/health_care_insurance/009789.html.

20. Matthew K. Wynia, "Oversimplifications I: Physicians Don't Do Public Health," *American Journal of Bioethics,* 5 (2005): 4–5.

21. Marion Gibbon, Ronald Labonte, and Glenn Laverack, "Evaluating Community Capacity," *Health and Social Care in the Community,* 10 (2002): 485–91.

22. René Bowser and Lawrence O. Gostin, "Managed Care and the Health of a Nation," *Southern California Law Review,* 72 (1999): 1209–95 (arguing for closer public-private partnerships and proposing economic incentives for managed care organizations to assume traditional public health functions); Mark

Wolfson, Mary Hourigan, and Todd Johnson, "Managed Care, Population Health, and Public Health," in *Research in the Sociology of Health Care,* ed. J. J. Kronenfeld (Greenwich, CT: JAI Press, 1998): 217–31, 229; Paul A. Simon and Jonathan E. Fielding, "Public Health and Business: A Partnership That Makes Cents," *Health Affairs,* 25 (2006): 1029–39 (noting that in 2003 businesses paid more than one quarter of the $1.7 trillion in aggregate health care costs).

23. Dean M. Hashimoto, "The Future Role of Managed Care and Capitation in Workers' Compensation," *American Journal of Law and Medicine,* 22 (1996): 233–61.

24. Elizabeth M. Armstrong, Daniel P. Carpenter, and Marie Hojnacki, "Whose Death Matters? Mortality, Advocacy, and Attention to Disease in the Mass Media," *Journal of Health Politics, Policy and Law,* 31 (2006): 729–72.

25. Institute of Medicine, *Who Will Keep the Public Healthy? Educating Public Health Professionals for the Twenty-first Century* (Washington, DC: National Academies Press, 2003).

26. *Black's Law Dictionary,* 6th ed. (New York: West Group, 1990): 721. The Supreme Court determined in *Whitman v. American Trucking Ass'ns,* 531 U.S. 457, 465–66 (2001), that the ordinary meaning of the term *public health* is "health of the community" or "health of the public."

27. Geoffrey Rose, "Sick Individuals and Sick Populations," *International Journal of Epidemiology,* 14 (1985): 32–38, 37.

28. Roger Detels, "Epidemiology: The Foundation of Public Health," in *Oxford Textbook of Public Health,* 4th ed., ed. Roger Detels, James McEwen, Robert Beaglehole, et al. (New York: Oxford University Press, 2002): 485–91, 485.

29. *Id.*

30. Judith S. Mausner and Shira Kramer, *Mausner and Bahn Epidemiology: An Introductory Text,* 2d ed. (Philadelphia: W. B. Saunders Company, 1985).

31. Rose, "Sick Individuals," 37.

32. Dan E. Beauchamp and Bonnie Steinbock, eds., *New Ethics for the Public's Health* (New York: Oxford University Press, 1999). See Ronald Bayer, Lawrence O. Gostin, Bruce Jennings, et. al., eds., *Public Health Ethics: Theory, Policy, and Practice* (New York: Oxford University Press, 2007).

33. Michael Marmot and Richard G. Wilkinson, eds., *Social Determinants of Health,* 2d ed. (New York: Oxford University Press, 2005).

34. Nancy Kari, Harry C. Boyte, Bruce Jennings, et al., "Health as a Civic Question," *Center for Democracy and Citizenship,* November 28, 1994, http://www.cpn.org/topics/health/healthquestion.html.

35. Judith Summers, *Soho: A History of London's Most Colourful Neighbourhood* (London: Bloomsbury Publishing, 1989): 113–17.

36. J. Michael McGinnis and William H. Foege, "Actual Causes of Death in the United States," *JAMA,* 270 (1993): 2207–12. The data in the McGinnis and Foege article were updated in Ali H. Mokdad, James S. Marks, Donna F. Stroup, et al., "Actual Causes of Death in the United States, 2000," *JAMA,* 291 (2003): 1238–45.

37. Ahmedin Jemal, Elizabeth Ward, Yongping Hao, et al., "Trends in the Leading Causes of Death in the United States, 1970–2002," *JAMA,* 294 (2005): 1255–59 (describing age-standardized deaths from each of the six leading causes

of death: heart disease, stroke, cancer, chronic obstructive pulmonary disease, accidents, and diabetes mellitus).

38. Dan E. Beauchamp, "Public Health as Social Justice," in *New Ethics for the Public's Health,* ed. Dan E. Beauchamp and Bonnie Steinbock (New York: Oxford University Press, 1999): 105–14.

39. John Rawls, *A Theory of Justice* (Cambridge, MA: Harvard University Press, 1971).

40. Lawrence O. Gostin and Madison Powers, "What Does Justice Require for the Public's Health? Public Health Ethics and Policy Imperatives of Social Justice," *Health Affairs,* 25 (2006): 1053–60.

41. Madison Powers and Ruth Faden, *Social Justice: The Moral Foundations of Public Health and Health Policy* (New York: Oxford University Press, 2006).

42. Lawrence O. Gostin and Benjamin E. Berkman, "Pandemic Influenza: Ethics, Law, and the Public Health," *Administrative Law Review,* 59 (2007): 121–75; Lawrence O. Gostin, "Medical Countermeasures for Pandemic Influenza: Ethics and the Law (Part I)," *JAMA,* 295 (2006): 554–57; Lawrence O. Gostin, "Public Health Strategies for Pandemic Influenza: Ethics and the Law (Part II)," *JAMA,* 295 (2006): 1700–1704; Institute of Medicine, *Threat of Pandemic Influenza: Are We Ready?: Workshop Summary* (Washington, DC: National Academies Press, 2005).

43. Richard H. Weisler, James G. Barbee, and Mark H. Townsend, "Mental Health and Recovery in the Gulf Coast after Hurricanes Katrina and Rita," *JAMA,* 296 (2006): 585–88. For similar problems after the South Asian tsunami on December 26, 2004, see Frits van Griensven, M. L. Somchai Chakkraband, Warunee Thienkrua, et al., "Mental Health Problems among Adults in Tsunami-Affected Areas in Southern Thailand," *JAMA,* 296 (2006): 537–48. See also Amy L. Fairchild, James Colgrove, and Marian Moser Jones, "The Challenge of Mandatory Evacuation For and Deciding For," *Health Affairs,* 25 (2006): 958–67 (outlining ethical and policy justifications for mandatory evacuation during emergencies).

44. Grad, *Public Health Law Manual,* 4.

45. Institute of Medicine, *The Future of Public Health* (Washington, DC: National Academies Press, 1988): 19.

46. Institute of Medicine, *Future of the Public's Health,* 4–5.

47. Public Health Statute Modernization National Excellence Collaborative, *Model State Public Health Act: A Tool for Assessing Public Health Laws* (Seattle, WA: Turning Point National Program Office, 2003).

48. See, e.g., Stephen Monaghan, Dyfed Huws, and Marie Navarro, *The Case for a New UK Health of the People Act* (London: Nuffield Trust, 2003).

49. James G. Hodge, Jr., Lawrence O. Gostin, Kristine Gebbie, et al., "Transforming Public Health Law: The Turning Point Model State Public Health Act," *Journal of Law, Medicine, and Ethics,* 34 (2006): 77–84.

50. Scott Burris, "The Invisibility of Public Health: Population-Level Measures in a Politics of Market Individualism," *American Journal of Public Health,* 87 (1997): 1607–10.

51. For an excellent discussion of different legal tools available to promote the public's health, as well as their advantages and disadvantages, see Roger

Brownsword, "Public Health, Private Right: Constitution and Common Law," *Medical Law International,* 7 (2006): 201–18.

52. U.S. Const., Art. I, § 8, cl. 1.

53. *South Dakota v. Dole,* 483 U.S. 203, 206 (1987) (upholding Congress's power to set terms and conditions "to further broad policy objectives" that must be complied with for "receipt of federal moneys").

54. See, e.g., Jonathan Weisman, "Businesses Jump on an SUV Loophole: Suddenly $100,000 Tax Deduction Proves a Marketing Bonanza," *Washington Post,* November 7, 2003; David Kiley, "Bush Plan Gives Huge Tax Break to Buyers of Big SUVs," *USA Today,* January 21, 2003.

55. Conservative scholars voice yet another objection to high tobacco taxes: promoting a black market in cigarette sales. Patrick Fleenor, "Cigarette Taxes, Black Markets, and Crime: Lessons from New York's Fifty-Year Losing Battle," *Cato Institute,* February 16, 2003, http://www.cato.org/pubs/pas/pa468.pdf.

56. See, e.g., *44 Liquormart, Inc. v. Rhode Island,* 517 U.S. 484 (1996) (finding that the state's ban on advertising liquor prices was not related to consumer protection and therefore subject to strict review).

57. Wendy C. Perdue, Lesley A. Stone, and Lawrence O. Gostin, "The Built Environment and Its Relationship to the Public's Health: The Legal Framework," *American Journal of Public Health,* 93 (2003): 1390–94.

58. Virginia Postrel, "The Pleasantville Solution: The War on 'Sprawl' Promises 'Livability' but Delivers Repression, Intolerance—and More Traffic," *Reason,* 30 (1999): 4–11.

59. Andres Duany, Elizabeth Plater-Zyberk, and Jeff Speck, *Suburban Nation: The Rise of Sprawl and the Decline of the American Dream* (New York: North Point Press, 2000).

60. Eugene Rogot, Paul Sorlie, Norman Johnson, et al., eds., *A Mortality Study of 1.3 Million Persons by Demographic, Social and Economic Factors: 1979–1985 Follow-Up* (Bethesda, MD: National Institutes of Health, 1992); S. Leonard Syme, "Social and Economic Disparities in Health: Thoughts about Intervention," *Milbank Quarterly,* 76 (1998): 493–505. In 2005, the WHO established a Commission on Social Determinants of Health with the mission of linking knowledge with action. Michael Marmot, "Social Determinants of Health Inequalities," *Lancet,* 365 (2005): 1099–1104; Barbara Starfield, "State of the Art in Research on Equity in Health," *Journal of Health Politics, Policy and Law,* 31 (2006): 11–32.

61. Michael Marmot, *The Status Syndrome: How Social Standing Affects Our Health and Longevity* (New York: Owl Books, 2005).

62. Angus Deaton, "Policy Implications of the Gradient of Health and Wealth," *Health Affairs,* 21 (2002): 13–30.

63. Evelyn M. Hauser and Philip M. Kitagaqa, *Differential Mortality in the United States: A Study of Socio-Economic Epidemiology* (Cambridge, MA: Harvard University Press, 1973); Michael G. Marmot and G. D. Smith, "Health Inequalities among British Civil Servants: The Whitehall II Study," *Lancet,* 337 (1991): 1387–93; Donald Acheson, ed., *Independent Inquiry into Inequalities in Health* (London: Stationery Office Books, 1998); Stephen J. Kunitz, with Irena Pesis-Katz, "Mortality of White Americans, African Americans, and Canadians:

The Causes and Consequences for Health of Welfare State Institutions and Policies," *Milbank Quarterly,* 83 (2005): 5–39 (finding that the life expectancy of African Americans has been substantially lower than that of White Americans for as long as records are available and that life expectancy of all Americans has been lower than that of all Canadians since the beginning of the twentieth century); Johan P. Mackenbach, "Health Inequalities: Europe in Profile," *UK Presidency of the EU* (February 2006), http://www.dh.gov.uk/assetRoot/04/12/15/84/04121584.pdf (finding "substantial inequalities" in health in all European countries based on education, occupational class, and income); Ken Judge, Stephen Platt, Caroline Costongs, et al., "Health Inequalities: A Challenge for Europe," *UK Presidency of the EU* (2006), http://www.dh.gov.uk/assetRoot/04/12/15/83/04121583.pdf (reviewing European efforts to reduce health disparities, including programs for social justice, social inclusion, and poverty reduction). For a comparison of health disparities outcomes and politics across states and countries, see "Special Issue: Comparative Perspectives on Health Disparities," *Journal of Health Politics, Policy and Law,* 31 (2006): 1–281. Health disparities in the United States are vast even by international standards, and cannot be explained by race, income, or health care access alone. Christopher J. L. Murray, Sandeep C. Kulkarni, Catherine Michaud, et al., "Eight Americas: Investigating Mortality Disparities across Races, Counties, and Race-Counties in the United States," *PLoS Medicine,* 3 (2006), http://medicine.plosjournals.org/perlserv/?request=get-document&doi=10.1371/journal.pmed.0030260 (showing that a Black man living in a high-crime city can expect to live twenty-one fewer years than an Asian woman).

64. Richard G. Wilkinson, *Unhealthy Societies: The Afflictions of Inequality* (London: Routledge, 1996).

65. Norman Daniels, Bruce Kennedy, and Ichiro Kawachi, "Justice Is Good for Our Health," *Boston Review,* 25 (2000): 6–15; Dan E. Beauchamp, "Public Health as Social Justice," *Inquiry,* 13 (1976): 3–14; Norman Daniels, "Equity and Population Health: Toward a Broader Bioethics Agenda," *Hastings Center Report,* 36 (2006): 22–35.

66. Gerald F. Anderson, Peter S. Hussey, Bianca K. Frogner, et al., "Health Spending in the United States and the Rest of the Industrialized World," *Health Affairs,* 24 (2005): 903–14.

67. UN Development Programme, *Human Development Report 2005* (New York: United Nations, 2005).

68. John Lynch, George D. Smith, Sam Harper, et al., "Is Income Inequality a Determinant of Population Health? Part 1. A Systematic Review," *Milbank Quarterly,* 82 (2004): 5–99; James Banks, Michael Marmot, Zoe Oldfield, et al., "Disease and Disadvantage in the United States and in England," *JAMA,* 295 (2006): 2037–45.

69. Critics of the public health case for redistributive policies also note that the explanatory variables for the relationship between SES and health are not entirely understood. Some deny the existence of a causal relationship between SES and health, suggesting instead that people who are ill tend not to attain high SES. The SES gradient probably does involve multiple pathways. These include material disadvantage (e.g., diminished access to food, shelter, and health care),

toxic physical environments (e.g., poor conditions at home, at work, and in the community); psychosocial stressors (e.g., financial or occupational insecurity and lack of control); and social contexts that encourage risk behaviors (e.g., smoking, physical inactivity, poor diet, and excessive alcohol consumption). Finding the exact pathways or causal relationships presents many challenges, but available data support the conclusion that SES is, in the main, a cause, not a consequence, of health status. Mitchell D. Wong, Martin F. Shapiro, W. John Boscardin, et al., "Contribution of Major Diseases to Disparities in Mortality," *New Engl. J. of Med.*, 347 (2002): 1585–92; Nancy E. Adler and Katherine Newman, "Socioeconomic Disparities in Health: Pathways and Policies," *Health Affairs*, 21 (2002): 60–76; Jonathan Klick and Sally Satel, *The Health Disparities Myth* (Washington, DC: AEI Press, 2006); Tina Rosenberg, "The Scandal of 'Poor People's Diseases,'" *New York Times*, March 29, 2006 (arguing that drug companies do not invest in treatments for diseases that primarily affect poor populations).

70. Nicholas Eberstadt and Sally Satel, *Health and the Income Inequality Hypothesis: A Doctrine in Search of Data* (Jackson, TN: AEI Press, 2004): 11–14.

71. Richard A. Epstein, "Let the Shoemaker Stick to His Last: A Defense of the 'Old' Public Health," *Perspectives in Biology and Medicine*, 46 (2003): S138–59.

72. Nathaniel C. Briggs, "Seat Belt Law Enforcement and Racial Disparities in Seat Belt Use," *American Journal of Preventive Medicine*, 31 (2006) (showing that Blacks have a lower prevalence of seat-belt use compared with Whites, but seat-belt use among both Blacks and Whites was more than 15 percent higher in states with primary, rather than secondary, law enforcement, indicating that such preventive legal interventions increase seat-belt use and reduce motor vehicle crash morbidity and mortality); David J. Houston and Lilliard E. Richardson, Jr., "Safety Belt Use and the Switch to Primary Enforcement, 1991–2003," *American Journal of Public Health*, 96 (2006): 1949–54 (arguing that states with secondary enforcement laws could increase belt use by 10 percent by upgrading to primary enforcement).

73. See my defense of the MSEHPA in the Dunwoody Distinguished Lecture in Law, with critical commentaries by four leading scholars. Lawrence O. Gostin, "When Terrorism Threatens Health: How Far Are Limitations on Personal and Economic Liberties Justified?" *Florida Law Review*, 55 (2003): 1–65.

74. *Compare* Epstein, "Shoemaker," S138–59, *with* Lawrence O. Gostin and M. Gregg Bloche, "The Politics of Public Health: A Reply to Richard Epstein," *Perspectives in Biology and Medicine*, 46, supp. 3 (Summer 2003): S160–75.

75. Karen Jochelson, "Nanny or Steward? The Role of Government in Public Health," *King's Fund*, October 2005, http://www.kingsfund.org.uk/resources/publications/nanny_or.html (arguing that paternalism can be viewed not as nanny statist but as a form of "stewardship"—part of government's responsibility to protect national health).

76. *City of Chicago v. Beretta Corp.*, 821 N.E. 2d 1099 (Ill. 2004) (suing on the theory that gun manufacturers' "conduct in designing, manufacturing, distributing, and selling certain models of handguns is done with the knowledge . . .

that a significant number of the guns will ultimately find their way into an illegal secondary gun market").

77. *Pelman v. McDonald's Corp.*, 396 F.3d 508 (2d Cir. 2005) (holding that a claim alleging McDonald's was deceptive in making and selling its products, causing minors to eat the products and injure their health by becoming obese, was sufficient to survive a motion to dismiss) (discussed in chapter 6).

78. *Class Action Fairness Act of 2005,* Pub. L. No. 109–2, 119 Stat. 4 (2005) (requiring class-action lawsuits with plaintiffs living in a state different from the defendant or those seeking more than $5 million in damages be removed from state to federal courts).

79. *Comprehensive Medical Malpractice Reform Act of 2006,* H.R. 4838, 109th Cong. (referred to committee on March 17, 2006) (proposing to limit noneconomic damages in medical malpractice suits).

80. *Protection of Lawful Commerce in Arms Act,* 15 U.S.C. § 7901 (2005) (immunizing firearms manufacturers, wholesalers, and dealers from civil liability in lawsuits alleging that they recklessly or negligently supplied guns to criminals) (discussed in chapter 6); Jon S. Vernick and Julia Samia Mair, "State Laws Forbidding Municipalities from Suing the Firearm Industry: Will Firearm Immunity Laws Close the Courthouse Door?" *Journal of Health Care Law and Policy,* 4 (2000): 126–57.

81. *Personal Responsibility in Food Consumption Act,* H.R. 554, 109th Cong. (preventing civil liability actions brought against food manufacturers, marketers, distributors, advertisers, sellers, and trade associations for claims of injury relating to a person's weight gain or obesity); *Commonsense Consumption Act of 2005,* S. 908, 109th Cong. (allowing Congress, state legislatures, and regulatory agencies to determine appropriate laws, rules, and regulations to address the problems of weight gain, obesity, and health conditions). See Trust for America's Health, *F as in Fat: How Obesity Policies Are Failing in America* (Washington, DC: Trust for America's Health, 2004).

82. Lawrence O. Gostin, *The AIDS Pandemic: Complacency, Injustice, and Unfulfilled Expectations* (Chapel Hill: University of North Carolina Press, 2004).

83. Government ambivalence around such policies as condom and sterile needle distribution is seen in national as well as foreign policy initiatives. The U.S. government reinstituted a policy that requires nongovernmental organizations to refrain from performing or promoting abortions as a condition for receipt of federal aid. Memorandum on Restoration of the Mexico City Policy, 37 *Weekly Comp. Pres. Doc.* 216, January 22, 2001; Editorial, "Ideology and AIDS," *New York Times,* February 26, 2005.

84. William J. Novak, "Public Economy and the Well-Ordered Market: Law and Economic Regulation in the Nineteenth Century," *Law and Social Inquiry,* 18 (1993): 1–32.

85. Lawrence Wallack and Regina Lawrence, "Talking about Public Health: Developing America's 'Second Language,'" *American Journal of Public Health,* 95 (2005): 567–70.

86. Sally Satel, "Public Health? Forget It: Cosmic Issues Beckon," *Wall Street Journal,* December 13, 2001; Richard Epstein, "Shoemaker," S138–59.

87. Dan Beauchamp has proposed that a second language of public health is necessary because "we are not only individuals, we are also a community and a body politic, and . . . we have shared commitments to one another and promises to keep." Dan Beauchamp, "Community: The Neglected Tradition in Public Health," *Hastings Center Report,* 15 (1985): 28–36, 34.

88. Ilan H. Meyer and Sharon Schwartz, "Social Issues as Public Health: Promise and Peril," *American Journal of Public Health,* 90 (2000): 1189–91.

89. Vicky Cattell, "Poor People, Poor Places, and Poor Health: The Mediating Role of Social Networks and Social Capital," *Social Science and Medicine,* 52 (2000): 1501–16.

90. Institute of Medicine, *Future of the Public's Health,* 46–95; Lawrence O. Gostin, Jo Ivey Boufford, and Rose Marie Martinez, "The Future of the Public's Health: Vision, Values, and Strategies," *Health Affairs,* 23 (2004): 96–107.

91. Mokdad et al., "Actual Causes," 1238. Even the presentation of data on the root causes of sickness and death can be politically charged. The authors of this seminal article from the CDC admitted later that "through an error in our computations, we overestimated the number of deaths caused by poor diet and physical inactivity. Our principal conclusions, however, remain unchanged: tobacco use and poor diet and physical inactivity contributed to the largest number of deaths, and the number of deaths related to poor diet and physical inactivity is increasing." Ali H. Mokdad, James S. Marks, Donna F. Stroup, et al., "Correction: Actual Causes of Death in the United States, 2000," *JAMA,* 293 (2005): 293. See Katherine M. Flegal, Barry I. Graubard, David F. Williamson, et al., "Excess Deaths Associated with Underweight, Overweight, and Obesity," *JAMA,* 293 (2005): 1861–67 (finding about 112,000 obesity-attributable deaths in 2000, far lower than the 414,000 estimated by Mokdad et al.). Conservative commentators attributed this error to overly zealous and careless advocacy by public health officials. See Daniel Henninger, "From Spin City to Fat City," *Wall Street Journal,* May 6, 2005.

92. M. Gregg Bloche and Lawrence O. Gostin, "Health Law and the Broken Promise of Equity," in *Law and Class in America: Trends since the Cold War,* ed. Paul Carrington and Trina Jones (New York: New York University Press, 2006): 310–30.

2. PUBLIC HEALTH REGULATION: A SYSTEMATIC EVALUATION

SOURCES FOR CHAPTER EPIGRAPHS: Amartya Sen, "Freedoms and Needs: An Argument for the Primacy of Political Rights," *New Republic,* 210 (1994): 31–38, 32; John Stuart Mill, *On Liberty* (New York: Penguin Books, 1985): 13; Mary Ann Glendon, *Rights Talk: The Impoverishment of Political Discourse* (New York: Free Press, 1991): 45; National Research Council, *Understanding Risk: Informing Decisions in a Democratic Society* (Washington, DC: National Academies Press, 1996): 215–16; Frank B. Cross, "The Public Role in Risk Control," *Environmental Law,* 24 (1994): 887–88; Oscar Wilde, *Lady Windermere's Fan* (Mineola, NY: Dover Publications, 1998): 38; Michael Kinsley, "As through a Glass Darkly," *Los Angeles Times,* March 6, 2005; Albert Einstein, Letter, March 3, 1954 (the quote is inscribed on a memorial statue of the scientist on the Institute of Medicine building in Washington, D.C.); UN Environment Programme, *Rio Declaration on Environment and Development,* June 14, 1992, http://www.unep.org/Documents/Default.asp?DocumentID=78&ArticleID=1163; His Holiness the Dalai Lama, *The Path to Tranquility: Daily Wisdom* (New York: Viking Arkana, 1999): 9, quoted in Dale Jamieson and Daniel Wartenberg, "The Precautionary Principle and Electric and Magnetic Fields," *American Journal of Public Health,* 91 (2001): 1355–58.

1. Norman Daniels, "Health-Care Needs and Distributive Justice," *Philosophy and Public Affairs,* 10 (1981): 146–79; Norman Daniels, *Just Health Care* (New York: Cambridge University Press, 1985); Lawrence O. Gostin, "Securing Health or Just Health Care? The Effect of the Health Care System on the Health of America," *St. Louis University Law Journal,* 39 (1994): 7–43.

2. Joel Feinberg, in a series of influential books, *The Moral Limits of the Criminal Law,* examines the sorts of conduct that the state may appropriately proscribe. Among the "liberty-limiting" principles he discusses are harm to others (the "harm principle") and offense to others (the "offense principle"). The "liberal position" holds that the harm and offense principles between them exhaust the class of good reasons for legal prohibitions. Liberals exclude harm to the person himself (paternalism) as a sufficient justification for legal prohibitions. Joel Feinberg, *The Moral Limits of the Criminal Law,* vol. 3, *Harm to Self* (New York: Oxford University Press, 1986): 27.

3. John Stuart Mill argues that, subject to background duties of justice and fair contribution, state coercion is justified only to prevent or punish acts causing harms to other persons, not harm to self. Mill, *On Liberty,* 68. Harm to others can be found in almost any type of behavior; indirect harm is thus subject to limitless expansion. Those who support paternalistic policies often identify financial and social harms to others with the risk behavior. For an example of the application of the harm principle to smoking regulations, see Thaddeus Mason Pope, "Balancing Public Health against Individual Liberty: The Ethics of Smoking Regulations," *University of Pittsburg Law Review,* 61 (1999–2000): 419–98.

4. Derived from the Greek *autos* ("self") and *nomos* ("law," "rule," or "governance"), meaning "the having or making of one's own laws."

5. Tom L. Beauchamp and James F. Childress, *Principles of Biomedical Ethics,* 5th ed. (New York: Oxford University Press, 2001).

6. Bernard Gert, Charles M. Culver, and K. Danner Clouser, *Bioethics: A Return to Fundamentals* (New York: Oxford University Press, 1997): 77–79.

7. Immanuel Kant, *Critique of Practical Reason and Other Writings in Moral Philosophy* (Chicago: University of Chicago Press, 1949).

8. Most liberal philosophers believe the state has no warrant for interfering with behavior that affects the individual herself. Consequently, liberals reject public health paternalism in the form of, for example, regulation of motorcycle helmets, seat belts, smoking bans, and safe sex campaigns. Lawrence O. Gostin, "When Terrorism Threatens Health: How Far Are Limitations on Personal and Economic Liberties Justified?" *Florida Law Review,* 55 (2003): 1105–70.

9. Mill, *On Liberty,* 13. Some modern liberals disagree, however, with the inflexibility of Mill's harm principle. See, e.g., H. L. A. Hart, *Law, Liberty, and*

Morality (Stanford, CA: Stanford University Press, 1972); Bernard E. Harcourt, "The Collapse of the Harm Principle," *Journal of Criminal Law and Criminology,* 90 (1999): 109–94.

10. Joel Feinberg, *Rights, Justice, and the Bounds of Liberty: Essays in Social Philosophy* (Princeton, NJ: Princeton University Press, 1980): 45.

11. Gostin, "When Terrorism Threatens Health"; Robert Nozick, *Anarchy, State, Utopia* (New York: Basic Books, 1974): 34 (endorsing the use of "force in defense against another party who is a threat, even though he is innocent and deserves no retribution").

12. Stanley S. Herr, Lawrence O. Gostin, and Harold Hongju Koh, eds., *The Human Rights of Persons with Intellectual Disabilities: Different but Equal* (Oxford: Oxford University Press, 2003).

13. See, e.g., *Simon v. Sargent,* 409 U.S. 1020 (1972), *aff'g* 346 F. Supp. 277 (D. Mass. 1972) (finding that the state can constitutionally require unwilling motorcyclists to wear protective headgear); *Everhardt v. City of New Orleans,* 217 So. 2d 400, 402 (La. 1968) (holding that "driving upon public streets and highways is a privilege and not a right; and, in the field of public safety, the [city] council" can regulate motorcycle helmets); *Benning v. State,* 641 A.2d 757, 761 (Vt. 1994) (finding that the motorcycle helmet regulation did not violate the state constitutional right of "enjoying and defending liberty").

14. See, e.g., *People v. Kohrig,* 498 N.E.2d 1158 (Ill. 1986) (holding that the legislature could rationally determine that a seat-belt use law would serve public safety and welfare); *State v. Batsch,* 541 N.E.2d 475 (Ohio Ct. App. 1988) (finding that seat belts promote the state's interest in protecting the health, safety, and welfare of its citizens); *Wells v. State,* 495 N.Y.S.2d 591 (N.Y. Sup. Ct. 1985) (holding that seat belts save lives and therefore come within state police power).

15. See, e.g., *Lewis v. United States,* 348 U.S. 419 (1955) (upholding a tax affecting gamblers as a valid exercise of taxing power); *Martin v. Trout,* 199 U.S. 212 (1905) (holding valid the exercise of state power subjecting the owner of a building where gaming was carried on to payment of judgments for money lost in play).

16. See, e.g., *Whalen v. Roe,* 429 U.S. 589 (1977) (upholding a state controlled-substances law that required people to register with the state if they had received a prescription for a drug for which there were both legitimate and illegal uses); *Randall v. Wyrick,* 441 F. Supp. 312 (W.D. Mo. 1977) (holding that the state's classification of marijuana as a controlled substance was a valid exercise of power to address the continuing social and health problems posed by the drug).

17. See, e.g., *Minn. State Board of Health v. City of Brainerd,* 241 N.W.2d 624, 629–30 (Minn. 1976) (holding that it is not the court's function to second-guess the scientific accuracy of legislation based on the fact that fluoridation prevents dental caries); *Readey v. St. Louis County Water Co.,* 352 S.W.2d 622, 631 (Mo. 1961) (finding that fluoridation of water did not deny residents freedom of choice in matters relating to bodily care and health); *Froncek v. City of Milwaukee,* 69 N.W.2d 242, 247 (Wis. 1955) (upholding fluoridation of the city's water supply in the interest of promoting public health and welfare).

18. Compulsory vaccination laws are sometimes classified as paternalistic, but vaccination prevents infection that can be transmitted to others.

19. Daniel I. Wikler, *Ethical Issues in Governmental Efforts to Promote Health* (Washington, DC: National Academy of Sciences, 1978).

20. Gerald Dworkin, "Paternalism," in *Philosophy of Law,* 6th ed., ed. Joel Feinberg and Jules Coleman (Belmont, CA: Wadsworth Publishing, 2000): 107–36; Roger B. Dworkin, "Getting What We Should from Doctors: Rethinking Patient Autonomy and the Doctor-Patient Relationship," *Health Matrix* 13 (2003): 235–96; Thaddeus Mason Pope, "Monstrous Impersonation: A Critique of Consent-Based Justifications for Hard Paternalism," *University of Missouri-Kansas City Law Review,* 73 (2005): 681–84.

21. Some commentators urge a distinction between "soft" and "hard" paternalism. The former is a limitation of liberty where the subject does not act substantially autonomously, while the latter is a limitation where the subject does act substantially autonomously. Soft paternalism entails restrictions on conduct where the person's decision is coerced, not factually informed, not adequately understood, or otherwise not substantially voluntary. Thaddeus Mason Pope, "Counting the Dragon's Teeth and Claws: The Definition of Hard Paternalism," *Georgia State University Law Review*, 20 (2004): 659–721. My discussion in the text is closest to the idea of hard paternalism. However, since I do not believe that a firm dichotomy can be drawn between fully autonomous and nonautonomous conduct, I do not employ the terms *hard* and *soft* paternalism.

22. Compare *Chevron U.S.A. Inc. v. Echazabal,* 536 U.S. 73 (2002) (finding that employers may lawfully fire an individual whose work poses a direct threat to that employee's health); with *International Union, U.A.W., v. Johnson Controls,* 499 U.S. 187 (1991) (rejecting paternalism as a justification for barring fertile women from a battery-making facility because of the effects of lead exposure on their reproductive systems and future offspring).

23. Ian Kennedy's definition exposes the problematic assumptions of paternalism: "Decisions concerning a particular person's fate are better made for him than by him, because others wiser than he are more keenly aware of his best interests than he can be." Ian Kennedy, "The Legal Effect of Requests by the Terminally Ill and Aged Not to Receive Further Treatment," *Criminal Law Review,* 1976 (1976): 217–32. In addition, restrictive laws not only forgo the individual's right to autonomous decision making, but can also prohibit owners from using their property as they otherwise would. For example, antismoking laws threaten the property rights of bar and restaurant owners and patrons. Nicholas A. Danella, "Smoked Out: Bars, Restaurants, and Restrictive Antismoking Laws as Regulatory Takings," *Notre Dame Law Review,* 81 (2006): 1095–1121.

24. Robert L. Rabin and Stephen D. Sugarman, eds., *Smoking Policy: Law, Politics, and Culture* (New York: Oxford University Press, 1993): 7.

25. For the philosophical perspective, see Dworkin, "Paternalism," 278 ("We are all aware of our irrational propensities, deficiencies in cognitive and emotional capacities, and avoidable and unavoidable ignorance, lack of will-power, and psychological and sociological pressures"). For the law and economics perspective, see Christine Jolls, Cass R. Sunstein, and Richard Thaler, "A Behavioral Approach to Law and Economics," *Stanford Law Review*, 50 (1998):

1471–1550 (arguing that individual capacity to pursue utility is constrained by "bounded rationality," "bounded willpower," and "bounded self-interest").

26. There are at least two possible social meanings in condom use. First, imagine a world where condom use is the exception, such that asking another to use it signals the belief that there is a special reason to use a condom and interrupt sex. Second, imagine a world where people ordinarily use condoms and where an ordinary part of sex is the use of a condom. Lawrence Lessig, "The Regulation of Social Meaning," *University of Chicago Law Review,* 62 (1995): 1022–23.

27. A negative externality is a "spillover" harm that extends outside the market and affects third parties. For example, activities that transmit an infectious disease are negative externalities. The burdens of behavior posing a risk of disease transmission are borne by other specific individuals (close contacts or sexual partners) or by the population at large. Individuals infected with a contagious disease have diminished incentives to reduce risk behaviors because the burdens of the unsafe activity do not affect them directly but fall primarily on others. W. Kip Viscusi, "Regulation of Health, Safety, and Environmental Risks," NBER Working Paper 11934 (Cambridge, MA: National Bureau of Economic Research, 2006).

28. Thaddeus Mason Pope, "Balancing Public Health against Individual Liberty: The Ethics of Smoking Regulations," *University of Pittsburg Law Review,* 61 (2000): 419–98.

29. Lawrence O. Gostin, "The Legal Regulation of Smoking (and Smokers): Public Health or Secular Morality?" in *Morality and Health,* ed. Allan M. Brandt and Paul Rozin (New York: Routledge, 1997): 331; Michael Brauer and Andrea 't Mannetje, "Restaurant Smoking Restrictions and Environmental Tobacco Smoke Exposure," *American Journal of Public Health,* 88 (1998): 1834–36; Ronald M. Davis, "Exposure to Environmental Tobacco Smoke: Identifying and Protecting Those at Risk," *JAMA,* 280 (1998): 1947–49.

30. *Everhardt v. City of New Orleans,* 217 So. 2d 400, 403 (La. 1968) ("Loose stones on the highway kicked up by passing vehicles . . . could so affect the operator of a motorcycle [without a helmet] as to cause him momentarily to lose control and thus become a menace to other vehicles on the highways"); *Benning v. Vermont,* 641 A.2d 757, 758 (Vt. 1994) ("An unprotected motorcycle operator could be affected by roadway hazards, temporarily lose control and become a menace to other motorists").

31. *Everhardt,* 217 So. 2d at 403 ("The legislature is [not] powerless to prohibit individuals from pursuing a course of conduct which could conceivably result in their becoming public charges"); *Benning,* 641 A.2d at 762 ("Whether in taxes or insurance rates, our costs are linked to the actions of others and are driven up when others fail to take preventive steps that would minimize health care consumption").

32. *Simon v. Sargent,* 346 F. Supp. 277, 279 (D. Mass. 1972) (declaring that a state law requiring motorcyclists to wear helmets was a valid exercise of police power).

33. Thaddeus Mason Pope, "Is Paternalism Really Never Justified? A Response to Joel Feinberg" (working paper, University of Memphis School of Law, 2005).

34. Dan E. Beauchamp, "Community: The Neglected Tradition of Public Health," in *New Ethics for the Public's Health,* ed. Dan E. Beauchamp and Bonnie Steinbock (New York: Oxford University Press, 1999): 57.

35. Andrew W. Siegel, "The Jurisprudence of Public Health: Reflections on Lawrence O. Gostin's *Public Health Law,*" *Journal of Contemporary Health Law and Policy,* 18 (2001): 359–72.

36. Richard J. Bonnie, "The Efficacy of Law as a Paternalistic Instrument," in *Nebraska Symposium on Motivation 1985: The Law as a Behavioral Instrument,* ed. Gary B. Melton (Lincoln: University of Nebraska Press, 1985): 131.

37. *Prion* is an acronym for "proteinaceous infectious particle." Prions cause a fatal, transmissible neurodegenerative disease often called prion disease or transmissible spongiform encephalopathy (TSE). This includes bovine spongiform encephalopathy (BSE) in cattle, scrapie in sheep and goats, and chronic wasting disease (CWD) in cervid species (deer and elk). Some humans who eat beef products containing the BSE agent have contracted variant Creutzfeldt-Jakob disease (vCJD). Institute of Medicine, *Advancing Prion Science: Guidance for the National Prion Research Program* (Washington, DC: National Academies Press, 2003).

38. National Research Council, *Understanding Risk.*

39. People face not only physical risks but also social risks, such as invasions of privacy, discrimination, or stigmatization. Scott Burris, "Law and the Social Risk of Health Care: Lessons from HIV Testing," *Albany Law Review,* 61 (1998): 821–96.

40. Risk analysis is the application of scientific and other methods to evaluate risk. Its aim is to increase understanding of the substantive qualities, seriousness, likelihood, and conditions of a hazard and the options for managing it. See, e.g., John J. Cohrssen and Vincent T. Covello, *Risk Analysis: A Guide to Principles and Methods for Analyzing Health and Environmental Risks* (Washington, DC: White House Council on Environmental Quality, 1989); National Research Council, *Issues in Risk Assessment* (Washington, DC: National Academies Press, 1993); Robert W. Hahn, Kenneth J. Arrow, Maureen L. Cropper, et al., *Benefit-Cost Analysis in Environmental, Health, and Safety Regulation: A Statement of Principles* (Washington, DC: AEI Press, 1996).

41. Risk perception is the study of the diverse ways that different communities perceive risk, and the use of these perceptions to select (and prioritize) a regulatory agenda to reduce risk. Many scholarly examinations of risk perception are concerned with differences between expert and lay perceptions of risk. See, e.g., Judith A. Bradbury, "The Policy Implications of Differing Concepts of Risk," *Science, Technology and Human Values,* 14 (1989): 380–99; Gerald. A. Cole and Stephen B. Withey, "Perspective on Risk Perception," *Risk Analysis,* 1 (1981): 143–63; Timothy McDaniels and Mitchell Small, *Risk Analysis and Society: An Interdisciplinary Characterization of the Field* (New York: Cambridge University Press, 2003); William R. Freudenburg, "Perceived Risk, Real Risk: Social Science and the Art of Probabilistic Risk Assessment," *Science,* 242 (1988): 44–49.

42. Risk characterization typically has been seen as a summary of scientific information as an aid to policy formulation. National Research Council, *Risk Assessment in the Federal Government: Managing the Process* (Washington, DC:

National Academies Press, 1983): 20. The National Research Council later emphasized the importance of consultation in a democratic society: "Risk characterization is a synthesis and summary of information about a potentially hazardous situation that addresses the needs and interests of decision makers and of interested and affected parties. Risk characterization is a prelude to decision-making and depends on an iterative, analytic-deliberative process." National Research Council, *Understanding Risk,* 215; Paul Slovic, *The Perception of Risk* (London: Earthscan, 2000).

43. Risk communication is the process by which policymakers explain the nature and seriousness of risks to the public. Risk communication is concerned with the effectiveness with which messages are presented to the public: Are they understandable? Do they over- or undersimplify? Do they accurately explain the scientific evidence or the scientific uncertainties? See, e.g., Peter Bennett and Kenneth Calman, eds., *Risk Communication and Public Health* (Oxford: Oxford University Press, 2001); National Research Council, *Improving Risk Communication* (Washington, DC: National Academies Press, 1989); Caron Chess, Kandice L. Salomone, and Billie Jo Hance, "Improving Risk Communication in Government: Research Priorities," *Risk Analysis,* 15 (1995): 127–35; Dorothy Nelkin, "Communicating Technological Risk: The Social Construction of Risk Perception," *Annual Review of Public Health,* 10 (1989): 95–113.

44. Risk management is the study of the various policies that could be adopted in response to risk. What policy options exist and how likely are they to prevent harm, reduce the probabilities that harm will occur, or ameliorate harms once they have occurred? Risk management may have to grapple with competing risks—for example, the risks of acting or not acting, and the risk from one source or another. See, e.g., Sheila Jasanoff, *Risk Management and Political Culture: A Comparative Analysis of Science* (New York: Russell Sage Foundation, 1986); Vlasta Molak, *Fundamentals of Risk Analysis and Risk Management* (New York: Lewis Publishers, 1996).

45. See, e.g., *Indus. Union Department v. American Petroleum Institute,* 448 U.S. 607, 644 (1980) (determining that lowering benzene exposure levels required proof of "a significant risk of harm and therefore a probability of significant benefits"). For an argument about the efficiency advantages of better information and evidence, see W. Kip Viscusi, *Risks by Choice: Regulating Health and Safety in the Work Place* (Cambridge, MA: Harvard University Press, 1983).

46. For historical works that chronicle the invidious discrimination and prejudiced attitudes regarding illness and disease, see, e.g., Susan Sontag, *Illness as Metaphor* (New York: Farrar, Straus and Giroux, 1988); Allan M. Brandt, *No Magic Bullet: A Social History of Venereal Disease in the United States since 1880* (New York: Oxford University Press, 1985).

47. In *Jacobson v. Massachusetts,* 197 U.S. 11 (1905), the Supreme Court articulated for the first time the requirement that the use of public health powers must be limited to real and significant threats. Public health powers should only be used in case of a public health necessity. See also *School Board of Nassau County v. Arline,* 480 U.S. 273, 285 (1987) (finding that because Congress intended to protect against "society's accumulated myths and fears about disability and disease," contagiousness alone is not a justification for employment dismissal).

48. Transgenic plants and animals have created concerns in Europe and North America despite the absence of scientific evidence about risks to human health. See, e.g., World Health Organization, Food Safety Department, *Modern Food Biotechnology, Human Health and Development: An Evidence-Based Study* (Geneva: WHO, 2005) (noting that genetically modified foods can enhance health and development but should undergo continued safety assessments before marketing to prevent risks to humans and the environment); National Research Council, *Genetically-Modified Pest-Protected Plants: Science and Regulation* (Washington, DC: National Academies Press, 2000); Royal Society of Medicine, *Genetically Modified Plants for Food Use* (London: Royal Society, 1998); Othmar Kappeli and Lillian Auberson, "How Safe Is Safe Enough in Plant Genetic Engineering?" *Trends in Plant Science,* 3 (1998): 276–81; Allison A. Snow and Pedro Moran Palma, "Commercialization of Transgenic Plants: Potential Ecological Risks," *BioScience,* 47 (1997): 86–96.

49. Public health officials are often justified in averting future as well as current risks. Consider a population comprised of asymptomatic persons infected with Mycobacterium tuberculosis (M.TB) who are not currently contagious but are likely to develop active disease in the future (e.g., persons dually infected with HIV and M.TB). Public health officials may be justified in imposing directly observed therapy on the entire population to avert the threat of individuals relapsing and posing a serious risk of TB transmission. Lawrence O. Gostin, "The Resurgent Tuberculosis Epidemic in the Era of AIDS: Reflections on Public Health, Law, and Society," *Maryland Law Review,* 54 (1995): 102–8.

50. For a perversion of the significant risk standard, see *Onishea v. Hopper,* 171 F.3d 1289 (11th Cir. 1999) (en banc) (upholding segregation of recreational, religious, and educational programs in state prison, based on inmates' HIV-positive status, because a "significant risk" of HIV transmission existed for any prison program in which HIV-positive inmates sought participation); *Davis v. Hopper,* 528 U.S. 1114 (2000) (holding that because HIV infection carries grave consequences, even a theoretical risk of transmission is sufficient to justify segregation of HIV-infected prisoners).

51. Harold P. Green, "The Law-Science Interface in Public Policy Decision Making," *Ohio State Law Journal* 51 (1990): 375–405.

52. Paul Slovic, "Trust, Emotion, Sex, Politics, and Science: Surveying the Risk Assessment Battlefield," *University of Chicago Legal Forum* (1997): 59–99; Paul Slovic, "Perception of Risk," *Science,* 236 (1987): 280–85.

53. For a discussion of the different uses of language by scientists and the public, see Lisa Randall, "Dangling Particles," *New York Times,* September 18, 2005 (arguing that scientific terminology has abstraction and complexity, while the lay public prefers a simple story); David C. Balderston, "Science and Uncertainty," *New York Times,* September 23, 2005 ("The appeal of the simple story is based in human nature and in the universal longing for security, certainty and predictability").

54. See, e.g., Howard Margolis, *Dealing with Risk: Why the Public and the Experts Disagree on Environmental Issues* (Chicago: University of Chicago Press, 1996): 1; Stephen Breyer, *Breaking the Vicious Circle: Toward Effective Risk Regulation* (Cambridge, MA: Harvard University Press, 1993): 35–39; Cass R. Sun-

stein, "Selective Fatalism," *Journal of Legal Studies,* 27 (1998): 799–823; Rick Kreutzer and Christine Arnesen, "The Scientific Assessment and Public Perception of Risk," *Current Issues in Public Health,* 1 (1995): 102; Viscusi, "Regulation of Health, Safety, and Environmental Risks."

55. *Compare* Cass R. Sunstein, "Misfearing: A Reply," *Harvard Law Review,* 119 (2006): 1110–25, 1110 ("In processing information, people use identifiable heuristics, which can produce severe and systematic errors. . . . As a result of various forms of bounded rationality, human beings are prone to what might be called 'misfearing': they fear things that are not dangerous, and they do not fear things that impose serious risks"), *with* Dan M. Kahan, Paul Slovic, Donald Braman, et al., "Fear of Democracy: A Cultural Evaluation of Sunstein on Risk," *Harvard Law Review,* 119 (2006): 1071–1109. See also Cass R. Sunstein, *Laws of Fear: Beyond the Precautionary Principle* (Cambridge, UK: Cambridge University Press, 2005).

56. Rachel Novak, "Flesh-Eating Bacteria: Not New, but Still Worrisome," *Science,* 264 (1994): 1665.

57. Eliot Marshall, "A Is for Apple, Alar, and . . . Alarmist? Two Years Ago Environmentalists Branded Alar the Most Dangerous Chemical Residue in Children's Food: Since Then, the Official Risk Estimates Have Fallen," *Science,* 254 (1991): 20–22.

58. The first U.S. case of BSE was identified in Washington state and was announced to the public on December 23, 2003. Shankar Vedantam, "Mad Cow Case Found in U.S. for First Time: Infected Animal Killed in Washington State," *Washington Post,* December 24, 2003.

59. Institute of Medicine, *Biological Threats and Terrorism: Assessing the Science and Response Capabilities* (Washington, DC: National Academies Press, 2002).

60. See, e.g., Breyer, *Breaking the Vicious Circle,* 9–10. Media coverage of negligible risks may lead regulators to undertake policy actions not warranted by actual risk levels. Viscusi, "Regulation of Health, Safety, and Environmental Risks."

61. These kinds of lay distinctions are far from simple. Cass R. Sunstein, "A Note on 'Voluntary' versus 'Involuntary' Risks," *Duke Environmental Law and Policy Forum,* 8 (1997): 173–80. Why, for example, is air travel thought to be involuntary, but automobile travel voluntary? Why do people feel that they can avert accidents through skillful and careful driving, even though the data show otherwise? See, e.g., Neil D. Weinstein, "Optimistic Biases about Personal Risks," *Science,* 246 (1989): 1232–33; Slovic, "Trust, Emotion, Sex, Politics, and Science."

62. Amartya Sen, "The Discipline of Cost-Benefit Analysis," in Matthew D. Adler and Eric A. Posner, eds., *Cost-Benefit Analysis: Legal, Economic, and Philosophical Perspectives* (Chicago: University of Chicago Press, 2000): 95–116 (arguing that current cost-benefit analyses are extraordinarily limited because of the insistence on doing the valuations entirely through market mechanisms and excluding important human values).

63. Public health policies may create not only health risks but also social risks. Stigmatization and economic punishments can be adverse effects of public health

regulation. Katherine Mayer, "An Unjust War: The Case against the Government's War on Obesity," *Georgetown Law Journal*, 92 (2004): 999–1006. And public health action entails trade-offs between benefits and risks. For example, crops genetically engineered to produce essential medicines and vaccines ("bio-pharming") create benefits but pose risks to the environment.

64. Lawrence O. Gostin, Zita Lazzarini, Verla S. Neslund, et al., "Water Quality Laws and Waterborne Diseases: *Cryptosporidium* and Other Emerging Pathogens," *American Journal of Public Health*, 90 (2000): 847–53.

65. World Health Organization, *Aide-Memoire for a Strategy to Protect Health Workers from Infection with Bloodborne Viruses* (Geneva: World Health Organization, 2003).

66. Cass R. Sunstein, "Health-Health Tradeoffs," *University of Chicago Law Review*, 63 (1996): 1533–71; Cass R. Sunstein, *Risk and Reason: Safety, Law, and the Environment* (Cambridge: Cambridge University Press, 2002): 133–52.

67. New York City launched an insecticide-spraying program in 1999 after residents became ill with West Nile virus. Environmental groups filed a lawsuit to stop the spraying, which they alleged was causing pollution in navigable waters, a violation of the federal Clean Water Act. The act requires a federal permit to discharge a pollutant into a navigable body of water and gives any citizen standing to bring suit to stop a violation. The U.S. Court of Appeals for the Second Circuit vacated a lower court decision, ruling that the Clean Water Act authorizes any citizen to bring suit to enforce its requirements. *No Spray Coalition, Inc. v. City of New York*, 351 F.3d 602 (2d Cir. 2003). The suit was remanded to the district court. Both parties sought to renew their summary judgment motions. The district court denied both motions because there were issues of material fact as to whether the city discharged pollutants into navigable waters without a permit. *No Spray Coalition Inc. v. City of New York*, No. 00 Civ. 5395, 2005 U.S. Dist. LEXIS 11097 (S.D.N.Y. June 7, 2005).

68. James F. Childress, Ruth R. Faden, Ruth D. Gaare, et al., "Public Health Ethics: Mapping the Terrain," *Journal of Law, Medicine, and Ethics*, 30 (2002): 170–81.

69. Institute of Medicine, *Improving Health in the Community: A Role for Performance Monitoring* (Washington, DC: National Academies Press, 1997); Institute of Medicine, *Health Performance Measurement in the Public Sector: Principles and Policies for Implementing an Information Network* (Washington, DC: National Academies Press, 1999); Institute of Medicine, *Using Performance Monitoring to Improve Community Health: Exploring the Issues* (Washington, DC: National Academies Press, 1996). See Centers for Disease Control and Prevention, "Framework for Program Evaluation in Public Health," *Morbidity and Mortality Weekly Report*, 48 (1999): 1–40.

70. See, e.g., Peter D. Jacobson and Matthew L. Kanna, "Cost-Effectiveness Analysis in the Courts: Recent Trends and Future Prospects," *Journal of Health Politics, Policy and Law*, 26, no. 2 (2001): 291–326.

71. Quality-adjusted life-years (QUALYs) are a measure of health needs that encompass not only length of life but also the quality of that life (e.g., in symptoms and ability to function). In the context of vaccines, see Institute of Medicine, *Vaccines for the Twenty-first Century: A Tool for Decisionmaking* (Wash-

ington, DC: National Academies Press, 1999) (reviewing cost-effectiveness and ethical concerns regarding QUALYs).

72. See, e.g., Cass R. Sunstein, *The Cost-Benefit State: The Future of Regulatory Protection* (Chicago: American Bar Association, 2002); W. Kip Viscusi, *Fatal Tradeoffs: Public and Private Responsibilities for Risk* (New York: Oxford University Press, 1992); Cass R. Sunstein, "Paradoxes of the Regulatory State," *University of Chicago Law Review,* 57 (1990): 407–41; Kenneth J. Arrow, Maureen L. Cropper, and George C. Eads, "Is There a Role for Benefit-Cost Analysis in Environmental, Health, and Safety Regulation?" *Science,* 272 (1996): 221–22; W. Kip Viscusi, "Regulating the Regulators," *University of Chicago Law Review,* 63 (1996): 1423–61; Douglas A. Kysar, "It Might Have Been: Risk, Precaution, and Opportunity Costs" (working paper, Cornell Law School, supported by the National Science Foundation's Nanotechnology and Interdisciplinary Research Award #0304483, 2006).

73. See, e.g., Jacobson and Kanna, *Cost-Effectiveness Analysis in the Courts;* Marthe R. Gold, Joanna E. Siegel, Louise B. Russel, et al., *Cost-Effectiveness in Health and Medicine,* ed. Marthe R. Gold (New York: Oxford University Press, 1996); Louise B. Russell, Marthe R. Gold, Joanna E. Siegel, et al., "The Role of Cost-Effectiveness Analysis in Health and Medicine," *JAMA,* 276 (1996): 1172–77; Joanna E. Siegel, Milton C. Weinstein, Louise B. Russell, et al., "Recommendations for Reporting Cost-Effectiveness Analyses," *JAMA,* 276 (1996): 1339–41; Milton C. Weinstein, J. E. Siegel, Marthe R. Gold, et al., "Recommendations of the Panel on Cost-Effectiveness in Health and Medicine," *JAMA,* 276 (1996): 1253–58.

74. John D. Graham, Phaedra S. Corso, Jill M. Morris, et al., "Evaluating the Cost-Effectiveness of Clinical and Public Health Measures," *Annual Review of Public Health,* 19 (1998): 125–52.

75. Steve P. Calandrillo, "Responsible Regulation: A Sensible Cost-Benefit, Risk versus Risk Approach to Federal Health and Safety Regulation," *Boston University Law Review,* 81 (2001): 957–1032.

76. *Whitman v. American Trucking Ass'n,* 531 U.S. 457, 467–68 (2001) (finding that the Clean Air Act bars the EPA from considering implementation costs in setting national ambient air quality standards).

77. Other sections of the Clean Air Act give explicit permission to engage in cost-benefit analysis. *Whitman,* 531 U.S. at 467.

78. Perhaps the most famous critique of the regulatory state was offered by Stephen Breyer before he was appointed to the Supreme Court. Breyer, *Breaking the Vicious Circle.*

79. Craig Gannett, "Congress and the Reform of Risk Regulation," *Harvard Law Review,* 107 (1994): 2095–104 (reviewing Breyer, *Breaking the Vicious Circle*).

80. *United States v. Ottati & Goss Inc.,* 900 F.2d 429 (1st Cir. 1990) (finding that the EPA should be held to a more stringent standard of review when addressing "not *whether* the site will be cleaned up, but rather . . . who should pay the added cost of making it extremely clean").

81. Here are some of the costs per lives saved (thousands) in John F. Morrall's famous table comparing various risk-reducing regulations: unvented space

heaters ($100), passive restraints/belts ($300), alcohol and drug control ($500), asbestos ($104,200), benzene/ethylbenzenol styrene ($483,000), formaldehyde ($72,000,000). John F. Morrall III, "A Review of the Record," *Regulation,* 10 (Nov./Dec. 1986): 25–34. For a powerful critique of Morrall's methods, see Lisa Heinzerling, "Regulatory Costs of Mythic Proportions," *Yale Law Journal,* 107 (1998): 1981–2070, 2042; Lisa Heinzerling, "The Rights of Statistical People," *Harvard Environmental Law Review,* 24 (2000): 189–207.

82. The value of human life can be reduced to a numerical ratio of costs and benefits only if that life is merely a statistic without a name and without a face. Once that life has an identity, human emotion negates such measures of worth. Society is thus more likely to refrain from using a cost-benefit analysis to evaluate life-saving regulatory programs when an identifiable person needs rescue. For further explication on the distinction between statistical and identified lives, see Heinzerling, "Rights of Statistical People," 203–6.

83. Heinzerling, "Regulatory Costs of Mythic Proportions."

84. Ellen K. Silbergeld, "The Risks of Comparing Risks," *New York University Environmental Law Journal,* 3 (1995): 405–30.

85. Heinzerling, "Regulatory Costs of Mythic Proportions" (arguing that the assumptions made in cost-benefit analyses are far from value-neutral).

86. Lisa Heinzerling and Frank Ackerman, "The Humbugs of the Anti-Regulatory Movement," *Cornell Law Review,* 87 (2002): 648–70.

87. Frank Ackerman and Lisa Heinzerling, "Pricing the Priceless: Cost-Benefit Analysis of Environmental Protection," *University of Pennsylvania Law Review,* 150 (2002): 1553–84.

88. Frank Ackerman and Lisa Heinzerling, *Priceless: On Knowing the Price of Everything and the Value of Nothing* (New York: New Press, 2004).

89. Despite costly regulation of cattle feed and cattle screening, there has not been a single documented case of variant Creutzfeldt-Jakob disease (vCJD) (the human disease caused by the infectious agent of BSE) contracted in the United States. Institute of Medicine, *Advancing Prion Science*; Ermias D. Belay and Lawrence B. Schonberger, "The Public Health Impact of Prion Diseases," *Annual Review of Public Health,* 26 (2005): 191–212.

90. Another way of thinking about fairness, advocated by many scholars in the fields of law and economics, is that costs and burdens might justifiably be placed not only on those who cause risk, but also on those who can best afford to incur regulatory costs or burdens.

91. Public Health Leadership Society, *Principles of the Ethical Practice of Public Health* (Washington, DC: American Public Health Association, 2002).

92. Something is transparent if it allows light to pass through with little or no interruption or distortion so that objects on the other side can be clearly seen. The secondary meaning, closer to the idea of transparency in the political sense, is: "Clearly recognizable as what it, he, or she really is, or completely open and frank." *Oxford English Dictionary,* 2d ed., s.v. "Transparent."

93. Childress et al., "Public Health Ethics."

94. Norman Daniels, "Accountability for Reasonableness," *British Medical Journal,* 321 (2000): 1300–1301.

95. Childress et al., "Public Health Ethics."

96. The Supreme Court has made it easier to discipline "whistle-blowers" by holding that when public employees speak pursuant to their official duties, they are not speaking as citizens and the First Amendment does not protect them from disciplinary action. *Garcetti v. Ceballos,* 547 U.S. 410 (2006) (upholding disciplinary action against an employee for reporting a sheriff's misrepresentation of facts in a murder case, since he made the statements pursuant to his official duties as a deputy district attorney).

97. Jayne Parry and John Wright, "Community Participation in Health Impact Assessments: Intuitively Appealing but Practically Difficult," *Bulletin of the World Health Organization,* 6 (2003): 388; CSIS Homeland Security and David Heyman, *Model Operational Guidelines for Disease Exposure Control* (Washington, DC: Center for Strategic and International Studies, 2005).

98. Kinsley, "As through a Glass Darkly."

99. Lawrence O. Gostin, Ronald Bayer, and Amy L. Fairchild, "Ethical and Legal Challenges Posed by Severe Acute Respiratory Syndrome," *JAMA,* 290 (2003): 3229–37.

100. Limited data exist on the effectiveness of the traditional methods used during the 2003 SARS outbreak. The value of social distancing, wearing masks, entry and exit screening, and educating travelers on the perceived risks remain unquantified. David M. Bell, "World Health Organization Working Group on Prevention of International and Community Transmission of SARS: Public Health Interventions and SARS Spread, 2003," *Emerging Infectious Diseases,* 10 (2004): 1900–1906; Ronald St. John, A. King, D. de Jong, et al., "Border Screening for SARS," *Emerging Infectious Diseases,* 11 (2005): 6–10.

101. As the epigraph from the Dalai Lama indicates, it is important to be careful about science and values when applying the precautionary principle. Taking precautions when the scientific evidence of future harm is highly suggestive but not definitive may make impeccable sense (e.g., to avert global warming). However, taking precautions when the scientific evidence of the *absence* of harm is suggestive but not definitive may undermine public health. For example, some parents argue that their children should not be vaccinated even though the Institute of Medicine found that there is no evidence that thimerosal (a mercury preservative in some vaccines) causes autism. Institute of Medicine, *Immunization Safety Review: Vaccines and Autism* (Washington, DC: National Academies Press, 2004).

102. American Public Health Association, "Policy Statement 200011: The Precautionary Principle and Children's Health," *American Journal of Public Health,* 91 (2001): 495–96.

103. The European Commission has issued perhaps the most detailed account of the precautionary principle. Communication from the Commission on the Precautionary Principle (COM [2000] 1) (arguing that precautionary regulation should be proportional, nondiscriminatory, consistent, cost-effective, subject to review, and part of more comprehensive risk assessment). See Dale Jamieson and Daniel Wartenberg, "The Precautionary Principle and Electric and Magnetic Fields," *American Journal of Law and Public Health,* 91 (2001): 1355–58; Nicolas De Sadeleer, "The Precautionary Principle in EC Health and Environmental Law," *European Law Journal,* 12 (2006): 139–72.

104. The roots of the precautionary principle can be traced to the concept of *vorsorgeprinzip* developed in Germany in the 1970s to prevent air pollution from damaging forests. Sonja Boehmer-Christiansen, "The Precautionary Principle in Germany," in *Enabling Government in Interpreting the Precautionary Principle,* ed. Tim O'Riordan and James Cameron (London: Earhtscan Publications, 1994): 36. *Vorsorge* means planning, foresight, and taking care by good husbandry. David Kriebel and Joel Tickner, "Reenergizing Public Health through Precaution," *American Journal of Public Health,* 91 (2001): 1351–55.

105. Carolyn Reffensperger and Joel A. Tickner, eds., *Protecting Public Health and the Environment: Implementing the Precautionary Principle* (Washington, DC: Island Press, 1999).

106. *World Charter for Nature,* G.A. Res. 37/7, U.N. GAOR, 37th Sess., Supp. No. 51, at 18, U.N. Doc. A/RES/37/7 and Add. 1 ("[Proponents of] activities which are likely to pose a significant risk to nature . . . shall demonstrate that the expected benefits outweigh potential damage"). For a history of the precautionary principle and analysis of its status as a legal rule or standard, see Sonia Boutillon, "The Precautionary Principle: Development of an International Standard," *Michigan Journal of International Law,* 23 (2002): 429–69.

107. Bill Durodie, "The True Cost of Precautionary Chemicals Regulation," *Risk Analysis,* 23 (2003): 389–98; Frank B. Cross, "Paradoxical Perils of the Precautionary Principle," *Washington and Lee Law Review,* 53 (1996): 851–925; Cass R. Sunstein, "The Laws of Fear," *Harvard Law Review,* 115 (2002): 1110–25, 1119.

108. A decision rule based on the precautionary principle is complex, requiring an assessment of at least four variables: (i) *the threat dimension*—to what types of hazards does the principle apply? (ii) *the uncertainty dimension*—what level of scientific evidence should be required? (iii) *the action dimension*—what types of measures against potential hazards are warranted? (iv) *the command dimension*—with what force are these measures implemented (voluntary, authorized, mandatory)? Per Sandin, "Dimensions of the Precautionary Principle," *Human and Ecological Risk Assessment,* 5 (1999): 889–907.

3. PUBLIC HEALTH LAW IN THE CONSTITUTIONAL DESIGN: PUBLIC HEALTH POWERS AND DUTIES

SOURCES FOR CHAPTER EPIGRAPHS: Nina Mendelson, "Bullies along the Potomac," *New York Times,* July 5, 2006 (noting that the National Uniformity for Food Act, passed by the House, would bar states from addressing a bevy of foodborne hazards); *DeShaney v. Winnebago County Dep't of Soc. Servs.,* 489 U.S. 189, 213 (1989) (Blackmun, J., dissenting); *Castle Rock v. Gonzales,* 545 U.S. 748 (2005); William Blackstone, *Public Wrongs,* vol. 4, *Commentaries on the Laws of England* (1769, rpt. Chicago: University of Chicago Press, 1979); *Mormon Church v. United States,* 136 U.S. 1, 57 (1890); Thomas M. Cooley, *A Treatise on Constitutional Limitations, Which Rest upon the Legislative Power of the States of the American Union,* 6th ed. (Boston: Little, Brown, 1890): 587.

1. "At least as far back as *Martin v. Hunter's Lessee* (1816), the Court has resolved questions 'of great importance and delicacy' in determining whether par-

ticular sovereign powers have been granted to the Federal Government or have been retained by the States." *New York v. United States,* 505 U.S. 144, 155 (1992) (internal citation omitted).

2. Erwin Chemerinsky, *Constitutional Law: Principles and Policies,* 2d ed. (New York: Aspen, Law and Business, 2002): 1–6.

3. Lawrence O. Gostin, Judith Areen, Patricia A. King, et. al., *Law, Science and Medicine,* 3d ed. (New York: Foundation Press, 2005): 440–43.

4. James G. Hodge, Jr., "Implementing Modern Public Health Goals through Government: An Examination of New Federalism and Public Health Law," *Journal of Contemporary Health Law and Policy,* 14 (1997): 93–126.

5. Tribal governments are also an important aspect of American federalism, although tribal sovereignty is keenly debated in political circles. Hope M. Babcock, "A Civic-Republican Vision of 'Domestic Dependent Nations' in the Twenty-first Century: Tribal Sovereignty Re-envisioned, Reinvigorated, and Re-empowered," *Utah Law Review,* 2 (2005): 443–573.

6. Michael J. Sandel, *Democracy's Discontent: America in Search of a Public Philosophy* (Cambridge, MA: Belknap Press of Harvard University Press, 1996): 347 (arguing that federalism is not just a "theory of intergovernmental relations" but a "political vision" that "self-government works best when sovereignty is dispersed and citizenship formed across multiple sites of civic engagement").

7. *McCulloch v. Maryland,* 17 U.S. 316 (1819) (holding that the "Necessary and Proper" Clause of the Constitution permits Congress to incorporate a bank).

8. "The constitution gives nothing to the States or to the people. Their rights existed before it was formed, and are derived from the nature of sovereignty and the principles of freedom." *Gibbons v. Ogden,* 22 U.S. 1, 87 (1824) (holding that a state law prohibiting vessels from navigating the waters of the state was repugnant to the Constitution and void).

9. *Gade v. Nat'l Solid Waste Mgmt. Ass'n,* 505 U.S. 88, 98 (1992) (holding that the federal Occupational Health and Safety Act implicitly preempts unapproved state regulations regarding trade association members' handling of hazardous waste).

10. David C. Vladeck, "Preemption and Regulatory Failure," *Pepperdine Law Review,* 33 (2005): 95–132; Richard C. Ausness, "Preemption of State Tort Law by Federal Safety Statutes: Supreme Court Preemption Jurisprudence since Cipollone," *Kentucky Law Journal,* 92 (2003–4): 913–78.

11. *The Cigarette Labeling and Advertising Act,* 15 U.S.C.A. §§ 1334–41 (2005), bars states from imposing requirements or prohibitions on tobacco manufacturers based on "smoking and health." See e.g., *Lorillard Tobacco Co. v. Reilly,* 533 U.S. 525 (2001) (invalidating a Massachusetts law aimed at preventing youth exposure to cigarette advertising, on grounds of preemption); *Cipollone v. Liggett Group,* 505 U.S. 504 (1992) (holding some state failure-to-warn and fraudulent misrepresentation claims are preempted). Federal preemption of state tobacco control laws can occur under other statutes as well, such as the Federal Aviation Administration Authorization Act of 1994. See *N.H. Motor Transp. Ass'n v. Rowe,* 448 F.3d 66 (1st Cir. 2006) (preempting a Maine law aimed at

preventing youth access to tobacco from Internet and mail-order sales by requiring carriers to ensure that cigarettes were delivered only to adults).

12. *The Occupational Safety and Health Act of 1970* (OSHA), 29 U.S.C.A. §§ 651–78 (2005), preempts states from establishing an occupational health and safety standard on an issue for which OSHA has already promulgated a standard, unless the state has obtained the Secretary's approval for the state's plan. See, e.g., *Chao v. Mallard Bay Drilling, Inc.*, 534 U.S. 235 (2002) (holding that OSHA preempted general marine safety regulations over working conditions on uninspected vessels conducting inland drilling operations where the Coast Guard regulations did not address the occupational safety and health risks posed by such drilling operations).

13. *Geier v. American Honda Motor Co.*, 529 U.S. 861 (2000) (holding that manufacturers of cars made before federal law required airbags cannot be sued under state negligence laws for failing to have the safety devices).

14. *The Employee Retirement Income Security Act of 1974* (ERISA), 29 U.S.C.A. § 1132(a) (2005), preempts state regulation of risk retention plans. See, e.g., *Aetna Health Inc. v. Davila*, 542 U.S. 200 (2004) (holding petitioners' claims that they suffered injuries due to a health care administrator's decision not to provide coverage for physician-recommended treatments were preempted by ERISA).

15. *Colaciccio v. Apotex, Inc.*, 432 F. Supp. 2d 514 (E.D. Penn. 2006) (holding that common law tort claims for failure to warn about the suicide risk from Paxil are preempted by the labeling requirements of the Food, Drug, and Cosmetic Act). See also Mary J. Davis, "Discovering the Boundaries: Federal Preemption of Prescription Drug Labeling Product Liability Actions," *Social Science Research Network*, May 22, 2006, http://papers.ssrn.com/sol3/papers.cfm?abstract_id=903757 (stating that the FDA directive represents the first time in the agency's hundred-year history that it has sought to preempt common law prescription drug labeling claims). But see *Jackson v. Pfizer, Inc.*, 432 F. Supp. 2d 964 (D. Neb. 2006) (rejecting a drug manufacturer's argument that the Food, Drug, and Cosmetic Act preempted state failure to warn claimants regarding the suicide risk of Zoloft); Thomas Ginsburg, "Litigation Inoculation," *Philadelphia Inquirer*, July 9, 2006 (reporting that most drug manufacturer dismissal attempts on preemption grounds have been denied).

16. Henry Waxman, *Congressional Preemption of State Laws and Regulations* (House Committee on Government Reform, Minority Office, June 2006), http://www.democrats.reform.house.gov/Documents/20060606095331–23055.pdf.

17. The Supreme Court's preemption cases have not been uniformly antiregulatory. The judiciary, due to its respect for principles of federalism, is sometimes reluctant to infer federal preemption in the absence of clearly expressed congressional intent. Consequently, courts have sustained state and local public health regulation, despite federal preemption claims, in spheres such as licensing of nuclear power plants, state tort actions for radiation exposure or faulty medical devices, smoking abatement, and permits for pesticide application to private land. See, e.g., *Sprietsma v. Mercury Marine*, 537 U.S. 51 (2002) (holding

that the express preemption clause of the Federal Boat Safety Act did not preempt a state tort claim arising out of manufacturer's failure to install proper propeller guards); *Wisconsin Public Intervenor v. Mortier,* 501 U.S. 597 (1991) (holding that express preemption of state labeling requirements in the Federal Insecticide, Fungicide, and Rodenticide Act did not supersede other types of state or local regulation); *Silkwood v. Kerr-McGee Corp.,* 464 U.S. 238 (1984) (holding that an award of punitive damages under state law for exposure to nuclear material was not preempted by the Atomic Energy Act); *Bates v. Dow Agrosciences LLC,* 544 U.S. 431 (2005) (holding claims for defective design, defective manufacture, negligent testing, breach of express warranty, and violation of the Texas Deceptive Trade Practice Act were not preempted by the Federal Insecticide, Fungicide, and Rodenticide Act); *Pharmaceutical Research & Manufacturers of America v. Walsh,* 538 U.S. 644 (2003) (holding that a state prescription drug rebate program was not preempted by federal Medicaid law); *Medtronic v. Lohr,* 518 U.S. 470 (1996) (holding that the federal Medical Device Amendment does not preempt state law defective design claims or defective labeling and marketing claims, thus allowing consumers injured by faulty medical devices to seek damages under state law against the manufacturers even if the devices comply with federal regulations).

18. Whereas all federal judges are appointed to lifetime tenures, many state judges are periodically elected.

19. Although public health commentators sometimes complain about judicial emphasis on the rights of individuals, much of this text demonstrates that, more often than not, the courts are highly deferential to public health decision making.

20. Lawrence O. Gostin, "The Formulation of Health Policy by the Three Branches of Government," in *Society's Choices: Social and Ethical Decision Making in Biomedicine,* ed. Ruth Ellen Bulger, Elizabeth Meyer Bobby, and Harvey V. Fineberg (Washington, DC: National Academies Press, 1995): 335.

21. Lawrence O. Gostin, Scott Burris, Zita Lazzarini, et. al., *Improving State Law to Prevent and Treat Infectious Disease* (New York: Milbank Memorial Fund, 1998); Lawrence O. Gostin, Scott Burris, and Zita Lazzarini, "The Law and the Public's Health: A Study of Infectious Disease Law in the United States," *Columbia Law Review,* 99 (1999): 59–128.

22. Randy E. Barnett, *Restoring the Lost Constitution: The Presumption of Liberty* (Princeton, NJ: Princeton University Press, 2004): 53–88.

23. U.S. Const. amend. VI ("In all criminal prosecutions, the accused shall enjoy the right to a speedy and public trial, by an impartial jury . . . ; to be informed of the nature and cause of the accusation; to be confronted with the witnesses against him; to have compulsory process for obtaining witnesses in his favor, and to have the Assistance of Counsel for his defense").

24. Susan Bandes, "The Negative Constitution: A Critique," *Michigan Law Review,* 88 (1990): 2271–2347; Mark Tushnet, "Symposium: A Critique on Rights," *Texas Law Review,* 62 (1984): 1363–1403.

25. See, e.g., *Jones v. Reynolds,* 438 F.3d 685 (6th Cir. 2006) (holding that police officers' failure to stop a drag race was not an affirmative act that increased the risk to a spectator who was killed); *Willhauck v. Town of Mansfield,* 164 F. Supp. 2d 127, 132 (2001) (holding that, even if a custodial special relationship

between school and student gives rise to an affirmative duty to protect, the duty terminates at the end of the school day).

26. *Estelle v. Gamble,* 429 U.S. 97, 103–4 (1976) (holding that the government has an obligation to provide medical care for incarcerated individuals).

27. *Youngberg v. Romeo,* 457 U.S. 307, 317 (1976) (holding that when a person is institutionalized, it becomes the duty of the state to provide certain services and care).

28. For a discussion of government duties to act in other contexts, such as when a child is in foster care or in school, or when a police officer witnesses other officers abusing an individual, see Erwin Chemerinsky, "Government Duty to Protect: Post-DeShaney Developments," *Touro Law Review,* 19 (2003): 679–706.

29. *Farmer v. Brennan,* 511 U.S. 825 (1994) (holding that prison officials have a duty under the Eighth Amendment to provide humane conditions of confinement, and prison officials can be liable for failing to protect an inmate from violence by other prisoners if the officials did not act when they knew of a "substantial risk of serious harm").

30. The test frequently used by the lower courts is: (1) does the government have a duty to the individual (the duty is not easily inferred), and (2) did the government act with "deliberate indifference" (mere negligence is insufficient)? *David v. Brady,* 143 F.3d 1021, 1026 (6th Cir. 1998), *cert. denied,* 525 U.S. 1093 (1999) (finding that the police acted with deliberate indifference to the safety of an intoxicated man who was hit by a car and rendered a quadriplegic after the police drove him outside the city and kicked him out of the car).

31. See, e.g., *David,* 143 F.3d at 1026; *Wood v. Ostrander,* 879 F.2d 583 (9th Cir. 1989), *cert. denied,* 498 U.S. 938 (1990) (finding "deliberate indifference" to the safety of a female passenger who was raped when the police left her in the car alone without the keys after the driver was arrested for intoxication); *Munger v. Glasgow Police Dep't,* 227 F.3d 1082 (9th Cir. 2000) (finding that the state affirmatively placed an intoxicated man "in a position of danger" when he died of hypothermia after being left on the streets overnight); *Currier v. Doran,* 242 F.3d 905 (10th Cir. 2001), *cert. denied,* 534 U.S. 1019 (2001) (finding the police acted with deliberate indifference to the foreseeable harm to a child who was killed after social workers transferred him from his mother to his abusive father).

32. *Johnson v. Dallas Independent School District* 38 F.3d 198 (5th Cir. 1994), *cert. denied,* 514 U.S. 1017 (1995) (finding that students have no constitutional right to affirmative protection from violence at school); *Archie v. City of Racine,* 847 F.2d 1211 (7th Cir. 1988), *cert. denied,* 489 U.S. 1065 (1989) (denying liability when a 911 dispatcher gave incorrect advice and failed to dispatch an ambulance for a caller who then died); *Gilmore v. Buckley,* 787 F.2d 714 (1st Cir. 1986), *cert. denied,* 479 U.S. 882 (1986) (finding no liability when state officials released a dangerous mental patient they knew had threatened a particular person, leading to her murder).

33. *DeShaney v. Winnebago County Dep't of Soc. Servs.,* 489 U.S. 189, 195 (1989) (holding that the state does not have a constitutional duty, absent a special relationship, to protect its citizens against deprivation of life, liberty, or property committed by private actors). "Nothing in the language of the Due Process Clause itself requires the State to protect the life, liberty, and property of its cit-

izens against invasion by private actors. The clause is phrased as a limitation on the State's power to act, not as a guarantee of certain minimal levels of safety and security. It forbids the State itself to deprive individuals of life, liberty, or property without 'due process of law,' but its language cannot fairly be extended to impose an affirmative obligation on the State to ensure that those interests do not come to harm through other means. Nor does history support such an expansive reading of the constitutional text. . . . Its purpose was to protect the people from the State, not to ensure that the State protected them from each other. The Framers were content to leave the extent of governmental obligation in the latter area to the democratic political processes." See *Bright v. Westmoreland County, PA*, 443 F.3d 276 (3d Cir. 2006) (holding that a substantive due process claim based on the state-created danger theory must allege misuse of state authority, not a mere failure to use it, that creates a foreseeable harm).

34. *Webster v. Reprod. Health Servs.*, 492 U.S. 490 (1989).

35. Laurence H. Tribe, "The Abortion Funding Conundrum: Inalienable Rights, Affirmative Duties, and the Dilemma of Dependence," *Harvard Law Review*, 99 (1985): 330–43.

36. *Webster*, 492 U.S. at 507.

37. *Id.* at 510.

38. *Board of Regents v. Roth*, 408 U.S. 564, 577 (1972) (holding that the plaintiff had no reasonable expectation to a property interest of receiving tenure), discussed in chapter 4.

39. "A well-established tradition of police discretion has long coexisted with apparently mandatory arrest statutes." *Castle Rock*, 545 U.S. 748 (2005).

40. *Gonzales v. City of Castle Rock*, 366 F.3d 1093,1101 (10th Cir. 2004) (en banc). Normally, the Supreme Court pays deference to the views of a federal court as to the law of a state within its jurisdiction. See, e.g., *Phillips v. Washington Legal Found.*, 524 U.S. 156, 167 (1998).

41. Justice Stevens, joined in dissent by Justice Ginsburg, drew attention to the nationwide movement of enacting laws directing police to arrest violators of domestic abuse protective orders. *Castle Rock*, 545 U.S. 748 (2005). Approximately two dozen states, in response to increased concern about domestic violence during the 1990s, made arrest mandatory for violating protective orders. "It is clear that the elimination of police discretion was integral to Colorado and its fellow States' solution to the problem of under enforcement in domestic violence cases." *Castle Rock*, 125 S. Ct. at 2818 (Stevens, J., dissenting).

42. *Roth*, 408 U.S. at 577.

43. *DeShaney*, 489 U.S. at 213 (Blackmun, J., dissenting).

44. *Osman v. United Kingdom* (87/1997/871/1083), 95 Eur. Ct. H.R. 3125, 29 Eur. H.R. Rep. 245, 5 B.H.R.C. 293 (1998) (the European Court of Human Rights finding that the government violated the right to life by not protecting a person whose life had been imminently and repeatedly threatened by a mentally ill man); *D v. United Kingdom*, 1997-III Eur. Ct. H.R. 777, 24 Eur. H.R. Rep. 423 (1997) (the European Court of Human Rights finding that it would constitute inhuman and degrading treatment to deport an immigrant with AIDS to his home country, where his health would likely deteriorate quickly).

45. Jenna MacNaughton, "Comment: Positive Rights in Constitutional Law:

No Need to Graft, Best Not to Prune," *University of Pennsylvania Journal of Constitutional Law,* 3 (2001): 750–82.

46. Seth F. Kreimer, "Allocational Sanctions: The Problem of Negative Rights in a Positive State," *University of Pennsylvania Law Review,* 132 (1984): 1293–1398.

47. Louis M. Seidman and Mark V. Tushnet, *Remnants of Belief: Contemporary Constitutional Issues* (New York: Oxford University Press, 1996): 52.

48. See Leroy Parker and Robert H. Worthington, *The Law of Public Health and Safety, and the Power and Duties of Boards of Health* (New York: Bender, 1892) for an early treatise on public health law that posted the maxim on its cover page. *Salus populi* was often used by the courts to uphold police regulations during the nineteenth century. William J. Novak, "Public Economy and the Well-Ordered Market: Law and Economic Regulation in Nineteenth-Century America," *Law and Social Inquiry,* 18 (1993): 1–32.

49. *Webster's Third New International Dictionary, Unabridged,* 3d ed., s.v. "Politia," "Polis," and "Politeia."

50. *Oxford English Dictionary,* 2d ed., s.v. "Police." For related meanings, see "Polity" and "Policy."

51. Clinton Rossiter, ed., *The Federalist Papers,* nos. 17, 34 (New York: Signet Books, 1961), quoted in Wendy E. Parmet, "From Slaughter-House to Lochner: The Rise and Fall of the Constitutionalization of Public Health," *American Journal of Legal History,* 40 (1996): 476–505, 478.

52. Pasquale Pasquino, "Theatrum Politicum: The Genealogy of Capital Police and the State of Prosperity," in *The Foucault Effect: Studies in Governmentality,* ed. Graham Burchell, Colin Gordon, and Peter Miller (Chicago: University of Chicago Press, 1991): 105, 108–11 ("police" as the "science of happiness" and the "science of government").

53. Ruth Locke Roettinger, *The Supreme Court and State Police Power: A Study in Federalism* (Washington, DC: Public Affairs Press, 1957): 10–22 (cataloguing Supreme Court statements on police power).

54. *Gibbons v. Ogden,* 22 U.S. 1, 249 (1824).

55. Frank P. Grad, *The Public Health Law Manual,* 3d ed. (Washington, DC: American Public Health Association, 2005): 11–12.

56. But see Randy E. Barnett, "The Proper Scope of the Police Power," *Notre Dame Law Review,* 79 (2004): 429–95 (concluding that there exist structural limits on state police power).

57. *Commonwealth v. Alger,* 61 Mass. 53, 96 (1851) (holding constitutional a state statute that established, to protect the common good, harbor lines beyond which owners of flats or wharves may not build).

58. William J. Novak, *The People's Welfare: Law and Regulation in Nineteenth-Century America* (Chapel Hill: University of North Carolina Press, 1996): 14.

59. See, e.g., Ernst Freund, *The Police Power, Public Policy, and Constitutional Rights* (Chicago: Callaghan, 1904); W. P. Prentice, *Police Powers Arising under the Law of Overruling Necessity* (Littleton, CO: Fred. B. Rothman, 1993): 38–41.

60. *Gibbons v. Ogden,* 22 U.S. 1, 203 (1824).

61. *Slaughter-House Cases,* 83 U.S. (16 Wall.) 36, 62 (1873) (holding that

regulation of the slaughter of meat "is, in its essential nature, one which has been . . . in the constitutional history of this country, always conceded to belong to the States").

62. Tom Chistoffel and Stephen P. Teret, *Protecting the Public: Legal Issues in Injury Prevention* (New York: Oxford University Press, 1993): 25–28.

63. 61B Am. Jur. 2D *Pollution Control* § 150 (2006).

64. *Zucht v. King*, 260 U.S. 174 (1922) (holding that a municipality may constitutionally vest in its officials broad discretion in matters affecting the enforcement of health law, specifically vaccinations).

65. Angie A. Welborn, *Federal and State Isolation and Quarantine Authority* (Washington, DC: CRS Report for Congress, updated January 18, 2005), http://www.fas.org/sgp/crs/RL31333.pdf.

66. See, e.g., *Givner v. State*, 124 A.2d 764 (Md. 1956) (upholding inspection of commercial and residential premises as a valid exercise of the police power); *See v. Seattle*, 387 U.S. 541, 550–52 (1967) (listing historical examples of state inspection) (Clark, J., dissenting).

67. See, e.g., *Jones v. State ex rel. Indiana Livestock Sanitary Board*, 163 N.E.2d 605, 606 (Ind. 1960) (finding that in the exercise of police powers, states may take the legislative steps necessary to eliminate nuisances); *Francis v. Louisiana State Livestock Sanitary Board*, 184 So. 2d 247, 253 (La. Ct. App. 1966) (upholding a statute giving the State Livestock Sanitary Board plenary power to deal with contagious and infectious diseases in animals).

68. *State ex rel. Corp. Commission v. Texas County Irrigation & Water Resources Ass'n*, 818 P.2d 449 (Okla. 1991) (upholding the state's police power to protect fresh groundwater from pollution).

69. *Strandwitz v. Board of Dietetics*, 614 N.E.2d 817, 824 (Ohio Ct. App. 1992) (finding that in the interest of protecting the health and safety of its citizens, a state may, pursuant to its police powers, regulate businesses regarding food and nutrition).

70. *Finkelstein v. City of Sapulpa*, 234 P. 187 (Okla. 1925) (holding an ordinance was not arbitrary or wrongful after the city declared a junkyard a public nuisance); *Devines v. Maier*, 728 F.2d 876 (7th Cir. 1984) (holding the city's order to temporarily vacate an uninhabitable dwelling did not constitute a Fifth Amendment taking).

71. *Safe Water Ass'n v. City of Fond du Lac*, 516 N.W.2d 13, 15 (Wis. Ct. App. 1994) (upholding the city council's adoption of a water fluoridation program as a valid exercise of state police power). See, e.g., Douglas A. Balog, "Fluoridation of Public Water Systems: Valid Exercise of State Police Power or Constitutional Violation?" *Pace Environmental Law Review*, 14 (1997): 645–90.

72. *State v. Otterholt*, 15 N.W.2d 529, 531 (Iowa 1944) (upholding state licensing requirements for chiropractors).

73. *Kassel v. Consol. Freightways Corp.*, 450 U.S. 662, 670 (1981) (holding unconstitutional an Iowa statute that purported to promote safety by diverting truck traffic to other states because the statute interfered with interstate commerce).

74. *Slaughter-House Cases*, 83 U.S. (16 Wall.) 36, 62 (1873).

75. *Pacific States Box & Basket Co. v. White*, 296 U.S. 176, 181 (1935) (hold-

ing that food regulation "is a part of the inspection laws; [and] was among the earliest exertions of the police power in America").

76. *Hillsborough County v. Automated Med. Labs. Inc.*, 471 U.S. 707, 719 (1985) (holding that federal regulations governing collection of blood plasma from paid donors did not preempt local ordinances).

77. *Rice v. Santa Fe Elevator Corp.*, 331 U.S. 218, 230 (1947), quoted with approval in *Medtronic, Inc. v. Lohr*, 518 U.S. 470, 471 (1996) (holding that in enacting the Medical Device Amendment, it was not Congress's intent to preempt general common law duties enforced by damages actions).

78. *West Virginia v. Chas. Pfizer & Co.*, 440 F.2d 1079, 1089 (2d Cir. 1971) (defining *parens patriae* theory as that which traditionally refers to the role of the state as sovereign and guardian of persons under a legal disability to act for themselves, such as juveniles or the mentally ill); for further discussion, see Daniel B. Griffith, "The Best Interests Standards: A Comparison of the State's Parens Patriae Authority and Judicial Oversight in Best Interests Determinations for Children and Incompetent Patients," *Issues in Law and Medicine*, 7 (1991): 283–338.

79. United Kingdom, *The Report of the Royal Commission on the Law Relating to Mental Illness and Mental Deficiency 1954–57* (Cmnd. 169, Her Majesty's Stationery Office: London, 1957), paras. 146, 255, 776–77, 846–52.

80. *The Statute de Prerogative Regis*, 1339, 17 Edw. II, St. I. cc. 9, 10.

81. *Alfred L. Snapp & Son, Inc. v. Puerto Rico*, 458 U.S. 592, 600 (1982) (quoting J. Chitty, *Prerogatives of the Crown* 155 [1820], explaining that the *parens patriae* action has its roots in the common law concept of the "royal prerogative," which included the right or responsibility to take care of persons who are legally incapable on account of mental incapacity).

82. *In re Estate of Longeway*, 549 N.E.2d 292 (Ill. 1989) (holding that the Probate Act implicitly authorizes a guardian to exercise the right to refuse artificial sustenance on a ward's behalf).

83. *Hawaii v. Standard Oil Co. of California*, 405 U.S. 251, 257 (1972) (holding that the Clayton Act section authorizing action for treble damages did not authorize states to sue for damages for injury to its general economy because of alleged antitrust law violations).

84. *Santosky v. Kramer*, 455 U.S. 745, 746 (1982) (requiring due process safeguards before a state could irrevocably sever a natural parent's right in her child).

85. Decision makers with total authority over the ward's personal and financial matters are commonly called plenary guardians; decision makers with authority over financial matters solely are called guardians of the estate or conservators; and decision makers with control over personal (e.g., medical and placement) questions only are guardians of the person. Marshall B. Kapp, "Ethical Aspects of Guardianship," *Clinics in Geriatric Medicine*, 10 (1994): 501–12.

86. See, e.g., Lawrence O. Gostin and Robert Weir, "Life and Death Choices after Cruzan: Case Law and Standards of Professional Conduct," *Milbank Quarterly*, 69 (1991): 143–73; Lawrence O. Gostin, "Ethics, the Constitution, and the Dying Process," *JAMA*, 293 (2005): 2403–7.

87. *Addington v. Texas*, 441 U.S. 418, 426 (requiring procedural due process requirements for use in commitment of persons with mental illness); *In re S.L.*,

94 N.J. 128, 136 (N.J. 1983) (holding that "the authority of the state to civilly commit citizens is said to be an exercise of its police power to protect the citizenry and its parens patriae authority to act on behalf of those unable to act in their own best interests"); "Developments in the Law—Civil Commitment of the Mentally Ill," *Harvard Law Review,* 87 (1974): 1190–1406.

88. *O'Connor v. Donaldson,* 422 U.S. 563, 583 (1975) (Burger, C.J., concurring) (holding that a state could not constitutionally confine a nondangerous individual who was capable of surviving safely outside of confinement).

89. See, e.g., *In re Raymond S.,* 623 A.2d 249 (N.J. Super. Ct. App. Div. 1993) (finding that sufficient evidence must exist to support involuntary commitment); *Addington,* 441 U.S. at 426.

90. *Specht v. Patterson,* 386 U.S. 605 (1967) (holding that involuntary confinement of an individual for any reason must be accomplished with due process of law).

91. Norman L. Cantor, "The Relation between Autonomy-Based Rights and Profoundly Mentally Disabled Persons," *Annals of Health Law,* 13 (2004): 37–80.

92. *Addington,* 441 U.S. at 426.

93. For a state to maintain a *parens patriae* action, it must have an interest separate from that of the private parties. *Alfred L. Snapp & Son, Inc. v. Puerto Rico ex rel. Barez,* 458 U.S. 592, 593 (1982). That is, a state cannot enter a controversy as a nominal party to forward the claims of individual citizens. *Oklahoma ex rel. Johnson v. Cook,* 304 U.S. 387 (1938). However, if a state is pursuing its own interests and, in the process, advances the interests of others, it can sue in *parens patriae.* The state's interests are expressed as "quasi-sovereign," which are those interests that a state has in the well-being of its populace; the state's interests must be sufficiently concrete to engender a conflict between the state and a defendant. A state's "quasi-sovereign" interests have two general characteristics: (1) they affect the economic or physical health and well-being of its residents, and (2) a state has an interest in not being discriminated against and denied its rightful status in the federal system. Although the courts have not delineated a quantifiable formula for determining what part of a state's population must be affected to reach a substantial segment and, therefore, trigger *parens patriae,* in making its claim, a state is allowed to consider, in addition to direct harm, the indirect effects on its population. *Alfred L. Snapp & Son,* 458 U.S. at 602.

94. A state's ability to bring an action under the doctrine of *parens patriae* is not conditioned upon whether private individuals in that state would have standing to bring suit. Larry W. Yackle, "Worthy Champion for Fourteenth Amendment Rights: The United States in Parens Patriae," *Northwestern University Law Review,* 92, no. 1 (1997): 111–72, 115. As a result, a state can redress public menaces in situations where private individuals would be unable to sue because of a lack of specific injury.

95. Yackle, "Worthy Companion," 143. The federal government also has a claim to *parens patriae* capacity where its interests in national welfare establish standing similar to that of a state.

96. *Louisiana v. Texas,* 176 U.S. 1, 19 (1900) (rejecting Louisiana's attempt to enjoin a quarantine maintained by Texas; however, Louisiana was granted standing as *parens patriae* because the quarantine affected its citizens at large).

97. *Missouri v. Illinois,* 180 U.S. 208 (1901) (holding that Missouri was permitted to sue the Chicago sanitation district on behalf of Missouri citizens to enjoin the discharge of sewage into the Mississippi River).

98. *Kansas v. Colorado,* 206 U.S. 46 (1907) (holding that Kansas was permitted to sue as *parens patriae* to enjoin the diversion of water from an interstate stream).

99. *Georgia v. Tennessee Copper Co.,* 206 U.S. 230 (1907) (holding that Georgia was entitled to sue to enjoin fumes from a copper plant across the state border from damaging land in five Georgia counties).

100. *New York v. New Jersey,* 256 U.S. 296 (1921) (holding that New York could sue to enjoin the discharge of sewage from New Jersey into the New York harbor).

101. *Support Ministries for Persons with AIDS, Inc. v. Village of Waterford,* 799 F. Supp. 272 (N.D.N.Y. 1992).

102. *McCulloch v. Maryland,* 17 U.S. 316, 421.

103. U.S. Const. art. I, § 8.

104. *Merck KGaA v. Integra Lifesciences I Ltd.,* 125 S. Ct. 2372, 2380 (2005) (finding that the drug research safe harbor in the patent statute "provides a wide berth" for the use of patented drugs in the pharmaceutical regulatory process).

105. U.S. Const. art. II, § 2. The World Health Organization's Framework Convention on Tobacco Control and the Kyoto Protocol to the United Nations Framework Convention on Climate Change were both signed but not ratified by the United States.

106. *Helvering v. Davis,* 301 U.S. 619, 640–41 (1937) (finding that Congress has discretion to determine whether taxing and spending advances the general welfare, and that its discretion will be upheld unless clearly wrong or arbitrarily exercised).

107. *United States v. Butler,* 297 U.S. 1, 65 (1936) (finding that the taxing and spending power "confers a power separate and distinct from those later enumerated").

108. *Black Lung Benefits Act,* 30 U.S.C. § 901 (1994). Consider excise taxes that have a trust fund with a related public health purpose; for example, the tax on the sale or use of domestically mined coal goes to the Black Lung Disease Trust Fund for Miners.

109. Office of Management and Budget, *Budget of the U.S. Government: Analytical Perspectives, Fiscal Year 2006* (Washington: OMB, 2005). Over the same period, the tax credit for orphan drug research will cost $1.47 billion and the deductibility of medical expenses will cost $54.77 billion. See John Sheils and Randall Haught, "The Cost of Tax-Exempt Health Benefits in 2004," *Health Affairs,* February 5, 2004, http://content.healthaffairs.org/cgi/reprint/hlthaff.w4.106v1 for a discussion of the government's tax expenditure for health benefits and its cost.

110. "No Capitation, or other direct, Tax shall be laid, unless in Proportion to the Census." This "apportionment" requirement made it burdensome for the federal government whenever the Supreme Court ruled that a tax, for constitutional purposes, was "direct." U.S. Const. art. I, § 9, cl. 4.

111. *Pollock v. Farmers' Loan & Trust Co.,* 157 U.S. 429 (1895) (holding

that the income tax, because the source of income is, in part, property, is unconstitutional unless apportioned).

112. *United States v. Constantine,* 296 U.S. 287, 295 (1935) (holding that a federal tax that punishes liquor dealers who violate state liquor laws is unconstitutional); *Bailey v. Drexel Furniture Co.,* 259 U.S. 20, 37 (1922) (holding that a federal tax imposed on violators of federal child labor regulations has a "prohibitory and regulatory effect and purpose [that is] palpable").

113. *United States v. Sanchez,* 340 U.S. 42, 44 (1950) (citing *Sonzinsky v. United States,* 300 U.S. 506, 513–14 [1937]. The earlier case upheld a federal tax on firearms capable of concealment; *United States v. Sanchez* upheld a federal tax on distribution or prescription of marijuana).

114. *United States v. Kahriger,* 345 U.S. 22 (1953) (holding the Gamblers' Occupational Tax Act, which levied a tax on persons engaged in the business of accepting wagers, thereby having a regulatory effect, was constitutional).

115. Daniel M. Fox and Daniel C. Schaffer, "Tax Policy as Social Policy: Cafeteria Plans, 1978–1985," *Journal of Health Politics, Policy and Law,* 12 (1987): 609–64, 610; see Daniel M. Fox and Daniel C. Schaffer, "Tax Administration as Health Policy: Hospitals, the Internal Revenue Service, and the Courts," *Journal of Health Politics, Policy and Law,* 16 (1991): 251–79; Lee R. Alton, *A History of Regulatory Taxation* (Lexington: University of Kentucky Press, 1973): 1–11.

116. *Child and Dependent Care Tax Credit,* I.R.C. § 21(a) (1996) (allowing taxpayers to subtract a percentage of money spent on child care from overall tax liability); I.R.C. § 21 (1989).

117. *Low Income Housing Credit,* I.R.C. § 42 (1989).

118. *Clinical Testing Expenses for Certain Drugs for Rare Diseases or Conditions,* I.R.C. § 45C (1989).

119. *Charitable Contributions,* I.R.C. § 170 (1989).

120. For a more complete discussion, see Jendi B. Reiter, "Citizens or Sinners? The Economic and Political Inequity of 'Sin Taxes' on Tobacco and Alcohol Products," *Columbia Journal of Law and Social Problems,* 29 (1996): 443–68.

121. I.R.C. § 5701 (2000) (tobacco).

122. I.R.C. §§ 5051 (1991) (beer); 5001 (1995) (distilled spirits); 5041 (1998) (wines).

123. I.R.C. § 5821 (1989) (making firearms).

124. I.R.C. § 4401 (1989) (wagering).

125. I.R.C. § 4081 (2006) (gas).

126. I.R.C. § 4681 (1997) (ozone-depleting chemicals).

127. *United States v. Butler,* 297 U.S. 1, 66 (1936) (holding that Congress's power to tax is expressly conferred by the General Welfare Clause of the Constitution).

128. *Helvering v. Davis,* 301 U.S. 619, 641 (1937) (upholding Title II of the Social Security Act, which provides for old-age benefits, as a valid exercise of the spending power).

129. *Pennhurst State Sch. & Hosp. v. Halderman,* 451 U.S. 1, 17 (1981) (holding that the Developmentally Disabled Assistance and Bill of Rights Act, which conditioned federal funding to aid states in creating programs to care for

the developmentally disabled, was a legitimate exercise of Congress's spending power).

130. *South Dakota v. Dole,* 483 U.S. 203, 211 (1987) (upholding the constitutionality of a federal statute conditioning states' receipt of federal funds on adoption of a minimum drinking age of twenty-one).

131. *Speiser v. Randall,* 357 U.S. 513, 526 (1958) (invalidating a statute that denied tax exemptions to those who could not prove they did not advocate the violent overthrow of the government); *United States v. American Library Ass'n,* 539 U.S. 194, 210 (2003) (finding that government may not deny a benefit on a basis that infringes the First Amendment even if the person has no entitlement to that benefit). Supreme Court cases on the unconstitutional conditions doctrine are difficult to reconcile. For example, compare *Rust v. Sullivan,* 500 U.S. 173 (1991) (allowing the federal government to condition aid to Planned Parenthood clinics on the requirement that they not provide abortion counseling or referrals); with *Legal Services Corp. v. Velazquez,* 531 U.S. 533 (2001) (invalidating a federal law that prevented recipients of legal services funds from challenging the validity of welfare laws and regulations). Most recently, see *Rumsfeld v. Forum for Academic and Institutional Rights, Inc,* 547 U.S. 47 (2006) (upholding the Solomon Amendment's requirement that universities grant military recruiters access to students on the basis that a funding condition cannot be unconstitutional if it could be constitutionally imposed directly).

132. *Halderman,* 451 U.S. at 17 (finding that states must be cognizant of the consequences in advance of their participation in a federal grant program).

133. *Halderman,* 451 U.S. at 17; *Barnes v. Gorman,* 536 U.S. 181 (2002) (holding that the provisions in the federal Rehabilitation Act and ADA, which prohibit discrimination in programs that receive federal funds, did not provide for punitive damages suits because if Congress wanted to condition federal funds, the recipients of the funds must have notice that by accepting federal funds they are exposing themselves to those conditions).

134. *Gonzaga Univ. v. Doe,* 536 U.S. 273 (2002) (holding that the Family Educational Rights and Privacy Act (FERPA), which conditions grants to state agencies and educational institutions upon compliance with requirements to keep student records private, did not create individual, enforceable rights).

135. *Sanchez v. Johnson,* 416 F.3d 1051 (9th Cir. 2005) (finding that the Medicaid provision, 42 U.S.C. § 1396a[a][30][A], did not create rights enforceable under 42 U.S.C. § 1983 for developmentally disabled Medicaid beneficiaries).

136. *Chas. C. Steward Mach. Co. v. Davis,* 301 U.S. 548, 590 (1937) (holding that a provision of the Social Security Act that enabled employers who paid taxes to a federally approved state unemployment compensation fund to credit those payments toward the federal payroll tax on employers was not overly coercive).

137. *Sabri v. United States,* 541 U.S. 600 (2004) (upholding a federal statute that criminalized accepting bribes by any organization, government, or agency that receives federal assistance, without requiring any showing of a connection between the bribes and the federal funds, because the statute promoted general welfare by ensuring taxpayer dollars were spent for general welfare); *United States v. American Library Ass'n, Inc.,* 539 U.S. 194 (2003) (upholding the Children's

Internet Protection Act [CIPA], which required public libraries receiving federal funds for Internet access to install software to block pornography).

138. *South Dakota v. Dole,* 483 U.S. 203 (1987) (holding that the indirect imposition of a minimum drinking age was a valid exercise of Congress's spending power, reasonably calculated to advance the general welfare and that national concern of interstate travel, and the Twenty-first Amendment was not violated because the statute did not induce the petitioner to engage in unconstitutional activities).

139. Albert J. Rosenthal, "Conditional Federal Spending and the Constitution," *Stanford Law Review,* 39 (1987): 1103–64.

140. 42 U.S.C. § 3756(f) (1994) (requiring involuntary postconviction testing of sex offenders); *Act of Oct. 28, 1991,* Pub. L. No. 102–141, Title VI, § 633, 1991 U.S.C.C.A.N. (105 Stat.) 834, 876–77, reprinted in note to 42 U.S.C. § 300ee-2 (1994) (requiring adoption of CDC guidelines or their "equivalent" for preventing transmission of infection during invasive medical procedures); *Ryan White CARE Act Amendments of 1996,* Pub. L. No. 104–146, § 7, 110 Stat. 1346, 1369 (codified at 42 U.S.C. § 300 ff [1994]) (requiring acceptance of CDC guidelines for counseling and testing of pregnant women). For general discussion, see Lawrence O. Gostin, *The AIDS Pandemic: Complacency, Injustice, and Unfulfilled Expectations* (Chapel Hill: University of North Carolina Press, 2004).

141. 42 U.S.C. § 1396a (1994) (enumerating Medicaid requirements for establishment of state plans; 42 U.S.C. § 1395i-4 (requiring state grants for planning and implementation of rural health care networks to be based on eligibility as defined in the statute).

142. *Rust v. Sullivan,* 500 U.S. 173 (1991) (permitting federal regulations prohibiting use of Title X funds in programs where abortion is used as a means of family planning).

143. *Coastal Zone Management Act of 1972,* 16 U.S.C. §§ 1451–65 (1994); *Federal Water Pollution Control Act,* 33 U.S.C. §§ 1251–1387 (1994); *Resource Conservation and Recovery Act,* 42 U.S.C. § 6901 (1994).

144. Large SUVs qualify for an expense allowance for small businesses, have preferred tax treatment for depreciation, and are excluded from the gas-guzzler excise tax. Gary Guenther, *Tax Preferences for Sport Utility Vehicles (SUVs): Current Law and Legislative Initiatives in the 109th Congress* (Washington: CRS Report for Congress, updated June 19, 2006), http://www.ncseonline.org/NLE/CRS/abstract.cfm?NLEid = 249.

145. *New York v. United States,* 505 U.S. 144, 159 (1992) (upholding monetary and access incentives but invalidating commandeering provisions of the Low-Level Radioactive Waste Policy Act).

146. *National Labor Relations Board. v. Jones & Laughlin Steel Corp.,* 301 U.S. 1, 37 (1937) (holding that a provision of the National Labor Relations Act, which assured employees the right to organize and bargain collectively, was a valid exercise of Congress's commerce power).

147. *United States v. Darby,* 312 U.S. 100, 115 (1941) (upholding Congress's commerce power to create a federally prescribed minimum wage for workers whose goods are shipped interstate).

148. *New York,* 505 U.S. at 159–60; *GDF Realty Invs., Ltd. v. Norton,* 326 F.3d 622 (5th Cir. 2003) (holding that a "take" provision of the Endangered Species Act of 1973 [ESA] was within Congress's commerce power because the regulation was part of a larger regulation of endangered species that is national in scope); *Rancho Viejo, LLC v. Norton,* 323 F.3d 1062 (D.C. Cir. 2003) (also upholding application of the ESA, under the Commerce Clause, to protect an animal species located entirely within one state).

149. *United States v. Sullivan,* 332 U.S. 689 (1948) (upholding Congress's commerce power to regulate the labeling of medicine shipped interstate and being held for future sales in purely local or intrastate commerce); *McDermott v. Wisconsin,* 228 U.S. 115 (1913) (upholding the Pure Food and Drugs Act of 1906 against a challenge under the Commerce Clause).

150. In *Hodel v. Virginia Surface Mining & Reclamation Ass'n,* 452 U.S. 264, 277 (1981), for example, the Supreme Court sustained federal regulation of surface mining, even though regulation of land use is a traditional state function. Congress's intent was to prevent "hazards dangerous to life," such as soil erosion and water pollution, and to "conserve soil, water, and other natural resources."

151. Department of Health and Human Services, Control of Communicable Diseases (Proposed Rule), 42 CFR Parts 70 and 71 (November 30, 2005) (justifying regulations based on the power to control the channels of foreign and interstate commerce [by protecting against the introduction and transmission of communicable diseases] and the instrumentalities of foreign and interstate commerce [e.g., flights arriving into the United States or traveling from one state into another]).

152. *United States v. Lopez,* 514 U.S. 549 (1995).

153. *United States v. Morrison,* 529 U.S. 1062 (2000).

154. In *Solid Waste Agency of Northern Cook County v. United States Army Corps of Engineers,* 531 U.S. 159, 173 (2001), the Court invalidated the Corps' assertion of jurisdiction over isolated wetlands, including seasonal ponds and small lakes that are not connected to navigable interstate waterways but serve as habitats for migratory birds. The Court avoided the Commerce Clause question but reiterated that "the grant of authority to Congress under the Commerce Clause, though broad, is not unlimited." The Court failed to provide hoped-for guidance for deciding when wetlands qualify as "waters of the United States," protected by the Clean Water Act in *Rapanos v. United States,* 547 U.S. 715 (2006), with a plurality saying that a wetland must be a relatively permanent body of water bearing "a continuous surface connection to 'waters of the United States,'" but Justice Kennedy stating that there needs to be only a "nexus" between wetlands and navigable waters. See also *United States v. Jones,* 529 U.S. 848 (2000) (stating that allowing a federal law criminalizing arson of property in interstate commerce to apply to arson of a residence would raise constitutional doubts as to whether Congress had exceeded the scope of its commerce power); *United States v. Smith,* 402 F.3d 1303 (11th Cir. 2005) (holding that purely intrastate possession of child pornography was not subject to congressional regulation under the Commerce Clause even though some of the disks on which the pornography was copied traveled through interstate commerce).

155. *Reno v. Condon,* 528 U.S. 141 (2000) (holding that the Driver's Pri-

vacy Protection Act [DPRA] is a proper exercise of Congress's authority to regulate interstate commerce because drivers' information is an article of commerce and its sale or release into the interstate stream of business is sufficient to support congressional regulation).

156. *Pierce County, WA v. Guillen,* 537 U.S. 129 (2003) (upholding a federal statute that protected reports and surveys compiled by state agencies after auto accidents as part of a federal program to identify potential accident sites from discovery under the reasoning that it protected channels of interstate commerce).

157. *Gonzales v. Raich,* 545 U.S. 1 (2005). For a more thorough discussion, see Lawrence Gostin, "Medical Marijuana, American Federalism, and the Supreme Court," *JAMA,* 294 (2005): 842–44.

158. *Raich,* 125 S. Ct. at 2209.

159. The Court found "striking similarities" between *Raich* and *Wickard v. Filburn,* 317 U.S. 111 (1942) (upholding a federal prohibition on a farmer growing wheat for his own consumption). "Like the farmer in *Wickard,* respondents are cultivating, for home consumption, a fungible commodity for which there is an established, albeit illegal, interstate market." *Raich,* 125 S. Ct. at 2206.

160. Lawrence O. Gostin, "The Supreme Court's Impact on Medicine and Health: The Rehnquist Court, 1986–2005," *JAMA,* 294 (2005): 1685–87.

161. The Supreme Court has long held that, in all but the narrowest circumstances, state laws violate the Commerce Clause if they mandate "differential treatment of in-state and out-of-state economic interests that benefits the former and burdens the latter." *Oregon Waste Systems, Inc. v. Department of Environmental Quality,* 511 U.S. 93, 99 (1994). Even when the states are acting under express constitutional powers to regulate the sale of alcoholic beverages (U.S. Const. amend. XXI), the Court has held that discriminatory action violates the Dormant Commerce Clause. *Granholm v. Heald,* 544 U.S. 460 (2005) (holding that a Michigan statute which prohibited out-of-state wineries from shipping wine directly to in-state consumers, but permitted in-state wineries to do so if licensed, discriminated against interstate commerce).

162. *Hillside Dairy, Inc. v. Lyons,* 539 U.S. 59 (2003) (rejecting the lower court's holding that California's milk pricing and pooling laws were exempt from Commerce Clause scrutiny); *West Lynne Creamery v. Healy,* 512 U.S. 186 (1994) (holding that a Massachusetts milk pricing order that subjected all milk sold to Massachusetts retailers to assessment, with the entire assessment distributed to Massachusetts dairy farmers, violated the Commerce Clause); *Dean Milk Co. v. City of Madison,* 340 U.S. 349 (1951) (holding that a local ordinance denying a corporation the right to sell its products within the city due to the distance of its pasteurization plants violated the Commerce Clause because it imposed an undue burden on interstate commerce).

163. *Bacchus Imp., Ltd. v. Dias,* 468 U.S. 263 (1984) (holding that a Hawaii local liquor tax exemption violated the Commerce Clause).

164. *Granholm v. Heald,* 544 U.S. 460 (2005) (holding that state laws which allow in-state wineries to sell directly to customers but force out-of-state wineries to use distributors violate the Commerce Clause).

165. *Sporhase v. Nebraska ex rel. Douglas,* 458 U.S. 941, 958–60 (1982) (in-

validating state regulation of ground water because it posed an unreasonable burden on interstate commerce).

166. *C & A Carbone, Inc. v. Clarkstown,* 511 U.S. 383 (1994) (invalidating a local requirement that solid waste be processed at the town's transfer station because it deprived out-of-state firms access to the local market); *Fort Gratiot Sanitary Landfill, Inc. v. Michigan Dep't of Natural Res.,* 504 U.S. 353 (1992) (holding that a state prohibition on private landfill operators from accepting solid waste that originated outside the county in which their facilities are located violated the Commerce Clause).

167. *City of Philadelphia v. New Jersey,* 437 U.S. 617 (1978) (invalidating a New Jersey statute prohibiting the importation of most solid or liquid waste that originated outside the state, because it attempted to regulate out-of-state commercial interests in violation of the Commerce Clause).

168. *Chemical Waste Mgmt v. Hunt,* 504 U.S. 334 (1992) (holding that an Alabama statute imposing an added fee on hazardous waste generated outside the state violated the Commerce Clause).

169. See, e.g., *Arkansas v. Oklahoma,* 503 U.S. 91, 101 (1992) (holding that the EPA was authorized to issue water quality regulations in Arkansas that affected Oklahoma).

170. *Gade v. Nat'l Solid Waste Mgmt. Ass'n,* 505 U.S. 88, 97 (1992) (holding that the federal Occupational Health and Safety Act implicitly preempts unapproved state regulations regarding the trade association members' handling of hazardous waste).

171. *United States Dep't of Energy v. Ohio,* 503 U.S. 607, 611–612 (1992) (holding that the national government's immunity from liability for civil fines imposed by a state for past violations of the Clean Water Act is not waived); *Kenaitze Indian Tribe v. Alaska,* 860 F.2d 312, 314 (9th Cir. 1988), *cert. denied,* 491 U.S. 905 (1989) (finding that a state's definition of "rural area" was in conflict with the federal definition under the Alaska National Interest Land Conservation Act).

172. One rationale for national minimum standards is to prevent states from relaxing environmental protection to attract industry. This "race-to-the-bottom" rationale is thought to help states resist local economic pressures, but it has been criticized. Richard L. Revesz, "Rehabilitating Interstate Competition: Rethinking the "Race-to-the-Bottom" Rationale for Federal Environmental Regulation," *New York University Law Review,* 67 (1992): 1210–54.

173. U.S. Const. amend. XI ("The Judicial power of the United States shall not be construed to extend to any suit . . . commenced or prosecuted against one of the United States by Citizens of another State or by Citizens or Subjects of any Foreign State"); *Lapides v. Bd of Regents of the Univ. Sys. of Georgia,* 535 U.S. 613 (2002) (holding that a state's removal of a suit to federal court constitutes waiver of its Eleventh Amendment immunity); *Fed. Mar. Comm'n v. South Carolina State Ports Auth.,* 535 U.S. 743 (2002) (holding that the state's sovereign immunity precludes the Federal Maritime Commission [FMC], created under Article I, from adjudicating suits against the state).

174. *Kansas v. Colorado,* 533 U.S. 1 (2003) (holding that Kansas's recovery of monetary damages from Colorado due to Colorado's violation of the Arkansas

River Compact did not violate the Eleventh Amendment because Kansas was protecting its own interest in the suit and not just that of its individual citizens).

175. *Alden v. Maine,* 527 U.S. 706, 709 (1999) (holding that Congress could not subject the state to suit in state court without its consent).

176. *College Sav. Bank v. Florida Prepaid Postsecondary Educ. Expense Board,* 527 U.S. 666 (1999); *Jim C. v. United States,* 235 F.3d 1079 (8th Cir. 2000) (holding that § 504 of the Rehabilitation Act was a valid exercise of Congress's spending power and that Arkansas waived its immunity to § 504 suits by accepting federal funds).

177. *Atascadero State Hosp. v. Scanlon,* 473 U.S. 234 (1983) (holding that Congress had not been sufficiently explicit in the Rehabilitation Act of 1974 to subject a state hospital to suit for refusing to hire a handicapped applicant); *Dellmuth v. Muth,* 491 U.S. 223 (1989) (holding that in enacting the Education of the Handicapped Act, Congress had not evinced "an unmistakably clear intention to abrogate the State's constitutionally secured immunity from suit").

178. *Seminole Tribe v. Florida,* 517 U.S. 44 (holding that Congress could not authorize an Indian tribe to sue the state in a dispute over gaming activities); Carlos Manuel Vazques, "What Is Eleventh Amendment Immunity?" *Yale Law Journal,* 106 (1997): 1683–1806.

179. The Court has similarly held that Congress cannot abrogate state immunity under its Article I powers. *Federal Mar. Comm'n,* 535 U.S. 743.

180. *Alden,* 527 U.S. at 709.

181. *Florida Prepaid,* 527 U.S. 627 (holding that the Patent and Plant Protection Remedy Clarification Act, which amended the patent laws to expressly abrogate the state's sovereign immunity, was unconstitutional).

182. *Florida Prepaid,* 527 U.S. 666 (holding that the Trademark Remedy Clarification Act [TRCA] did not abrogate the state's sovereign immunity).

183. *Kimel v. Florida Board of Regents,* 528 U.S. 62 (2000) (holding that the Age Discrimination in Employment Act [ADEA] did not validly abrogate states' Eleventh Amendment immunity from suit by private individuals).

184. *Fitzpatrick v. Bitzer,* 427 U.S. 445 (1976) (holding that Congress could abrogate the state's sovereign immunity pursuant to its enforcement power under the Fourteenth Amendment to remedy sex discrimination).

185. U.S. Const. amend. XIII, § 5.

186. U.S. Const. amend. XIV, § 5.

187. U.S. Const. amend. XV, § 5.

188. *Kimel,* 528 U.S. 62.

189. *Board of Trs. of the Univ. of Alabama v. Garrett,* 531 U.S. 356 (2001) (holding that Title I of the Americans with Disabilities Act [ADA], barring disability discrimination in employment, did not validly abrogate states' Eleventh Amendment immunity, citing lack of evidence of disability bias against state employees, but leaving open whether Title II [public services] is a valid exercise of Congress's section 5 enforcement power). The Court noted that the "overwhelming majority" of evidence of disability discrimination pertained to public services (Title II) and public accommodations (Title III). See Judith Olans Brown and Wendy E. Parmet, "The Imperial Sovereign: Sovereign Immunity and the ADA," *University of Michigan Journal of Law Reform,* 35 (2001): 1–36. In *Ten-*

nessee v. Lane, 541 U.S. 509 (2004), the Court held that a suit brought under Title II of the ADA was not barred by the Eleventh Amendment, because Title II, as applied to cases involving access to judicial services, was valid legislation under section 5 of the Fourteenth Amendment because it implicated a constitutional right. See Michael E. Waterstone, "Lane, Fundamental Rights, and Voting," *Alabama Law Review,* 56 (2005): 793–850, for a more thorough discussion.

190. *Nevada Dep't of Human Res. v. Hibbs,* 538 U.S. 721 (2003) (finding that the Family and Medical Leave Act aimed to prevent unconstitutional gender discrimination, and hence suits were not barred by the Eleventh Amendment because Congress can abrogate a state's sovereign immunity when it does so pursuant to a valid exercise of its power under section 5 of the Fourteenth Amendment).

191. *Tennessee v. Lane,* 541 U.S. 509 (2004) (involving a horrific set of facts in which a person in a wheelchair was able to gain access to the courtroom only by crawling or being carried up the stairs). In its 2005–6 term, the Supreme Court decided another ADA Title II case involving a paraplegic prisoner who claimed that he was kept in his cell for twenty-three hours per day as a result of his disability and denied access to medical treatment and privileges. *United States v. Georgia,* 126 S. Ct. 877 (2006) (holding that because Title II permits private lawsuits for damages against states for violations of the Fourteenth Amendment, the statute validly abrogates state sovereign immunity).

192. *Ex parte Young,* 209 U.S. 123 (1908) (reasoning that unconstitutional conduct by a state officer should not be considered state action on the ground that the state may not authorize unconstitutional action, and therefore, the Eleventh Amendment is not a bar to injunctive relief). The "legal fiction" of *Young* allowed federal courts in the twentieth century to implement federal constitutional protections against the states.

193. *Milliken v. Bradley (Milliken II),* 433 U.S. 267 (1977) (holding that a federal court requirement that state defendants pay one-half of the additional costs for remedial services under a school desegregation plan did not violate the Eleventh Amendment because it involved "compliance in the future with a substantive federal question determination"). But see *Edelman v. Jordan,* 415 U.S. 651 (1974) (holding that even in a suit directed against a public official, if relief involves a charge on the general revenues of the state and cannot be distinguished from an award of damages, the Eleventh Amendment bars the award).

194. The only other case in that half-century to invalidate a federal statute on Tenth Amendment grounds was later overruled. *Nat'l League of Cities v. Usery,* 426 U.S. 833 (1976), was overruled by *Garcia v. San Antonio Metro. Transit Auth.,* 469 U.S. 528 (1985).

195. *New York v. United States,* 505 U.S. 144 (1992).

196. Congress, of course, may offer incentives to the states to influence their policy choices, through, for instance, conditional spending or cooperative federalism. In both of these two methods, however, the electorate retains the ultimate authority to decide whether the state will comply. See *City of Abilene v. United States Envtl. Prot. Agency,* 325 F.3d 657 (5th Cir. 2003) (holding that although the Tenth Amendment bars federal government from compelling a city to implement a federal regulatory program, it may give the city a choice of im-

plementing the program, so long as the offered alternative does not exceed the federal government's constitutional authority).

197. *New York,* 505 U.S. at 169.

198. *Printz,* 521 U.S. 898 (holding that interim provisions of the Brady Act violated the Constitution by compelling states to enact or enforce a federal regulatory program).

199. The lower courts have not always been hospitable to challenges to federal regulation based on the reserved powers doctrine. See *City of Abilene,* 325 F.3d at 657 (holding that EPA permits imposing conditions on cities' discharge of pollutants from their storm sewer systems into U.S. waters did not violate the Tenth Amendment because alternatives to implementing the federal regulatory scheme existed, even if the alternatives were expensive or unappealing); *United States v. Milstein,* 401 F.3d 53 (2nd Cir. 2005) (holding the Prescription Drug Marketing Act of 1987 [PDMA] requiring states to have a federally mandated scheme for licensing wholesale drug distributors engaged in interstate commerce did not violate the Tenth Amendment because the PDMA allows a state to choose between creating a licensing framework pursuant to federal guidelines and not distributing through interstate commerce).

200. Frank Goodman, ed., "The Supreme Court's Federalism: Real or Imagined," *Annals of the American Academy of Political and Social Science,* 574 (2001): 9–23.

4. CONSTITUTIONAL LIMITS ON THE EXERCISE OF PUBLIC HEALTH POWERS: SAFEGUARDING INDIVIDUAL RIGHTS AND FREEDOMS

SOURCES FOR CHAPTER EPIGRAPHS: *New York v. Budd,* 22 N.E. 670, 676 (N.Y. 1889); editorial, *New York Times,* Feb. 22, 1905, p. 6.

1. Early public health law texts are dominated by discussions of compulsory powers. "It needs no argument to prove that the highest welfare of the State is subserved by protecting the life and health of its citizens by laws which will compel the ignorant, the selfish, the careless and the vicious, to so regulate their lives and use their property, as not to be a source of danger to others. If this be so, then the State has the right to enact such laws as shall best accomplish this purpose, even if their effect is to interfere with individual freedom and the untrammeled enjoyment of property." Leroy Parker and Robert H. Worthington, *The Law of Public Health and Safety and the Powers and Duties of Boards of Health* (Albany, NY: M. Bender, 1892): xxxviii.

2. U.S. Const. amends. I–X. The first eight amendments prohibit the federal government from invading individual rights; the Ninth Amendment provides that the enumeration of certain rights in the Constitution shall not be construed to deny other rights retained by the people; and the Tenth Amendment reserves to the states, or to the people, those powers not delegated to the federal government.

3. Constitutional entitlements also exist outside the Bill of Rights: Article I guarantees the availability of habeas corpus (to test the legality of the detention) and prohibits bills of attainder (a special legislative act that inflicts

punishment on a particular person), ex post facto laws (allowing criminal conviction of a person for an act done that was not a criminal offense when it was committed), and impairments in contractual obligations. Article III guarantees trial by jury and establishes the basic elements of the crime of treason. Article IV provides an entitlement to all privileges and immunities of citizens in the several states. Article VI prohibits the use of religious tests as a qualification for elected office.

4. Prior to the twentieth century, there was considerable uncertainty as to whether the Bill of Rights constrained the states. See, e.g., *Barron v. Baltimore,* 32 U.S. 243, 248 (1833) (holding that the Takings Clause of the Fifth Amendment did not apply to the city of Baltimore and the state of Maryland by extension, and noting that the Fifth Amendment "must be understood as restraining the power of the general government, not as applicable to the states").

5. *Planned Parenthood of Southeastern Pennsylvania v. Casey,* 505 U.S. 833, 848 (1992) ("We have held that the Due Process Clause of the Fourteenth Amendment incorporates most of the Bill of Rights against the States"). See Mark D. Rosen, "The Surprisingly Strong Case for Tailoring Constitutional Principles," *University of Pennsylvania Law Review,* 153 (2005): 1513–1637.

6. The amendments that have not been incorporated are the second (right to bear arms), third (right not to have soldiers quartered in a person's home), fifth (grand jury), seventh (civil jury), and eighth (prohibition of excessive fines).

7. *Shelley v. Kraemer,* 334 U.S. 1 (1948) (holding that judicial enforcement of racially discriminatory restrictive covenants constituted state action). See *The Civil Rights Cases,* 109 U.S. 3, 17 (1883) (constitutional rights "cannot be impaired by the wrongful acts of individuals, unsupported by State authority in the shape of laws, customs, or judicial or executive proceedings").

8. However, certain government actions are not considered to be official state action for constitutional purposes, such as the discipline of government employees. *Garcetti v. Ceballos,* 547 U.S. 410 (2006) (holding that discipline of a government employee for his speech did not violate the First Amendment).

9. *Adickes v. S. H. Kress & Co.,* 398 U.S. 144 (1970) (holding that the plaintiff had a claim under a statute affording civil action for deprivation of rights by showing the existence of a state-enforced custom of segregating races in public eating places).

10. Though I attempt to impose clarity with respect to public health activities, multiple, complicated relationships exist between health authorities and private entities. As the Supreme Court observed, to "fashion and apply a precise formula for recognition of state responsibility . . . is an impossible task." *Burton v. Wilmington Parking Authority,* 365 U.S. 715, 722 (1961) (holding that the exclusion of an individual, solely on account of race, from a restaurant in a building operated by public funds violated the Equal Protection Clause of the Fourteenth Amendment).

11. *Jackson v. Metropolitan Edison Co.,* 419 U.S. 345, 352 (1974) (holding that actions of a regulated business, providing arguably essential goods and services "affected with a public interest," are not, absent more, actions of the state for purposes of the Fourteenth Amendment Due Process Clause).

12. *Jackson,* 419 U.S. at 351.

13. *Rendell-Baker v. Kohn,* 457 U.S. 830 (1982) (finding no state action when a private school, receiving over 90 percent of its funds from the state, fired a teacher because of her speech).

14. *National Collegiate Athletic Ass'n v. Tarkanian,* 488 U.S. 179 (1988) (holding that the NCAA, in regulating collegiate athletics, does not perform a traditional or exclusive state function). But see *Brentwood Academy v. Tennessee Secondary School Athletic Ass'n,* 531 U.S. 288 (2001) (holding that pervasive entwinement of state school officials in an ostensibly private organization that regulated school sports suggested state action).

15. *Jacobson v. Massachusetts,* 197 U.S. 11 (1905) (upholding state compulsory vaccination law).

16. James A. Tobey, *Public Health Law,* 2d ed. (New York: Commonwealth Fund, 1939): 355 ("This famous decision is reproduced here in its entirety . . . because it is a noteworthy statement of the constitutional principles underlying public health administration").

17. *Lochner v. New York,* 198 U.S. 45 (1905) (holding that a state law limiting employment in bakeries to a specified number of hours unconstitutionally interferes with the freedom to contract guaranteed by the Fourteenth Amendment).

18. Wendy Parmet, Richard Goodman, and Amy Farber, "Individual Rights versus the Public's Health—One Hundred Years after *Jacobson v. Massachusetts,*" *New England Journal of Medicine,* 352 (2005): 652–54; Lawrence O. Gostin, "*Jacobson v. Massachusetts* at One Hundred Years: Police Power and Civil Liberties in Tension," *American Journal of Public Health,* 95 (2005): 576–81; James Colgrove and Ronald Bayer, "Manifold Restraints: Liberty, Public Health, and the Legacy of *Jacobson v. Massachusetts,*" *American Journal of Public Health,* 95 (2005): 571–76; Wendy K. Mariner, George J. Annas, and Leonard H. Glantz, "*Jacobson v. Massachusetts:* It's Not Your Great-Great-Grandfather's Public Health Law," *American Journal of Public Health,* 95 (2005): 581–90. See also "Symposium: Lochner Centennial Conference," *Boston University Law Review,* 85 (2005): 671–1015.

19. *Jacobson,* 197 U.S. at 26.

20. *Viemeister v. White,* 72 N.E. 97 (N.Y. 1904) (holding that laws requiring vaccination of children as a condition of their attendance in public schools are a valid exercise of the state police powers).

21. *Jacobson,* 197 U.S. at 34.

22. *Id.* at 38.

23. Michael Albert, Kristen Ostheimer, and Joel Breman, "The Last Smallpox Epidemic in Boston and the Vaccination Controversy, 1901–1903," *New Engl. J. Med.,* 344 (2001): 375–79.

24. "Vaccine Is Attacked: English Lecturer Denounces Inoculation for Smallpox," *Washington Post,* February 25, 1909.

25. "Vaccination a Crime: Porter Cope, of Philadelphia, Claims It Is the Only Cause of Smallpox," *Washington Post,* July 29, 1905 (discussing Porter F. Cope, who devoted his life to fighting the "delusion").

26. Editorial, *New York Times,* September 26, 1885.

27. "The Anti-Vaccinationists' Triumph," *New York Times,* August 18, 1898.

28. Editorial, *New York Times,* September 26, 1885.

29. "The Anti-Vaccinationists' Triumph," *New York Times*, August 18, 1898.

30. "Topic of the Times," *New York Times*, June 19, 1901.

31. "Smallpox: Vaccination and Tetanus," *Current Literature*, 32 (1902): 484–87, 485.

32. "Compulsory Vaccination," *New York Law Notes* (1901): 224–28; *Blue v. Beach*, 56 N.E. 89, 91 (Ind. 1900) ("With the wisdom or policy of vaccination, or as to whether it is or is not a preventive of . . . smallpox, courts . . . have no concern").

33. See, e.g., "Compulsory Vaccination," *New York Law Notes; Bissell v. Davison*, 32 A. 348 (Conn. 1894) (holding that a school may require that every child be vaccinated before being permitted to attend public school).

34. *Morris v. City of Columbus*, 30 S.E. 850, 851–52 (Ga.1898) ("The right to enforce vaccination . . . is derived from necessity," and the requirement of necessity is met where smallpox is prevalent in nearby towns).

35. *Potts v. Breen*, 47 N.E. 81 (Ill. 1897) (holding that where the board of health's duties under the authorizing statute were "purely ministerial," it lacked the power to compel school vaccinations absent an emergency).

36. *Potts*, 47 N.E. 81.

37. *Bissell*, 32A. at 349 (rejecting assertion that school vaccination laws deny "the privileges of the common schools . . . to those who do not" believe in vaccination).

38. *In re Walters*, 32 N.Y.S. 322 (N.Y. Gen. Term 1895).

39. "The legislature has a discretion which will not be reviewed by the courts; for it is not a part of the judicial functions to criticize the propriety of legislative action in matters which are within the authority of the legislative body." Parker and Worthington, *The Law of Public Health and Safety.*

40. *State ex rel. McBride v. Superior Court*, 174 P. 973, 976 (Wash. 1918) (the quarantine of a person diagnosed with syphilis is a lawful exercise of the police power).

41. Wendy Parmet, "From Slaughter-House to Lochner: The Rise and Fall of the Constitutionalization of Public Health," *American Journal of Legal History*, 40 (1996): 476–505.

42. *Jacobson*, 197 U.S. at 26–27.

43. *Price v. Illinois*, 238 U.S. 446 (1915) (upholding a state prohibition on the sale of certain food preservatives to protect the public health).

44. *New York ex rel. Lieberman v. Van de Carr*, 199 U.S. 552 (1905) (upholding a state prohibition on the sale of milk without a health board permit).

45. *California Reduction Co. v. Sanitary Reduction Works*, 199 U.S. 306 (1905) (upholding an ordinance requiring refuse to be cremated or destroyed at the owner's expense).

46. *Jacobson*, 197 U.S. at 28.

47. Judy Pearsall, *The Concise Oxford Dictionary*, 10th ed. (New York: Oxford University Press, 1999), s.v. "Necessity."

48. *Jacobson*, 197 U.S. at 31. Even though, under *Jacobson*, the government is permitted to act only in the face of a demonstrable threat to health, the Court did not appear to require the state to produce credible scientific, epidemiologic,

or medical evidence of that threat. Justice Harlan said that "what the people believe is for the common welfare must be accepted as tending to promote the common welfare, whether it does in fact or not." *Jacobson,* 197 U.S. at 35 (quoting *Viemeister,* 72 N.E. at 99).

49. *Jacobson,* 197 U.S. at 31; *Nebbia v. New York,* 291 U.S. 502, 510–11 (1933) (holding that public welfare regulation must not be "unreasonable, arbitrary, or capricious, and the means selected shall have a real and substantial relation to the object sought to be attained").

50. *Jacobson,* 197 U.S. at 38.

51. *Id.* at 39.

52. *Id.* ("We are not to be understood as holding that the statute was intended to be applied to such a case [involving an unfit subject], or, if it was so intended, that the judiciary would not be competent to interfere and protect the health and life of the individual concerned"). It is interesting to note that Henning Jacobson did allege that, when a child, a vaccination had caused him "great and extreme suffering." *Id.* at 36. Jacobson's claim of potential harm was not without merit. In Jenner's original publication in the *Inquiry* in 1799, he noted in case IV a severe adverse reaction to vaccination, now termed anaphylaxis. Harry Bloch, "Edward Jenner (1749–1823): The History and Effects of Smallpox, Inoculation, and Vaccination," *American Journal of Diseases and Children,* 147 (1993): 772–74.

53. *Jew Ho v. Williamson,* 103 F. 10, 22 (C.C.N.D. Cal. 1900) ("It must necessarily follow that, if a large . . . territory is quarantined, intercommunication of the people within that territory will rather tend to spread the disease than to restrict it").

54. *Kirk v. Wyman,* 83 S.C. 372 (S.E. 1909) (statutes requiring the removal or destruction of property, or the isolation of infected persons, when necessary to protect public health, do not violate the Constitution).

55. *Jew Ho,* 103 F. at 22.

56. *Lochner,* 198 U.S. 45.

57. Howard Gillman, *The Constitution Besieged: The Rise and Demise of Lochner Era Police Powers Jurisprudence* (Durham, NC: Duke University Press, 1993).

58. *Lochner,* 198 U.S. at 58 ("There is . . . no reasonable foundation for holding this to be necessary or appropriate as a health law to safeguard the public health, or the health of the individuals who are following the trade of a baker").

59. *Lochner,* 198 U.S. at 69 (Harlan, J., dissenting).

60. *Lochner,* 198 U.S. at 71 (Harlan, J., dissenting).

61. *Lochner,* 198 U.S. at 73 (Harlan, J., dissenting). Ironically, the Court's insistence that government demonstrate a close connection between the intervention and the protection of public health led to better public interest lawyering. In *Muller v. Oregon,* 208 U.S. 412 (1908), Louis Brandeis wrote a richly empirical brief demonstrating the relationship between excessive labor and reproductive health. The extensive use of social and medical science in judicial briefs, often called "Brandeis briefs," therefore originated during the *Lochner* period.

62. *Coppage v. Kansas,* 236 U.S. 1 (1915) (invalidating federal and state legislation forbidding employers to require employees to agree not to join a union).

63. *Adkins v. Children's Hospital,* 261 U.S. 525 (1923) (invalidating a law establishing minimum wages for women).

64. *Weaver v. Palmer Bros.,* 270 U.S. 402 (1926) (striking down a law that prohibited use of rags and debris in mattresses, enacted to protect the public health).

65. *New State Ice Co. v. Liebmann,* 285 U.S. 262 (1932) (striking down a statute forbidding a state commission to license the sale of ice except on proof of necessity).

66. *West Coast Hotel Co. v. Parrish,* 300 U.S. 379, 391 (1937) (upholding a minimum wage law for women).

67. See, e.g., *Williamson v. Lee Optical of Oklahoma,* 348 U.S. 483 (1955) (upholding a statute prohibiting an optician from selling lenses without a prescription); *Turner v. Elkhorn Mining Co.,* 428 U.S. 1 (1976) (upholding a federal statute providing compensation to coal miners who suffered from pneumoconiosis, or black lung disease).

68. Cass Sunstein, "Lochner's Legacy," *Columbia Law Review,* 87 (1987): 873–919.

69. *Cruzan v. Director, Missouri Department of Health,* 497 U.S. 261 (1990) (citing *Jacobson* for finding a liberty interest in refusing unwanted medical treatment and for using a balancing test to determine that the state's interest in preservation of life outweighs the individual right to refuse life-sustaining treatment).

70. *Zucht v. King,* 260 U.S. 174, 176 (1922) ("*Jacobson v. Massachusetts* had settled that it is within the police power of the State to provide for compulsory vaccination").

71. Steve Calandrillo, "Vanishing Vaccinations: Why Are So Many Americans Opting Out of Vaccinating Their Children?" *University of Michigan Journal of Law Reform,* 37 (2004): 353–440 ("Compulsory vaccination laws thus enjoy broad judicial and constitutional support").

72. *Boone v. Boozman,* 217 F.Supp. 2d 938, 953 (E.D. Ark. 2002) ("Because the immunization statute is a neutral law of general applicability, heightened scrutiny is not required even though compulsory immunization may burden plaintiff's right to free exercise"), appeal dismissed, *McCarthy v. Ozark School District,* 359 F. 3d 1029 (8th Cir. 2004).

73. *Washington v. Glucksberg,* 521 U.S. 702 (1997) (holding that there is no right to assistance in committing suicide and that a Washington law banning assisted suicide was constitutional).

74. *Washington v. Harper,* 494 U.S. 210 (1990) (treatment of a prisoner against his will does not violate substantive due process where the prisoner was found to be dangerous to himself or others).

75. *Planned Parenthood of Southeastern Pennsylvania,* 505 U.S. 833.

76. However, the D.C. Circuit recently ruled that terminally ill patients have a substantive due process interest in deciding for themselves whether to accept the risk-benefit trade-offs of experimental medicines that have passed phase I safety trials. *Abigail Alliance for Better Access to Developmental Drugs v. Von Eschenbach,* 445 F.3d 470 (D.C. Cir. 2006) (holding that the FDA must present a compelling interest in order to maintain its present policy of denying access to

drugs that are not yet approved but have cleared phase I trials). See Susan Okie, "Access before Approval: A Right to Take Experimental Drugs?" *New Engl. J. Med.,* 355 (2006): 437–40. The following year, however, the decision of the Abigail Alliance panel was vacated by the circuit court sitting en banc. 495 F. 3d 695 (2007) (holding that terminally ill patients do not have a fundamental right to access such drugs).

77. *Mills v. Rogers,* 457 U.S. 291, 299 (1982) (recognizing a "liberty interest in avoiding the unwanted administration of antipsychotic drugs . . . as well as identification of the conditions under which competing state interests might outweigh it").

78. See, e.g., *Cruzan,* 497 U.S. at 261.

79. *Harper,* 494 U.S. 210.

80. *Sell v. United States,* 539 U.S. 166 (2003) (the Fifth Amendment Due Process Clause permits the government involuntarily to administer antipsychotic drugs to a mentally ill defendant facing serious criminal charges in order to render that defendant competent to stand trial, but only if the treatment is medically appropriate, is substantially unlikely to have side effects that may undermine the fairness of the trial, and taking account of less intrusive alternatives, is necessary significantly to further important governmental trial-related interests).

81. *Reynolds v. McNichols,* 488 F.2d 1378, 1383 (10th Cir. 1973) (upholding the enforcement of the city's "hold and treat" ordinance requiring testing and treatment of persons reasonably suspected of having an STI against a female sex worker, but not the john: "The ordinance is aimed at the primary source of venereal disease and the . . . prostitute was the potential source, not her would-be customer").

82. *City of New York v. Antoinette R.,* 630 N.Y.S.2d 1008 (App. Div. 1994) (enforcement of an order requiring forcible detention in a hospital setting of a person with active, infectious tuberculosis to allow for completion of an appropriate regime of medical treatment is constitutional).

83. Kathleen Stratton, Alicia Gable, and Marie McCormick, eds., *Immunization Safety Review: Thimerosal-Containing Vaccines and Neurodevelopmental Disorders* (Washington, D.C.: National Academies Press, 2001) (evaluating the scientific evidence concerning neurodevelopmental disorders in children receiving thimerosal-containing vaccines, given the growing public concern over thimerosal in the late 1990s).

84. Thomas May and Ross D. Silverman, "Clustering of Exemptions as a Collective Action Threat to Herd Immunity," *Vaccine,* 21 (2003): 1048–51.

85. *Doe v. Rumsfeld,* 341 F. Supp. 2d 1 (D.D.C. 2001) (enjoining the Department of Defense from administering the anthrax vaccine to service members without consent unless and until the FDA approves the vaccine), dismissed, 172 Fed. Appx. 327 (D.C. Cir. 2006) (FDA approval mooted the appeal and dissolved the injunction).

86. Institute of Medicine, *The Smallpox Vaccination Program: Public Health in an Age of Terrorism* (Washington, D.C.: National Academies Press, 2005); Institute of Medicine, *Review of the Centers for Disease Control and Prevention's Smallpox Vaccination Program Implementation: Letter Reports #1–6* (Washington, D.C.: National Academies Press, 2003–4).

87. Thomas B. Stoddard and Walter Rieman, "AIDS and the Rights of the

Individual: Toward a More Sophisticated Understanding of Discrimination," *Milbank Quarterly,* 68, supp. 1 (1990): 143–74.

88. Lawrence O. Gostin, "The Supreme Court's Impact on Medicine and Health: The Rehnquist Court, 1986–2005," *JAMA,* 294 (2005): 1685–87.

89. See, e.g., *Glucksberg,* 521 U.S. at 719 ("The Due Process Clause guarantees more than fair process, and the 'liberty' it protects includes more than the absence of physical restraint"); *Collins v. Harker Heights,* 503 U.S. 115, 125 (1992) (due process "protects individual liberty against certain government actions regardless of the fairness of the procedures used to implement them").

90. *Penny v. Wyoming Mental Health Professions Licensing Board,* 120 P.3d 152 (Wyo. 2005) (holding that a social worker received adequate procedural due process before an application for relicensure was denied); *Stono River Environmental Protection Ass'n v. South Carolina Department of Health & Environmental Control,* 406 S.E.2d 340 (S.C. 1991) (interveners in a water quality certification were entitled to due process rights of notice and an opportunity to be heard).

91. *Hutchinson v. City of Valdosta,* 227 U.S. 303, 308 (1913) ("It is the commonest exercise of the police power . . . to provide for a system of sewers and to compel property owners to connect therewith").

92. See, e.g., *Ewing v. Mytinger & Casselberry,* 339 U.S. 594, 599–600 (1950) ("One of the oldest examples is the summary destruction of property without prior notice or hearing for the protection of public health"); *Hodel v. Virginia Surface Mining & Reclamation Ass'n,* 452 U.S. 264, 299–300 (1981) (regulating surface mining to protect society and the environment from adverse effects); *North American Cold Storage Co. v. City of Chicago,* 211 U.S. 306 (1908) (upholding emergency seizure of contaminated food).

93. *Cleveland Board of Education v. Loudermill,* 470 U.S. 532 (1985) (finding that public employees cannot be denied their property right in continued employment without due process).

94. *United States v. Cardiff,* 344 U.S. 174 (1952) (holding that an industry that processes apples is entitled to written notice of the intention to inspect).

95. *Penny,* 120 P.3d at 175 (holding that a social worker has a constitutionally protected property interest in license); *Lowe v. Scott,* 959 F.2d 323, 335 (1st Cir. 1992) (a physician enjoys a protected property interest in a license to practice medicine); *Caine v. Hardy,* 943 F.2d 1406 (5th Cir. 1991), *cert. denied* 503 U.S. 936 (1992) (procedural due process can be accomplished by using a "post-suspension remedy," especially if the physician poses a health risk).

96. *Women's Medical Professional Corp. v. Baird,* 438 F.3d 595 (6th Cir. 2006) (holding that an abortion clinic had a property interest in continued operation that was violated by a lack of hearing); *St. Agnes Hospital, Inc. v. Riddick,* 748 F. Supp. 319, 337 (D.Md. 1990) (holding that the procedures utilized in withdrawing the accreditation of a hospital comported with due process and fairness standards).

97. *Fair Rest Home v. Commonwealth Department of Health,* 401 A.2d 872 (Pa. Commw. Ct. 1979) (requiring the health department to hold a hearing before revoking a rest home's license). But see *O'Bannon v. Town Court Nursing Center,* 447 U.S. 773 (1980) (finding that residents had no due process right before their nursing home was decertified, but the nursing home itself may have had a due process right).

98. *Contreras v. City of Chicago*, 920 F. Supp. 1370, 1392–94 (N.D. Ill. 1996), *aff'd in part* 199 F.3d 1286 (7th. Cir. 1997) (finding that a postdeprivation hearing comports with procedural due process because there is a reduced expectation of privacy for closely regulated businesses such as restaurants).

99. *Driscoll v. Stucker*, 893 So. 2d. 32 (La. 2005) (holding that a residency program director's revocation, without a hearing, of a recommendation that a graduate be eligible to take medical boards violated due process); *Darlak v. Bobear*, 814 F.2d 1055, 1061 (5th Cir. 1987) ("It is well-settled . . . that a physician's staff privileges may constitute a property interest protected by the due process clause").

100. *Board of Regents v. Roth*, 408 U.S. 564, 577 (1972) (holding that the plaintiff had no reasonable expectation of a property interest of receiving tenure).

101. *Goldberg v. Kelly*, 397 U.S. 254 (1970) (finding a property interest in the receipt of welfare and holding that due process is therefore applicable to the termination of such benefits).

102. See, e.g., *Roth*, 408 U.S. at 577; *American Manufacturers Mutual Insurance Co. v. Sullivan*, 526 U.S. 40 (1999) (finding that a Pennsylvania law which allowed insurance companies to withhold payment for medical treatment pending a utilization review did not violate due process).

103. *Kentucky Department of Corrections v. Thompson*, 490 U.S. 454, 462–63 (1989) (holding that prison regulations setting forth categories of visitors who might be excluded from visitation did not give inmates a liberty interest in receiving visitors that is protected by due process).

104. *Castle Rock v. Gonzales*, 545 U.S. 748 (2005) (holding that benefit created by state law that a third party may receive from having someone else arrested for a crime does not trigger protections under the Due Process Clause, neither in its procedural nor in its substantive manifestations).

105. *Id.* at 766.

106. *Kansas v. Hendricks*, 521 U.S. 346, 356 (1997).

107. *Hamdi v. Rumsfeld*, 542 U.S. 507 (2004) (holding that the Due Process Clause entitles U.S. citizens detained as "enemy combatants" to a hearing to contest the lawfulness of their detention). See also *Hamdan v. Rumsfeld*, 548 U.S. 577 (2005) (holding that military commissions established by President Bush to conduct criminal trials for alleged alien and terrorist detainees lacked the power to do so).

108. *Roth*, 408 U.S. at 572.

109. In cases where quick action is required, a postdeprivation hearing, or even a common law tort remedy for erroneous deprivation, satisfies due process. See, e.g., *Logan v. Zimmerman Brush Co.*, 455 U.S. 422, 436 (1982) (holding that an employee's right to use the Fair Employment Practices Act's adjudicatory procedure is a property interest protected by the Due Process Clause).

110. *Mathews v. Eldridge*, 424 U.S. 319, 335 (1976); *Hamdi v. Rumsfeld*, 124 S. Ct. 2633, 2646 (2004) (due process is a flexible concept requiring that the level of process granted be commensurate with the degree of deprivation and the circumstances). See, e.g., *Morales v. Turman*, 562 F.2d 993, 998 (5th Cir. 1977), *denying reh'g*, 565 F.2d 1215 (5th. Cir. 1977) ("The interests of the individual and of society in the particular situation determine the standards for due process"); *Harper*, 494 U.S. at 229–30.

111. Lesser deprivations of liberty (e.g., directly observed therapy) may require a more relaxed procedural standard.

112. See, e.g., *Olivier v. Robert L. Yeager Mental Health Center,* 398 F.3d 183 (2d Cir. 2005) (requiring due process in civil commitment proceedings); *In re Ballay,* 482 F.2d 648 (D.C. Cir. 1973) (same).

113. *Souvannarath v. Hadden,* 116 Cal. Rptr. 2d 7 (Cal. Ct. App. 2002) (outlining the process that must be completed before a recalcitrant patient can be detained for tuberculosis treatment under state law); *Greene v. Edwards,* 263 S.E.2d 661 (W.Va. 1980) (entitling a patient to a new hearing because counsel was not appointed until after commencement of an involuntary commitment hearing).

114. Involuntary civil commitment to a mental institution, for example, is a "massive curtailment of liberty." *Vitek v. Jones,* 445 U.S. 480, 491–92 (1980).

115. *Parham v. J. R.,* 442 U.S. 584, 609 (1979) (holding a juvenile commitment decision when made by a "neutral factfinder" is sufficient to satisfy due process requirements).

116. *Wilkinson v. Austin,* 125 S. Ct. 2384 (2005) (holding that informal, nonadversarial procedures for reviewing placement in a supermax prison satisfied the three-part test in *Mathews v. Eldridge* and therefore did not violate due process); *Neinast v. Board of Trustees of Columbus Metropolitan Library,* 346 F.3d 585 (6th Cir. 2003) (no due process violation found when a patron received notice and an opportunity to be heard prior to his one-day eviction from the library for failure to wear shoes).

117. *City of Cuyahoga Falls v. Buckeye Community Hope Foundation,* 538 U.S. 188 (2003) (holding that the city's subjection of a low-income housing ordinance to a referendum did not constitute arbitrary government conduct in violation of substantive due process).

118. See, e.g., *Troxel v. Granville,* 530 U.S. 57, 65 (2000) (the Fourteenth Amendment's Due Process Clause has a substantive component that "provides heightened protection against government interference with certain fundamental rights and liberty interests," quoting *Washington v. Glucksberg,* 521 U.S. 702, 720 [1997]).

119. *State Farm Mutual Automobile Insurance Co. v. Campbell,* 538 U.S. 408, 409 (2003) (holding that a punitive damage award of $145 million, where compensatory damages are $1 million, is excessive; the Due Process Clause "prohibits the imposition of grossly excessive or arbitrary punishments on a tortfeasor").

120. *Romer v. Evans,* 517 U.S. 620 at 635; see *Cleburne v. Cleburne Living Center, Inc.,* 473 U.S. 432 (1985) (invalidating a zoning ordinance that prevented the construction of a group home for the mentally retarded). Even though *Romer* and *Cleburne* were decided on equal protection grounds, they illustrate the Court's insistence on a valid public interest.

121. *Collins v. Harker Heights,* 503 U.S. 115, 125 (1992) (holding the city's alleged failure to train or warn employees about workplace hazards did not violate the Due Process Clause).

122. *Glucksberg,* 521 U.S. at 712.

123. *Id.* at 713.

124. *Lawrence v. Texas,* 539 U.S. 558, 568 (2003) (invalidating a law crim-

inalizing sodomy because it violated the due process right of consenting adults in the privacy of their homes).

125. *Bowers v. Hardwick*, 478 U.S. 186 (1986) (upholding a statute prohibiting sodomy).

126. The Court held the statute invalid under substantive due process: "Were we to hold the statue invalid under the Equal Protection Clause some might question whether a prohibition would be valid if drawn differently, say, to prohibit the conduct both between same-sex and different-sex participants." *Lawrence*, 539 U.S. at 575.

127. *Lawrence*, 539 U.S. at 567.

128. *Dudgeon v. United Kingdom*, 45 Eur. Ct. H.R. 52 (1981) (holding that the criminalization in Northern Ireland of homosexual acts between consenting adults was a violation of Article 8 of the European Convention of Human Rights and Fundamental Freedoms).

129. *Bolling v. Sharpe*, 347 U.S. 497 (1954) (holding that equal protection applies to the federal government through the Due Process Clause of the Fifth Amendment).

130. *Romer*, 517 U.S. at 631.

131. *Shaw v. Hunt*, 517 U.S. 899 (1996) (holding that race was the predominant factor motivating a legislative decision to gerrymander a voting district, thus triggering strict scrutiny).

132. *Plyler v. Doe*, 457 U.S. 202, 216 (1982) ("The Constitution does not require things which are different in fact or opinion to be treated in law as though they were the same").

133. *Jew Ho*, 103 F. at 24; *Yick Wo v. Hopkins*, 118 U.S. 356 (1886) (finding unlawful discrimination when an ordinance prohibiting washing of clothes in public laundries after 10 P.M. was enforced only against Chinese owners).

134. *Berman v. Parker*, 348 U.S. 26 (1954) (holding that aesthetic considerations were validly taken into account when the city condemned property under the Takings Clause).

135. *Railway Express Agency, Inc. v. New York*, 336 U.S. 106 (1949) (upholding regulation of vehicle advertising as a traffic safety measure).

136. *Williamson*, 348 U.S. 483.

137. *Jacobson*, 197 U.S. at 11.

138. *Heller v. Doe*, 509 U.S. 312, 321 (1993) (directing that the courts accept "a legislature's generalizations even when there is an imperfect fit between means and ends").

139. *Berger v. City of Mayfield Heights*, 154 F.3d 621 (6th Cir. 1998) (invalidating as arbitrary an ordinance requiring certain lots to be clear-cut of all vegetation over eight inches).

140. See, e.g., *Village of Euclid v. Ambler Realty Co.*, 272 U.S. 365, 395 (1926) (finding that persons adversely affected by public health regulation carry the burden of proving that the law is "arbitrary and unreasonable, having no substantial relation to the public health, safety, morals, or general welfare"); *Lehnhausen v. Lake Shore Auto Parts Co.*, 410 U.S. 356, 364 (1973) ("The burden is on the one attacking the legislative arrangement to negate every conceivable basis which might support it").

141. *FCC v. Beach Communications,* 508 U.S. 307, 313 (1993) (upholding distinctions among cable facilities under rational basis review). See also *Aida Food and Liquor, Inc. v. City of Chicago,* 439 F.3d 397 (7th Cir. 2006) (holding that building inspections that allegedly singled out a particular liquor store did not violate equal protection under rational basis review).

142. *Nordlinger v. Hahn,* 505 U.S. 1, 11 (1992) (holding the California taxing system to be constitutional).

143. *Beach Communications,* 508 U.S. at 313.

144. *Heller,* 509 U.S. at 320.

145. *Beach Communications,* 508 U.S. at 307.

146. *Metropolis Theatre Co. v. City of Chicago,* 228 U.S. 61, 69 (1913) (holding that grading of municipal licensing fees for theaters based on the selling prices of seats did not violate the Equal Protection Clause).

147. *Local 1812, American Federation of Government Employees v. United States Department of State,* 662 F. Supp. 50 (D.D.C. 1987) (upholding the government's mandatory HIV testing program for foreign service personnel).

148. *Reynolds,* 488 F.2d at 1378.

149. *Leuz v. Secretary of Health and Human Services,* 63 Fed. Cl. 602 (2005) (finding that a shorter statute of limitations for deaths than illnesses under the National Childhood Vaccine Injury Act did not violate equal protection under rational basis review).

150. *Pro-Eco v. Board of Commissioners* 57 F.3d 505 (7th Cir. 1995), *cert. denied,* 516 U.S. 1028 (1995) (holding that depositing garbage in landfills is not a fundamental right, and concern for public health is a sufficient reason to regulate landfills).

151. *New York State Trawlers Ass'n v. Jorling,* 16 F.3d 1303 (2d Cir. 1994) (upholding a conservation law that prohibited trawlers from possessing lobsters in Long Island Sound).

152. *United States v. Carolene Products Co.,* 304 U.S. 144, 152, n.4 (1938): "It is unnecessary to consider now whether legislation which restricts those political processes which can ordinarily be expected to bring about repeal of undesirable legislation, is to be subjected to more exacting scrutiny. . . . Nor need we enquire . . . whether prejudice against discrete and insular minorities may be a special condition, which tends seriously to curtail the operation of those political processes ordinarily to be relied upon to protect minorities, and which may call for a correspondingly more searching judicial inquiry."

153. See, e.g., *Kansas v. Limon,* 112 P.3d 22 (Kan. 2005) (holding that disparate sentencing for heterosexual and homosexual sex with underage minors failed to satisfy a heightened rational basis test).

154. *Cleburne,* 473 U.S. at 432 (holding the requirement of special use permits for a proposed group home for the mentally retarded unconstitutional under equal protection analysis); but see *Heller,* 509 U.S. at 312 (finding that the higher standard of proof for involuntary commitment of the mentally ill, as opposed to the mentally retarded, had a rational basis).

155. *Romer,* 517 U.S. at 620 (1996).

156. *Id.* at 632.

157. *Id.*

158. *United States Department of Agriculture v. Moreno,* 413 U.S. 528, 534 (1973) (finding denial of food stamps if a household includes unrelated persons unconstitutional under rationality review).

159. Scott Burris, "Rationality Review and the Politics of Public Health," *Villanova Law Review,* 34, no. 5 (1989): 933–82.

160. *United States v. Virginia,* 518 U.S. 515 (1996) (using intermediate scrutiny to invalidate the maintenance of an all-male military college).

161. *New Jersey Welfare Rights Organization v. Cahill,* 411 U.S. 619 (1973) (using intermediate scrutiny to strike down a law that limited benefits to families with two individuals of the opposite sex "ceremoniously married").

162. See, e.g., *Mississippi University for Women v. Hogan,* 458 U.S. 718 (1982) (using intermediate scrutiny to invalidate the policy of excluding men from state nursing school); *Nguyen v. Immigration & Naturalization Service,* 533 U.S. 53 (2001) (holding that a statute making it more difficult to enter the United States for a child born abroad and out of wedlock to an American father, as opposed to an American mother, did not violate equal protection because it served an important objective and the means employed were substantially related to that objective).

163. *Craig v. Boren,* 429 U.S. 190, 197 (1976) (holding that gender-based classifications on legal drinking age must serve state interests and be substantially related to achievement of state objectives).

164. *Virginia,* 518 U.S. at 526.

165. See, e.g., *Reynolds* 488 F.2d at 1383; *Illinois v. Adams,* 597 N.E.2d 574 (Ill. 1992) (finding that mandatory HIV testing of prostitutes does not violate equal protection because it draws no distinction between male and female offenders and the legislature had no intent to disadvantage females).

166. However, such an effort might violate the Fourth Amendment's prohibition on unreasonable searches and seizures. See *Ferguson v. City of Charleston,* 532 U.S. 67 (2001) (overturning on search and seizure grounds a state law mandating testing of pregnant women who appear to have used drugs).

167. See, e.g., *Loving v. Virginia,* 388 U.S. 1 (1967) (invalidating Virginia's miscegenation law, which made it a crime for a White person to marry outside the Caucasian race); *Johnson v. California,* 125 S. Ct. 1141 (2005) (holding that placing cellmates of the same race together was subject to the strict scrutiny standard of review).

168. See, e.g., *Korematsu v. United States,* 323 U.S. 214 (1944) (applying strict scrutiny, but nonetheless upholding the internment of persons of Japanese descent during World War II).

169. Classifications based on alienage involve discrimination against persons who are not U.S. citizens. See, e.g., *Bernal v. Fainter,* 467 U.S. 216 (1984) (invalidating a law requiring that a notary public be a U.S. citizen).

170. So-called positive discrimination benefiting racial minorities also triggers strict scrutiny. See, e.g., *Regents of University of California v. Bakke,* 438 U.S. 265 (1978) (invalidating the University of California's affirmative action program for medical school admission).

171. *Skinner v. Oklahoma,* 316 U.S. 535 (1942) (striking down a statute authorizing the sterilization of habitual criminals).

172. *Loving,* 388 U.S. at 1.

173. *Shapiro v. Thompson,* 394 U.S. 618 (1969) (invalidating the residency requirements for welfare programs).

174. See, e.g., *Stanley v. Illinois,* 405 U.S. 645, 651 (1972) (holding that an unwed father was entitled to a hearing on his fitness as a parent before his children could be taken from him in a dependency proceeding instituted by the State of Illinois after the death of the children's natural mother); *Troxel,* 530 U.S. at 59.

175. *Planned Parenthood of Southeastern Pa. v. Casey,* 505 U.S. 833, 848 (1992) (finding unconstitutional state regulations that have the purpose or effect of placing a substantial obstacle in the path of a woman seeking an abortion of a nonviable fetus).

176. Compare *Stenberg v. Carhart,* 530 U.S. 914 (2000) (striking down a Nebraska law that barred "partial birth" abortions which lacked a health exception for the mother) with *Gonzales v. Carhart,* 127 S. Ct. 1610 (2007) (upholding a federal ban on "deliberate" use of "partial birth" abortion, as Congress found this technique is never medically necessary).

177. See, e.g., *Cruzan,* 497 U.S. at 278 ("The principle that a competent person has a constitutionally protected liberty interest in refusing unwanted medical treatment may be inferred from our prior decisions"); *Harper,* 494 U.S. at 221–22 (finding that a mentally ill prisoner has a "significant liberty interest in avoiding the unwanted administration of antipsychotic drugs").

178. *Planned Parenthood of Southeastern Pennsylvania,* 505 U.S. at 851.

179. *Glucksberg,* 521 U.S. at 720–21.

180. *New York City Transit Authority v. Beazer,* 440 U.S. 568, 575 (1979) (upholding an ordinance that excluded persons in methadone maintenance from employment with the transit authority despite the substantial overinclusiveness).

181. *Gratz v. Bollinger,* 539 U.S. 244 (2003) (finding a university's admission policy violated the Equal Protection Clause because its use of race was not narrowly tailored to achieve the respondent's asserted compelling interest in diversity).

182. *Grutter v. Bollinger,* 539 U.S. 306 (2003) (finding a law school admission policy did not violate the Equal Protection Clause because the policy was narrowly tailored to serve the school's compelling interest in obtaining the educational benefits that flow from a diverse student body).

183. *Grutter,* 539 U.S. at 343.

184. *Parents involved in Community Schools v. Seattle School District* No. 1, 127 S. Ct. 2738 (2007). In his concurring opinion, which provided the necessary fifth vote to reverse the court of appeals, Justice Kennedy expressed concern that the plurality opinion "impl[ies] an all-too-unyielding insistence that race cannot be a factor in instances where, in my view, it may be taken into account" (127 S. Ct. at 2791).

185. See, e.g., *San Antonio Independent School District v. Rodriguez,* 411 U.S. 1, 109–10 (1973) (Marshall, J., dissenting) (finding that a principled constitutional analysis would apply a spectrum of standards depending on the nature of the right and the discriminatory effects).

186. *Fullilove v. Klutznick,* 448 U.S. 448 (1980) (Marshall, J., concurring) (holding unconstitutional a requirement to hire a percentage of minority workers for public works projects).

187. *Bowers,* 478 U.S. 186.

188. See, e.g., *Heller,* 509 U.S. at 312 (1993); *Cleburne,* 473 U.S. at 432.

189. *Rodriguez,* 411 U.S. at 1.

190. *Banner v. United States,* 428 F.3d 303 (D.C. Cir. 2005) (holding that District of Columbia residency does not constitute a suspect class for purposes of analyzing a commuter tax on nonresidents who work in the district).

191. *Whalen v. Roe,* 429 U.S. 589 (1977) (upholding a state statute requiring that the state be provided with every prescription for certain types of drugs).

192. *Glucksberg,* 521 U.S. at 711.

5. PUBLIC HEALTH GOVERNANCE: DIRECT REGULATION FOR THE PUBLIC'S HEALTH AND SAFETY

SOURCES FOR CHAPTER EPIGRAPHS: James A. Tobey, "Public Health and the Police Power," *New York University Law Review,* 4 (1927): 126–33, 126; William J. Novak, *The People's Welfare: Law and Regulation in Nineteenth-Century America* (Chapel Hill: University of North Carolina Press, 1996); Franklin D. Roosevelt, *Public Health in New York State, Report of the New York State Commission,* quoted in James A. Tobey, *Public Health Law* (New York: Commonwealth Fund, 1939): 57; Herbert Hoover, "Message Endorsing the Children's Charter," *The American Presidency Project,* December 2005, http://www.presidency.ucsb.edu/ws/index.php?pid=22593; Paul A. Samuelson and William D. Nordhaus, *Economics,* 17th ed. (Boston: McGraw-Hill, 2004) (describing "public choice" theory).

1. Daniel M. Fox, "The Politics of Physicians' Responsibility in Epidemics: A Note on History," *Hastings Center Report,* 18 (1988): S5–S10.

2. Editorial, "Tolerating Death in the Mines," *New York Times,* February 5, 2006 (noting that West Virginia enacted laws requiring that miners be equipped with wireless communication and location devices, better oxygen supplies, and more organized rescue crews). In May 2006 the West Virginia Mine Safety Task Force, per West Virginia Code § 56-4-4, released a report on mine safety recommendations in direct response to the fourteen deaths at the Sago and Aracoma mines. West Virginia Mine Safety Task Force, *Mine Safety Recommendations: Report to the Director of the Office of Miners' Health, Safety and Training* (May 29, 2006): ii. Shortly after the release of the West Virginia Task Force report, President Bush signed the Mine Improvement and New Emergency Response Act (MINER) into law. The act requires that covered mines develop and update written emergency response plans, which are to be reviewed and recertified every six months. Sean Ruppert, "Mine Act to Become Federal Law," *Daily Athenaeum,* May 14, 2006, http://www.da.wvu.edu/XMLParser/printstory.phtml?id=22879.

3. Orly Lobel, "The Renew Deal: The Fall of Regulation and the Rise of Governance in Contemporary Legal Thought," *Minnesota Law Review,* 89 (2004–5): 342–470 (characterizing new governance as increased participation of nonstate actors, stakeholder collaboration, diversity and competition, decentralization, integration of policy domains, flexibility and noncoerciveness, and adaptability and dynamic learning).

4. Institute of Medicine, *The Future of the Public's Health in the Twenty-first Century* (Washington, D.C.: National Academies Press, 2002).

5. Neil Gunningham and Peter Grabosky, *Smart Regulation: Designing Environmental Policy* (Oxford: Clarendon Press, 1998); Roger Brownsword, "Public Health, Private Right: Constitution and Common Law," *Medical Law International,* 7 (2006): 201–18.

6. Some agencies, particularly at the federal level, are placed within the legislative or even the judicial branch, and some are so-called independent agencies that are insulated from executive control (e.g., quasi-autonomous commissions and boards, sometimes referred to as the "fourth branch" of government). The Supreme Court upholds the constitutionality of independent agencies. See, e.g., *Morrison v. Olson,* 487 U.S. 654 (upholding the constitutionality of independent counsel).

7. Eleanor D. Kinney, "Administrative Law and the Public's Health," *Journal of Law, Medicine and Ethics,* 30 (2002): 212–23, 213 ("Government regulation of any type necessarily implicates the discipline of administrative law—a discipline concerned with the procedures by which agencies of government discharge their statutory responsibilities and reviewing courts oversee the legality of agency actions").

8. Elizabeth Fee, "The Origins and Development of Public Health in the United States," in *Oxford Textbook of Public Health*, ed. Roger Detels, Walter W. Holland, James McEwen, et al., 3d ed. (New York: Oxford University Press, 1997): 35–54.

9. John B. Blake, *Public Health in the Town of Boston, 1630–1822* (Cambridge, MA: Harvard University Press, 1959): 13–14.

10. John Duffy, *The Sanitarians: A History of American Public Health* (Urbana: University of Illinois Press, 1990): 12–13.

11. Elizabeth C. Tandy, "The Regulation of Nuisances in the American Colonies," *American Journal of Public Health,* 13 (1923): 810–13.

12. John Duffy, *A History of Public Health in New York City, 1625–1866* (New York: Russell Sage Foundation, 1968): 10–15.

13. For a critique of the idea that early American governance embraced a laissez-faire political economy, see Frank P. Bourgin, *The Great Challenge: The Myth of Laissez Faire in the Early Republic* (New York: George Braziller, 1989).

14. Barbara Gutmann Rosenkrantz, "Cart before Horse: Theory, Practice and Professional Image in American Public Health, 1870–1920," *Journal of the History of Medicine and Allied Sciences,* 29 (1974): 55–73, 57 ("The field of public health exemplified a happy marriage of engineers, physicians and public spirited citizens providing a model of complementary comportment under the banner of sanitary science").

15. Lemuel Shattuck, *Report of a General Plan for the Promotion of General and Public Health, Devised, Prepared, and Recommended by the Commissioners Appointed under a Resolve of the Legislature of Massachusettes, Relating to a Sanitary Survey of the State* (1850; rpt., Cambridge, MA: Harvard University Press, 1948); John H. Griscom, *The Sanitary Condition of the Laboring Population of New York, with Suggestions for Its Improvement* (1845; rpt., New York: Arno, 1970); Benjamin W. McCready, *On the Influence of Trades,*

Professions, and Occupations in the United States, in the Production of Disease (1837; rpt., Baltimore, MD: Johns Hopkins University Press, 1943).

16. George Rosen, *A History of Public Health* (Baltimore, MD: Johns Hopkins University Press, 1993): 168–226; Duffy, *The Sanitarians,* 175.

17. Shattuck, *Report of a General Plan,* 9–10.

18. Norton T. Horr and Alton A. Bemis, *A Treatise on the Power to Enact, Passage, Validity and Enforcement of Municipal Police Ordinances* (Cincinnati, OH: R. Clarke, 1887): §§ 211–62 (classifying ordinances according to their subject matter, ranging from food, markets, and fire to care of streets, buildings, and public infrastructure [e.g., sewerage and water], general nuisances, inspection, and licenses); Christopher G. Tiedeman, *A Treatise on State and Federal Control of Persons and Property in the United States: Considered from Both a Civil and Criminal Standpoint,* 2 vols. (St. Louis: F. H. Thomas, 1900): chs. 9 (regulation of trades and occupations), 10–11 (regulation of real and personal property), and 15 (police regulation of corporations).

19. William J. Novak, *The People's Welfare: Law and Regulation in Nineteenth-Century America* (Chapel Hill: University of North Carolina Press, 1996): 21.

20. Nancy Frank, *From Criminal Law to Regulation: A Historical Analysis of Health and Safety Law* (New York: Garland, 1986): 1.

21. Edwin H. Sutherland, *White-Collar Crime* (New York: Dryden Press, 1949): 42–50.

22. Tobey, *Public Health Law,* 76.

23. Fee, "The Origins and Development of Public Health in the United States," 38.

24. Rosen, *A History of Public Health,* 210; Ernest S. Griffith, *History of American City Government* (New York: Oxford University Press, 1938): 289 ("The modern health department and all save a negligible number of its several activities were completely missing").

25. Duffy, *The Sanitarians,* 148.

26. *Laws of the State of New York,* 89th Sess., I, chap. 74 (Albany, 1866); Charles E. Rosenberg, *The Cholera Years: The United States in 1832, 1849, and 1866* (Chicago: University of Chicago Press, 1962): 190–91 (stating that the board "would be needed [because] New York's streets were almost impassable with a mixture of snow, ice, dirt, and garbage").

27. Horr and Bemis, *A Treatise on the Power to Enact, Passage, Validity and Enforcement of Municipal Police Ordinances,* § 215.

28. R. G. Paterson, ed., *Historical Directory of State Health Departments in the United States of America* (Columbus: Ohio Public Health Association, 1939).

29. The first reported county health departments were in Jefferson County, Kentucky, in 1908 (see *Jefferson County v. Jefferson County Fiscal Court,* 108 S.W.2d 181 [Ky. Ct. App. 1938]); Guilford County, North Carolina, and Yakima County, Washington, in 1911; and Robeson County, North Carolina, in 1912. John Atkinson Ferrell and P. A. Mead, "History of County Health Organizations in the United States, 1908–1933," *Public Health Bulletin,* no. 222 (Washington, DC: Government Printing Office, 1936); Allen Weir Freeman, *A Study of Rural Public Health Service* (New York: Commonwealth Fund, 1933); Harry S. Mustard, *Rural Health Practice* (New York: Commonwealth Fund, 1936).

30. Charles V. Chapin, "Pleasures and Hopes of the Health Officer," in *Papers of Charles V. Chapin, M.D.*, ed. Frederic P. Gorham and Clarence L. Scamman (New York: Commonwealth Fund, 1934): 11.

31. For a detailed description of the U.S. public health system, see Glen P. Mays, "Organization of the Public Health Delivery System," in *Public Health Administration for Population-Based Management,* ed. Lloyd F. Novick and Glen P. Mays (Gaithersburg, MD: Aspen Publishers, 2001): 63–116.

32. Novick and Mays, *Public Health Administration,* 244–46; Stephen Breyer, *Administrative Law and Regulatory Policy,* 3d ed. (Boston: Little Brown, 1992); Duffy, *The Sanitarians.*

33. *Federal Food Drug and Cosmetic Act,* 21 U.S.C. §§ 301–99.

34. Lawrence O. Gostin, Zita Lazzarini, Verla S. Neslund, et. al., "Water Quality Laws and Waterborne Diseases: *Cryptosporidium* and Other Emerging Pathogens," *American Journal of Public Health,* 90 (2000): 847–53.

35. Lawrence O. Gostin and James G. Hodge, Jr., "Piercing the Veil of Secrecy in HIV/AIDS and Other Sexually Transmitted Diseases: Theories of Privacy and Disclosure in Partner Notification," *Duke Journal of Gender Law and Policy,* 5 (1998): 9–88.

36. *Social Security Act,* 42 U.S.C. §§ 301–1397.

37. Karen Davis and Cathy Schoen, *Health and the War on Poverty: A Ten Year Appraisal* (Washington, DC: Brookings Institution, 1978).

38. Exec. Order No. 12,291, 46 *Fed. Reg.* 13,193 (February 17, 1981). See Eleanor D. Kinney, "Administrative Law and the Public's Health," *Journal of Law, Medicine and Ethics,* 30 (2002): 212–23.

39. Although the scope of federal regulatory power is broad, many federal health and safety regulations are antiquated. Most food safety laws date back to 1908–38, and were formulated in response to adulteration of meat (e.g., dirt, feces) rather than biological contaminants (e.g., *E. coli, salmonella*). The Federal Meat Inspection Act of 1907, for example, has never been updated to reflect what we have learned about pathogens such as *salmonella, E. coli,* bovine spongiform encephalopathy, and *listeria.*

It is doubtful whether the USDA can regulate biological threats under that statute. *Supreme Beef Processors v. USDA,* 275 F.3d 432 (5th Cir., Tex., 2001) (holding that *salmonella* is not an adulterant and thus is beyond the scope of the USDA's regulatory authority).

40. See, e.g., *State Board of Health v. City of Greenville,* 98 N.E. 1019, 1021 (Ohio 1912) ("It is now settled law that the legislature of the State possesses plenary power to deal with [health]").

41. I am grateful to one of America's most experienced health officers, Lloyd Novick, for help in developing this discussion of state and local public health agencies and for drafting figures 18 and 19. See Susan Dandoy, "The State Public Health Department," in *Principles of Public Health Practice,* ed. Nancy Rawding and Martin Wasserman (Albany, NY: Delmar Publishers, 1997): 68; Bernard Turnock, *Public Health: What It Is and How It Works* (Gaithersberg, MD: Aspen Publishers, 2001): 145–56; Kristine M. Gebbie, "Steps to Changing State Public Health Structures," *Journal of Public Health Management and Practice,* 4 (1998): 33–41.

42. D. J. Gossert and C. Arden Miller, "State Boards of Health, Their Mem-

bers and Commitments," *American Journal of Public Health,* 63 (1973): 486–93; J. W. Kerr and A. A. Moll, "Organization, Powers, and Duties of Health Authorities," *Public Health Bulletin,* no. 54 (1912).

43. Association of State and Territorial Health Officials, *Directory of State Public Health Agencies* (Washington, DC: ASTHO, 1998).

44. Benjamin Gilbert, Merry-K. Moos, and C. Arden Miller, "State Level Decision Making for Public Health: The Status of Boards of Health," *Journal of Public Health Policy,* 3 (1982): 51–63.

45. Centers for Disease Control and Prevention, *Profile of State and Territorial Public Health Systems: United States* (Atlanta: CDC, 1999).

46. A large number of cases supporting the preeminence of public health powers in local government are presented in Eugene McQuillin, *The Law of Municipal Corporations,* 3d ed. (Wilmette, IL: Callaghan, 1978), §§ 24.219–22.

47. Leslie M. Beitsch, Meade Grigg, Nir Menachemi, et al., "Roles of Local Public Health Agencies within the State Public Health System," *Journal of Public Health Management Practice,* 12 (2006): 232–42 (noting that several functions, such as epidemiology and surveillance and licensing, were most often state responsibilities).

48. Glen P. Mays, C. Arden Miller, and Paul K. Halverson, eds., *Local Public Health Practice: Trends and Models* (Washington, DC: American Public Health Association, 2000); F. Douglas Scutchfield and C. William Keck, *Principles of Public Health Practice* (Albany, NY: Delmar Publishers, 1997).

49. *Zullo v. Board of Health,* 88 A.2d 625 (N.J. 1952); *Fort Smith v. Roberts,* 9 S.W.2d 75 (Ark. 1928); see C. Arden Miller, Benjamin Gilbert, David G. Warren, et al., "Statutory Authorization for the Work of Local Health Departments," *American Journal of Public Health,* 67 (1977): 940–45.

50. National Association of County and City Health Officials, *Profile of Local Health Departments, 1992–1993* (1995); Thomas L. Milne, "The Local Health Department," in *Principles of Public Health Practice,* ed. Scutchfield and Keck; Thomas B. Richards, Charles M. Croner, and Lloyd F. Novick, eds., "Toward a GIS Sampling Frame for Surveys of Local Health Departments and Local Boards of Health," *Journal of Public Health Management and Practice,* 5 (1999): 65–75; Glen P. Mays, P. K. Halverson, and C. A. Miller, "Assessing the Performance of Local Public Health Systems: A Survey of State Health Agency Efforts," *Journal of Public Health Management and Practice,* 4 (1998): 63–78.

51. Turnock, *Public Health,* 160–61.

52. Beitsch et al., "Roles of Public Health Agencies" (finding that 43 percent of states had an intermediate administrative structure between the state-level agency and local health departments).

53. *Id.* (finding that local boards or councils of health were present in 69 percent of the states); Rawding and Wasserman, *Principles of Public Health Practice,* 91–92.

54. See, e.g., *Zucht v. King,* 260 U.S. 174 (1922) (upholding local discretion in compulsory vaccination—see chapter 7); *Ellingwood v. City of Reedsburg,* 64 N.W. 885 (Wis. 1895) (holding that the power to establish a water system is implied from the grant of general police power, since a good water system is important to the community's health).

55. *Harrison v. Baltimore,* 1 Gill 264 (Md. 1843).

56. Special districts are typically created to bypass government borrowing limitations, to insulate public health activities from traditional political influence, and to ensure sufficient expertise for a specialized task.

57. Classically, states possess plenary power over local government and may create, dissolve, or deny them power, except as limited by the state constitution. *Hunter v. City of Pittsburgh,* 207 U.S. 161, 178–79 (1907). The federal Constitution does not protect municipal corporations against state interference with their personal property or rights. *City of Newark v. New Jersey,* 262 U.S. 192 (1923); *Williams v. Mayor of Baltimore,* 289 U.S. 36, 40 (1933).

58. In a few states, such as California, home rule charters are thought of not as grants of power but as limitations on the reservoir of constitutionally delegated governing authority.

59. Home rule has been granted either by constitutional provision or by statute in forty-three states. Sandra M. Stevenson, *Antieau on Local Government Law,* 2d ed., § 21.01 (Newark, NJ: Matthew Bender, 2006). See, e.g., *People ex rel. Metropolitan Street Railway v. State Board of Tax Commissioners,* 67 N.E. 69, 70–71 (N.Y. 1903), *aff'd,* 199 U.S. 1 (1905) ("The principle of home rule, or the right of self-government as to local affairs, existed before we had a constitution").

60. Ill. Const. art. VII, § 6.

61. John Forrest Dillon, *Treatise on the Law of Municipal Corporations,* § 55 (Chicago: J. Cockcroft, 1872).

62. See Hendrik Hartog, *Public Property and Private Power: The Corporation of the City of New York in American Law, 1730–1870* (Chapel Hill: University of North Carolina Press, 1983): 235 (stating that the strict construction of delegations to local governments "provided an [important] technique for justifying judicial intervention" to block actions judges regarded as unwarranted).

63. Stevenson, *Antieau on Local Government Law,* §§ 24.01–24.04.

64. James G. Hodge, Jr., "The Role of New Federalism and Public Health Law," *Journal of Law and Health,* 12 (1998): 309–57.

65. Contra Costa County Health Servs. Dep't Prevention Program, *Taking Aim at Gun Dealers: Contra Costa's Public Health Approach to Reducing Firearms in the Community* (1995) (stating that forty-one states preempt local regulation of gun sales). But see *Great Western Shows Inc. v. County of Los Angeles,* 27 Cal.4th 853 (Cal. 2002) (holding [1] that state law did not preempt a county ordinance because the ordinance was not expressly preempted by state statutes, it did not duplicate or contradict state statutes, and it was not the manifest legislative intent of these statutes to occupy the field, and [2] that a county may regulate the sale of firearms on its own property located within a city when the county ordinance does not conflict with city law); *Nordyke v. King,* 27 Cal. 4th 875 (Cal. 2002) (holding that state law did not preempt a county's prohibition of gun shows held on its property).

66. *Suter v. City of Lafayette,* 67 Cal. Rptr. 2d 420 (Cal. Ct. App. 1997) (upholding against preemption challenge a city ordinance requiring firearm dealers to obtain land use and police permits in addition to licenses already required by state and federal law); Marice Ashe, David Jernigan, Randalph Kline, et al., "Land Use Planning and the Control of Alcohol, Tobacco, Firearms, and Fast Food

Restaurants," *American Journal of Public Health,* 93 (2003): 1404–8; Daniel W. Webster, Jon S. Vernick, and Lisa M. Hepburn, "The Relationship between Licensing, Registration, and Other Gun Sales Laws and the Source State of Crime Guns," *Injury Prevention,* 7 (2001): 184–89.

67. See, e.g., *Industrial Union Department, AFL-CIO v. American Petroleum Institute* 448 U.S. 607 (1980) (holding that by empowering OSHA to promulgate standards that are "reasonably necessary or appropriate to provide safe or healthful employment," Congress intended that it must first find that the workplaces are not safe and that "safe" is not the equivalent of "risk-free"); *American Textile Manufacturers Institute v. Donovan,* 452 U.S. 490 (1981) (finding that the OSHA statute itself balances costs and benefits, and that Congress did not intend for the agency to conduct its own cost-benefit analysis before promulgating a toxic material-agent standard).

68. *FDA v. Brown & Williamson Tobacco Corp.,* 529 U.S. 120 (2000).

69. See *Massachusetts v. EPA,* 127 S. Ct. 1438 (2007); *Environmental Defense v. Duke Energy Corp.,* 127 S. Ct. 1423 (2007). In these two companion cases, the Supreme Court rebuked the EPA for failing to regulate auto emissions and factory air pollutants, respectively. While the Court fell just short of requiring the agency to act, the decision strongly suggested that a continued failure to act would have to be supported by strong scientific evidence and reasoning.

70. Another pertinent illustration is the federal Meat Inspection Act of 1907, passed a year after the publication of Upton Sinclair's *The Jungle* to address the cleanliness and purity of meat. In *Supreme Beef Processors, Inc. v. USDA,* 275 F.3d 432 (5th Cir. 2001), the Court of Appeals struck down USDA regulation of *salmonella* in raw meat because the agency had no statutory authority to regulate levels of "non-adulterant pathogens." However, after a series of high-profile food contamination events in 2006, the issue of food safety has moved up the congressional policy agenda, with the introduction of proposed legislation to enhance agency authority. Adam Cohen, "One Hundred Years Later, the Food Industry Is Still 'The Jungle,'" *New York Times,* Jan. 2, 2007.

71. *Occupational Safety and Health Act (OSHA) of 1970,* 29 U.S.C. § 651.

72. Unless specified by statute, state administrative procedure acts generally have been held not to apply to local government agencies. *Arthur D. Little, Inc. v. Commissioner of Health & Hospitals,* 481 N.E.2d 441 (Mass. 1985). But see, e.g., *Justewicz v. Hamtramck Civil Service Commission,* 237 N.W.2d 555 (Mich. 1975).

73. *Vermont Yankee Nuclear Power Corp. v. NRDC,* 435 U.S. 519, 523–25 (1978).

74. In rulemaking, agencies set general standards that apply to classes of people, whereas in adjudication, agencies adjudicate the claims of individuals, which may involve a deprivation of liberty or property. Compare *Londoner v. Denver,* 210 U.S. 373 (1908) (requiring an evidentiary hearing for assessment of an individual owner's property), with *Bi-Metallic Investment Co. v. State Board of Equalization,* 239 U.S. 441 (1915) (finding no due process was required when agency regulation increased the valuation of all taxable property).

75. The exemptions are for interpretive rules, policy statements, procedural rules, certain substantive rules (e.g., pertaining to the military, foreign affairs, agency management, loans, grants, benefits, or contracts), and where notice and

comment procedures are "impracticable, unnecessary, or contrary to the public interest." 5 U.S.C. § 553(a).

76. 5 U.S.C § 553.

77. *Automobile Parts & Accessories Ass'n v. Boyd,* 407 F.2d 330, 338 (D.C. Cir. 1968) (holding that a standard requiring installation of seat belts in cars is a "concise general statement" under the Administrative Procedure Act).

78. 5 U.S.C. §§ 553(c), 556, 557.

79. *National Nutritional Foods Ass'n v. FDA,* 504 F.2d 761, 792–99 (2nd Cir. 1974); see Robert W. Hamilton, "Rulemaking on the Record by the Food and Drug Administration," *Texas Law Review,* 50 (1972): 1132–94 (discussing the FDA hearings where experts were cross-examined on whether peanut butter should contain 87 percent or 90 percent peanuts).

80. Michael Asimow, ed., *A Guide to Federal Agency Adjudication* (Chicago: Section of Administrative Law and Regulatory Practice, American Bar Association, 2003).

81. 5 U.S.C. § 553(c).

82. 5 U.S.C. §§ 554, 556, 557.

83. *Withrow v. Larkin,* 421 U.S. 35, 47 (1975) ("A fair trial in a fair tribunal is a basic requirement of due process"). See *In re Murchison,* 349 U.S. 133, 136 (1955). This rule applies to adjudicating administrative agencies as well as courts. *Gibson v. Berryhill,* 411 U.S. 564, 579 (1973) (holding that licensing board members with a pecuniary interest in the outcome is constitutionally unacceptable).

84. Nondelegation is a constitutional law doctrine based on the exclusive grant of legislative powers to the Congress (U.S. Const. art. 1) and judicial powers to the courts (U.S. Const. art. 3).

85. Since 1935, the Supreme Court has rarely, if ever, invalidated health and safety regulation as an impermissible delegation of lawmaking power to the executive. For the early twentieth-century view, see *A.L.A. Schechter Poultry Corp. v. United States,* 295 U.S. 495 (1935) (invalidating agency rules regarding maximum hours and minimum wages because the legislature did not provide clear standards). For a more modern view, see, e.g., *Touby v. United States,* 500 U.S. 160 (1991) (rejecting a nondelegation doctrine challenge to congressional authorization of the attorney general to criminalize distribution of any drug that posed a risk to public health).

86. *Whitman v. American Trucking Ass'ns,* 531 U.S. 457 (2001).

87. Michael Asimow, Arthur Earl Bonfeld, and Ronald M. Levine, *State and Federal Administrative Law* (St. Paul, MO: West Group, 1988): 451–61.

88. *Howe v. City of St. Louis,* 512 S.W.2d 127, 133 (Mo. 1974) (noting a modern tendency toward greater liberality in permitting grants of discretion to administrative officials as the complexity of government increases).

89. *People v. Tibbitts,* 305 N.E.2d 152 (Ill. 1973) (striking down a statute allowing absolute and unguided discretion to an administrative agency as an unlawful delegation of power).

90. *Boreali v. Axelrod,* 517 N.E.2d 1350, 1356 (N.Y. 1987). Following *Boreali,* several counties and New York City enacted antismoking legislation. In 2003, the state legislature amended the New York Clean Indoor Air Act (Public Health Law, Article 13-E), prohibiting smoking in virtually all workplaces, in-

cluding restaurants and bars. The act contains a "floor" preemption that supersedes local laws which are less strict than the state statute.

91. *Industrial Union Department, v. Am. Petrol. Inst.*, 448 U.S. 607 (construing congressional grant of authority as requiring OSHA to find significant risk of harm to workers, which the agency had not found in issuing the rule).

92. *Skidmore v. Swift & Co.*, 323 U.S. 134 (1944) (creating a sliding scale of deference based on the "thoroughness evident in its [the administrator's] consideration, the validity of its reasoning, its consistency with earlier and later pronouncements, and all those factors which give it power to persuade").

93. *Chevron v. NRDC*, 467 U.S. 837 (1984). *Chevron* grants deference to an agency's interpretation of an ambiguous enabling statute. *Auer v. Robbins*, 519 U.S. 452, 461–63 (1997), similarly grants deference to an administrative rule interpreting the issuing agency's own ambiguous regulation.

94. *Chevron*, 467 U.S. at 842. See, e.g., *Friends of the Earth Inc. v. EPA*, 446 F.3d. 140 (D.C. Cir. 2006) (finding that a Clean Air Act directive requiring "daily" limits on effluent discharges into highly polluted waters means what it says and does not authorize the EPA to craft seasonal or annual limits).

95. *Chevron*, 467 U.S. at 843.

96. *United States v. Mead Corp.*, 533 U.S. 218, 226–27 (2001). See Eric R. Womack, "Into the Third Era of Administrative Law: An Empirical Study of the Supreme Court's Retreat from *Chevron* Principles in *United States v. Mead*," *Dickinson Law Review*, 107 (2002): 289–341.

97. *Skidmore v. Swift & Co.*, 323 U.S. at 140.

98. *Gonzales v. Oregon*, 546 U.S. 243 (2006). See Lawrence O. Gostin, "Physician-Assisted Suicide: A Legitimate Medical Practice?" *JAMA*, 295 (2006): 1941–43.

99. Public choice theory uses economic reasoning to explain collective decision making—i.e., people act primarily out of self-interest. The theory posits the idea of "government failure"—inbuilt reasons why government intervention does not achieve the desired effect. Government regulators, the theory holds, do not have strong incentives to promote the common good, while interest groups are strongly motivated to achieve their goals. See James M. Buchanan and Gordon Tullock, *The Calculus of Consent* (Indianapolis, IN: Liberty Fund, 1999).

100. Lobel, "The Renew Deal," at 344; Jody Freeman, "Public Values in an Era of Privatization: Extending Public Law Norms through Privatization," *Harvard Law Review*, 116 (2003): 1285–1352 (arguing that privatization could extend public law norms to private actors, a process called "publicization").

101. Orly Lobel, "Setting the Agenda for New Governance Research," *Minnesota Law Review*, 89 (2004–5): 498–509.

102. The 2006 *E. coli* outbreak in spinach demonstrated how all of these actors play a role in addressing foodborne disease. Food and Drug Administration, "FDA Statement on Foodborne E. coli O157: H7 Outbreak in Spinach," *FDA News*, October 10, 2006, http://www.fda.gov/bbs/topics/NEWS/2006/NEW01486.html (describing the roles of government, industry, consumers, and the media in responding to the *E. coli* outbreak).

103. The Salzburg Seminar on the Global Governance of Health, *Conference Report,* December 5–8, 2005.

104. 40 C.F.R §§ 72–78 (2002).

105. United Nations, *Kyoto Protocol to the United Nations Framework Convention on Climate Change,* December 11, 1997, http://unfccc.int/resource/docs/convkp/kpeng.pdf. In 2005, twenty-three multinational corporations formed a business group at the G8 Climate Change Roundtable, stressing the importance of market-based solutions to climate change. World Economic Forum in Collaboration with Her Majesty's Government, United Kingdom, *Statement of the G8 Climate Change Roundtable,* June 9, 2005, http://www.weforum.org/pdf/g8_climatechange.pdf.

106. Philip J. Harter, "Negotiated Regulations: A Cure for Malaise," *Georgetown Law Journal,* 71 (1982): 1–118.

107. Cornelius M. Kerwin, *Rulemaking: How Government Agencies Write Law and Make Policy* (Washington, DC: CQ Press, 1994): 185–91.

108. *Negotiated Rulemaking Act of 1990,* 5 U.S.C. § 561, reauthorized in 1996 and now incorporated into the *Administrative Procedure Act,* 5 U.S.C. §§ 561–570 ("To encourage agencies to use [negotiated rulemaking] when it enhances the informal rulemaking process"). See Exec. Order No. 12,866 on Regulatory Planning and Review (September 30, 1993), issued by President Clinton, directing agencies to consider consensual mechanisms for developing regulations, including "reg-neg."

109. *Administrative Dispute Resolution Act of 1996,* 5 U.S.C. §§ 571–583.

110. David M. Pritzker and Deborah S. Dalton, *Negotiated Rulemaking Sourcebook* (Washington, DC: U.S. Government Printing Office, 1990): 3–5.

111. *USA Group Loan Services, Inc. v. Riley,* 82 F.3d 708 (7th Cir. 1996) (Posner, C.J.) (holding that the Secretary's promise to abide by the consensus reached in reg-neg was unenforceable).

112. Richard B. Stewart, "The Reformation of American Administrative Law," *Harvard Law Review,* 88 (1975): 1667–1813.

113. Agency proposals to subsidize interveners in the absence of explicit statutory authority have encountered judicial resistance. *Pacific Legal Foundation v. Goyan,* 664 F.2d 1221 (4th Cir. 1981) (holding that the FDA lacked authority to reimburse interveners).

114. Federal Trade Commission, *Self-Regulation in the Alcohol Industry: A Review of Industry Efforts to Avoid Promoting Alcohol to Underage Consumers,* September 1999, http://www.ftc.gov/reports/alcohol/alcoholreport.htm.

115. American Beverage Association, *School Beverage Guidelines,* 2006, http://www.ameribev.org/industry-issues/beverages-in-schools/school-beverage-guidelines/index.aspx (announcing the new school beverage policy of the American Beverage Association, PepsiCo, Coca-Cola, and Cadbury Schweppes). See Caroline E. Mayer, "Sugary Drinks to Be Pulled from Schools: Industry Agrees to Further Limit Availability to Children," *Washington Post,* May 3, 2006. A similar initiative, negotiated by former president Clinton, was launched by five large snack food manufacturers to discourage schools from stocking vending machines with unhealthy foods. David B. Caruso, "Firms to Tout Healthy Snacks in Schools," *Boston Globe,* October 6, 2006.

116. Johathan Panter, letter to the editor, *New York Times,* May 15, 2006.

117. Timothy Jost, "Medicare and the Joint Commission on Accreditation of Healthcare Organizations," *Law and Contemporary Problems,* 15 (1994): 15–45.

118. It can also be argued that too much self-regulation has the potential to result in a dangerously lax enforcement environment. See Stephen Labaton, "OSHA Leaves Worker Safety Largely in the Hands of Industry," *New York Times,* April 25, 2007 (arguing that under the Bush administration, OSHA has wiped out dozens of existing regulations and has avoided adopting many others, favoring a voluntary compliance strategy that has led to potentially dangerous workplace situations).

119. Furthermore, the lack of enforcement inherent in self-regulation creates a risk that companies will not perform their promised behavior. For example, a recent report suggests that beer and liquor companies are not complying with a self-imposed ban on advertising to teenagers. Centers for Disease Control and Prevention, "Youth Exposure to Advertising on Radio—United States, June–August 2004," *Morbidity and Mortality Weekly Report,* 55 (2006): 937–40.

120. Federal Trade Commission, *Self-Regulation in the Alcohol Industry.*

121. Federal Trade Commission and Department of Health and Human Services, *Perspectives on Marketing, Self-Regulation, and Childhood Obesity: A Report on a Joint Workshop of the Federal Trade Commission and the Department of Health and Human Services,* April 2006, http://www.ftc.gov/os/2006/05/PerspectivesOnMarketingSelf-Regulation&ChildhoodObesityFTCandHHSReportonJointWorkshop.pdf.

122. Mayer, "Sugary Drinks."

123. Campaign for a Commercial-Free Childhood, *Frequently Asked Questions about the Lawsuit against Viacom and Kellogg,* 2004, http://www.commercialexploitation.org/pressreleases/lawsuitfaq.htm.

124. *Financial Disclosure by Clinical Investigators,* 21 C.F.R. §§ 54.1 to 54.6.

125. Steven P. Croley, *Regulation and Public Interests: The Possibility of Good Regulatory Government* (Princeton, NJ: Princeton University Press, 2007).

126. Consider this example of the demonstrable need for bright-line regulation: In response to the energy crisis of 2006, President Bush proposed an expansion of tax credits for hybrid cars—at first glance, a sure winner for market-based incentives. But paradoxically, more hybrids are unlikely to reduce overall oil consumption unless there is a concurrent increase in fuel economy standards. The standard for cars—27.5 miles per gallon in 2006—is a fleetwide average. So if carmakers sold more high-mileage hybrids, they could also ignore fuel efficiency in gas-guzzling cars. And this market-based incentive also fails to address the added problem that car fuel-efficiency standards do not even apply to SUVs and light trucks. Editorial, "Less Than Meets the Eye," *New York Times,* May 15, 2006.

6. TORT LAW AND THE PUBLIC'S HEALTH: INDIRECT REGULATION

SOURCES FOR CHAPTER EPIGRAPHS: Susan Rose-Ackerman, "Tort Law in the Regulatory State," in *Tort Law and the Public Interest,* ed. Peter H. Schuck (New York: W.W. Norton, 1991): 80–81; *Donoghue v. Stevenson* [1932] A.C. 562,

580 (H.L.) (appeal taken from Scot.) (U.K.); *Rylands v. Fletcher* (1868) 3 L.R.E. and I. App. 330 (H.L.); David Hume, *A Treatise of Human Nature* (Amherst, MA: Prometheus Books, 1992): 91; *San Diego Bldg. Trades Council v. Garmon,* 359 U.S. 236, 247 (1959); *Haines v. Liggett,* 975 F.2d 81 (3d Cir. 1992); William E. Townsley and Dale K. Hanks, "The Trial Court's Responsibility to Make Cigarette Disease Litigation Affordable and Fair," *California Western Law Review,* 25 (1989): 275–322, 277; *Haines v. Liggett Group, Inc.,* 814 F. Supp. 414, 421 (D.N.J. 1993) (quoting J. Michael Jordan, defending R. J. Reynolds Tobacco); *McLaughlin v. United States,* 476 U.S. 17, 17 (1986).

1. For an excellent illustration in the context of tobacco litigation, see Peter D. Jacobson and Soheil Soliman, "Litigation as Public Health Policy: Theory or Reality?" *Journal of Law, Medicine, and Ethics,* 30 (2002): 224–38; see also Richard A. Posner, "A Theory of Negligence," *Journal of Legal Studies,* 1 (1972): 29–96.

2. Private rights of action are also created by statutes such as the *Clean Air Act,* 42 U.S.C. §§ 7401–7671q (2005) and the *Clean Water Act,* 33 U.S.C. §§ 1251–1387 (2005), which authorize citizen suits to abate pollution.

3. *K-Mart Corp. v. Ponsock,* 732 P.2d 1364, 1368 (Nev. 1987). Note that this is an imperfect definition, as some civil actions for monetary damages are not torts, such as remedies afforded in environmental statutes; some torts have elements of contract, for example breach of warranty; and some torts provide nonmonetary damages, such as an injunction to cease the continuation of a nuisance.

4. Controversy remains over just what the goals of the tort system should be. See Heidi L. Feldman, "Science and Uncertainty in Mass Exposure Litigation," *Texas Law Review,* 74 (1995): 1–48; Steven Shavell, *Economic Analysis of Accident Law* (Cambridge, MA: Harvard University Press, 1987): 7; Guido Calabresi, *The Costs of Accidents: A Legal and Economic Analysis* (New Haven, CT: Yale University Press, 1970): 16.

5. Jon S. Vernick, Jason W. Sapsin, Stephen P. Teret, et al., "How Litigation Can Promote Product Safety," *Journal of Law, Medicine, and Ethics,* 32 (2004): 551–55; Jon S. Vernick, Julie Samia Mair, Stephen P. Teret, et al., "The Role of Litigation in Preventing Product-Related Injuries," *Epidemiologic Reviews,* 25 (2003): 90–98; Peter D. Jacobson and Soliman, "Litigation as Public Health Policy"; Wendy E. Parmet and Richard A. Daynard, "The New Public Health Litigation," *Annual Review of Public Health,* 21 (2000): 437–54; Stephen P. Teret, "Prevention and Torts: The Role of Litigation in Injury Control," *Law, Medicine, and Health Care,* 17 (1989); Stephen P. Teret, "Litigating for the Public's Health," *American Journal of Public Health,* 76 (1986): 1027–29.

6. See, e.g., *St. Bernard Citizens for Envtl. Quality, Inc. v. Chalmette Ref., LLC,* 354 F. Supp. 2d 697 (E.D. La. 2005) (finding valid a suit by environmental groups against a petroleum refinery for violations of the Clean Air Act).

7. See, e.g., *Sierra Club v. El Paso Gold Mines, Inc.,* 421 F.3d 1133 (10th Cir. 2005) (finding that a gold mine owner could be liable under the Clean Water Act for discharges of pollutants from an abandoned mine shaft even though the owner had never conducted any mining operations on the property).

8. See, e.g., *Villari v. Terminix Int'l, Inc.,* 692 F. Supp. 568 (E.D. Pa. 1988) (regarding pesticide contamination of home).

9. See, e.g., *Allen v. United States,* 588 F. Supp. 247 (D. Utah 1984), *rev'd,* 816 F.2d 1417 (10th Cir. 1987) (regarding radiation exposure from atmospheric testing of nuclear devices).

10. See, e.g., *In re Agent Orange Prod. Liab. Litig.,* 597 F. Supp. 740 (E.D.N.Y. 1984), *aff'd,* 818 F.2d 145 (2d Cir. 1987) (regarding dioxin spraying in Vietnam); see also Peter H. Schuck, *Agent Orange on Trial: Mass Toxic Disasters in the Courts,* enlarged ed. (Cambridge, MA: Belknap Press, 2006).

11. *Sindell v. Abbott Laboratories,* 607 P.2d 924 (Cal. 1980) (regarding market share liability for DES); *Bichler v. Eli Lilly & Co.,* 436 N.E.2d 182 (N.Y. 1988) (regarding liability for cancer caused by DES).

12. See, e.g., *Reyes v. Wyeth Lab.,* 498 F.2d 1264 (5th Cir. 1974) (holding the manufacturer liable for marketing polio vaccine with insufficient warnings); *Fraley v. American Cyanamid Co.,* 570 F. Supp. 497 (D. Colo. 1983) (holding the manufacturer liable for inadequate warnings when a vaccinated child contracted polio).

13. See, e.g., *Wooderson v. Ortho Pharm. Corp.,* 681 P.2d 1038 (Cal. 1984) (finding the manufacturer had a duty to warn a physician of the inherent dangers of oral contraceptives); *In re A. H. Robins Co.,* 88 B.R. 742 (E.D. Va. 1988), *aff'd,* 880 F.2d 694 (4th Cir. 1989) (establishing a manufacturer's trust fund to settle 300,000 claims of women who had been injured by the Dalkon Shield, an intrauterine contraceptive device); see also Kenneth R. Feinberg, "The Dalkon Shield Claimants Trust," *Law and Contemporary Problems,* 53 (1990): 79–112.

14. See, e.g., *Grand Aerie Fraternal Order of Eagles v. Carneyhan,* 169 S.W.3d 840 (Ky. 2005) (finding that a chapter of a national fraternal order could be held liable for the drunk driving death of a minor who was served alcohol when already clearly intoxicated); *Batten v. Bobo,* 528 A.2d 572 (N.J. 1986) (holding that an intoxicated minor guest involved in a car accident can bring a cause of action against his or her social host). The courts have refused to hold alcoholic beverage manufacturers liable for failing to warn consumers about the adverse effects of alcohol. See, e.g., *Greif v. Anheuser-Busch Co.,* 114 F. Supp. 2d 100 (D. Conn. 2000) (finding the brewing company not liable for failure to warn about the dangers of alcohol-related accidents).

15. See, e.g., *Moning v. Playskool Inc.,* 30 F.3d 459 (3d Cir. 1994) (regarding building blocks); *Moning v. Alfono,* 254 N.W.2d 759 (Mich. 1977) (regarding pogo sticks); *Cunningham v. Quaker Oats Co.,* 639 F. Supp. 234 (W.D.N.Y. 1986) (regarding toy figurines).

16. See, e.g., *Fiske v. MacGregor,* 464 A.2d 719 (R.I. 1983) (regarding football helmets); *AMF v. Victor J. Andrew High School,* 526 N.E. 2d 584 (Ill. App. Ct. 1988) (regarding trampolines).

17. See, e.g., *Goodwin v. MTD Products, Inc.,* 232 F.3d 600 (7th Cir. 2000) (holding a lawn mower manufacturer liable for eye injury); *Parsons v. Honeywell, Inc.,* 929 F.2d 901 (2d Cir. 1991) (regarding a water heater); *Bean v. Bic Corp.,* 597 So. 2d 1350 (Ala. 1992) (regarding a cigarette lighter).

18. *Losee v. Buchanan,* 51 N.Y. 476, 491 (N.Y. 1873).

19. Percy H. Winfield, "The History of Negligence in the Law of Torts," *Law Quarterly Review,* 42 (1926): 184–201; Charles O. Gregory, "Trespass to Negligence to Absolute Liability," *Virginia Law Review,* 37 (1951): 359–97. But see

Robert L. Rabin, "The Historical Development of the Fault Principle: A Reinterpretation," *Georgia Law Review,* 15 (1980–81): 925–61, 927 ("I view it as a serious mistake to characterize the pre-industrial era as one of strict liability").

20. Chief Justice Lemuel Shaw is often credited with first imposing fault-based liability for unintentionally caused harm. *Brown v. Kendall,* 60 Mass. (6 Cush.) 292, 296 (1850) (articulating a standard of "ordinary care" as "that kind and degree of care, which prudent and cautious men would use, such as is required by the exigency of the case, and such as is necessary to guard against probable danger").

21. William Lloyd Prosser, W. Page Keeton, Dan B. Dobbs, et al., *Prosser and Keeton on Torts,* 5th ed. (St. Paul, MN: West Group, 1984): § 30; 57 *Am. Jur.* 2d *Negligence* § 78 (1989); *Restatement (Second) of Torts* § 281 (1965).

22. Barry R. Furrow, "Forcing Rescue: The Landscape of Health Care Provider Obligations to Treat Patients," *Health Matrix,* 3 (1993): 31–87.

23. Prosser et al., *Prosser and Keeton on Torts,* § 56.

24. See, e.g., *The Nitro-Glycerine Case,* 82 U.S. 524, 536–37 (1872) (the law does "not charge culpable negligence upon anyone who takes the usual precautions against accident, which careful and prudent men are accustomed to take under similar circumstances").

25. Marshall S. Shapo, *Basic Principles of Tort Law* (St. Paul, MN: West Group, 1999), § 19.01.

26. Oliver Wendell Holmes, *The Common Law* (Boston: Little, Brown, 1881; ed. by Mark DeWolfe Howe, Boston: Little, Brown, 1963).

27. Troyen A. Brennan, "Environmental Torts," *Vanderbilt Law Review,* 46 (1993): 1–74, 56.

28. *Geier v. American Honda Motor Co.,* 529 U.S. 861 (2000) (finding that the plaintiff's claim for defective design due to lack of an airbag was preempted by Department of Transportation safety regulations).

29. *Riegel v. Medtronic, Inc.,* 128 S. Ct. 999 (2008) (finding that a product liability claim against the manufacturer of a balloon catheter is preempted by the federal Food, Drug, and Cosmetic Act).

30. *Colaciccio v. Apotex, Inc.,* 432 F. Supp. 2d 514 (E.D. Penn. 2006) (holding that common law tort claims for failure to warn about the suicide risk from Paxil are preempted by the labeling requirements of the Food, Drug, and Cosmetic Act). See also Mary J. Davis, "Discovering the Boundaries: Federal Preemption of Prescription Drug Labeling Product Liability Actions," *Social Science Research Network,* May 22, 2006, http://papers.ssrn.com/sol3/papers.cfm?abstract_id=903757 (stating that the FDA directive represents the first time in the agency's hundred-year history that it has sought to preempt common law prescription drug labeling claims).

31. Prosser et al., *Prosser and Keeton on Torts,* § 41. If two causes concur to bring about an injury and either one of them, operating alone, would have been sufficient to cause the same result, the courts ask whether the defendant's conduct was a "substantial factor" in causing the injury.

32. *Ornstein v. New York City Health & Hosp. Corp,* 806 N.Y.S.2d 566 (App. Div. 2006) (finding that a nurse could not recover for emotional distress due to fear of contracting HIV after a needlestick, based on the low probability of trans-

mission); see also Lawrence O. Gostin and David W. Webber, "The AIDS Litigation Project, Part I: HIV/AIDS in the Courts in the 1990s," *AIDS and Public Policy Journal,* 12 (1997): 105–21.

33. *United States v. Carroll Towing Co.,* 159 F.2d 169 (2d Cir. 1947).

34. A private nuisance is different from but not inconsistent with the concept of trespass. Trespass protects an interest in the exclusive possession of land, while a private nuisance protects an interest in the use and enjoyment of land; trespass requires a physical entry, while private nuisance does not. James A. Henderson, Richard N. Pearson, and John A. Siliciano, *The Torts Process,* 6th ed. (New York: Aspen, 2003).

35. Scholars often associate nuisances with the full spectrum of tort culpability, ranging from "intentional" conduct and negligence to strict liability for abnormally dangerous activity. See, e.g., *Restatement (Second) of Torts* § 822 (1965); Marshall S. Shapo, *Basic Principles of Tort Law* (St. Paul, MN: West Group, 1999): § 36.01. Conceptually, it may be better to think of these as independent sources of liability.

36. Prosser et al., *Prosser and Keeton on Torts,* § 88.

37. Guido Calabresi and Douglas A. Melamed, "Property Rules, Liability Rules, and Inalienability: One View of the Cathedral," *Harvard Law Review,* 85 (1972): 1089–1128; A. Mitchell Polinsky, "Resolving Nuisance Disputes: The Simple Economics of Injunctive and Damage Remedies," *Stanford Law Review,* 32 (1980): 1075–1112.

38. One way of thinking about nuisance actions is that they require the payment of compensation to those injured in exchange for the right to pollute. See, e.g., *Boomer v. Atl. Cement Co.,* 257 N.E.2d 870 (N.Y. 1970) (awarding damages despite the company's positive effect on local employment); *Restatement (Second) of Torts* § 826 (1965) (stating that the industry may have to compensate for unreasonable interferences even if a favorable balance of benefits and burdens exists).

39. *United States v. Reserve Mining Co.,* 380 F. Supp. 11, 55–56 (D. Minn. 1974). Though this case is a public nuisance case, the standard for obtaining an injunction is the same in private nuisance. Cf. *City of Harrisonville v. W. S. Dickey Clay Mfg. Co.,* 289 U.S. 334 (1933) (finding that an injunction was not appropriate in a nuisance case for sewage discharge because monetary compensation was available).

40. *Laird v. Nelms,* 406 U.S. 797 (1972) (regarding the sonic boom generated by aircraft).

41. *Rylands,* L.R. 3 H.L. at 339–40 (per Lord Cairns).

42. *Rylands,* 3 H.L. at 340 (per Lord Cairns).

43. *Restatement (Second) of Torts* §§ 519–20 (1965).

44. *Id.* § 520, cmt. i.

45. See Charles E. Cantu, "Distinguishing the Concept of Strict Liability in Tort from Strict Product Liability: Medusa Unveiled," *University of Memphis Law Review,* 33 (2003): 829–72.

46. *Department of Envtl. Prot. v. Ventron Corp.,* 468 A.2d 150 (N.J. 1982) (regarding disposal of mercury); *T & E Indus. v. Safety Light Corp.,* 587 A.2d

1249 (N.J. 1991) (regarding disposal of radium tailings); *Prospect Indus. Corp. v. Singer Co.*, 569 A.2d 908 (N.J. Super. Ct. 1989) (regarding leaking of PCBs).

47. *In re Hanford Nuclear Reservation Litig.*, 350 F. Supp. 2d 871 (E.D. Wash. 2004) (finding that the chemical separation process used in the production of plutonium is abnormally dangerous, triggering strict liability). See also Prosser et al., *Prosser and Keeton on Torts*, § 78.

48. Marshall S. Shapo, *Basic Principles of Tort Law* (St. Paul, MN: West Group, 1999): 166–67.

49. *MacPherson v. Buick Motor Co.*, 111 N.E. 1050 (N.Y. 1916).

50. See, e.g., *Henningsen v. Bloomfield Motors*, 161 A.2d 69 (N.J. 1960) (finding implied warranty liability against a nonprivity car manufacturer whose car ran off the road, causing personal injuries).

51. *Greenman v. Yuba Power Prods.*, 377 P.2d 897 (Cal. 1963) (finding strict tort liability for a manufacturer that places a product on the market "knowing that it is to be used without inspection for defects, [which] then proves to have a defect that causes injury").

52. *Restatement (Second) of Torts* § 402A (1965) (stating that a seller of a product "in a defective condition unreasonably dangerous to the consumer is liable for physical harm thereby caused to the ultimate user or consumer if . . . it is expected to and does reach the user or consumer without substantial change in the condition in which it is sold").

53. Product liability has extended to include intangibles such as electricity. See *Houston Lighting & Power Co. v. Reynolds*, 765 S.W.2d. 784 (Tex. 1988) (finding that electricity is a product once it is delivered to the consumer).

54. See, e.g., *Richardson v. Volkswagenwerk, A.G.*, 552 F. Supp. 73 (W.D. Mo. 1982) (finding a Volkswagen model to be defectively designed).

55. See, e.g., *Ferdig v. Melitta, Inc.*, 320 N.W.2d 369 (Mich. Ct. App. 1981) (finding a coffee-filtering apparatus defective based on express warranty and negligence theories when hot water spilled on the plaintiff's legs).

56. See, e.g., *Roe v. Deere & Co.*, 855 F.2d 151 (3d Cir. 1988) (allowing the plaintiff to present a theory of liability based upon the lack of crashworthiness of a tractor).

57. See, e.g., *Everett v. Bucky Warren, Inc.*, 380 N.E.2d 653 (Mass. 1978) (finding a hockey helmet to be defectively designed).

58. See, e.g., *Shanks v. Upjohn Co.*, 835 P.2d 1189 (Alaska 1992) (refusing to exempt prescription drugs from strict liability design defect claims).

59. See, e.g., *Jones v. Lederle Lab.*, 695 F. Supp. 700 (E.D.N.Y. 1988) (holding that the claim of defective design of whole-cell pertussis vaccine was not preempted by federal law).

60. See, e.g., *Medtronic, Inc. v. Lohr*, 518 U.S. 470 (1996) (finding that FDA approval of an allegedly defective heart pacemaker did not preempt product liability claims); *Goodlin v. Medtronic, Inc.*, 167 F.3d 1367 (11th Cir. 1999) (same); *Haudrich v. Howmedica, Inc.*, 662 N.E.2d 1248 (Ill. 1996) (finding that a knee prosthesis could be found defective when it failed three years after it had been implanted).

61. *Cavan v. General Motors Corp.*, 571 P.2d 1249, 1251–52 (Or. 1977).

62. See, e.g., *Weishorn v. Miles-Cutter,* 721 A.2d 811 (Pa. Super. Ct. 1998) (holding that the blood shield statute precludes strict liability and breach of warranty claims); see also Eric Feldman and Ronald Bayer, eds., *Blood Feuds: AIDS, Blood, and the Politics of Medical Disaster* (New York: Oxford University Press, 1999).

63. *Barker v. Lull Engineering Co.,* 573 P.2d 443, 545 (Cal. 1978).

64. The factors in the risk-utility calculation are product utility for the consumer and the public; likelihood of risk and severity of harm; alternative products with the same function; manufacturer's ability to reduce the risk without impairing usefulness or creating inordinate expense; the user's awareness of the risk and ability to avoid it by exercising care; and feasibility of the manufacturer spreading the loss through price increases or liability insurance. John Wade, "On the Nature of Strict Tort Liability for Products," *Mississippi Law Journal,* 44 (1973): 825–51, 837–38.

65. *Restatement (Third) of Torts: Prod. Liab.* § 2 (1998).

66. But see *American Tobacco Co., Inc. v. Grinnell,* 951 S.W.2d 420 (Tex. 1977) (finding that pesticide residue, unintentionally but "normally" found in the defendant's tobacco after fumigation, was a manufacturing rather than a design defect).

67. *Restatement (Third) of Torts: Prod. Liab.* § 2(a) (1998).

68. *Id.*

69. The Product Liability Restatement relegates the "consumer expectation" test to a minor role as one of several factors to be considered. Aaron Arnold, "Rethinking Design Defect Law: Should Arizona Adopt the Restatement (Third) of Torts: Product Liability?" *Arizona Law Review,* 45 (2003): 173–95, 186. Note that the "reasonable design alternative" standard may not be required if the product has low social utility and high risk. E.g., *Potter v. Chicago Pneumatic Tool Co.,* 694 A.2d 1319, 1331 (Conn. 1997).

70. Pharmaceutical companies and others sometimes use the "learned intermediary" defense, arguing that parties with superior knowledge, notably the physician, had the responsibility to warn the user of the product's hazards. See, e.g., *Swayze v. McNeil Lab., Inc.,* 807 F.2d 464 (5th Cir. 1987) (applying the learned intermediary defense where a drug manufacturer only warned the prescribing physician); *Mazur v. Merck & Co.,* 964 F.2d 1348 (3d Cir. 1992) (finding that the CDC was a learned intermediary when Merck sold the MMRII vaccine to the CDC for a mass immunization program).

71. However, courts sometimes hold that relatively lax regulatory requirements, demanding only that dangerous products bear warning labels, preempt failure to warn claims. This is similar to the proposition that meeting a low safety standard can preempt a negligence claim. See, e.g., *Colaciccio v. Apotex, Inc.,* 432 F. Supp. 2d 514 (E.D. Penn 2006) (holding that common law tort claims for failure to warn about the suicide risk from Paxil are preempted by the labeling requirements of the Food, Drug, and Cosmetic Act).

72. *Restatement (Third) of Torts: Prod. Liab.* § 2(c) (1998).

73. *Beshada v. Johns-Manville Products Corp.,* 447 A.2d 539, 546–49 (N.J. 1982) (regarding the danger of asbestos).

74. *Restatement (Second) of Torts* § 402B (1965) (stating that a seller who

"makes to the public a misrepresentation of a material fact . . . is subject to liability for physical harm to a consumer . . . caused by justifiable reliance upon the misrepresentation").

75. See, e.g., *Ladd v. Honda Motor Co.*, 939 S.W.2d 83 (Tenn. Ct. App. 1996) (holding that a plaintiff may recover based on advertisements for an entire product line).

76. Frank J. Vandall, "Constructing a Roof before the Foundation Is Prepared: The Restatement (Third) of Torts: Product Liability Section 2(b) Design Defect," *University of Michigan Journal of Law Reform*, 30 (1996–97): 261–79, 261. See George W. Conk, "Is There a Design Defect in the Restatement (Third) of Torts: Product Liability?" *Yale Law Journal*, 109 (2000): 1087–1133.

77. Ellen Wertheimer, "The Bitter Bit: Unknowable Dangers, the Third Restatement, and the Restatement of Liability without Fault," *Brooklyn Law Review*, 70 (2004–5): 889–938, 892 (codification of a negligence-based standard into failure to warn and design defects in the Product Liability Restatement caused states to "remember why they had adopted strict product liability in the first place and returned to the doctrine"). See, e.g., *Freeman v. Hoffman-LaRoche, Inc.*, 618 N.W.2d 827, 840 (Neb. 2000) (declining to adopt *Third Restatement*, §6[c], in favor of *Second Restatement*, §402[a]).

78. Learned Hand, "Historical and Practical Considerations regarding Expert Testimony," *Harvard Law Review*, 15 (1901): 40–58.

79. "Developments in the Law: Confronting the New Challenges of Scientific Evidence," *Harvard Law Review*, 108 (1995): 1481–1605, 1484; see also Sheila Jasanoff, *Science at the Bar: Law, Science and Technology in America* (Cambridge, MA: Harvard University Press, 1995); Peter H. Schuck, "Multi-Culturalism Redux: Science, Law, and Politics," *Yale Law and Policy Review*, 11 (1993): 1–46; Margaret G. Farrell, "*Daubert v. Merrell Dow Pharmaceuticals, Inc.*: Epistemology and Legal Process," *Cardozo Law Review*, 15 (1994): 2183–2217.

80. Tom Christoffel and Stephen P. Teret, "Epidemiology and the Law: Courts and Confidence Intervals," *American Journal of Public Health*, 81 (1991): 1661–66, 1665 ("The scientist's conclusion is achieved when truth is illuminated, and the level of certainty or proof required is very high. The court's conclusion is achieved when the best decision, given the weight of the evidence, is made for that case . . . [and the resolution] is socially acceptable"); Leon Gordis, "Scientific Methodology and Epidemiology," *Kansas Journal of Law and Public Policy*, 9 (2000): 89–104.

81. *In re Union Carbide Gas Plant Disaster at Bhopal, India in Dec. 1984*, 809 F.2d 195 (2d Cir. 1987).

82. Causality is easier to prove with "signature" diseases, which are rare in the absence of specific exposure. Kenneth S. Abraham, "Individual Action and Collective Responsibility: The Dilemma of Mass Tort Reform," *Virginia Law Review*, 73 (1987): 845–907. For example, vaginal adenocarcinoma of the cervix is a rare condition except in women exposed to diethylstilbestrol (DES).

83. *Allen v. United States*, 588 F. Supp. 247 (D. Utah 1984), *rev'd*, 816 F.2d 1417 (10th Cir. 1987).

84. *Mancuso v. Consol. Edison Co. of New York*, 967 F. Supp. 1437, 1445–46 (S.D.N.Y. 1997) ("Numerous courts have followed this method . . . (1) deter-

mine the dosage of the toxin to which the plaintiff was exposed . . . (2) establish general causation by demonstrating that . . . levels of the toxin comparable to those received by the plaintiff can cause the specific types of injuries; and . . . (3) establish specific causation by demonstrating that, more likely than not, the toxin caused the plaintiff's injuries").

85. *Wright v. Willamette Industries Inc.*, 91 F.3d 1105, 1107–8 (8th Cir. 1996) (holding that the dose is necessary to address the issue of general causation).

86. Christopher H. Buckley, Jr., and Charles H. Haake, "Separating the Scientist's Wheat from the Charlatan's Chaff: *Daubert's* Role in Toxic Tort Litigation," *Environmental Law Reporter,* 28 (1998): 10293–305, 10298.

87. Christoffel and Teret, "Epidemiology and the Law," 1662–63.

88. Troyen Brennan, "Causal Chains and Statistical Links: The Role of Scientific Uncertainty in Hazardous-Substance Litigation," *Cornell Law Review,* 73 (1987–88): 469–533.

89. For an account of the salience of probabilistic thinking, see Daniel M. Fox, "Epidemiology and the New Political Economy of Medicine," *American Journal of Public Health,* 89 (1999): 493–96, 495.

90. Kenneth J. Rothman and Sander Greenland, "Causation and Causal Inference," in *Oxford Textbook of Public Health,* vol. 2, ed. Roger Detels, James McEwen, Robert Beaglehole, et al. (New York: Oxford University Press, 1997); Laurens Walker and John Monahan, "Sampling Liability," *Virginia Law Review,* 85 (1999): 329–51.

91. See generally Clark C. Havighurst, Peter Barton Hutt, Barbara J. McNeil, et. al., "Special Issue: Evidence: Its Meanings in Health Care and in Law," *Journal of Health Politics and Policy,* 26 (2001): 191–446.

92. *Frye v. United States,* 293 F. 1013, 1014 (D.C. Cir. 1923) (holding that while courts will go a long way in admitting expert testimony deduced from a well-recognized scientific principle or discovery, the fact from which the deduction is made must be sufficiently established to have gained general acceptance in its particular field).

93. *Fed. R. Evid.* 702.

94. The Supreme Court in 1983 endorsed this idea in *Barefoot v. Estelle,* 463 U.S. 880, 901 (1983) ("We are unconvinced . . . that the adversary process cannot be trusted to sort out the reliable from the unreliable evidence"); see also Michael H. Gottesman, "From *Barefoot* to *Daubert* to *Joiner:* Triple Play or Double Error?" *Arizona Law Review,* 40 (1998): 753–80.

95. Peter W. Huber, *Galileo's Revenge: Junk Science in the Courtroom* (New York: Basic Books, 1991).

96. Marcia Angell, *Science on Trial: The Clash of Medical Evidence and Law in the Breast Implant Case* (New York: W. W. Norton, 1997); see Institute of Medicine, *Safety of Silicone Breast Implants* (Washington, DC: National Academies Press, 1999) (showing no evidence associating implants with adverse health outcomes); Zena A. Stein, "Silicone Breast Implants: Epidemiological Evidence of Sequelae," *American Journal of Public Health,* 89 (1999): 484–87 (reviewing epidemiologic evidence).

97. *Daubert v. Merrell Dow Pharm., Inc.,* 509 U.S. 579 (1993).

98. See Federal Judicial Center, *Reference Manual on Scientific Evidence,* 2d

ed. (Washington, DC: Federal Judicial Center, 2000); see also John M. Conley and David W. Paterson, "The Science of Gatekeeping: The Federal Judicial Center's New Reference Manual on Scientific Evidence," *North Carolina Law Review,* 74 (1995–96): 1183–1223.

99. Consider Prof. Feldman's critique of the Court's "shift to science": "The more closely legal standards hew to scientific ones for selecting information worth considering, the more often it will be apparent that science is severely uncertain about the causal effects of [toxic] substances. . . . When scientists are severely uncertain, . . . legal factfinders will lack a basis [for decision making]." See Heidi L. Feldman, "Science and Uncertainty in Mass Exposure Litigation," *Texas Law Review,* 74 (1995): 1–48, 2–3.

100. *Daubert,* 509 U.S. at 589. For post-*Daubert* cases, see, e.g., *Allen v. Penn. Engineering Corp.,* 102 F.3d 194 (5th Cir. 1996) (finding expert testimony that exposure to ethylene oxide caused cancer to be not scientifically valid under *Daubert*).

101. *Daubert,* 509 U.S. at 592–94. On remand, the Ninth Circuit added an additional factor: whether the expert has conducted research independent of the litigation. The court reasoned that research conducted for the purpose of the litigation was more likely to be biased. *Daubert v. Merrell Dow Pharm., Inc.,* 43 F.3d 1311, 1317 (9th Cir. 1995) ("*Daubert II*").

102. *Kumho Tire Co. v. Carmichael,* 526 U.S. 137, 141 (1999) (holding that *Daubert* factors do not constitute a definitive checklist or test).

103. *United States v. Brown,* 415 F.3d 1257 (11th Cir. 2005) (finding that expert evidence that does not meet three of the four *Daubert* factors nevertheless can be admitted); *Larson v. Kempker,* 414 F.3d 936, 941 (8th Cir. 2005) (allowing evidence of environmental tobacco exposure in a prison using a broad standard of admissibility—so long as it is not so "unsupported that it can offer no assistance to the jury"); *Clausen v. M/V New Carissa,* 339 F.3d 1049 (9th Cir. 2003) (allowing evidence that was not peer-reviewed or published so long as the methods are scientifically acceptable).

104. *Daubert,* 509 U.S. at 591.

105. *Daubert II,* 43 F.3d at 1315.

106. *In re Paoli Railroad Yard PCB Litigation,* 35 F.3d 717, 745 (3d Cir. 1994) (finding an expert's extrapolation from animal studies to humans inadmissible).

107. *Schudel v. General Electric Co.,* 120 F.3d 991, 997 (9th Cir. 1997) (ruling that testimony did not satisfy *Daubert*'s reliability requirements because conclusions were based on extrapolations from studies involving other chemicals and because of inability to testify to a specific causal relationship).

108. *Schudel,* 120 F.3d 991.

109. *Gen. Elec. Co. v. Joiner,* 522 U.S. 136, 141 (1997).

110. Buckley and Haake, "Separating the Scientist's Wheat from the Charlatan's Chaff," 10297.

111. *Joiner,* 522 U.S. 136.

112. *Kumho Tire Co. v. Carmichael,* 526 U.S. 137 (1999).

113. *Carmichael,* 526 U.S. at 152.

114. Gottesman, "From *Barefoot* to *Daubert* to *Joiner,*" 759; Adina Schwartz, "A 'Dogma of Empiricism' Revisited: *Daubert v. Merrell Dow Pharmaceuticals, Inc.* and the Need to Resurrect the Philosophy of Insight of *Frye v. United*

States," Harvard Journal of Law and Technology, 10 (1996–97): 149–237, 151. Similar problems have arisen in foreign courts. See *McTear v. Imperial Tobacco Ltd.* (2005) ScotCS CSOH 69 (finding that causality cannot usually be found using only epidemiologic data); see also Alexander Danne, "*McTear v. Imperial Tobacco:* Understanding the Role and Limitations of Expert Epidemiological Evidence in Scientific Litigation," *Journal of Law and Medicine,* 13 (2006): 471–78.

115. *Hollander v. Sandoz Pharmaceuticals Corp.,* 289 F.3d 1193, 1209 (10th Cir. 2002).

116. *Merrell Dow Pharmaceuticals, Inc. v. Havnor,* 953 S.W.2d 706 (Tex. 1997) (finding that a relative risk of 2.0 or greater is needed to demonstrate causality). Relative risk, or incidence rate ratio, is the ratio of disease incidence in an exposed population to disease incidence in an unexposed population. Bright-line rules excluding evidence with less than 2.0 risk ratio misinterpret epidemiology, which is concerned with the cumulative evidence from many studies and is population-based.

117. *Joiner,* 522 U.S. at 145–47.

118. David Egilman, Joyce Kim, and Molly Biklen, "Proving Causation: The Use and Abuse of Medical and Scientific Evidence inside the Courtroom—An Epidemiologist's Critique of the Judicial Interpretation of the *Daubert* Ruling," *Food and Drug Law Journal,* 58 (2003): 223–50.

119. Lisa Heinzerling, "Doubting *Daubert,*" *Journal of Law and Policy,* 14 (2006): 65–83, 81.

120. Jon S. Vernick, Julie Samie Mair, Stephen P. Teret, et al., "The Role of Litigation in Preventing Product-Related Injuries," *Epidemiologic Reviews,* 25 (2003): 90–98.

121. Jacobson and Soliman, "Litigation as Public Health Policy."

122. G. Edward White, *Tort Law in America: An Intellectual History* (New York: Oxford University Press, 1980): 220–23, 230; Scott Burris, "Law and the Social Risk of Health Care: Lessons from HIV Testing," *Albany Law Review,* 61 (1998): 831–95.

123. S. Chapman, "Blaming Tobacco's Victims," *Tobacco Control,* 11 (2002): 167–68 (arguing that smoker culpability is obviated by the tobacco industry: targeting children, selling an addictive product, and preventing consumers from actually knowing the risks of smoking).

124. My appreciation goes to my colleague Lisa Heinzerling for the idea that limitations of traditional tort doctrines can sometimes be helpful to public health advocates.

125. Jon Hanson, "Taking Behavioralism Seriously: Some Evidence of Market Manipulation," *Harvard Law Review,* 112 (1998–99): 1420–1572.

126. Edward Hammond and Daniel Horn, "Smoking and Death Rates: Report on Forty-four Months of Follow-up on 187,783 Men, I and II," *JAMA,* 166 (1958): 1159–72, 1294–1308; Richard Doll and A. Bradford Hill, "A Study of the Aetiology of Carcinoma of the Lung," *British Medical Journal,* 2 (1952): 1271–86; Ernest L. Wynder and Evarts A. Graham, "Tobacco Smoking as a Possible Etiologic Factor in Bronchiogenic Carcinoma: A Study of 684 Proved Cases," *JAMA,* 143 (1950): 329–36.

127. Roy Norr, "Cancer by the Carton," *Reader's Digest,* 61 (December

1952): 7–8; Lois Mattox Miller and James Monahan, "The Facts behind the Cigarette Controversy," *Reader's Digest,* 65 (July 1954): 1–6.

128. *Lowe v. R. J. Reynolds Tobacco Co.,* No. 9673(C) (E.D. Mo. filed March 10, 1954) (case subsequently dropped).

129. Robert Rabin, "A Socio-Legal History of the Tobacco Tort Litigation," *Stanford Law Review,* 44 (1991–92): 853–78, 857. See Wendy E. Parmet, "Tobacco, HIV, and the Courtroom: The Role of Affirmative Litigation in the Formation of Public Health Policy," *Houston Law Review,* 36 (1999): 1663–1712.

130. See, e.g., *Lartigue v. R. J. Reynolds Tobacco Co.,* 317 F.2d 19 (5th Cir. 1963); *Green v. American Tobacco Co.,* 154 So. 2d 169 (Fla. 1969).

131. Graham E. Kelder, Jr., and Richard A. Daynard, "The Role of Litigation in the Effective Control of the Sale and Use of Tobacco," *Stanford Law and Policy Review,* 8 (1997): 63–98, 71.

132. U.S. Department of Health, Education, and Welfare, *Smoking and Health: Report of the Advisory Committee to the Surgeon General of the Public Health Service* (Washington, DC: Government Printing Office, 1964) (marshaling scientific data on the health risks posed by tobacco).

133. *Restatement (Second) of Torts* § 402A, cmt. i (1965).

134. 15 U.S.C. § 1333 (1994).

135. Linda Greenhouse, "Court to Say If Cigarette Makers Can Be Sued for Smokers' Cancer," *New York Times,* March 26, 1991.

136. Lawrence O. Gostin, Allan M. Brandt, and Paul D. Cleary, "Tobacco Liability and Public Health Policy," *JAMA,* 266 (1991): 3178–82, 3179.

137. *Thayer v. Liggett and Myers Tobacco Co.,* No. 5314, slip op. (W.D. Mich., Feb. 20, 1970) (cataloguing in detail how the industry wore down plaintiffs). The industry was also strident in its opposition to direct regulation. See Peter S. Arno, Allan M. Brandt, Lawrence O. Gostin, et al., "Tobacco Industry Strategies to Oppose Federal Regulation," *JAMA,* 275 (1996): 1258–62.

138. Richard A. Daynard and Graham E. Kelder, Jr., "The Many Virtues of Tobacco Litigation," *Trial Products Liability,* 34 (1998): 34–43, 36.

139. Donald Janson, "Data on Smoking Revealed at Trial," *New York Times,* March 13, 1988.

140. 79 Stat. 282 (1965), *as amended,* 15 U.S.C. §§ 1331–40 (1965) ("No statement relating to smoking and health [other than the congressionally mandated warnings] shall be required on any cigarette package").

141. *Public Health Cigarette Smoking Act,* 84 Stat. 88 (1970), *as amended,* 15 U.S.C. §§ 1331–40 (1969) ("No requirement or prohibition based on smoking and health shall be imposed [by a state] with respect to the advertising or promotion of any cigarettes").

142. *Cipollone v. Liggett Group,* 505 U.S. 504 (1992).

143. *Id.* at 530–31.

144. Stanton A. Glantz, Deborah E. Barnes, Lisa A. Bero, et al., "Looking through a Keyhole at the Tobacco Industry: The Brown and Williamson Documents," *JAMA,* 274 (1995): 219–24; John Slade, Lisa A. Bero, Peter Hanauer, et al., "Nicotine and Addiction: The Brown and Williamson Documents," *JAMA,* 274 (1995): 225–33. To view the Brown and Williamson documents, see

University of California, San Francisco, *Tobacco Control Archives,* April 24, 2006, http://www.library.ucsf.edu/tobacco. Other online collections contain tobacco industry documents from a variety of sources; see, e.g., *Tobacco Documents Online,* 1999–2006, http://www.tobaccodocuments.org.

145. See, e.g., Philip J. Hilts and Glenn Collins, "Records Show Philip Morris Studies Influence of Nicotine," *New York Times,* June 8, 1995; Philip J. Hilts, "Tobacco Company Was Silent on Hazards," *New York Times,* May 7, 1994.

146. See, e.g., Richard D. Hurt and Channing R. Robertson, "Prying Open the Door to the Tobacco Industry's Secrets about Nicotine," *JAMA,* 280 (1998): 1173–81 (reviewing more than 39,000 internal documents disclosed in Minnesota's Medicaid recoupment suit).

147. *Mike Moore, ex rel. State v. American Tobacco Co.,* No. 94–1429 (Miss. Ch. Ct., Jackson County, filed May 23, 1994).

148. S. 1415, 105th Cong. (1998). See also John Schwartz and Saundra Torry, "Tobacco Targets the McCain Bill," *Washington Post,* April 11, 1998.

149. The text of these settlements is available at http://ag.ca.gov/tobacco/pdf/1msa.pdf#search=%22Master%20Settlement%20Agreement%22 (September 21, 2006). Minnesota settled on perhaps the most favorable terms. See *State v. Philip Morris, Inc.,* 551 N.W.2d 490 (Minn. 1996) (en banc); Settlement Agreement and Stipulation for Entry of Consent Judgment, *Minnesota v. Philip Morris,* No. CI-94–8565 (Minn. Dist. Ct. May 18, 1998).

150. National Association of Attorneys General, *Master Settlement Agreement,* Nov. 16,1998, http://www.naag.org/backpages/naag/tobacco/msa/msa-pdf/.

151. *Star Scientific, Inc., v. Beales,* 278 F.3d 339 (4th Cir. 2002) (holding that the MSA does not violate the Commerce Clause, the Equal Protection Clause, the Due Process Clause, or the Compact Clause of the Constitution).

152. *Mariana v. Fisher,* 338 F.3d 189 (3d Cir. 2003) (relying on the Noerr-Pennington doctrine ["a party who petitions the government for redress generally is immune from antitrust liability"] to reject claims that the MSA unreasonably restrains trade).

153. *Table Bluff Reservation v. Philip Morris, Inc.,* 256 F.3d 879 (9th Cir. 2001) (holding that Indian tribes did not have standing to contest their exclusion from MSA negotiations, because the tribes did not establish: (1) that they had made claims against the tobacco companies for health care costs which had been rejected, and (2) that their exclusion from the MSA injured their future ability to get reimbursement for health care costs or other relief from the tobacco companies).

154. *United States v. Philip Morris USA, Inc.,* 396 F.3d 1190 (D.C. Cir. 2005).

155. Michael Janofsky and David Johnston, "Limit for Award in Tobacco Case Sets Off Protest," *New York Times,* June 9, 2005.

156. *United States v. Philip Morris USA, Inc.,* 449 F. Supp. 2d 1 (D.D.C 2006). In *Schwab v. Philip Morris USA, Inc.* 449 F. Supp. 2d 992 (E.D.N.Y. 2006) the district court certified a class of light cigarette smokers, finding "substantial evidence" that manufacturers knew that light cigarettes were at least as dangerous as regular cigarettes. David Cay Johnston and Melanie Warner, "Tobacco Makers Lose Key Ruling on Latest Suits," *New York Times,* September 26, 2006. As of November 20, 2006, proceedings in the case had been formally stayed pend-

ing a Second Circuit Court of Appeals panel review of the lower court's decision. Staff reporter, "Stay Put on 'Light Cigarette' Suit," *Wall Street Journal,* November 20, 2006.

157. *Glover v. Philip Morris USA Inc.,* 380 F. Supp. 2d 1279 (M.D. Fla. 2005) (holding that individuals could not sue tobacco companies as private attorneys general under the Medicare Secondary Payer statute because the companies' underlying tort liability and responsibility to pay Medicare had not been established by a judgment).

158. See, e.g., *Empire Healthchoice Inc., v. Philip Morris USA Inc.,* 393 F.3d 312 (2d Cir. 2004) (holding that claims by a third-party payer of health care costs are too remote to permit suit under New York's consumer protection statute); *SEIU Health & Welfare Fund v. Philip Morris, Inc.,* 249 F.3d 1068 (D.C. Cir. 2001) (denying plaintiffs' RICO and fraud claims against the tobacco industry for failure to establish a sufficiently direct causal relationship between the alleged injury and wrongdoing).

159. *In re Tobacco Health Care Costs Litigation,* 83 F. Supp. 2d 125 (D.D.C. 1999) (dismissing the plaintiff's claim with prejudice because the injury was too remote to be proximately caused by the defendant's alleged misconduct); *Republic of Venezuela ex rel. Garrido v. Philip Morris Co.,* 827 So. 2d 339 (Fla., 2003) (dismissing the plaintiff's claim because the government of Venezuela did not have a direct cause of action against the tobacco companies to recover for smoking-related medical expenses incurred by its citizens); *SEIU Health & Welfare Fund v. Philip Morris, Inc.,* 249 F.3d 1068 (2001) (reversing a previous denial of motion to dismiss RICO and fraud claims because the harms alleged by plaintiffs were too far remote from defendant's alleged wrongdoings to allow for RICO or antitrust standing, and affirming dismissal of the plaintiffs' additional claims).

160. *Falise v. American Tobacco Co.,* 94 F. Supp. 2d 316 (E.D.N.Y. 2000); *Owens Corning v. R. J. Reynolds Tobacco Co.,* 868 So. 2d 331 (Miss. 2004) (deciding that tobacco companies were not liable to asbestos companies for costs of past and future smoking-related claims).

161. *Broin v. Philip Morris Co.,* 641 So. 2d 888 (Fla. Dist. Ct. App. 1994) (certifying a class defined as all nonsmoking flight attendants employed by U.S.-based airlines and suffering from diseases caused by exposure to secondhand smoke), *rev. denied,* 654 So. 2d 919 (Fla. 1995) (unpublished table opinion).

162. *Ramos v. Philip Morris Co.,* 743 So. 2d 24 (Fla. Dist. Ct. App. 1999).

163. *Castano v. American Tobacco Co.,* 84 F.3d 734 (5th Cir. 1996).

164. *Engle v. Liggett Group, Inc.,* No. SC03–1856 (Fla. July 6, 2006).

165. *Price v. Philip Morris, Inc.,* 848 N.E. 2d 1 (Ill. 2005). Plaintiffs sued as a class of consumers who had been deceived by tobacco company descriptions of "low tar," "ultra low tar," and "light" cigarettes. The trial court certified the class, finding the issue of consumer deception to pose common questions of fact that could be determined for the class as a whole. After plaintiffs won a $10 billion judgment, the Illinois Supreme Court reversed on the grounds that Philip Morris advertised its product in compliance with applicable FTC regulations. The $10 billion judgment against the company was thrown out. See also *Simon II Litigation v. Philip Morris USA Inc.,* 407 F.3d 125 (2d Cir. 2005) (decertifying a nationwide class of smokers seeking punitive damages, due to the lack of evi-

dence that individual actions could not be maintained); *Marrone v. Philip Morris USA, Inc.*, 850 N.E.2d 31 (Ohio 2006) (denying class certification to smokers of light cigarettes because the defendant did not have notice that its alleged conduct was deceptive).

166. *Williams v. Philip Morris Inc.*, 127 P.3d 1165 (Or. 2006) (awarding the plaintiff's estate $79.5 million in punitive damages), rev'd in part, 127 S. Ct. 1057 (2007) (holding punitive damages award was improperly based in part on jury's desire to punish defendent for harm to nonparties).

167. See, e.g., *Henley v. Philip Morris, Inc.*, 5 Cal. Rptr. 3d 42 (Cal. Ct. App. 2003) (awarding the plaintiff $25 million in punitive damages, reduced in later proceedings); *Boeken v. Philip Morris Inc.*, 26 Cal. Rptr. 3d 638 (Cal. Ct. App. 2005) (reducing a punitive damage award to $50 million).

168. Some individual actions are being dismissed because of the "common knowledge" that tobacco is harmful. See, e.g., *Tompkins v. R.J. Reynolds Tobacco Co.*, 92 F. Supp. 2d 70 (N.D.N.Y. 2000).

169. Melanie Warner, "Big Award on Tobacco Is Rejected by Court," *New York Times*, July 7, 2006.

170. *Engle*, 31 Fla. L. Weekly S464.

171. Edward L. Sweda, "Lawsuits and Secondhand Smoke," *Tobacco Control*, 13 (2004): i61–i66 (describing secondhand smoke litigation over the past quarter-century, in which nonsmoking litigants have prevailed).

172. Stephen D. Sugarman, "Mixed Results from Recent United States Tobacco Litigation," *Tort Law Review*, 10 (2002): 94–126 (noting that nonsmokers may struggle to establish a causal connection between exposure to secondhand smoke and injury).

173. U.S. Department of Health and Human Services, *The Health Consequences of Involuntary Exposure to Tobacco Smoke: A Report of the Surgeon General* (Washington, DC: Government Printing Office, 2006). Notably, R. J. Reynolds asserts that there are still legitimate scientific questions concerning the reported risks of secondhand smoke. See R. J. Reynolds Tobacco Co., *Smoking and Health: Summary of Opinions*, http://www.rjrt.com/smoking/summaryCover.aspx.

174. Work-product discovery allows plaintiffs to request materials from other plaintiffs or previous cases, which would normally be protected.

175. Milo Geyelin, "Behind Giant Tobacco Verdicts, a Legal SWAT Team," *Wall Street Journal*, April 12, 1999.

176. *State Farm Mutual Automobile Insurance Co. v. Campbell*, 538 U.S. 408, 425 (2003) (holding that a punitive damages award of $145 million, where full compensatory damages were $1 million, was neither reasonable nor proportionate to the wrong committed, and it was thus an irrational, arbitrary, and unconstitutional deprivation of the property of the insurer); see Sara D. Guardino and Richard A. Daynard, "Punishing Tobacco Industry Misconduct: The Case for Exceeding a Single Digit Ratio between Punitive and Compensatory Damages," *University of Pittsburgh Law Review*, 67 (2005): 1–66 (discussing when punitive damage awards should be allowed to exceed the *State Farm* single-digit ratio limit).

177. *Williams v. Philip Morris Inc.*, 127 P.3d 1165 (Or. 2006) (reinstating $79.5 million in punitive damages—ninety-nine times the $800,000 compensatory damage award in the case).

178. *Philip Morris USA v. Williams,* 127 S. Ct. 1057 (2007) (throwing out a $79.5 million verdict because it imposed punitive damages on the defendant for injuring persons not party to the suit).

179. Linda Greenhouse, "Judges Overturn $79.5 Million in Punitive Damages against Philip Morris," *New York Times,* February 20, 2007.

180. Danny David, "Three Paths to Justice: New Approaches to Minority Instituted Tobacco Litigation," *Harvard BlackLetter Law Journal,* 15 (1999): 185–226.

181. Frank A. Sloan, Emily Streyer Carlisle, John R. Rattliff, et al., "Determinants of States' Allocation of the Master Settlement Agreement Payments," *Journal of Health Politics, Policy, and Law,* 30 (2005): 643–86 (finding that the underallocation of funds for tobacco control is most severe in tobacco-producing states, states with a high proportion of conservative Democrats, and states with a high proportion of elderly, Black, Hispanic, or wealthy citizens); U.S. Government Accountability Office, *Tobacco Settlement: States' Allocations of Fiscal Year 2005 and Expected Fiscal Year 2006 Payments,* GAO-06–502 (April 2006) (reporting how the states allocated the $5.4 billion tobacco settlement funds they received in 2006).

182. Campaign for Tobacco-Free Kids, "A Broken Promise to Our Children: The 1998 State Tobacco Settlement Seven Years Later," November 30, 2005, http://www.tobaccofreekids.org/reports/settlements/2006/fullreport.pdf.

183. Lara Zwarun, "Ten Years and One Master Settlement Agreement Later: The Nature and Frequency of Alcohol and Tobacco Promotion in Televised Sports, 2000 through 2002," *American Journal of Public Health,* 96 (2006): 1492–97.

184. Pamela Prah, "Tobacco Money—Hard Habit for States to Kick," *Stateline.org,* February 8, 2007, http://www.stateline.org/live/details/story?contentId=178571 (discussing how states are spending the tobacco settlement money, and how the unexpected shortfall has affected their budgets).

185. Robert A. Hahn, Oleg O. Bilukha, Alex Crosby, et al., "First Reports Evaluating the Effectiveness of Strategies for Preventing Violence: Firearms Law," *Morbidity and Mortality Weekly Review,* 52 (2003): 11–20.

186. Tom Diaz, "The American Gun Industry: Designing and Marketing Increasingly Lethal Weapons," in *Suing the Gun Industry: A Battle at the Crossroads of Gun Control and Mass Torts,* ed. Timothy Lytton (Ann Arbor: University of Michigan Press, 2005): 84–104.

187. David Hemenway, *Private Guns, Public Health* (Ann Arbor: University of Michigan Press, 2004).

188. Deborah Azrael, Phillip J. Cook, and Matthew Miller, "State and Local Prevalence of Firearms Ownership: Measurement, Structure, Trends," *Journal of Quantitative Criminology,* 20 (2004): 43–62.

189. The two leading mechanisms causing fatal injury in the United States are motor vehicles and firearms. Institute of Medicine, *Reducing the Burden of Injury: Advancing Prevention and Treatment* (Washington, DC: National Academies Press, 1999); Sara B. Vyrostek, Joseph L. Annest, and George W. Ryan, "Surveillance for Fatal and Non-fatal Injuries—United States, 2001," *Morbidity and Mortality Weekly Report,* 53 (2004): 1–57.

190. Donna L. Hoyert, Melanie P. Heron, Sherry L. Murphy, et al., "Deaths:

Final Data for 2003," *National Vital Statistics Report,* 54 (2006): 1–120. Firearm deaths have remained stable since 1999, with a rate of approximately 10 per 100,000. This and other data suggest that firearm deaths have transitioned from an epidemic to an endemic condition. Katherine Kaufer Christoffel, "Firearm Injuries: Epidemic Then, Endemic Now," *American Journal of Public Health,* 97 (2007): 626–29.

191. Centers for Disease Control and Prevention, "Nonfatal and Fatal Firearm-Related Injuries—United States, 1993–1997," *JAMA,* 283 (2000): 47–48. See Jon S. Vernick and Stephen P. Teret, "New Courtroom Strategies regarding Firearms: Tort Litigation against Firearm Manufacturers and Constitutional Challenges to Gun Laws," *Houston Law Review,* 36 (1999): 1713–54.

192. See, e.g., Lois A. Fingerhut and Margy Warner, *Health, United States, 1996–1997 and Injury Chartbook* (Hyattsville, MD: National Center for Health Statistics, 1997); Darci Cherry, Joseph L. Annest, James A. Mercy, et al., "Trends in Nonfatal and Fatal Firearm-Related Injury Rates in the United States, 1985–1995," *Annals of Emergency Medicine,* 32 (1998): 51–59.

193. Out of all firearm injury deaths in 2003, homicide accounted for 39.6 percent and suicide accounted for 56.1 percent. Males incur firearm injuries at 6.8 times the rate of females, and African Americans incur such injuries at 2.1 times the rate of Whites. Hoyert et al., "Deaths: Final Data for 2003."

194. U.S. Department of Justice, "Nonfatal Firearm-Related Violent Crimes, 1993–2005," *Bureau of Justice Statistics,* September 10, 2006, http://www.ojp.usdoj.gov/bjs/glance/tables/firearmnonfataltab.htm.

195. See, e.g., Centers for Disease Control and Prevention, "Rates of Homicide, Suicide, and Firearm-Related Death among Children—Twenty-six Industrialized Countries," *Morbidity and Mortality Weekly Report,* 46 (1997): 101–5; Etienne G. Krug, K. E. Powell, and L. L. Dahlberg, "Firearm-Related Deaths in the United States and Thirty-five Other High and Upper-Middle-Income Countries," *International Journal of Epidemiology,* 27 (1998): 214–21.

196. Firearm and Injury Center at Penn, *Firearm Injury in the U.S.,* August 17, 2004, http://www.uphs.upenn.edu/ficap/resourcebook/pdf/monograph.pdf.

197. See, e.g., *McAndrew v. Mularchuk,* 162 A.2d 820 (N.J. 1960) (finding that the potential of a loaded revolver to inflict serious injury is such that the law imposes a duty to employ extraordinary care in its handling and use); but see *Miller v. Kennedy,* 241 Cal. Rptr. 472 (Cal. Ct. App.1987) (finding that, in an action against a police officer by a man accidentally shot, the standard is ordinary care); *Shaw v. Lord,* 137 P. 885 (Okla. 1914) (requiring ordinary negligence for liability for firearm use in self-defense).

198. Mark D. Polston and Douglas S. Weil, "Unsafe by Design: Using Tort Actions to Reduce Firearm-Related Injuries," *Stanford Law and Policy Review,* 8 (1997): 13–24.

199. American Psychological Association and American Academy of Pediatrics, *Raising Children to Resist Violence: What You Can Do* (Elk Grove Village, IL: American Academy, Division of Publications, 1995).

200. Yvonne D. Senturia, Katherine K. Christoffel, and Mark Donovan, "Gun Storage Patterns in U.S. Homes with Children," *Archives of Pediatrics and Adolescent Medicine,* 150 (1996): 265–69.

201. See, e.g., Philip J. Cook and Jens Ludwig, *Guns in America: Results of a Comprehensive National Survey on Firearms Ownership and Use* (Washington, DC: Police Foundation, 1997) (stating that 34 percent of owners keep their handguns loaded and unlocked); Douglas Weil and David Hemenway, "Loaded Guns in the Home: Analysis of a National Random Survey of Gun Owners," *JAMA,* 267 (1992): 3033–37; David Hemenway, Sara J. Solnick, and Deborah R. Azrael, "Firearm Training and Storage," *JAMA,* 273 (1995): 46–50.

202. See, e.g., *Cal. Penal Code* § 12035 (West 1991).

203. *Restatement (Second) of Torts* § 308, cmt. b (1965) (using a child's access to a firearm as an illustration of negligent entrustment).

204. See, e.g., *Butcher v. Cordova,* 728 P.2d 388 (Colo. Ct. App. 1986) (applying § 308 to child access to a firearm); *Reida v. Lund,* 96 Cal. Rptr. 102 (Cal. Ct. App. 1971) (imposing liability even though the rifle was kept locked, since the son knew the location of the key); but see *Robertson v. Wentz,* 232 Cal. Rptr. 634 (Cal. Ct. App. 1986) (failing to impose liability when the parent had no ability to restrain a minor's access to firearms kept in the house). For a detailed discussion of negligent entrustment, see L. S. Rogers, "Liability of Person Permitting Child to Have a Gun, or Leaving Gun Accessible to Child, for Injury Inflicted by the Latter," *American Law Reports,* 68 (2004): 782–837.

205. Centers for Disease Control and Prevention, "Motor-Vehicle Safety: A Twentieth Century Public Health Achievement," *Morbidity and Mortality Weekly Report,* 48 (1999): 369–74 (reduction of the death rate from motor vehicle crashes due to technological advancement represents one of the great public health achievements); David Hemenway, "Regulation of Firearms," *New Engl. J. Med.,* 339 (1998): 843–45, 844 ("Injury control experts recognized that to increase the safety of driving, it would be more cost effective to change the vehicle and highway environment than to change human behavior").

206. An argument can be made that firearm dealers are also in a good position to limit access to guns. Unfortunately, current federal regulation of dealers is not effective, and state regulatory regimes are uneven, often providing for only minimal oversight. Jon Vernick, Daniel Webster, Maria Bulzacchelli, et al., "Regulation of Firearm Dealers in the United States: An Analysis of State Law and Opportunities for Improvement," *Journal of Law, Medicine, and Ethics,* 34 (2005): 765–75; Jon S. Vernick and Daniel Webster, "Policies to Prevent Firearm Trafficking," *Injury Prevention,* 13 (2007): 78–79.

207. Julia Samia Mair, Stephen Teret, and Shannon Frattaroli, "A Public Health Perspective on Gun Violence Prevention," in *Suing the Gun Industry: A Battle at the Crossroads of Gun Control and Mass Torts,* ed. Timothy Lytton (Ann Arbor: University of Michigan Press, 2005): 39–61.

208. James Dao, "Under Legal Siege, Gunmaker Agrees to Accept Curbs," *New York Times,* March 18, 2000.

209. *Protection of Lawful Commerce in Arms Act,* Pub. L. No. 109–92, 119 Stat. 2095 (2005) (to be codified at 15 U.S.C. §§ 7901–3, 18 U.S.C. §§ 922, 924 [2005]).

210. "Recent Legislation: Tort Law—Civil Immunity—Congress Passes Prohibition of Qualified Civil Claims against Gun Manufacturers and Distributors," *Harvard Law Review,* 19 (2006): 1939–45.

211. Lytton, *Suing the Gun Industry,* 5.

212. General Accounting Office, *Accidental Shootings: Many Deaths and Injuries Caused by Firearms Could Be Prevented* (Washington, DC: General Accounting Office, 1991) (stating that 31 percent of deaths occurred either because a child was able to fire the gun or because it was fired by a person unaware that the gun was loaded).

213. Stephen P. Teret, Susan DeFrancesco, Stephen W. Hargarten, et al., "Making Guns Safer," *Issues in Science and Technology,* 14 (1998): 37–40; Garen J. Wintemute, "The Relationship between Firearm Design and Firearm Violence," *JAMA,* 275 (1996): 1749–53.

214. Lytton, *Suing the Gun Industry,* 5.

215. John P. McNicholas and Matthew McNicholas, "Ultrahazardous Product Liability: Providing Victims of Well-Made Firearms Ammunition to Fire Back at Gun Manufacturers," *Loyola of Los Angeles Law Review,* 30 (1997): 1557–99, 1559 ("There is no other reason [but mass killing] to allow the gun to swivel from the hip in a spray-fire fashion, to . . . permit the user to fire thirty-two rounds without reloading, or to adjust the trigger so that the product can empty its hail of fire at a fully automatic rate").

216. See *Patterson v. Rohm Gesellschaft,* 608 F. Supp. 1206, 1211 (N.D. Tex. 1987).

217. Lytton, *Suing the Gun Industry,* 7.

218. *Id.* at 8.

219. The following cases involving failure to provide a loaded chamber indicator or a magazine safety were not allowed to proceed to trial: *Bolduc v. Colt's Manufacturing Co., Inc.,* 968 F. Supp. 16 (D. Mass. 1997); *Wasylow v. Glock, Inc.* 975 F. Supp. 370 (D. Mass. 1996); *Raines v. Colt Industries,* 757 F. Supp 819 (E.D. Mich. 1991); *Crawford v. Navegar,* 453 Mich. 891 (1996).

220. *Richman v. Charter Arms Corp.,* 571 F. Supp 192 (E.D. La. 1983) (holding that criminal use of a handgun was a "normal" use and marketing to the public was not an "unreasonably dangerous activity").

221. See, e.g., *Perkins v. F.I.E. Corp.,* 762 F.2d 1250 (5th Cir. 1985) (denying strict liability as an available remedy where guns functioned as designed and dangers were obvious and well known); *Raines,* 757 F. Supp. at 819 (stating that the manufacturer was absolved from liability because the risks of firearms are known and expected).

222. See, e.g., *Moore v. R. G. Industries, Inc.,* 789 F.2d 1326 (9th Cir. 1986) (refusing to impose strict liability on the manufacturer of a .25 caliber automatic handgun for injuries to a woman shot by her husband, because the product "performed as intended"); but see *Kelley v. R. G. Indus.,* 497 A.2d 1143 (Md. 1985) (holding the manufacturer of a "Saturday Night Special" handgun strictly liable). The court's reasoning was later rejected by the legislature; see *Md. Ann. Code* art. 27 § 36-I(h) (1992).

223. Dan B. Dobbs, *The Law of Torts* (St. Paul, MN: West Publishing Company, 2000): § 330.

224. See, e.g., *Kitchen v. K-Mart Corp.,* 697 So. 2d 1200 (Fla. 1997) (holding the seller of a firearm to an intoxicated buyer liable to an injured person under the theory of negligent entrustment).

225. See, e.g., *City of Chicago v. Beretta U.S.A. Corp.*, 821 N.E.2d 1099 (Ill. 2004) (finding that plaintiffs' allegations of negligent conduct were not supported by any recognized duty).

226. *Hamilton v. Beretta U.S.A. Corp.*, 750 N.E. 2d 1055 (N.Y. 2001).

227. *Id.* at 1061.

228. *Id.* at 1064.

229. *Ileto v. Glock*, 349 F.3d 1191 (9th Cir. 2003).

230. See, e.g., *City of Chicago v. Beretta U.S.A. Corp.*, 821 N.E.2d 1099 (Ill. 2004) (stating that plaintiffs could not establish probable cause for either negligence or public nuisance claims).

231. John G. Culhane and Jean Macchiaroli Eggen, "Public Nuisance Claims against Gun Sellers: New Insights and Challenges," *University of Michigan Journal of Law Reform*, 38 (2004): 1–56.

232. *Restatement (Second) Torts* § 821B (1977).

233. Eric L. Kintner, "Bad Apples and Smoking Barrels: Private Actions for Public Nuisance against the Gun Industry," *Iowa Law Review*, 90 (2005): 1163–1240. Note that public nuisance suits brought by individuals are distinct from private nuisance suits. Private nuisance refers to nontrespassory interference with an individual's use and enjoyment of their land.

234. *City of Chicago v. Beretta U.S.A. Corp.*, 821 N.E.2d 1099 (Ill. 2004).

235. Lytton, *Suing the Gun Industry*, 11.

236. James Dao, "Under Legal Siege, Gunmaker Agrees to Accept Curbs," *New York Times*, March 18, 2000.

237. *Protection of Lawful Commerce in Arms Act*, 15 U.S.C § 7901 *et. seq.* (2005).

238. *Id.* at § 7903(5)(A).

239. Negligent entrustment suits are not precluded, but except for *Ileto*, they have met with little success.

240. *City of New York v. Beretta U.S.A., Corp.*, 401 F. Supp. 2d 244 (E.D.N.Y. 2005).

241. See New York P.L. 240.45 (defining criminal nuisance in the second degree as a person who "by conduct either unlawful in itself or unreasonable under all the circumstances, . . . knowingly or recklessly creates or maintains a condition which endangers the safety or health of a considerable number of persons").

242. 15 U.S.C. § 7903(5)(A)(3). See William K. Rashbaum, "Judge Clears Way for City to Sue Gun Companies," *New York Times*, December 3, 2005.

243. *Ileto v. Glock*, 421 F. Supp. 2d 1274 (C.D. Cal. 2006).

244. Jacobson and Soliman, "Litigation as Public Health Policy."

245. Council of Economic Advisors, *Who Pays for Tort Liability Claims? An Economic Analysis of the U.S. Tort Liability System*, April 2002, http://www.whitehouse.gov/cea/tortliabilitysystem_apr02.pdf (finding that tort claims cost $650 per capita, which "amounts to a 2 percent tax on consumption, a three percent tax on wages or a five percent tax on corporate income," and that most costs are passed on to consumers and workers).

246. 28 U.S.C. §§ 1332(d), 1453, 1711–15 (allowing removal of a class action to federal courts even when the great majority of class members are from the same state as the defendant, and restricting the use of coupon settlements).

247. John F. Harris, "Victory for Bush on Suits," *Washington Post,* February 18, 2005 ("Waging class-action lawsuits amid a patchwork of state laws . . . invites abuse by plaintiffs' attorneys filing lawsuits in certain courts known to be sympathetic to the cases").

248. "Class Action Lawsuits," *New York Times,* February 2, 2005.

249. Tort costs may be viewed as much higher than they actually are, but if companies have inflated views of these costs, they may respond in the same way as if the costs were real.

250. W. Kip Viscusi, "The Social Costs of Punitive Damages against Corporations in Environmental and Safety Torts," *Georgetown Law Journal,* 87 (1998–99): 285–346 (arguing that innovative products often are not developed for fear of liability).

251. Derry Ridgway, "No-Fault Vaccine Insurance: Lessons from the National Vaccine Injury Compensation Program," *Journal of Health Politics, Policy and Law,* 24 (1999): 59–90.

252. For example, Merrell Dow withdrew the morning sickness drug Bendectin from the market due to escalating insurance and litigation costs, even though there was no scientific evidence of a causal relationship between the drug and birth defects. See Joseph Sanders, *Bendectin on Trial: A Study of Mass Tort Litigation* (Ann Arbor: University of Michigan Press, 1998); Kenneth R. Foster and Peter W. Huber, *Judging Science: Scientific Knowledge and the Federal Courts* (Cambridge, MA: MIT Press, 1997): 1–7.

253. However, many authors argue that medical malpractice liability has not significantly increased medical costs. See Jordyn K. McAfee, "Medical Malpractice Crisis Factional or Fictional? An Overview of the GAO Report as Interpreted by the Proponents and Opponents of Tort Reform," *Journal of Medicine and Law,* 9 (2005): 161–90.

254. Wendy E. Parmet and Richard A. Daynard, "The New Public Health Litigation," *Annual Review of Public Health,* 21 (2000): 437–54.

255. In the silicone breast implant litigation discussed above, Dow Corning filed for bankruptcy as part of a $3.2 billion settlement, although the jury verdicts appeared to fly in the face of the scientific evidence. Does the deterrent signal in this litigation teach corporations to engage in reasonable safety checks before putting a product on the market or does it simply retard innovation? See Ruth Macklin, "Ethics, Epidemiology, and Law: The Case of Silicone Breast Implants," *American Journal of Public Health,* 89 (1999): 487–89.

7. GLOBAL HEALTH LAW: HEALTH IN A GLOBAL COMMUNITY

SOURCES FOR CHAPTER EPIGRAPHS: Aristotle, *The Nicomachean Ethics,* trans. J. E. C. Welldon (New York: Prometheus Books, 1987); N. R. Kleinfield, "Modern Ways Open India's Door to Diabetes," *New York Times,* September 13, 2006; Eleanor Roosevelt, Remarks at the United Nations, March 27, 1953.

1. Derek Yach and Douglas Bettcher, "The Globalization of Public Health I: Threats and Opportunities," *American Journal of Public Health,* 88 (1998): 735–38, 735.

2. David P. Fidler, "The Globalization of Public Health: Emerging Infec-

tious Diseases and International Relations," *Indiana Journal of Global Legal Studies*, 5 (1997): 11–51.

3. There are many other areas of international law that are important to global health, including environmental law, humanitarian law, arms control, and disaster relief.

4. Early foundational work in international public health law can be found in Valentin S. Mikhailov, *History of International Health Law* (in Russian) (Vladivostok: Far Eastern University Publishing House, 1984); Michel Bélanger, *Droit international de la santé* (Paris: Economica, 1983); Norman Howard-Jones, "Origins of International Health Work," *British Medical Journal*, 1 (1950): 1032–37. For excellent accounts of contemporary international public health law, see Obijiofor Aginam, *Global Health Governance: International Law and Public Health in a Divided World* (Toronto: University of Toronto Press, 2005); David P. Fidler, *International Law and Public Health* (Ardsley, NY: Transnational Publishers, 2000); David P. Fidler, *International Law and Infectious Diseases* (Oxford: Clarendon Press, 1999); Allyn L. Taylor, Douglas W. Bettcher, Sev S. Fluss, et al., "International Health Instruments: An Overview," in *Oxford Textbook of Public Health*, ed. Roger Detels et al. (Oxford: Oxford University Press, 2002): 359–86.

5. Laurie Garrett and Scott Rosenstein, "Missed Opportunities: Governance of Global Infectious Diseases," *Harvard International Review*, 27 (2005): 64–69.

6. Approximately half of the world's population lives in urban centers, and by 2030 nearly two-thirds will live in urban areas. Melinda Moore, Phillip Gould, and Barbara S. Keary, "Global Urbanization and Impact on Health," *International Journal of Hygiene and Environmental Health*, 206 (2003): 269–78; UN Department of Economic and Social Affairs, *World Urbanization Prospects: The 2005 Revision* (New York: United Nations, 2006); David Vlahav, S. Galea, and N. Freudenberg, "The Urban Health 'Advantage,'" *Journal of Urban Health*, 82 (2005): 1–4.

7. Ronald Waldman, "Public Health in War," *Harvard International Review*, 27 (2005): 60–63; World Health Organization, *International Migration, Health and Human Rights*, Health and Human Rights Publication Series, no. 4 (December 2003).

8. Samantha L. Thomas and Stuart D. M. Thomas, "Displacement and Health," *British Medical Bulletin*, 69 (2004): 115–27 (describing health needs of refugees and the stress concentrated and traumatized populations place on health care infrastructures).

9. William B. Karesh, Robert A. Cook, Elizabeth L. Bennett, et al., "Wildlife Trade and Global Disease Emergence," *Emerging Infectious Diseases*, 11 (2005): 1000–1002 (describing global movement of infectious pathogens as a result of contact between wildlife and humans).

10. More than 60 percent of known infectious diseases are capable of infecting both humans and animals; most of these diseases, including HIV/AIDS, SARS, and Ebola virus, originated in animals but have crossed the species barrier to infect humans. William B. Karesh and Robert A. Cook, "The Human-Animal Link," *Foreign Affairs*, 84 (2005): 38–50 (explaining that no national agency or IGO focuses on diseases that threaten people, domestic animals, and wildlife; FAO monitors livestock and crops but not wild plants and animals, while the

World Animal Health Organization considers wildlife-related disease but has few powers or resources).

11. The Writing Committee of the World Health Organization, "Avian Influenza A (H5N1) Infection in Humans," *New Eng. J. Med.,* 353 (2005): 1374–85.

12. For example, Chinese farmers tried to suppress the 2005 A (H5N1) influenza outbreaks by feeding chickens an antiviral drug used for humans. As a result, the antiviral is unlikely to protect humans in the case of a pandemic. Alan Sipress, "Bird Flu Drug Rendered Useless: Chinese Chickens Given Medication Made for Humans," *Washington Post,* June 18, 2005; see also David P. Fidler, "Legal Challenges Posed by the Use of Antimicrobials in Food Animal Production," *Microbes and Infection,* 1 (1999): 29–38.

13. When a cow in Washington state was found to be infected with bovine spongiform encephalopathy (BSE, or mad cow disease) in 2003, fifty countries put a ban on American beef, which cost the U.S. cattle industry $1.7 billion and forced beef prices to rise by 20 percent. "The Madness of Herds," *Wall Street Journal,* July 18, 2005.

14. T. Kuiken, F. A. Leighton, R. A. M. Fouchier, et al., "Pathogen Surveillance in Animals," *Science,* 309 (2005): 1680–81.

15. The Millennium Ecosystem Assessment, a comprehensive study of the natural environment commissioned by the United Nations, examined the interdependence of humans and ecosystems; preliminary reports warn about severe depletion of the natural environment and the inability of ecosystems to support future generations. Millennium Ecosystem Assessment, "Living beyond Our Means: Natural Assets and Human Well-Being" (prepublication draft, 2005).

16. "How Bad Is the Environment for Our Health," *Bulletin of the World Health Organization,* 83 (2005): 327–28 (interview with Kerstin Leitner, Assistant Director-General of WHO's Sustainable Development and Healthy Environment cluster of departments).

17. F. Michael Willis, "Economic Development, Environmental Protection, and the Right to Health," *Georgetown International Environmental Law Review,* 9 (1996): 195–220.

18. Joint Learning Initiative, *Human Resources for Health: Overcoming the Crisis* (Cambridge, MA: Harvard University Press, 2004).

19. See generally Dean T. Jamison, Joel G. Breman, Anthony R. Measham, et al., eds., *Disease Control Priorities in Developing Countries,* 2d ed. (New York: Oxford University Press, 2006).

20. Abdesslam Boutayeb and Saber Boutayeb, "The Burden of Non Communicable Diseases in Developing Countries," *International Journal for Equity in Health,* 4 (2005); David Crawford and Robert W. Jeffrey, eds., *Obesity Prevention and Public Health* (Oxford: Oxford University Press, 2005).

21. In recognition of this dangerous trend, the WHO embarked in 2004 on a Global Strategy on Diet, Physical Activity and Health designed to identify and implement preventive strategies to control risk factors such as tobacco, alcohol, obesity, diet, and inactivity. World Health Organization, *Global Strategy on Diet, Physical Activity, and Health* (Geneva: World Health Organization, 2004); see also Derek Yach, Corinna Hawkes, Linn Gould, et al., "The Global Burden of

Chronic Diseases: Overcoming Impediments to Prevention and Control," *JAMA,* 291 (2004): 2616–22.

22. Derek Yach and Robert Beaglehole, "Globalization of Risks for Chronic Diseases Demands Global Solutions," *Perspectives on Global Development and Technology,* 3 (2004): 213–33.

23. World Health Organization, Commission on Macroeconomics and Health, *Macroeconomics and Health: Investing in Health for Development* (Geneva: World Health Organization, 2001); Food and Agriculture Organization of the United Nations, "Ethical Issues in Food and Agriculture," *FAO Corporate Document Repository,* 2001, http://www.fao.org/docrep/003/X9601E/X9601E00.HTM.

24. N. R. Kleinfield, "Modern Ways Open India's Door to Diabetes," *New York Times,* September 13, 2006.

25. Geoffrey Rose, *The Strategy of Preventive Medicine* (Oxford: Oxford University Press, 1992).

26. Political leaders are beginning to understand the need for collective action. The G8 Summit in 2000 recognized that health is the "key to prosperity" and that "poor health drives poverty." G8 Information Centre, "G8 Communiqué Okinawa 2000," July 23, 2000, and May 26, 2004, http://www.g8.utoronto.ca/summit/2000okinawa/finalcom.htm. The G8 leaders also agreed to mobilize resources, which eventually led to the creation of the Global Fund for HIV/AIDS, Tuberculosis, and Malaria. The Global Fund, "Investing in Our Future: The Global Fund to Fight AIDS, Tuberculosis and Malaria," July 16, 2006, http://www.theglobalfund.org/en/. See also Michael Marmot, "Social Determinants of Health Inequalities," *Lancet,* 365 (2005) 1099–1104; World Commission on the Social Dimension of Globalization, *A Fair Globalization: Creating Opportunities for All* (Geneva: International Labor Organization, 2004).

27. Lawrence O. Gostin, "Meeting Basic Survival Needs of the World's Least Healthy People: Toward a Framework Convention on Global Health," *Georgetown Law Journal* (forthcoming 2007).

28. David P. Fidler, "Architecture amidst Anarchy: Global Health's Quest for Governance," *Global Health Governance,* 1 (2007), available at http://diplomacy.shu.edu/academics/global_health/journal/PDF/Fidler-article.pdf; Allyn L. Taylor, "Governing the Globalization of Public Health," *Journal of Law, Med. and Ethics,* 32 (2004): 500–508; Scott Burris, "Governance, Microgovernance and Health," *Temple Law Review,* 77 (2004): 335–61; David P. Fidler, "A Globalized Theory of Public Health Law," *Journal of Law, Med. and Ethics,* 30 (2002): 150–61; Lawrence O. Gostin, "World Health Law: Toward a New Conception of Global Health Governance for the Twenty-first Century," *Yale Journal of Health Policy and Ethics,* 5 (2005): 413–24.

29. The GHSI, launched in 2001, is an informal international partnership of countries to strengthen health preparedness and response globally to threats of biological, chemical, and radio-nuclear terrorism, and pandemic influenza. Available at http://www.ghsi.ca/english/index.asp.

30. UNITAID, established in 2006, is an innovative funding mechanism to accelerate access to drugs and diagnostics for HIV/AIDS, malaria, and TB in coun-

tries with a high burden of disease. Available at http://www.who.int/mediacentre/news/statements/2006/s15/en/index.html.

31. IFFIm, an idea presented by U.K. chancellor Gordon Brown at the 2003 G8 Summit, is designed to accelerate the availability of funds for health and immunization programs through the GAVI Alliance (formerly Global Alliance for Vaccines and Immunization) in seventy of the poorest countries. Available at http://www.iff-immunisation.org/. See also Ernst R. Berndt, Rachel Glelnnerster, and Michael Kremer, "Advance Market Commitments for Vaccines: Working Paper and Spread Sheet," available at http://ssrn.com/abstract=982966 (describing and evaluating a G8 proposal to commit to purchase vaccines against diseases concentrated in low-income countries to spur research and development; sponsors would commit to a minimum price to be paid per person immunized, up to a certain number of individuals immunized, and for additional purchases, the price would eventually drop to close to marginal cost; if no suitable product were developed, no payments would be made).

32. Gian Luca Burci and Claude-Henri Vignes, *World Health Organization* (2004); Allyn L. Taylor, Douglas W. Bettcher, Sev S. Fluss et al., "International Health Instruments: An Overview," in *Oxford Textbook of Public Health,* ed. Roger Detels et al. (Oxford: Oxford University Press, 2002): 359–86.

33. The World Health Assembly, by a two-thirds vote, may adopt conventions or agreements (Art. 19). Though these are not binding on member governments until accepted by them, WHO members have to "take action" leading to their acceptance within eighteen months. Thus, each member government must act, even if its delegation voted against a convention in the assembly. For example, it must submit the convention to its legislature for ratification. It must then notify WHO of the action taken. If the action is unsuccessful, it must notify WHO of the reasons for nonacceptance (Art. 20).

34. Arts. 20, 62.

35. WHO, *History of the International Classification of Diseases (ICD),* available at http://www.who.int/classifications/icd/en/.

36. WHO, FCTC, WHO Doc. A56/VR/4, May 21, 2003, http://www.who.int/gb/ebwha/pdf_files/WHA56/ea56r1.pdf.

37. Allan M. Brandt, *The Cigarette Century: The Rise, Fall, and Deadly Persistence of the Product That Defined America* (Cambridge, MA: Harvard University Press, 2007).

38. Allyn Lise Taylor, "Making the World Health Organization Work: A Legal Framework for Universal Access to the Conditions for Health," *American Journal of Law and Medicine,* 18 (1992): 301–46; David P. Fidler, "The Future of the World Health Organization: What Role for International Law?" *Vanderbilt Journal of Transnational Law,* 31 (1998): 1079–1126.

39. Norman Howard-Jones, *The Scientific Background of the International Sanitary Conferences, 1851–1938* (Geneva: World Health Organization, 1975). I am grateful to Prof. David Fidler for our collaborative work, which is reflected in the discussion of the IHR in our published work. David P. Fidler and Lawrence O. Gostin, "The New International Health Regulations: An Historic Development for International Law and Public Health," *Journal of Law, Medicine, and Ethics,* 34 (2006): 85–94.

40. Lawrence O. Gostin, "International Infectious Disease Law: Revision of the World Health Organizations' International Health Regulations," *JAMA,* 291 (2004): 2623–27.

41. World Health Organization, "Global Crises—Global Solutions: Managing Public Health Emergencies of International Concern through the Revised International Health Regulations," *International Health Regulations Revision Project,* WHO Doc. WHO/CDS/CSR/GAR/2002.4 (2002), 2002, http://www.who.int/csr/resources/publications/ihr/whocdsgar20024.pdf.

42. *International Sanitary Convention,* December 3, 1903, 35 Stat. 1770, 1 Bevans 359.

43. Agreement between the World Health Organization and the Pan American Health Organization, Res. WHA2.91 (June 30, 1949), in *World Health Organization Basic Documents,* 44th ed. (Geneva: World Health Organization, 2003).

44. Fidler, *International Law and Infectious Diseases.*

45. The Covenant of the League of Nations, Art. 23(f).

46. Article 55 of the UN Charter states that a primary objective of the United Nations is to promote "higher standards of living" and "solutions of international . . . health." UN Charter, Art. 55.

47. Y. Arai-Takahashi, "The Role of International Health Law and WHO in the Regulation of Public Health," in *Law and the Public Dimension of Health,* ed. Martin R. Johnson and L. Johnson, 113–41 (London: Cavendish Publishing, 2001).

48. Frank P. Grad, "The Preamble of the Constitution of the World Health Organization," *Bulletin of the World Health Organization,* 80 (2002): 981.

49. World Health Organization, *Basic Texts,* "Forty-Fourth Edition: Constitution of the World Health Organization," *WHO Policy System,* March 2004, http://policy.who.int/cgi-bin/om_isapi.dll?hitsperheading=on&infobase=basicdoc&record={21}&softpage=Document42.

50. World Health Organization, *International Health Regulations (IHR),* WHO Res. WH22.46 (July 25, 1969).

51. World Health Organization, *International Health Regulations (IHR),* WHO Res. WHA34.14 (May 20, 1981).

52. The IHR entered into force on January 15, 2007. On December 13, 2006, the United States accepted the IHR, with the reservation that it will implement them according to the U.S. principles of federalism. The United States also made the following declarations about its understanding of the IHR: first, incidents that involve the natural, accidental, or deliberate release of chemical, biological, or radiological materials are notifiable under the IHR; second, countries that accept the IHR are obligated to report potential public health emergencies that occur outside their borders to the extent possible; and third, the IHR do not create any separate private right to legal action against the federal government. U.S. Department for Health and Human Services, "United States Officially Accepts New International Health Regulations," news release, December 13, 2006, http://www.hhs.gov/news/press/2006pres/20061213.html.

53. David P. Fidler and Lawrence O. Gostin, *Biosecurity in the Global Age: Biological Weapons, Public Health, and the Rule of Law* (Stanford, CA: Stanford University Press, 2008).

54. World Health Organization, *Revision and Updating of the International Health Regulations,* W.H.A. Res. 48.7 (May 12, 1995).

55. Lawrence O. Gostin, *The AIDS Pandemic: Complacency, Injustice, and Unfulfilled Expectations* (Chapel Hill: University of North Carolina Press, 2004).

56. Angela McLean, Robert May, John Pattison, et al., *SARS: A Case Study in Emerging Infections* (Oxford: Oxford University Press, 2005); Lawrence Gostin, Ronald Bayer, and Amy L. Fairchild, "Ethical and Legal Challenges Posed by Severe Acute Respiratory Syndrome: Implications for the Control of Severe Infectious Disease Threats," *JAMA,* 290 (2003): 3229–37; World Health Organization, *Severe Acute Respiratory Syndrome (SARS): Status of the Outbreak and Lessons for the Immediate Future* (Geneva: World Health Organization, 2003).

57. Peter Aldhous and Sarah Tomlin, "Avian Flu: Are We Ready?" *Nature,* 435 (2005): 399–402; David P. Fidler, "Global Outbreak of Avian Influenza A (H5N1) and International Law," *ASIL Insights,* January 2004, http://www.asil.org/insights/insigh125.htm. In 2006, the WHO directed member states to comply with specific IHR provisions relevant to prevention of avian and pandemic flu. World Health Organization, *Application of the International Health Regulations,* Agenda Item 11.1 (May 26, 2006).

58. N. Ndayimirije and M. K. Kindhauser, "Marburg Hemorrhagic Fever in Angola—Fighting Fear and a Lethal Pathogen," *New Eng. J. Med.,* 352 (2005): 2155–57.

59. Lawrence O. Gostin, Jason W. Sapsin, Stephen P. Teret, et al., "The Model State Emergency Health Powers Act: Planning and Response to Bioterrorism and Naturally Occurring Infectious Diseases," *JAMA,* 288 (2002): 622–28; David P. Fidler, "Bioterrorism, Public Health, and International Law," *Chicago Journal of International Law,* 3 (2002): 7–26; Laurie Garrett, "The Nightmare of Bioterrorism," *Foreign Affairs,* 80 (2001): 76–89.

60. For a definitive account of the IHR (2005), see David P. Fidler, "From International Sanitary Conventions to Global Health," *Chinese Journal of International Law,* 4 (2005): 325–92. See also Michelle Forrest, "Using the Power of the World Health Organization: The International Health Regulations and the Future of International Health Law," *Columbia Journal of Law and Social Problems,* 33 (2000): 153–79; Allyn L. Taylor, "Controlling the Global Spread of Infectious Diseases: Toward a Reinforced Role for the International Health Regulations," *Houston Law Review,* 33 (1997): 1327–62.

61. A public health risk is defined as "a likelihood of an event that may affect adversely the health of human populations, with emphasis on one which may spread internationally or may present a serious and direct danger." *IHR,* Art. 1.

62. A public health emergency of international concern is defined as "an extraordinary event which is determined: (i) to constitute a public health risk to other States through the international spread of disease and (ii) to potentially require a coordinated international response." *IHR,* Art. 1.

63. Since WHO's new jurisdiction overlaps with several international or-

ganizations, it was necessary to harmonize their various roles (Arts. 6[1], 10[3], 14, 17[f], 57). WHO is required to coordinate its activities with other intergovernmental organizations and international bodies, including the United Nations, International Labor Organization, Food and Agriculture Organization, International Atomic Energy Agency, International Civil Aviation Organization, International Maritime Organization, and International Committee of the Red Cross. *International Health Regulations,* W.H.A. Res. 58.3, ¶ 4 (May 23, 2005).

64. The IHR requires that in determining whether to implement health measures, States Parties must rely on scientific principles and scientific evidence; before implementing health measures that significantly interfere with international traffic, States Parties must provide the WHO with the relevant public health rationale and scientific evidence for it. *IHR,* Art. 43 § 2–3.

65. Frederick M. Abbott, Christine Breining, and Thomas Cottier, eds., *International Trade and Human Rights: Foundations and Conceptual Issues* (Ann Arbor: University of Michigan Press, 2005).

66. World Health Organization, *The World Health Report 2000* (Geneva: World Health Organization, 2000), Annex Table 8 (latest available data from 1997).

67. World Health Organization, Fifty-eighth World Health Assembly, *Third Report of Committee A,* W.H.A. Doc. A58/55 (May 23, 2005).

68. "When requested by WHO, States Parties should provide, to the extent possible, support to WHO-coordinated response activities." *IHR,* Art. 13(5).

69. "States Parties shall undertake to collaborate with each other, to the extent possible, in: (a) the detection and assessment of, and response to, events as provided under these Regulations; (b) the provision or facilitation of technical cooperation and logistical support, particularly in the development, strengthening and maintenance of the public health capacities required under these Regulations; (c) the mobilization of financial resources to facilitate implementation of their obligations under these Regulations; and (d) the formulation of proposed laws and other legal and administrative provisions for the implementation of these Regulations." *IHR,* Art. 44(1).

70. *IHR,* Arts. 5(3), 13(3), and 13(6).

71. World Health Organization, *The Three by Five Initiative,* 2006, http://www.who.int/3by5/en/.

72. World Health Organization, *Achievement of Health-Related Millennium Development Goals: Report by the Secretariat,* WHO Doc. A58/5 (May 13, 2005).

73. States parties have a similar duty to inform WHO of public health risks outside their territory (Art. 9[2]).

74. Listed diseases are automatically notifiable: smallpox, polio, SARS, and a new subtype of influenza. For other listed diseases (cholera, pneumonic plague, yellow fever, viral hemorrhagic fevers, West Nile fever, and other diseases of special concern such as dengue fever, Rift Valley fever, and meningococcal disease), States Parties must use the algorithm. Finally, the algorithm must be used for any other event of potential international concern. The algorithm utilizes criteria such as the seriousness of the public health impact, the unusual or unexpected char-

acter of the event, the risk of international spread, and the risk of international travel or trade restrictions. *IHR,* Annex 2.

75. However, notably absent from the IHR are detailed specifications for information, lab specimens, and on-the-ground assistance in the event of a suspected terrorist event.

76. World Health Organization, *Global Crises—Global Solutions;* see "Statement for the Record by the Government of the United States of America concerning the World Health Organization's Revised International Health Regulations," delivered by David Hohman, member of the U.S. Delegation to the World Health Assembly, May 23, 2005.

77. David P. Fidler, "Emerging Trends in International Law concerning Global Infectious Disease Control," *Emerging Infectious Diseases,* 9 (2003): 285–90; World Health Organization, *Global Defense against the Infectious Disease Threat* (Geneva: World Health Organization, 2002).

78. Lawrence O. Gostin, "National Health Information Privacy: Regulations under the Health Insurance Portability and Accountability Act," *JAMA,* 285 (2001): 3015–21.

79. Tamara K. Hervey and Jean V. McHale, "Law, Health and the European Union," *Legal Studies,* 25 (2005): 228–59; Deryck Beyleveld, David Townend, Ségolène Rouillé-Mirza, et al., *The Data Protection Derivative and Medical Research across Europe* (Burlington, VT: Ashgate Publishing, 2004); T. Hervey and J. McHale, *Health Law and the European Union* (Cambridge: Cambridge University Press, 2004); "European Directive on Data Protection," Symposium Issue, 95/46/EC, *European Journal of Health Law,* 9 (2002).

80. Criteria for issuing recommendations include consideration of the views of States Parties and the Emergency or Review Committee, scientific evidence, and international standards. *IHR,* Art. 17.

81. A "suspect" is a person considered to have been exposed or possibly exposed to a public health risk capable of transmission. *IHR,* Art. 1.

82. Bruce Jay Plotkin and Ann Marie Kimball, "Designing an International Policy and Legal Framework for the Control of Emerging Infectious Diseases: First Steps," *Emerging Infectious Diseases,* 3 (1997): 1–9.

83. United Nations, Economic and Social Council, UN Sub-Commission on Prevention of Discrimination and Protection of Minorities, *Siracusa Principles on the Limitation and Derogation of Provisions in the International Covenant on Civil and Political Rights,* Annex, U.N. Doc. E/CN.4/1985/4 (1985).

84. World Health Organization, *FCTC,* May 21, 2003, http://www.who.int/gb/ebwha/pdf_files/WHA56/ea56r1.pdf.

85. For the history of the FCTC process, see Ruth Roemer, Allyn Taylor, and Jean Lariviere, "Origins of the WHO Framework Convention on Tobacco Control," *American Journal of Public Health,* 95 (2005): 936–38; World Health Organization, *FCTC,* Annex 2; Allyn L. Taylor and Douglas Bettcher, "Sustainable Health Development: Negotiation of the WHO Framework Convention on Tobacco Control," *Development Bulletin,* 54 (2001): 6–10.

86. World Health Organization, *An International Strategy for Tobacco Control,* W.H.A. Res. WHA 48.11 (May 12, 1995) (requesting WHO Director-General

to report on the feasibility of developing an international instrument on tobacco control).

87. World Health Organization, *WHO Framework Convention on Tobacco Control,* W.H.A. Res. WHA 56.1 (May 21, 2003) (adopting FCTC).

88. As of September 2006, there were 168 signatories and 140 parties to the WHO FCTC. The United States signed on May 10, 2004, but has not ratified the treaty. World Health Organization, "Updated Status of the WHO Framework Convention on Tobacco Control," *Tobacco Free Initiative,* September 27, 2006, http://www.who.int/tobacco/framework/countrylist/en/index.html.

89. Judith Mackay and Michael Erikson, *The Tobacco Atlas* (Geneva: World Health Organization, 2002).

90. World Health Organization, "Why Is Tobacco a Public Health Priority?" *Tobacco Free Initiative,* 2006, http://www.who.int/tobacco/health_priority/en/index.html.

91. Kenneth E. Warner, "The Role of Research in International Tobacco Control," *American Journal of Public Health,* 95 (2005): 976–84; Allyn Taylor, Frank J. Chaloupka, Emmanuel Guindon, et al., "The Impact of Trade Liberalization on Tobacco Consumption," in *Tobacco Control in Developing Countries,* ed. Prabhat Jha and Frank Chaloupka (New York: Oxford University Press, 2000): 343–64.

92. Frank A. Sloan et al., *The Price of Smoking* (Cambridge, MA: MIT Press, 2004).

93. Jeff Collin, Kelley Lee, and Karen Bissell, "The Framework Convention on Tobacco Control: The Politics of Global Health Governance," *Third World Quarterly,* 23 (2002): 265.

94. Garrett Mehl, Heather Wipfli, and Peter Winch, "Controlling Tobacco: The Vital Role of Local Communities," *Harvard International Review,* 27 (2005): 54–58.

95. Arthur D. Little, Inc., *Public Finance Balance of Smoking in the Czech Republic* (Prague: Arthur D. Little International, Inc., 2001).

96. Altria, Philip Morris Companies, Inc., "Comments regarding Czech Study," July 26, 2001, http://www.altria.com/media/press_release/03_02_pr_2001_07_26_01.asp.

97. Allyn L. Taylor, Douglas W. Bettcher, and Richard Pect, "International Law and the International Legislative Process: The WHO Framework Convention on Tobacco Control," in *Global Public Health Goods for Health: Health Economic and Public Health Perspectives,* ed. Richard Smith, Robert Beaglehole, David Woodward, et al. (Oxford: Oxford University Press, 2003): 212–29; M. Lyndon Haviland, "Global Brands, Global Priorities," *American Journal of Public Health,* 95 (2005): 935.

98. Benjamin Mason Meier, "Breathing Life into the Framework Convention on Tobacco Control: Smoking Cessation and the Right to Health," *Yale Journal of Health, Policy, Law and Ethics,* 5 (2005): 137–92, 149.

99. Melissa E. Crow, "Smokescreens and State Responsibility: Using Human Rights Strategies to Promote Global Tobacco Control," *Yale Journal of International Law,* 29 (2004): 209–50.

100. Gregory F. Jacob, "Without Reservation," *Chicago Journal of Interna-*

tional Law, 5 (2004): 287–302 (quoting Tommy Thompson, U.S. Secretary of Health and Human Services: "I'm going to support [the FCTC]—much to the surprise of many around the world . . . . We have no reservations"). Unusually, the FCTC had a "no reservations" clause inserted into Article 30 over the United States' objection.

101. Sajjad Ahmad, "Increasing Excise Taxes on Cigarettes in California: A Dynamic Simulation of Health and Economic Impacts," *Preventive Medicine,* 41 (2005): 276–83; J. M. Lee, D. S. Liao, C. Y. Ye, et al., "Effect of Cigarette Tax Increase on Cigarette Consumption in Taiwan," *Tobacco Control,* 14, supp. 1 (2005): 71–75; Thomas R. Frieden, Farzad Mostashari, Bonnie Kerker, et al., "Adult Tobacco Use Levels after Intensive Tobacco Control Measures: New York City, 2002–2003," *American Journal of Public Health,* 95 (2005): 1016–23; Carey Conly Thomson, Laurie Fisher, Jonathan P. Winickoff, et al., "State Tobacco Excise Taxes and Adolescent Smoking Behaviors in the United States," *Journal of Public Health Management and Practice,* 10 (2004): 490–96.

102. *RJR-MacDonald Inc. v. Canada,* [1995] 3 S.C.R. 199 (Can.).

103. The European Parliament banned all forms of tobacco advertising and sponsorship in 1998, but the European Court of Justice struck down the law, holding that its measures went beyond the European Union's proper scope of powers. Case C-376/98, *Federal Republic of Germany v. European Parliament and Council of the European Union,* 2001 E.C.R. I-2247. The Court of Justice did allow for a more limited form of advertising regulation, and in 2003 the European Parliament—adhering to the guidelines laid out in the 2001 decisions—passed a directive banning tobacco advertising in print media, on radio, and over the Internet. 2003 O.J. (L 152) 16–19.

104. Each day, 4,400 young people in the United States between the ages of twelve and seventeen start smoking. Substance Abuse and Mental Health Administration, *2001 National Household Survey on Drug Abuse: Trends in Initiation of Substance Abuse* (Rockville, MD: Substance Abuse and Mental Health Services Administration, 2003).

105. Short-term consequences of smoking by young people include lower levels of lung function, higher rates of lung cancer, addiction to nicotine, and associated risk of other drug use. Long-term consequences of youth smoking are reinforced by the fact that most young people who smoke regularly continue to smoke throughout adulthood. Centers for Disease Control and Prevention, National Center for Chronic Disease Prevention and Health Promotion, Tobacco Information and Prevention Source (TIPS), *Health Effects of Smoking among Young People,* January 26, 2005, http://www.cdc.gov/tobacco/research_data/youth/stspta5.htm.

106. For a history of tobacco litigation in the United Kingdom, see Stephen Davis, "Smoke Screen," *New Statesman,* 18 (2005): 10–12. For a history of tobacco litigation in the United States, see D. Douglas Blanke, *Towards Health with Justice: Litigation and Public Inquiries as Tools for Tobacco Control* (Geneva: World Health Organization, 2002): 16–32.

107. The FCTC, however, has been criticized for failing to give enough at-

tention to smoking cessation. Meier, "Breathing Life into the Framework Convention on Tobacco Control," 149.

108. I am grateful to Lesley Stone, Katrina Pagonis, and Helena Nygren-Krug for our collaborative work, which is reflected in the discussion of international trade, as well as the subsequent discussion on human rights.

109. Ronald Labonte and Matthew Sanger, "Glossary of the World Trade Organization and Public Health: Part 1," *Journal of Epidemiology and Community Health,* 60 (2006): 655–61. Richard D. Smith, "Trade and Public Health: Facing the Challenges of Globalization," *Journal of Epidemiology and Community Health,* 60 (2006): 650–51.

110. WHO Secretariat and WTO Secretariat, *WTO Agreements and Public Health* (Geneva: World Trade Organization, 2002) (recognizing the inexorable, yet resolvable, link between international trade and public health). But see Robert Howse, "The WHO/WTO Study on Trade and Public Health: A Critical Assessment," *Risk Analysis,* 24 (2004): 501–7 (presenting a less optimistic view of society's ability to resolve conflicts between trade and health).

111. World Trade Organization, *Understanding the WTO: Principles of the Trading System,* 2006, http://www.wto.org/english/thewto_e/whatis_e/tif_e/fact2_e.htm.

112. World Trade Organization, *Legal Texts: The WTO Agreements,* 2006, http://www.wto.org/english/docs_e/legal_e/ursum_e.htm#mAgreement (regarding "The Final Act Embodying the Results of the Uruguay Round of Multilateral Trade Negotiations," signed by ministers in Marrakesh on April 15, 1994, which is 550 pages long and contains legal texts that spell out the results of the negotiations since the round was launched in Punta del Este, Uruguay, in September 1986).

113. Marrakesh Agreement Establishing the World Trade Organization, April 15, 1994, 33 I.L.M. 1144 (1994).

114. Before the WTO was formed, there were several multilateral and bilateral treaties on trade, including the General Agreement on Tariffs and Trade (GATT 1947). The original GATT envisioned the creation of an International Trade Organization (ITO), but the ITO was never ratified. Today, the GATT 1947 has been superseded by the substantially similar GATT 1994, part of the WTO "package" of trade agreements that took effect in 1995. Konstantinos Adamantopoulos, ed., *An Anatomy of the World Trade Organization,* Anatomy Series of International Institutions (London: Kluwer Law International, 1997).

115. The GATS has important implications for health. It treats health and human services, such as medical care, professional licensure, water, and sanitation, as subject to trade rules. The GATS is not as prescriptive as other WTO agreements. It allows members to choose which service sectors to open and to negotiate the applicability of trade rules. GATS exempts services supplied in the exercise of governmental authority (e.g., governmental public health services), but not health services supplied by the private sector. World Trade Organization, *The General Agreement on Trade in Services (GATS): Objectives, Coverage, and Disciplines,* 2006, http://www.wto.org/english/tratop_e/serv_e/gatsqa_e.htm. See also David P. Fidler, Carlos Correa, and Obijiofor Aginam, "Draft Legal Re-

view of the General Agreement on Trade in Service (GATS) from a Health Policy Perspective," *World Health Organization,* 2006, http://www.who.int/trade/resource/GATS_Legal_Review_15_12_05.pdf.

116. Ellen R. Shaffer, Howard Waitzkin, Joseph Brenner, et al., "Global Trade and Public Health," *American Journal of Public Health,* 95 (2005): 23–34.

117. The Agreement on Technical Barriers to Trade (TBT) is also relevant to health. The TBT agreement governs "technical" barriers to trade, which arise as a result of technical specifications concerning product quality, packaging, labeling, and safety. The TBT reiterates the basic trade principles. Technical regulations must not create unnecessary barriers to trade or have trade-restrictive effects that are greater than necessary to fulfill a legitimate objective such as protection of health safety or the environment (Art. 2). Members must use international standards as a basis for their domestic regulation unless these standards would be ineffective. The agreement provides rules for conformity assessment procedures—e.g., certification of product safety (Art. 5). Agreement on Technical Barriers to Trade, April 15, 1994; Marrakesh Agreement Establishing the World Trade Organization, Annex 1A, April 15, 1994, 33 I.L.M. 1145 (1994).

118. The ultimate goal for proponents of such regional agreements is the Free Trade Area of the Americas (FTAA), which would liberalize trade among all nations in the western hemisphere with the exception of Cuba. Free Trade Area of the Americas, *Antecedents of the FTAA Process,* http://www.ftaa-alca.org/View_e.asp.

119. General Agreement on Tariffs and Trade (GATT) 1994, Art. 1, April 15, 1994; Marrakesh Agreement Establishing the World Trade Organization, Annex 1A, April 15, 1994, 33 I.L.M. 1153 (1994) ("Any advantage, favour, privilege or immunity granted by any contracting party to any product originating in or destined for any other country shall be accorded immediately and unconditionally to the like product originating in or destined for the territories of all other contracting parties"). The issue of what is a "like" product is often contested, and disputes often turn on the meaning adopted for this term.

120. The national treatment principle is not yet fully extended to trade in services; under GATS, member states may negotiate with each other over which foreign services will be covered. Shaffer et al., "Global Trade and Public Health," 23–24.

121. Appellate Body Report, *European Communities—Measures Affecting Asbestos and Asbestos-Containing Products,* ¶ 172, WT/DS135/AB/R (Mar. 12, 2001).

122. Similar rights are given to nations to enact health regulation of services under the GATS (Art. XIV[b]).

123. *Measures Affecting Asbestos,* ¶ 61 (stating that WTO members have the "right to determine the level of protection of health that they consider appropriate in a given situation").

124. Appellate Body Report, *United States—Standards for Reformulated and Conventional Gasoline*, WT/DS2/AB/R (May 20, 1996).

125. *Measures Affecting Asbestos,* ¶ 178 (stating that countries are free to rely on "divergent, but qualified and respected" scientific opinions in formulating the public health regulations).

126. Panel Report, *Thailand—Restrictions on Importation of and Internal Taxes on Cigarettes,* WT/DS10/R-37S/200 (Nov. 7, 1990).

127. The Codex Alimentarius Commission was created in 1963 by the UN Food and Agriculture Organization and WHO to develop food standards. The main purposes are to protect consumer health and ensure fair trade practices in the food trade. UN Food and Agriculture Organization (FAO), *Codex Alimentarius,* 2006, http://www.codexalimentarius.net/web/index_en.jsp. See also Fritz K. Kaferstein, "Food Safety in Food Security and Food Trade," *2020 Vision for Food, Agriculture, and the Environment,* Brief No. 2 (September 2003).

128. Appellate Body Report, *Japan—Measures Affecting Agricultural Products,* WT/DS76/AB/R (Feb. 22, 1999) (upholding WTO Panel's findings that Japan's requirement of testing the efficacy of quarantine for each variety of certain agricultural products was not supported by sufficient scientific evidence, within the meaning of Art. 2.2 of the SPS).

129. Appellate Body Report, *European Communities—Measures concerning Meat and Meat Products (Hormones),* WT/DS26/AB/R, WT/DS48/AB/R (Feb. 13, 1998).

130. Jason W. Sapsin, Theresa M. Thompson, Lesley Stone, et al., "International Trade, Law, and Public Health Advocacy," *Journal of Law, Medicine and Ethics,* 31 (2003): 546–56, 549; David P. Fidler, "Trade and Health: The Global Spread of Diseases and International Trade," *German Yearbook of International Law,* 40 (1997): 301–35.

131. Request for Consultations by the United States, *European Communities—Measures Affecting the Approval and Marketing of Biotech Products,* WT/DS291/1 (May 13, 2003) (unresolved).

132. Institute of Medicine and National Research Council of the National Academies, *Safety of Genetically Modified Foods: Approaches to Assessing Unintended Health Effects* (Washington, DC: National Academies Press, 2004).

133. Council Directive 2001/18/EC, 2001 O.J. (L 106) 1 (EC).

134. WTO Report, *European Communities—Measures Affecting the Approval and Marketing of Biotech Products,* WT/DS291/R, WT/DS292/R, WT/DS293/R (September 29, 2006).

135. Oren Perez, "Abnormalities at the Precautionary Kingdom: Reflections on the GMO Panel's Decision," Hebrew University International Law Research Paper No. 13–06, http://ssrn.com/abstract=940907.

136. For discussions of trade and health, see, e.g., World Health Organization, *Public Health: Innovation and Intellectual Property Rights: Report of the Commission on Intellectual Property Rights, Innovation and Public Health,* April 1, 2006, http://www.who.int/intellectualproperty/documents/thereport/; symposium, "How Do International Trade Agreements Influence the Promotion of Public Health?" *Yale Journal of Health Policy, Law, and Ethics,* 4 (2004): 339–73; Sapsin, "International Trade"; M. Gregg Bloche and Elizabeth R. Jungman, "Health Policy and the WTO," *Journal of Law, Medicine and Ethics,* 31 (2003): 529–45.

137. John H. Barton and Ezekiel J. Emanuel, "The Patents-Based Pharmaceutical Development Process: Rationale, Problems, and Potential Reforms," *JAMA,* 294 (2005): 2075–82.

138. When the WTO agreements took effect on January 1, 1995, developing countries were given five years to ensure that their laws and practices conform to the TRIPS agreement. Least-developed countries had eleven years, until 2006—now extended to 2016 for pharmaceutical patents under the Doha Declaration issued in 2001.

139. Public health advocates urged WHO in February 2005 to consider an alternative international framework that does not rely on intellectual property—the Medical Research and Development Treaty (MRDT), February 7, 2005, http://www.cptech.org/workingdrafts/rndtreaty4.pdf. At the core of MRDT is an obligation to finance qualified medical research and development tied to country GDP. The preamble states: "The State Parties to this Treaty seek to create a new global framework for supporting medical research and development that is based upon equitable sharing of the costs of research and development, incentives to invest in useful research and development in the areas of need and public interest, and which recognizes human rights and the goal of all sharing in the benefits of scientific advancement."

140. J. Michael Finger, *The Doha Agenda and Development: A View from the Uruguay Round* (Manila, Philippines: Asian Development Bank, 2002). (The $60 billion is composed of $40 billion in patent payments and $20 billion in copyright royalties); see also J. Michael Finger and Philip Schuler, eds., *Poor People's Knowledge: Promoting Intellectual Property in Developing Countries* (Washington, DC: World Bank and Oxford University Press, 2004).

141. WTO rules allow members to negotiate additional bilateral and multilateral trade agreements that include obligations beyond those required by WTO agreements—so-called TRIPS-plus agreements. Countries with strong pharmaceutical industries such as the U.S. have negotiated trade agreements with heightened IP protections. Without the TRIPS tools of compulsory licensing and parallel importation, TRIPS-plus countries are constrained in their ability to improve access to medicines.

142. To qualify for a patent, an invention must be new (novel), an inventive step (not obvious), and have "industrial application" (be useful). TRIPS, Art. 27.

143. Daniel Gervais, *The Trips Agreement: Drafting History and Analysis*, 2d ed. (London: Sweet and Maxwell, 2003).

144. *Bipartisan Trade Promotion Act of 2002,* 19 U.S.C. § 3802(b)(4)(A)(i)(II) (2004).

145. Senator Kennedy and Representative Waxman have requested an investigation into the Bush administration's trade negotiation practices and their negative effects on developing countries' access to medicine. Edward Kennedy and Henry Waxman, "Call for Investigation of U.S. Trade Agreements and International Health," *Committee on Government Reform Minority Office,* October 13, 2006, http://www.democrats.reform.house.gov/Documents/20061013141056-59889.pdf.

146. World Trade Organization, *Ministerial Declaration on the TRIPS Agreement and Public Health,* WT/MIN(01)/DEC/2, 41 I.L.M. 746 (2002); see Carlos M. Correa, *Implications of the Doha Declaration on the TRIPS Agreement and Public Health,* WHO/EDM/PAR/2002.3 (World Health Organization, EDM Series, no. 12, 2002).

147. Médecins sans Frontières, "U.S. Action at WTO Threatens Brazil's Successful AIDS Programme," press release, February 1, 2001, http://www.accessmed-msf.org/prod/publications.asp?scntid=218200122823 2&contenttype=PARA&.

148. Pat Sidley, "Drug Companies Withdraw Suit against South Africa," *British Journal of Medicine,* 357 (2001): 1011; Editorial, "South Africa's Moral Victory," *Lancet,* 357 (2001): 1303.

149. The conditions are: (i) the waiver applies only to pharmaceutical products (including necessary diagnostic kits); (ii) the members must notify the Council on TRIPS; (iii) the exporting member can license only the amount necessary to meet the needs of the importing member, and the importing member must confirm that it has insufficient manufacturing capabilities to make the drug; and (iv) the drugs must be specifically labeled or marked as being the product of a compulsory license, and member states agree to ensure the availability of legal means to prevent unauthorized importation.

150. World Health Organization, *Intellectual Property Rights, Innovation and Public Health,* WHO Doc. WHA56.27 (May 28, 2003); World Health Organization, *Scaling Up Treatment and Care within a Coordinated and Comprehensive Response to HIV/AIDS,* WHA57.14 (May 22, 2004).

151. As of January 2006, no country had actually exported generic drugs pursuant to the agreement. Frederick M. Abbott and Rudolf V. Van Puymbroeck, *Compulsory Licensing for Public Health: A Guide and Model Documents for Implementation of the Doha Declaration Paragraph 6 Decision* (New York: World Bank, 2005): 2 (noting that Canada and Norway had amended their national laws to facilitate implementation of drug exports, and that the United Kingdom and European Union had expressed support).

152. Keith Maskus and Jerome Reichman, eds., *International Public Goods and the Transfer of Technology after TRIPS* (Cambridge: Cambridge University Press, 2005); Frederick M. Abbott, "The Doha Declaration on the TRIPS Agreement and Public Health: Lighting a Dark Corner at the WTO," *Journal of International Economic Law,* 5 (2002): 469–505.

153. Shankar Vedantam and Terence Chea, "Drug Firm Plays Defense in Anthrax Scare: For Now, U.S. Declines to Suspend Bayer's Patent and Authorize Generic Cipro," *Washington Post,* October 21, 2001. The avian influenza A (H5N1) outbreaks in 2005 also caused a controversy over compulsory licensing. Advocates called on the U.S. government to compulsorily license the antiviral drug Tamiflu to ensure sufficient supplies in the event of an influenza pandemic. Dennis J. Kucinich, letter to the editor, *New York Times,* November 5, 2005 (advocating the issuance of a compulsory license to grant manufacturers the right to produce Tamiflu, with the patent holder, Roche, receiving a royalty).

154. Louis B. Sohn, "The New International Law: Protection of the Rights of Individuals Rather than States," *American University Law Review,* 32 (1982): 1–64.

155. Eleanor Roosevelt, "My Day," August 13, 1943. In his 1941 State of the Union address, as the nation prepared for war, President Franklin D. Roosevelt spelled out "Four Freedoms" as a reminder of what we must fight for: freedom of speech and expression, freedom of every person to worship God, freedom from want, and freedom from fear. The president specified that freedom

from want "means economic understandings which will secure to every nation a healthy peacetime life for its inhabitants—everywhere in the world." "The 'Four Freedoms,' Franklin D. Roosevelt's Address to Congress, January 6, 1941," *World Civilizations,* 1997, http://www.wwnorton.com/college/history/ralph/workbook/ralprs36b.htm.The right to adequate medical care and the opportunity to achieve and enjoy good health was a core entitlement in FDR's vision. Cass Sunstein, *The Second Bill of Rights: FDR's Unfinished Revolution and Why We Need It More Than Ever* (New York: Basic Books, 2004): ix.

156. Sofia Gruskin and Daniel Tarantola, "Health and Human Rights," Working Paper Series No. 10 (Cambridge, MA: François-Xavier Bagnoud Center for Health and Human Rights, 2000).

157. Louis B. Sohn and Thomas Buergenthal, *International Protection of Human Rights* (Indianapolis, IN: Bobbs-Merrill, 1973).

158. *International Convention on the Elimination of All Forms of Racial Discrimination,* G.A. Res. 2106 (XX), annex, U.N. Doc. A/6014 (Dec. 21, 1965); *International Covenant on Civil and Political Rights,* G.A. Res. 2200A (XXI), U.N. Doc. A/6316 (Dec. 16, 1966); *International Covenant on Economic, Social and Cultural Rights,* G.A. Res. 2200A (XXI), U.N. Doc. A/6316 (Dec. 16, 1966); *Convention on the Elimination of All Forms of Discrimination against Women,* G.A. Res. 34/180, U.N. Doc. A/34/46 (Dec. 18, 1979); *Convention against Torture and Other Cruel, Inhuman or Degrading Treatment or Punishment,* G.A. Res. 39/46, annex, U.N. Doc. A/39/51 (Dec. 10, 1984); *International Convention on the Protection of the Rights of All Migrant Workers and Members of Their Families,* G.A. Res. 45/158, annex, U.N. Doc. A/45/49 (Dec. 18, 1990).

159. *Convention for the Protection of Human Rights and Fundamental Freedoms,* 213 U.N.T.S. 222 (Nov. 4, 1950); *African [Banjul] Charter on Human and Peoples' Rights,* OAU Doc. CAB/LEG/67/3 (June 27, 1981); *American Convention on Human Rights,* O.A.S. Treaty Series No. 36, 1144 U.N.T.S. 123 (Nov. 22, 1969).

160. *Restatement (Third) of Foreign Relations Law of the United States* § 702 (1987) (listing the following state practices as violating CIL: genocide; slavery; murder or causing the disappearance of individuals; torture or other cruel, inhuman, or degrading treatment or punishment; prolonged arbitrary detention; systematic racial discrimination; and consistent patterns of gross violations of internationally recognized human rights).

161. The covenants have some common provisions, but each treaty establishes a distinct set of rights and international enforcement systems. The common provisions are the right of a "people" (indicating a collective right) to self-determination (Art. 1[1]) and not to be deprived of its own means of subsistence (Art. 1[2]); and the right not to be discriminated against based on race, color, sex, language, religion, political or other opinion, national or social origin, property or birth (ICCPR, Art 2[1] and ICESCR, Art. 2[2]).

162. The HRC periodically issues general comments to provide guidance to States Parties in discharging their reporting obligations and interpreting the treaty.

163. Committee on Economic, Social and Cultural Rights, 5th Sess., *General Comment No. 3,* U.N. Doc. E/1991/23 (1990).

164. ECOSOC Res. 1985/17, U.N. Doc. S/RES/1985/17 (May 22, 1985).

165. For example, ICCPR permits "limitations" or "restrictions" on the freedom of movement, religion, expression, assembly, and association (Arts. 12[3], 18[3], 19[3], 21, 22[2]).

166. All limitation clauses should be interpreted strictly and in favor of the human right at issue. "Symposium on the Siracusa Principles on the Limitation and Derogation Provisions in the International Covenant on Civil and Political Rights," *Human Rights Quarterly,* 7 (1985): 1–157.

167. UN Economic and Social Council, *Siracusa Principles on the Limitation and Derogation Provisions in the International Covenant on Civil and Political Rights,* Annex, U.N. Doc. E/CN.4/1985/4 (1985).

168. *Enhorn v. Sweden* [2005] E.C.H.R. 56529/00 (finding a violation of Art. 5[1] of the European Convention of Human Rights because the government had not sought "less severe measures" before isolating a person living with HIV/AIDS). See also Robyn Martin, "The Exercise of Public Health Powers in Cases of Infectious Disease: Human Rights Implications," *Medical Law Review,* 14 (2006): 130–43.

169. The language of Article 4 suggests that cultural, economic, or social rights can be limited on grounds of the public's health. The Committee on Economic, Social and Cultural Rights, however, stresses that states have the burden of justifying each element of Article 4: powers must be in accordance with the law, including international human rights, in the interest of legitimate aims, and strictly necessary for the general welfare in a democratic society. Public health powers also must be the least restrictive, of limited duration, and subject to review. Committee on Economic, Social and Cultural Rights, 22d Sess., *General Comment No. 14: The Right to the Highest Attainable Standard of Health,* E/C.12/2000/4 (Aug. 11, 2000).

170. Jonathan M. Mann, Lawrence Gostin, Sofia Gruskin, et al., "Health and Human Rights," *Health and Human Rights,* 1 (1994): 6–23 (explaining that health and human rights are both powerful, modern approaches to defining and advancing human well-being). This seminal article posited three relationships: the impact of health policies, programs, and practices on human rights; the health impact resulting from violations of human rights; and the synergistic nature of health and human rights—each inextricably linked to the other. See Sofia Gruskin, Michael A. Grodin, George J. Annas, et al., eds., *Perspectives on Health and Human Rights: A Reader* (New York: Routledge, 2005); Lawrence O. Gostin, "Public Health, Ethics, and Human Rights: A Tribute to the Late Jonathan Mann," *Journal of Law, Medicine, and Ethics,* 29 (2001): 121–30. In a later article, Mann and colleagues offered a human rights impact assessment that systematically evaluated the effects of health policies on human rights. Lawrence O. Gostin and Jonathan Mann, "Towards the Development of a Human Rights Impact Assessment for the Formulation and Evaluation of Health Policies," *Health and Human Rights,* 1 (1994): 58–81.

171. Countries can incorporate a right to health by making the ICESCR "self-executing" so that treaty duties are directly enforceable by national courts and administrative tribunals. Mary Ann Torres, "The Human Right to Health, National Courts, and Access to HIV/AIDS Treatment: A Case Study from Vene-

zuela," *Chicago Journal of International Law,* 3 (2002): 105–14, 109. Countries can also enshrine the right to health in their national constitutions. Eleanor D. Kinney and Brian Alexander Clark, "Provisions for Health and Health Care in the Constitutions of the Countries around the World," *Cornell International Law Journal,* 37 (2004): 285–355, 287 (reporting that 67.5 percent of national constitutions surveyed included provisions regarding the right to health or health care). The South African Constitutional Court, for example, held that the government's plan to limit pregnant women's access to the antiretroviral Nevaripine violated the constitution, which granted access to health care services. *Treatment Action Campaign v. Minister of Health,* 2002 (4) BCLR 356 (T) (CC) (S. Afr.); see Roger Philips, "South Africa's Right to Health Care: International and Constitutional Duties in Relation to the HIV/AIDS Epidemic," *Human Rights Brief,* 11 (2004): 9. For more on essential medicines and human rights, see Hans V. Hogerzeil, "Essential Medicines and Human Rights: What Can They Learn from Each Other?" *World Health Organization Bulletin,* 84 (2006): 371–75; Hans V. Hogerzeil, Melanie Samson, Jaume Vidal Casanovas, et al., "Is Access to Essential Medicines as Part of the Fulfillment of the Right to Health Enforceable through the Courts?" *Lancet,* 368 (2006): 305–11.

Some courts find health rights in constitutional protections of life, liberty, or security of the person. *Chaoulli v. Quebec (Attorney General)* [2005] SCC 35 (Can.) (finding a violation of the right to personal security in the Canadian and Quebec Charters when provincial legislation prohibited Quebec residents from taking out private health insurance in the face of long waiting times for Medicare services). *Chaoulli* appears to proclaim an economic right to purchase private medical services rather than actually affording the whole population (poor and rich alike) a right to personal security. If a human right to personal security is violated by long waiting times for health services, why would this right attach only to those financially able to purchase private insurance? See generally, Colleen M. Flood, Kent Roach, and Lorne Sossin, eds., *Access to Care, Access to Justice: The Legal Debate over Private Health Insurance in Canada* (Toronto: University of Toronto Press, 2005); Alicia Ely Yamin, "The Right to Health under International Law and Its Relevance to the United States," *American Journal of Public Health,* 95 (2005): 1156–61; Steven D. Jamar, "The International Human Right to Health," *Southern University Law Review,* 22 (1994): 1–68.

172. Jennifer Prah Ruger, "Democracy and Health," *Quarterly Journal of Medicine,* 98 (2006): 299–304 (exploring the complex relationship between health, its determinants, and political systems); Benjamin Mason Meier and Larisa M. Mori, "The Highest Attainable Standard: Advancing a Collective Human Right to Public Health," *Columbia Human Rights Law Review,* 37 (2005): 101–46; Debbie Fox and Alex Scott Samuel, eds., *Human Rights, Equity and Health: Proceedings from a Meeting of the Health Equity Network Held at the London School of Economics, March 28, 2003* (London: Nuffield Trust, 2004).

173. For example, in *D. v. United Kingdom* the European Court of Human Rights held that the United Kingdom could not deport an end-stage HIV-positive alien, because in his home country he would not have access to antiretroviral treatment or support services. *D. v. United Kingdom,* 24 E.C.H.R. 423 (1997).

174. Committee on Economic, Social and Cultural Rights, 5th Sess., *General Comment No. 3,* U.N. Doc. E/1991/23 (1990).

175. See, e.g., Paul Hunt, "Report of Paul Hunt, Special Rapporteur on the Right of Everyone to the Enjoyment of the Highest Attainable Standard of Physical and Mental Health," U.N. Doc. E/CN.4/2005/51 (Feb. 11, 2005); Paul Hunt, "The Right of Everyone to the Enjoyment of the Highest Attainable Standard of Physical and Mental Health," U.N. Doc. E/CN.4/2004/49 (Feb. 16, 2004).

176. Lawrence O. Gostin, "Survival Needs of the World's Least Healthy People: A Proposal for a Framework Convention on Global Health," *JAMA* (forthcoming 2007).

8. SURVEILLANCE AND PUBLIC HEALTH RESEARCH: PERSONAL PRIVACY AND THE "RIGHT TO KNOW"

SOURCES FOR CHAPTER EPIGRAPHS: William Farr, *Vital Statistics: A Memorial Volume of Selections from the Reports and Writings with a Biographical Sketch* (Lanham, MD: Scarecrow Press, 1975); N. R. Kleinfield, "Living at an Epicenter of Diabetes, Defiance and Despair," *New York Times,* January 10, 2006; Thomas Parran, "The Eradication of Syphilis as a Practical Public Health Objective," *JAMA,* 92 (1931): 73; Marion C. Potter, "Venereal Prophylaxis," *American Journal of Nursing,* 7 (1907): 349–50; World Bank, "Public Health Surveillance Toolkit," *World Bank,* February 2002, http://web.worldbank.org/WBSITE/EXTERNAL/TOPICS/EXTHEALTHNUTRITIONANDPOPULATION/0,,contentMDK:20740013~pagePK:210058~piPK:210062~theSitePK:282511,00.html; Amy L. Fairchild, Ronald Bayer, James Colgrove, et al., *Searching Eyes: Privacy, the State, and Disease Surveillance in America* (Berkeley: University of California Press, 2007): 1.

1. Denis J. Protti, "The Application of Information Science, Information Technology, and Information Management to Public Health," in *Oxford Textbook of Public Health,* ed. Roger Detels, James McEwen, Robert Beaglehole, et al., 4th ed. (Oxford: Oxford University Press, 2002): 1, 419.

2. Institute of Medicine, *Health Data in the Information Age: Use, Disclosure, and Privacy* (Washington, DC: National Academies Press, 1994); National Research Council, *For the Record: Protecting Electronic Health Information* (Washington, DC: National Academies Press, 1997); John R. Lumpkin and Margaret S. Richards, "Transforming the Public Health Information Infrastructure," *Health Affairs,* 21 (2002): 45–56.

3. Patrick W. Carroll, William A. Yasnoff, M. Elizabeth Ward, et al., eds., *Public Health Informatics and Information Systems* (New York: Springer, 2003).

4. Jeff Luck, Carol Chang, E. Richard Brown, et al., "Using Local Health Information to Promote Public Health," *Health Affairs,* 25 (2006): 979–91; Lawrence O. Gostin, "Health Information Privacy," *Cornell Law Review,* 80 (1995): 482–84.

5. Lynne Bishop, with Bradford J. Holmes and Christopher M. Kelley, *National Consumer Health Privacy Survey 2005* (Oakland, CA: California Healthcare Foundation, 2005) (stating that 67 percent of national respondents

are "somewhat" or "very concerned" about the privacy of their personal health information).

6. *The Oxford English Dictionary,* 2d ed. (1989): 309 (stating that General Becker was the officer who was charged with the surveillance of Bonaparte); see Willy J. Eylenbosch and Norman D. Noah, *Surveillance in Health and Disease* (New York: Oxford University Press, 1988): 9; Ruth L. Berkelman, Donna F. Stroup, and James W. Buehler, "Public Health Surveillance," in *Oxford Textbook of Public Health,* ed. Detels et al., 1, 759–78.

7. Stephen B. Thacker and Ruth L. Berkelman, "Public Health Surveillance in the United States," *Epidemiologic Review,* 10 (1988): 164; Alexander D. Langmuir, "The Surveillance of Communicable Diseases of National Importance," *New Eng. J. Med.,* 268 (1963): 182.

8. Stephen B. Thacker, "Historical Development," in *Principles and Practice of Public Health Surveillance,* ed. Steven M. Teutsch and R. Elliott Churchill, 2d ed. (New York: Oxford University Press, 2000): 4.

9. Henry Ingersoll Bowditch, D. L. Webster, J. C. Hoadley, et al., "Letter from Massachusetts State Board of Health to Physicians," *Public Health Reports,* 30 (1915): 31.

10. National Office of Vital Statistics, *Vital Statistics of the United States, 1958* (Washington, DC: U.S. Government Printing Office, 1960).

11. Centers for Disease Control and Prevention, *Manual of Procedures for National Morbidity Reporting and Public Health Surveillance Activities* (Atlanta, GA: Public Health Service, 1985).

12. James A. Tobey, *Public Health Law: A Manual of Law for Sanitarians* (Baltimore, MD: Williams and Wilkins, 1926): 109.

13. Alexander D. Langmuir, "The Surveillance of Communicable Diseases of National Importance," *New Eng. J. Med.,* 268 (1963): 182–92.

14. Donald A. Henderson, "Surveillance of Smallpox," *International Journal of Epidemiology,* 5 (1976): 19.

15. Centers for Disease Control and Prevention, "Kaposi's Sarcoma and Pneumocystis Pneumonia among Homosexual Men—New York City and California," *Morbidity and Mortality Weekly Report,* 30 (1981): 305.

16. Brian Hjelle, Steven Jenison, Gregory Mertz, et al., "Emergence of Hanta-Viral Disease in the Southwestern United States," *Western Journal of Medicine,* 161 (1994): 467–73.

17. Stephanie J. Schrag, John T. Brooks, Chris Van Beneden, et al., "SARS Surveillance during Emergency Public Health Response, United States, March–July 2003," *Emerging Infectious Diseases,* 10 (2004): 185–94.

18. World Health Organization, *WHO Consultation on Priority Public Health Interventions before and during an Influenza Pandemic* (Geneva: World Health Organization, 2004) (proposing three surveillance principles: build integrated surveillance systems, concentrate on the interpandemic phase, and focus on detection of clusters).

19. See, e.g., Centers for Disease Control and Prevention, "Youth Risk Behavior Surveillance—United States, 1997," *Morbidity and Mortality Weekly Report,* 47 (1998): 1.

20. National Center for Chronic Disease Prevention and Health Promotion,

"BRFSS: Turning Information into Health," *Centers for Disease Control and Prevention*, July 5, 2006, http://www.cdc.gov/brfss/.

21. Institute of Medicine, *Implications of Genomics for Public Health* (Washington, DC: National Academies Press, 2005); Muin J. Khoury, "From Genes to Public Health: The Applications of Genetic Technology in Disease Prevention," *American Journal of Public Health*, 86 (1996): 1717–22.

22. Allyn L. Taylor, "Governing the Globalization of Public Health," *Journal of Law, Medicine, and Ethics*, 32 (2004): 500–502; Maude M. T. E. Huynen, Pim Martens, and Henk B. M. Hilderink, "The Health Impacts of Globalization: A Conceptual Framework," *Globalization and Health*, 1 (2005): 1–14.

23. David L. Heymann and Guénaël Rodier, "Global Surveillance, National Surveillance, and SARS," *Emerging Infectious Diseases*, 10 (2004): 173–75.

24. P. Formenty, C. Roth, F. Gonzalez-Martin, et al., "Les pathogènes emergents, la veille international et le règlement sanitaire international (2005)," *Médecine et maladies infectieuses*, 36 (2006): 9–15 (stating that over forty-five newly recognized diseases have emerged over the last three decades); David N. Durrheim and Rick Speare, "Communicable Disease Surveillance and Management in a Globalized World," *Lancet*, 363 (2004): 1339–40; Mike Mitka, "Global Pathogen Surveillance," *JAMA*, 295 (2006): 611–12.

25. World Health Organization, *International Health Regulations (IHR)*, Art. 1; see Michael G. Baker and David P. Fidler, "Global Public Health Surveillance under New International Health Regulations," *Emerging Infectious Diseases*, 12 (2006): 1058–65; World Health Organization, *Global Crises, Global Solutions: Managing Public Health Emergencies of International Concern through the Revised International Health Regulations* (Geneva: World Health Organization, 2002).

26. Public health agencies seek access to school health information to protect the health of children, families, and the public. However, some schools have refused access to health data (even reportable STIs), citing the Family Educational Rights and Privacy Act (FERPA), which safeguards the privacy of student educational records. Association of State and Territorial Health Officials, *Accessing School Health Information for Public Health Purposes: Position Statement* (Washington, DC: Association of State and Territorial Health Officials, 2006).

27. *Whalen v. Roe*, 429 U.S. 589 (1977) (upholding the New York reporting requirement for prescriptions for certain dangerous drugs).

28. Lawrence O. Gostin, Scott Burris, and Zita Lazzarini, "The Law and the Public's Health: A Study of Infectious Disease Law in the United States," *Columbia Law Review*, 99 (1999): 58–128.

29. *New York State Society of Surgeons v. Axelrod*, 572 N.E.2d 605 (N.Y. 1991).

30. Terence L. Chorba, Ruth L. Berkelman, Susan K. Safford, et al., "Mandatory Reporting of Infectious Diseases by Clinicians," *JAMA*, 262 (1989): 3018–26.

31. Centers for Disease Control and Prevention, "Mandatory Reporting of Infectious Disease by Clinicians," *Morbidity and Mortality Weekly Report*, 39 (1990): 1.

32. Centers for Disease Control and Prevention, "Nationally Notifiable Infectious Disease: United States 2006," *Centers for Disease Control and Prevention,* January 13, 2006, http://www.cdc.gov/EPO/DPHSI/phs/infdis2006.htm.

33. Council for State and Territorial Epidemiologists, "Reporting Requirements of Disease and Conditions under National Surveillance," *Council for State and Territorial Epidemiologists,* http://www.cste.org/nndss/ReportingRequirements.htm.

34. Centers for Disease Control and Prevention, "Case Definitions for Infectious Conditions under Public Health Surveillance," *Morbidity and Mortality Weekly Report,* 46 (1997): 1.

35. Daniel M. Fox, "Social Policy and City Politics: Tuberculosis Reporting in New York, 1889–1900," *Bulletin of the History of Medicine,* 49 (1975): 169–95.

36. Daniel M. Fox, "From TB to AIDS: Value Conflicts in Reporting Disease," *Hastings Center Report,* 11 (1986): 11–16.

37. Gerard Krause, Gwendolin Ropers, and Klaus Stark, "Notifiable Disease Surveillance and Practicing Physicians," *Emerging Infectious Diseases,* 11 (2005): 442–45 (finding that nearly 60 percent of physician respondents claimed not to have received any feedback on infectious disease surveillance); C. J. Allen and Mark J. Ferson, "Notification of Infectious Diseases by General Practitioners: A Quantitative and Qualitative Study," *Medical Journal of Australia,* 172 (2000): 325–28 (addressing low compliance of physicians with notification systems partly caused by insufficient feedback of surveillance data to physicians).

38. Timothy J. Doyle, M. Kathleen Glynn, and Samuel L. Groseclose, "Completeness of Notifiable Infectious Disease Reporting in the United States: An Analytical Literature Review," *American Journal of Epidemiology,* 155 (2002): 866–74 (stating completeness of reporting varied from 9 to 99 percent, with mean reporting completeness for AIDS, STIs, and TB significantly higher [79 percent] than for all other diseases combined [49 percent]).

39. Ronald Bayer, *Private Acts, Social Consequences: AIDS and the Politics of Public Health* (New Brunswick, NJ: Rutgers University Press, 1991): 117–23.

40. Lawrence O. Gostin, John W. Ward, and A. Cornelius Baker, "National HIV Case Reporting for the United States: A Defining Moment in the History of the Epidemic," *New Eng. J. Med.,* 337 (1997): 1162–67; Lawrence O. Gostin and James G. Hodge, Jr., "The 'Names Debate': The Case for National HIV Reporting in the United States," *Albany Law Review,* 61 (1998): 679–743.

41. American Civil Liberties Union, "HIV Surveillance and Name Reporting: A Public Health Case for Protecting Civil Liberties," *American Civil Liberties Union,* October 4, 1997, http://www.aclu.org/privacy/medical/14945pub19971004.html#credits.

42. Sue Landry, "AIDS List Is Out: State Investigating Breach," *St. Petersburg Times,* September 20, 1996.

43. Ill. Pub. Act 87–763, sec. 693.40(3)(A) (1991), codified at 410 *Ill. Comp Stat* 325/5.5.

44. AIDS Action Foundation, *Should HIV Test Results Be Reportable? A Discussion of the Key Policy Questions* (Washington, DC: AIDS Action Foundation, 1993).

45. Gail L. Dolbear and Linda T. Newell, "Consent for Prenatal Testing: A

Preliminary Examination of the Effects of Named HIV Reporting and Mandatory Partner Notification," *Journal of Public Health Management Practice,* 8 (2002): 69–72; Cari Cason, Nan Orrock, Karla Schmitt, et al., "Tools to Prevent Infectious Disease: The Impact of Laws on HIV and STD Prevention," *Journal of Law, Medicine, and Ethics,* 30 (2002): 139–44; Andrew B. Bindman, Dennis Osmond, Frederick M. Hecht, et al., "Multistate Evaluation of Anonymous HIV Testing and Access to Care," *JAMA,* 280 (1998): 1416–20.

46. Lynda Richardson, "AIDS Group Urges New York to Start Reporting of HIV," *New York Times,* January 13, 1998.

47. Centers for Disease Control and Prevention, "Evaluation of HIV Case Surveillance through the Use of Non-Name Unique Identifiers—Maryland and Texas, 1994–1996," *Morbidity and Mortality Weekly Report,* 46 (1998): 1254; David H. Osmond, Andrew B. Bindman, Karen Vranizan, et al., "Name-Based Surveillance and Public Health Interventions for Persons with HIV Infection," *Annals of Internal Medicine,* 131 (1999): 775–79.

48. Centers for Disease Control and Prevention, "Guidelines for National HIV Case Surveillance," *Morbidity and Mortality Weekly Report,* 48 (1999).

49. Reporting of CDC-defined AIDS has been well established since the beginning of the epidemic, but HIV reporting has only evolved gradually. The CDC and the WHO are currently considering revising their HIV case surveillance definition to categorize the disease in several—probably three to four—"levels" of the progression of the disease based on CD4 count and opportunistic infections.

50. Kaiser Family Foundation, "HIV Reporting Policy," *Kaiser Family Foundation,* April 2006, http://www.statehealthfacts.org/cgi-bin/healthfacts.cgi?action=comp.

51. Ronald Bayer and Amy L. Fairchild, *The Role of Name-Based Notification in Public Health and HIV Surveillance* (Geneva: UNAIDS, 2000); see also UNAIDS/WHO, *Opening up the HIV/AIDS Epidemic: Guidance on Encouraging Beneficial Disclosure, Ethical Partner Counselling and Appropriate Use of HIV Case-Reporting* (Geneva: UNAIDS, 2000).

52. Thomas R. Frieden, Moupali Das-Douglas, Scott E. Kellerman, et al., "Applying Public Health Principles to the HIV Epidemic," *New Eng. J. Med.,* 353 (2005): 2397–2402.

53. Thomas R. Frieden, "Asleep at the Switch: Local Public Health and Chronic Diseases," *American Journal of Public Health,* 94 (2004): 2059–61 (arguing for greater monitoring and control of chronic diseases by local public health agencies).

54. See the symposium on diabetes in the *American Journal of Public Health,* 95 (September 2005): 1493–1649.

55. The American Diabetes Association (ADA) recommends A_1C, also known as glycosylated (or glycated) hemoglobin, testing every three months for insulin-treated patients to ascertain if a patient's blood sugar is under control over time. Research shows that the lower the A_1C, the greater the chances of preventing the development of serious eye, kidney, and nerve disease. American Diabetes Association, "Standards of Medical Care in Diabetes—2006," *Diabetes Care* (2006): S4–S42.

56. Charles D. MacLean, Benjamin Littenberg, and Michael Gagnon, "Dia-

betes Decision Support: Initial Experience with the Vermont Diabetes Information System," *American Journal of Public Health,* 96 (2006): 593–95.

57. Robert Steinbrook, "Facing the Diabetes Epidemic: Mandatory Reporting of Glycosylated Hemoglobin Values in New York City," *New Eng. J. Med.,* 354 (2006): 545–48.

58. JoAnne Glisson, senior vice president of the American Clinical Laboratory Association, letter to Rena Bryant, secretary to the New York City Board of Health, August 16, 2005.

59. Amy L. Fairchild, "Diabetes and Disease Surveillance," *Science,* 313 (2006): 175–76.

60. New York City, N.Y., *Health Code* § 13.04 (2006).

61. For examples of diabetes-related employment discrimination, see N. R. Kleinfield, "Diabetics in the Workplace Confront a Tangle of Laws," *New York Times,* December 26, 2006.

62. Fairchild, "Diabetes and Disease Surveillance."

63. Ronald Bayer and Kathleen E. Toomey, "HIV Prevention and the Two Faces of Partner Notification," *American Journal of Public Health,* 82 (1992): 1158–64.

64. George Rosen, *A History of Public Health* (Baltimore, MD: Johns Hopkins University Press, 1993): 73; Vern L. Bullough, *The History of Prostitution* (New Hyde Park, NY: University Books, 1964): 166–72.

65. The Contagious Disease Acts of 1864 and 1866 adopted partner notification as a method of controlling STIs in the military. The statutes also ordered confinement for up to six months for prostitutes. See Michael J. Adler, "The Terrible Peril: A Historical Perspective on the Venereal Diseases," *British Medical Journal,* 281 (1980): 206.

66. Allan M. Brandt, *No Magic Bullet: A Social History of Venereal Disease in the United States since 1880* (New York: Oxford University Press, 1987).

67. *Army Appropriations Act,* 40 Stat. 855, 856 (1918), amended by the *National Venereal Disease Act,* 52 Stat. 439, 439–40 (1938); see *Public Health Service Act,* ch. 373, 58 Stat. 667, 693–94 (1944) (granting funds to the states for prevention, treatment, and control of venereal diseases).

68. Jon K. Andrus, D. W. Fleming, D. R. Harger, et al., "Partner Notification: Can It Control Syphilis?" *Annals of Internal Medicine,* 112 (1990): 539–43.

69. The Centers for Disease Control and Prevention require federally funded contact tracing programs to provide a comprehensive set of supplemental services, including testing, medical treatment, and counseling, in addition to notification assistance. Centers for Disease Control and Prevention, "HIV Partner Notification Support Services Operational Guidance Outline" (1997): 1–8.

70. For a table of state laws authorizing contact tracing, see Lawrence O. Gostin and James G. Hodge, Jr., "Piercing the Veil of Secrecy in HIV/AIDS and Other Sexually Transmitted Diseases: Theories of Privacy and Disclosure in Partner Notification," *Duke Journal of Gender Law and Policy,* 5 (1998): 9–88, 28–32.

71. Early federal law on the control of STIs did not mention contact tracing, but created a Division of Venereal Diseases within the Bureau of the Public Health Service. *Army Appropriations Act,* 40 Stat. 855, 856 (1918), amended by the

National Venereal Disease Act, 52 Stat. 439, 439–40 (1938); see *Public Health Service Act,* ch. 373, 58 Stat. 667, 693–94 (1944) (funding states for prevention, treatment, and control of venereal diseases).

72. Although Surgeon General Parran incorporated contact tracing into mainstream public health practice in the 1930s, the term was not enumerated in federal law until 1972, when Congress passed the *Communicable Disease Control Amendments Acts,* Pub. L. No. 92–449, sec. 203 § 318(d)(1)(B), 86 Stat. 751, 870–72 (1972) (authorizing the Secretary to fund case finding, including contact tracing). The acts were amended by the *Public Health Service Act of 1976,* Pub. L. 94–317, sec. 203 § d(1)(B), 90 Stat. 695, 703–4 (codified as amended 42 U.S.C. § 247c [1997]) (authorizing the Secretary to make project grants for routine testing). The acts were further amended by the *Preventative Health Amendments of 1984,* Pub. L. No. 98–555, sec. 3 § (d)(6)(A–B), 98 Stat. 2854, 2855 (1984) (adding STIs in addition to syphilis and gonorrhea, and replacing the antiquated term *venereal disease* with *sexually transmitted disease*).

73. *AIDS Emergency Act of 1990,* Pub. L. No. 101–381, title III, § 301(a), 104 Stat. 597, 602 (codified as 42 U.S.C. § 300[f][f]-46 [1994]).

74. Pub. L. No. 104–146, S41, 110 Stat. 1346 (codified at 42 U.S.C. § 201 [Supp. 1996]).

75. Centers for Disease Control and Prevention, "Advancing HIV Prevention: New Strategies for a Changing Epidemic—United States, 2003," *Morbidity and Mortality Weekly Report,* 52 (2003): 329–32; Centers for Disease Control and Prevention, "Incorporating HIV Prevention into the Medical Care of Persons Living with HIV," *Morbidity and Morality Weekly Report,* 52 (2003): 1–24 (advising physicians to discuss risk behaviors, facilitate testing, counseling, and partner notification, and treat other STIs).

76. Centers for Disease Control and Prevention, "1993 Sexually Transmitted Diseases Treatment Guidelines," *Morbidity and Morality Weekly Report,* 42 (1993); Frances M. Cowan, Rebecca French, and Anne M. Johnson, "The Role and Effectiveness of Partner Notification in STD Control: A Review," *Genitourinary Medicine,* 72 (1996): 247–52.

77. Chandler Burr, "The AIDS Exception: Privacy vs. Public Health," *Atlantic Monthly* (June 1997): 57–67.

78. Karen H. Rothenberg and Stephen J. Paskey, "The Risk of Domestic Violence and Women with HIV Infection: Implications for Partner Notification, Public Policy, and the Law," *American Journal of Public Health,* 85 (1995): 1569–76.

79. The evidence is accumulated in Gostin and Hodge, "Piercing the Veil of Secrecy," 72–82.

80. The duty to warn applies to physicians and psychotherapists but not necessarily to all health care professionals. See *Bradley v. Ray,* 904 S.W.2d 302 (Mo. Ct. App. 1995) (extending *Tarasoff* to cover other health care professionals); *In re Sealed Case,* 67 F.3d 965 (D.C. Cir. 1995) (refusing to extend the duty to warn third parties to a lab technician).

81. For an argument that no ethical dilemma exists and that physicians have an absolute duty of confidentiality, see Kenneth Kipnis, "A Defense of Unqualified Medical Confidentiality," *American Journal of Bioethics,* 6 (2006): 7–18.

82. See, e.g., *Alberts v. Devine,* 479 N.E.2d 113, 115 (Mass. 1985) (recognizing an exception to the duty of confidentiality where there is serious danger to the patient or others).

83. John C. Williams, *Annotation, Liability of One Treating Mentally Afflicted Patient for Failure to Warn or Protect Third Persons Threatened by Patient,* 83 A.L.R.3d 1201 (1995).

84. *Tarasoff v. Regents of Univ. of Cal.,* 551 P.2d 334 (Cal. 1976). Interestingly, the precedent for *Tarasoff* was from old infectious disease cases. See, e.g., *Davis v. Rodman,* 227 S.W. 612 (Ark. 1921) (upholding a physician's duty to advise family members likely to be exposed to a patient's typhoid fever); *Skillings v. Allen,* 173 N.W. 663 (Minn. 1919) (finding a physician negligent for advising the plaintiff's wife that it was safe to visit a child known to have scarlet fever). These cases, however, are different from *Tarasoff* because they involve *misdiagnosis* of an infectious condition so that family members were placed at risk, or *misinformation* so that physicians incorrectly informed the family that the disease was not infectious.

85. The case involved the murder of Tatiana Tarasoff, who was a former acquaintance of Prosenjit Poddar, a mentally deranged patient of psychotherapist Dr. Lawrence Moore. In therapy sessions Poddar conveyed to Dr. Moore his intent to kill a girl whom he did not specifically name, although it was evident to the doctor that the intended victim was Tarasoff. Dr. Moore did not warn Tarasoff or her parents but instead asked the campus police to pick up Poddar. Although the police detained Poddar initially, he was later released on his recognizance after being advised to stay away from Tarasoff. Two months later, Poddar murdered Tarasoff.

86. *Lipari v. Sears, Roebuck & Co.,* 497 F. Supp. 185 (D. Neb. 1980) (establishing liability by the existence of foreseeable danger to any member of a targeted class of people).

87. *Lemon v. Stewart,* 682 A.2d 1177 (Md. Ct. Spec. App. 1996) (denying recovery to a family who unknowingly cared for an HIV-infected man, because there was no possibility of transmission).

88. See, e.g., *Cairl v. State,* 323 N.W.2d 20, 26 (Minn. 1982) (finding that the duty required warning only insofar as latent dangers posed a risk to identifiable, specific persons).

89. See, e.g., *Garcia v. Santa Rosa Health Care Corp.,* 925 S.W.2d 372, 377 (Tex. App. 1996) (health care workers "who discover some disease . . . owe a duty to reasonably warn the third party").

90. *Gammill v. United States,* 727 F.2d 950 (10th Cir. 1984) (denying that a person has a duty to protect another except when a special relationship exists, or when the first person placed the other in peril); see *Derrick v. Ontario Comm. Hosp.,* 120 Cal. Rptr. 566 (Cal. Ct. App. 1975) (finding that a hospital has no duty to warn the general public that a patient with a contagious disease is being released).

91. *Hofmann v. Blackmon,* 241 So. 2d 752, 753 (Fla. Dist. Ct. App. 1970) (finding a doctor liable to persons infected by his patient for negligent failure to diagnose a contagious disease); contra see *Britton v. Soltes,* 563 N.E.2d 910 (Ill. App. 1990) (finding that negligent failure to diagnose tuberculosis does not

give rise to action by a third party who became infected through contact with the patient).

92. *Wojcik v. Aluminum Co. of America,* 183 N.Y.S.2d 351, 357–58 (N.Y. Sup. Ct. 1959) (placing a doctor under duty to warn members of the patient's family after diagnosing a contagious disease).

93. *Reisner v. Regents of University of California,* 37 Cal. Rptr. 2d 518, 523 (Ct. App. 1995) ("We believe that a doctor who knows he is dealing with the 20th Century version of Typhoid Mary ought to have a very strong incentive to tell his patient what she ought to do and not do and how she ought to comport herself in order to prevent the spread of her disease"); see also Lawrence O. Gostin, "Hospitals, Health Care Professionals, and AIDS: The 'Right to Know' the Health Status of Professionals and Patients," *Maryland Law Review,* 12 (1989): 48–50.

94. See, e.g., *Berner v. Caldwell,* 543 So.2d 686, 688 (Ala. 1989) ("For over a century, liability has been imposed on individuals who have transmitted communicable diseases that have harmed others"); *Meany v. Meany,* 639 So. 2d 229 (La. 1994); *McPherson v. McPherson,* 712 A.2d 1043 (Me. 1998); *Crowell v. Crowell,* 105 S.E. 206, 208 (N.C. 1920) ("It is a well-settled proposition of law that a person is liable if he negligently exposes another to a contagious or infectious disease"); *Mussivand v. David,* 544 N.E.2d 265 (Ohio 1989) (finding that people with an STI have a duty to use reasonable care to avoid infecting others with whom they have had sex); see also Eric L. Schulman, "Sleeping with the Enemy: Combating the Sexual Spread of HIV-AIDS through a Heightened Legal Duty," *John Marshall Law Review,* 29 (1996): 957–93.

95. *Christian v. Sheft,* No. C 574153 (Cal. Super. Ct. Feb. 17, 1989).

96. *Aetna Cas. & Surety Co. v. Sheft,* 989 F.2d 1105 (9th Cir. 1993) (holding that a man's misrepresentation that he did not have AIDS to induce his lover to engage in sex was inherently harmful conduct).

97. *Doe v. Johnson,* 817 F. Supp. 1382 (W.D. Mich. 1993) (sustaining the claim for negligent transmission of HIV if the defendant knew he was infected or that a prior sex partner was infected).

98. *John B. v. Superior Court,* 137 P.3d 153 (2006).

99. David W. Webber, "Self-Incrimination, Partner Notification, and the Criminal Law: Negatives for the CDC's 'Prevention for Positives' Initiative," *AIDS and Public Policy Journal,* 19 (2004): 54–66.

100. John M. Last, "Epidemiology and Ethics," *Law, Medicine and Health Care,* 19 (1991): 166.

101. Amy L. Fairchild, "Dealing with Humpty Dumpty: Research, Practice, and the Ethics of Public Health Surveillance," *Journal of Law, Medicine and Ethics,* 31 (2003): 615–23; Steven S. Coughlin, "Ethical Issues in Epidemiological Research and Public Health," *Emerging Themes in Epidemiology,* October 3, 2006, http://www.ete-online.com/content/3/1/16.

102. Paul J. Amoroso and John P. Middaugh, "Research vs. Public Health Practice: When Does a Study Require IRB Review?" *Preventive Medicine,* 36 (2003): 250–53.

103. Dale E. Hammerschmidt, "There Is No Substantive Due-Process Right to Conduct Human Subjects Research," *IRB,* 19 (1997): 13–15.

104. 45 C.F.R. § 46.102(d) (1993). Classifying an activity as research does

not automatically require IRB review. Once an activity is classified as research, two additional determinations must be made: Does the research involve "human subjects" and, if so, is the research "exempt" from IRB review? As to the meaning of *human subject,* see 45 C.F.R. § 46.102(f)(1)(2). As to the categories of research that are exempt from IRB review, see 45 C.F.R. § 46.101(b).

105. National Bioethics Advisory Commission, *Ethical and Policy Issues in Research Involving Human Participants* (Springfield, VA: National Technical Information Service, 2001): 1, 34.

106. Centers for Disease Control and Prevention, "Guidelines for Defining Public Health Research and Public Health Non-Research," *Centers for Disease Control and Prevention,* October 4, 1999, http://www.cdc.gov/od/ads/opspoll1.htm.

107. Centers for Disease Control and Prevention, "Guidelines for Defining Public Health Research."

108. National Commission for the Protection of Human Subjects of Biomedical and Behavioral Research, *Belmont Report: Ethical Principles and Guidelines for the Protection of Human Subjects of Research* (Washington, DC: DHEW, 1979).

109. James G. Hodge, Jr., "An Enhanced Approach to Distinguishing Public Health Practice and Human Subjects Research," *Journal of Law, Medicine, and Ethics,* 33 (2005): 125–40.

110. Hodge, "An Enhanced Approach to Distinguishing Public Health Practice"; James G. Hodge, Jr., and Lawrence O. Gostin, with the CSTE Advisory Committee, *Public Health Practice vs. Research: A Report for Public Health Practitioners Including Cases and Guidance for Making Distinctions,* May 24, 2004, http://www.publichealthlaw.net.

111. Dixie E. Snider and Donna F. Stroup, "Defining Research When It Comes to Public Health," *Public Health Reports,* 112 (1997): 29–32.

112. *Compare* Amy L. Fairchild and Ronald Bayer, "Ethics and the Conduct of Public Health Surveillance," *Science,* 303 (2004): 631–32, *with* John P. Middaugh, James G. Hodge, and Matthew L. Cartter, "The Ethics of Public Health Surveillance (Letter)," *Science,* 304 (2004): 681–82.

113. 45 C.F.R. §46.111(a)(7) (1993).

114. 45 C.F.R. §46.116(a)(5).

115. Department of Health and Human Services, *Protecting Personal Health Information in Research: Understanding the HIPAA Privacy Rule* (Washington, DC: DHHS, 2003).

116. 45 C.F.R. § 164.512(e).

117. Mark A. Rothstein, "Currents in Contemporary Ethics: Research Privacy under HIPAA and the Common Rule," *Journal of Law, Medicine, and Ethics,* 33 (2005): 154–58; Jennifer Kulynych and David Korn, "The Effect of the New Federal Medical-Privacy Rule on Research," *New Eng. J. Med.,* 346 (2002): 201–4.

118. 42 U.S.C. §241(d) (1994). Certificate of Confidentiality protection was originally limited to disclosure of subject data in research on the "use and effect of drugs." *Comprehensive Drug Abuse Prevention and Control Act of 1970,* Pub. L. No. 91–513, §3(a). In 1974 the act was expanded to cover "mental health, including research on the use and effect of alcohol and other psychoactive drugs."

Comprehensive Alcohol Abuse and Alcoholism Prevention, Treatment, and Rehabilitation Amendments of 1974, Pub. L. No. 93–282, §122(b). Another expansion (to cover health research generally) in 1988 authorized the current project. *Health Omnibus Programs Extension of 1988*, Pub. L. No. 100–607, §163; see Zachary N. Cooper, Robert M. Nelson, and Lainie Friedman Ross, "Certificates of Confidentiality," *Genetic Testing*, 8 (2004): 214–220.

119. Protection is available upon application for a named project and is conferred in the form of a "Certificate of Confidentiality" issued directly by the assistant secretary for health. The Certificate provides legal authority to resist compulsory demands for identifiable research subject information. An investigator with a Certificate has a legal defense against subpoena or court order similar to the physician-patient privilege. The defense applies only to information about individual subjects, not aggregate data. Assistant Secretary for Health, *Interim Policy Statement* (June 8, 1989), in *Office of Protection of Human Subjects Institutional Review Board Guidebook* (1993), A5–30.

120. However, if the researcher seeks a Certificate to avoid reporting a communicable disease, the assistant secretary requires a special demonstration of how the research would be impaired by the reporting. *Id.*

121. Peter M. Currie, "Balancing Privacy Protections with Efficient Research: Institutional Review Boards and the Use of Certificates of Confidentiality," *IRB: Ethics and Human Research*, 27 (2005): 7–13.

122. Leslie E. Wolf, J. Zandecki, and Bernard Lo, "The Certificate of Confidentiality Application: A View from the NIH Institutes," *IRB: Ethics and Human Research*, 26 (2004): 14–18.

123. M. Justin Coffey and Lainie Friedman Ross, "Human Subject Protection in Genetic Research," *Genetic Testing*, 8 (2003): 209–13.

124. *People v. Newman*, 298 NE. 2d 651 (N.Y. 1973). For a broader discussion of the "scholar's privilege" and judicial treatment of research data confidentiality, see *Journal of Law and Contemporary Problems*, 59 (1996): 1–191.

125. For a historical account, see James G. Hodge, Jr., and Kieran G. Gostin, "Challenging Themes in American Health Information Privacy and the Public's Health: Historical and Modern Assessments," *Journal of Law, Medicine, and Ethics*, 32 (2004): 670–79.

126. Lawrence O. Gostin, "Personal Privacy in the Health Care System: Employer-Sponsored Insurance, Managed Care, and Integrated Delivery Systems," *Kennedy Institute of Ethics Journal*, 7 (1997): 363–64.

127. Samuel D. Warren and Louis D. Brandeis, "The Right to Privacy," *Harvard Law Review*, 4 (1890): 193.

128. Information Infrastructure Task Force, Privacy Working Group, *Privacy and the National Information Infrastructure: Principles for Providing and Using Personal Information* (1995), available at http://nsi.org/Library/Comm/niiprive.htm.

129. Richard Saver, "Medical Research and Intangible Harm," *University of Cincinnati Law Review*, 74 (2006): 941–1012.

130. Amitai Etzioni, *The Limits of Privacy* (New York: Basic Books, 1999).

131. Seth F. Kreimer, "Sunlight, Secrets, and Scarlet Letters: The Tension between Privacy and Disclosure in Constitutional Law," *University of Pennsylva-*

nia Law Review, 140 (1991): 1–147; Francis S. Chlapowski, "The Constitutional Protection of Informational Privacy," *Boston University Law Review,* 71 (1991): 133–60.

132. *Whalen v. Roe,* 429 U.S. 589 (1977). In *Nixon v. Administrator of General Services,* 433 U.S. 425 (1977), decided four months after *Whalen,* the Court also hesitantly acknowledged a narrow right to privacy. See also *Planned Parenthood of Central Missouri v. Danforth,* 428 U.S. 52, 80 (1976) (recognizing the right to privacy but upholding reporting and record-keeping requirements that were reasonably directed to the preservation of maternal health and properly respected a patient's privacy).

133. *Whalen,* 429 U.S. at 605.

134. *Id.*

135. *Rasmussen v. South Florida Blood Service, Inc.,* 500 So. 2d 533 (Fla. 1987) (finding that a person with AIDS is not entitled to a subpoena to assist him in proving that he was infected during a blood transfusion).

136. 638 F.2d 570, 578 (3d Cir. 1980).

137. Individuals asserting a constitutional right to informational privacy are unlikely to obtain a remedy except in cases where the state fails to assert any significant interest or is particularly careless in disclosing highly sensitive information. See *Doe v. Borough of Barrington,* 729 F. Supp. 376 (D.N.J. 1990) (holding that a police officer violated the constitutional right to privacy by disclosing that a person was infected with HIV); *Woods v. White,* 689 F. Supp. 874 (W.D. Wis. 1988) (extending the constitutional right to privacy to disclosure of a prisoner's HIV status by prison medical service personnel), *aff'd,* 899 F.2d 17 (7th Cir. 1990).

138. Lawrence O. Gostin and James G. Hodge, Jr., "Personal Privacy and Common Goods: A Framework for Balancing under the National Health Information Privacy Rule," *Minnesota Law Review,* 86 (2002): 1439–79.

139. *Health Insurance Portability and Accountability Act of 1996,* Pub. L. No. 104–191, 110 Stat. 1936.

140. Department of Health and Human Services, "Standards for Privacy of Individually Identifiable Health Information, Final Rule," 45 C.F.R. §§ 160–64; see Lawrence O. Gostin, "National Health Information Privacy: Regulations under the Health Insurance Portability and Accountability Act," *JAMA,* 285 (2001): 3015–21.

141. Centers for Disease Control and Prevention, "HIPAA Privacy Rule and Public Health: Guidance from CDC and the U.S. Department of Health and Human Services," *Morbidity and Mortality Weekly Report,* 52 (2003): 1–12.

142. 45 C.F.R. § 160.203(c) (exempting from the Privacy Rule public health laws providing for "the reporting of disease or injury, child abuse, birth, or death, or for the conduct of public health surveillance, investigation, or intervention").

143. See generally U.S. Department of Health and Human Services, *HIPAA Questions and Answers* (August 28, 2003), available at http://www.hhs.gov/hipaafaq/index.html.

144. 45 C.F.R. § 164.501.

145. *Id.* at § 164.512(a).

146. *Standards for Privacy of Individually Identifiable Health Information,* 64 Fed. Reg. 59,918, 59,929 (Nov. 3, 1999) (codified at 45 C.F.R. §§ 160–64).

147. James G. Hodge, Jr., Erin Fuse Brown, and Jessica P. O'Connell, "The HIPAA Privacy Rule and Bioterrorism Planning, Prevention, and Response," *Biosecurity and Bioterrorism,* 2 (2004): 73–80.

148. 5 U.S.C. §§552(b)(1)–(3), (6) (1994).

149. *Id.* at §552a(a)(7). Health agencies have used this concept to justify many further uses of personally identifiable information. For example, the Health Care Financing Administration (HCFA) releases to researchers data collected from patient records by Medicare peer review organizations, with patient names and provider identifiers intact.

150. *Id.* at §552 (1994). In 1999 a rider, known colloquially as the Shelby Amendment, was attached to the Omnibus Appropriations Act for FY1999 directing the Office of Management and Budget to require federal agencies to ensure that "all data produced under an award will be made available to the public through the procedures established under the Freedom of Information Act (FOIA)" (*Omnibus Consolidated and Emergency Supplemental Appropriations Act,* Pub. L. No. 105–277, 112 Stat. 2681 [1998]). Enactment of the Shelby Amendment raised a number of issues and objections, including uncertainty over privacy protections for human research subjects. Defenders of the Shelby Amendment argued that it provided the public with both accountability and transparency. Although many concerns remain about privacy issues raised by the amendment, it has not yet been tested in court. See Institute of Medicine, *Access to Research Data in the Twenty-first Century: An Ongoing Dialogue among Interested Parties—Report of a Workshop* (Washington, DC: National Academies Press, 2002).

151. See, e.g., 13 U.S.C. §9 (1994) (regarding raw census data); 42 U.S.C. §290dd-2 (1994) (regarding drug abuse records); 38 U.S.C. §5701 (1994) (regarding claimants' medical and insurance records); 42 U.S.C. §242m(d) (Supp. V 1993) (regarding identifiable health statistics); and 42 U.S.C. §247c(e)(5) (1994) (regarding venereal disease records).

152. But see *Washington Post v. U.S. Dep't of Health & Hum. Servs.,* 690 F.2d 252, 258 (D.C. Cir. 1982) (finding that data exempt from disclosure under FOIA may still be subject to discovery). Courts balance privacy interests against the parties' interests in the administration of justice, and sometimes fashion creative protective orders that permit discovery while limiting privacy infringements. *Burka v. United States Department of Health & Hum. Services,* 87 F.3d 508 (D.C. Cir. 1996) (holding that questionnaires and data tapes relating to a survey undertaken as part of a federal study of smoking behavior were not exempt from FOIA disclosure requirements); *Rasmussen v. South Florida Blood Service, Inc.,* 500 So. 2d 533, 535 (Fla. 1987); *Lampshire v. Procter & Gamble Co.,* 94 F.R.D. 58, 60 (N.D. Ga. 1982); *Farnsworth v. Procter & Gamble Co.,* 101 F.R.D. 355, 357 (N.D. Ga. 1984), *aff'd,* 758 F.2d 1545 (11th Cir. 1985).

153. *United States Department of State v. Washington Post Co.,* 456 U.S. 595, 599 (1982) (exempting medical files from the FOIA because disclosure would invade privacy).

154. Lawrence O. Gostin, Zita Lazzarini, Verla S. Neslund, et al., "The Public Health Information Infrastructure: A National Review of the Law on Health Information Privacy," *JAMA,* 275 (1996): 1921–27.

155. Gostin et al., "The Public Health Information Infrastructure."

156. Workgroup for Electronic Data Interchange, Department of Health and Human Services, *Obstacles to EDI in the Current Health Care Infrastructure* (Washington, DC: DHHS, 1992): app. 4 at iii.

157. 42 U.S.C. §290dd-2 (1994) (upholding strict confidentiality for oral and written communications of "records of the identity, diagnosis, prognosis, or treatment").

158. Harold Edgar and Hazel Sandomire, "Medical Privacy Issues in the Age of AIDS: Legislative Options," *American Journal of Law and Medicine,* 16 (1990): 155–222.

159. Lawrence O. Gostin and James G. Hodge, Jr., "Genetics Privacy and the Law: An End to Genetics Exceptionalism," *Jurimetrics,* 40 (1999): 21–58.

160. Lawrence O. Gostin and James G. Hodge, Jr., "Model State Public Health Privacy Act," http://www.critpath.org/msphpa/privacy.htm; Lawrence O. Gostin, James G. Hodge, Jr., and Ronald O. Valdiserri, "Informational Privacy and the Public's Health," *American Journal of Public Health,* 91 (2001): 1388–92; Amy L. Fairchild, Lance Gable, Lawrence O. Gostin, et al., "Public Goods, Private Data: HIV and the History, Ethics, and Uses of Personally Identifiable Public Health Information," *Public Health Reports,* 122 (2007): 7–15.

9. HEALTH, COMMUNICATION, AND BEHAVIOR: FREEDOM OF EXPRESSION

SOURCES FOR CHAPTER EPIGRAPHS: Alexis de Tocqueville, *Democracy in America,* vol. 2 (New York: Random House, 1990): 106; *Abrams v. United States,* 250 U.S. 616, 630 (1919) (Holmes, J., dissenting); *American Booksellers Ass'n. v. Hudnut,* 771 F.2d 323, 327–28 (7th Cir. 1985) (quoting *West Virginia State Board of Education v. Barnette,* 319 U.S. 624, 642 [1943]); Rebecca M. Knight, "Helping Pollock Quit, Even Posthumously," *New York Times,* February 6, 1999; Dan E. Beauchamp, *The Health of the Republic: Epidemics, Medicine, and Moralism as Challenges to Democracy* (Philadelphia: Temple University Press, 1988): 147; *Virginia State Bd. of Pharmacy v. Virginia Citizens Consumer Council,* 425 U.S. 748, 763 (1976); *Riley v. National Federation of the Blind of North Carolina,* 487 U.S. 781, 796–97 (1988); J. Michael McGinnis, Jennifer Appleton Gootman, and Vivica I. Kraak, eds., *Food Marketing to Children and Youth: Threat or Opportunity?* (Washington, D.C.: National Academies Press, 2006).

1. Barbara A. Israel, Barry Checkoway, Amy Schulz, et al., "Health Education and Community Empowerment: Conceptualizing and Measuring Perceptions of Individual, Organizational, and Community Control," *Health Education Quarterly,* 149 (1994): 149.

2. See generally Nancy Signorielli, *Mass Media Images and Impact on Health: A Sourcebook* (Westport, CT: Greenwood Press, 1993) (stating that the success of health education campaigns depends on the broader cultural context and is shaped predominantly by mass media).

3. Steve Younger, "Alcoholic Beverage Advertising on the Airwaves: Alternatives to a Ban or Counter-Advertising," *University of California Los Angeles Law Review,* 34 (1987): 1139–93.

4. Erwin Chemerinsky, *Constitutional Law: Principles and Policies*, 3d ed. (New York: Aspen Law and Business, 2006): 751–56.

5. C. Edwin Baker, "Scope of the First Amendment Freedom of Speech," *University of California Los Angeles Law Review*, 25 (1978): 964–94.

6. Alexander Meiklejohn, *Free Speech and Its Relation to Self-Government* (New York: Harper and Brothers, 1948); Alexander Meiklejohn, *Political Freedom* (New York: Harper and Brothers, 1960); Alexander Meiklejohn, "The First Amendment Is an Absolute," *Supreme Court Review*, 1961 (1961): 245–66.

7. For an argument that political speech should be the foremost, if not the only, expression deserving of First Amendment protection, see Robert Bork, "Neutral Principles and Some First Amendment Problems," *Indiana Law Journal*, 47 (1971): 1–35; Cass R. Sunstein, *Democracy and the Problem of Free Speech* (New York: Free Press, 1993).

8. John Milton, *Areopagitica—A Speech for the Liberty of Unlicensed Printing, to the Parliament of England* (Philadelphia: John W. Moore, 1847): 42 ("And though all the winds of doctrine were let loose to play upon the earth, so Truth be in the field, we do injuriously, by licensing and prohibiting, to misdoubt her strength. Let her and Falsehood grapple; who ever knew Truth put to the worst, in a free and open encounter?").

9. John Stuart Mill, *On Liberty* (London: Penguin Books, 1974): 76 (stating the "peculiar evil of silencing the expression of an opinion is that it is robbing the human race, posterity as well as the existing generation—those who dissent from the opinion, still more than those who hold it").

10. Gerald Gunther and Kathleen M. Sullivan, *Constitutional Law* (New York: Foundation Press, 2004): 1025 (summarizing the Millian theory of free expression).

11. *Abrams v. United States*, 250 U.S. 616, 630 (1919) (Holmes, J., dissenting).

12. Ronald Bayer, Lawrence O. Gostin, and Devin McGraw, "Trades, AIDS, and the Public's Health: The Limits of Economic Analysis," review of *Private Choices and Public Health: The AIDS Epidemic in an Economic Perspective*, by Tomas J. Philipson and Richard A. Posner, *Georgetown Law Journal*, 83 (1994): 79–107, 82 ("Public health is therefore interventionist, taking the prevailing pattern of morbidity-related choices and their outcomes as both the beginning of the analysis and as the prod for public policy").

13. Baker, "Scope of the First Amendment Freedom of Speech," 964–1040 ("The marketplace of ideas appears improperly biased in favor of presently dominant groups"); Jerome A. Barron, "Access to the Press—A New First Amendment Right," *Harvard Law Review*, 80 (1967): 1641–78 ("A right of expression is somewhat thin if it can be exercised only at the sufferance of the managers of mass communications"); Stanley Ingber, "The Marketplace of Ideas: A Legitimizing Myth," *Duke Law Journal*, 1984 (1984): 1–91 (regulation is needed to correct "communicative market failures").

14. Laurence H. Tribe, *American Constitutional Law*, 3d ed. (New York: Associated Press, 2000): 827.

15. Space limitations prevent me from examining two additional areas of public health regulation that affect First Amendment values. First, government

regulation of public places implicates the right to freedom of expression and association. For example, courts have upheld the closure of bathhouses and adult cinemas or bookstores to control anonymous sex, which risks HIV or STI transmission. See, e.g., *Ben Rich Trading, Inc. v. City of Vineland,* 126 F.3d 155 (3d Cir. 1997) (finding that an ordinance requiring viewing booths in bookstores to be open and visible did not violate the patrons' freedom of expression); *New York v. New St. Mark's Baths,* 497 N.Y.S. 2d 974 (N.Y. Sup. Ct. 1986), *aff'd,* 505 N.Y.S. 2d 1015 (N.Y. App. Div. 1986) (finding that closure of a bathhouse did not violate the patrons' freedom of association). Second, the government controls access to public property ("public forums") for the presentation of health-related messages. For example, courts have required transportation authorities to provide nondiscriminatory access to condom advertisements to prevent HIV transmission. See, e.g., *AIDS Action Committee of Massachusetts v. Massachusetts Bay Transportation Authority,* 42 F.3d 1 (1st Cir. 1994). Similarly, the Supreme Court has heard a number of cases involving restricted access to the vicinity around abortion clinics (traditional public forums). See, e.g., *Madsen v. Women's Health Center,* 512 U.S. 753, 764–65 (1994) (denying that an injunction establishing a thirty-six-foot buffer zone around abortion clinic entrances violates the First Amendment).

16. For a definition of health communication campaigns, see William Paisley, "Public Communication Campaigns: The American Experience," in *Public Communication Campaigns,* ed. Ronald E. Rice and Charles K. Atkin, 2d ed. (Newbury Park, CA: Sage Publications, 1989): 7 ("Purposive attempts to inform, persuade, or motivate behavior changes in a relatively well-defined and large audience, generally for noncommercial benefits to the individuals and/or society at large, typically within a given time period, by means of organized communication activities involving mass media and often complemented by interpersonal support").

17. Pub. L. No. 100–102, § 514(a), 101 Stat. 1329–89 (1988) (the Helms Amendment).

18. Mark V. Tushnet, "Talking to Each Other: Reflections on Yudof's *When Government Speaks,*" review of *When Government Speaks,* by Mark G. Yudof, *Wisconsin Law Review,* 1984 (1984): 129–45, 132.

19. Lawrence Lessig, "The Regulation of Social Meaning," *University of Chicago Law Review,* 62 (1995): 943–1045 (regarding how government constructs social norms); Cass R. Sunstein, "Social Norms and Social Roles," *Columbia Law Review,* 96 (1996): 903–68; see also David Buchanan, *An Ethic for Health Promotion: Rethinking the Sources of Human Well-Being* (New York: Oxford University Press, 2000); Daniel Callahan, *Promoting Health Behavior: How Much Freedom? Whose Responsibility?* (Washington, DC: Georgetown University, 2000).

20. For example, health education campaigns may be designed to instill fear in people about the harmful effects of their behavior. R. F. Soames Job, "Effective and Ineffective Use of Fear in Health Promotion Campaigns," *American Journal of Public Health,* 78 (1988): 163.

21. Health communication campaigns can pose social risks in more subtle ways. For example, campaigns that associate smoking with impotence portray impotent men in mocking or derogatory ways. Campaigns can also imply that

people who fail to comply with the health message are stupid or antisocial (e.g., "Listen to a Dummy—Buckle Up").

22. Government health messages may be hurtful to discrete groups or populations. In 1995, the CDC revised guidelines that had recommended that women infected with HIV "should consider not having children" after community groups of women and African Americans protested that the recommendation was stigmatizing and insensitive. Centers for Disease Control and Prevention, "Revised Recommendations for HIV Screening of Pregnant Women," *Morbidity and Mortality Weekly Report,* 50 (2001): 59–86.

23. Ruth R. Faden, "Ethical Issues in Government Sponsored Public Health Campaigns," *Health Education Quarterly,* 14 (1987): 33–34.

24. Women's Health Initiative, *Postmenopausal Hormone Therapy,* April 13, 2006, http://www.nhlbi.nih.gov/whi/index.html.

25. Barbara V. Howard, JoAnn D. Manson, Marcia L. Stefanick, et al., "Low-Fat Dietary Pattern and Weight Change over Seven Years: The Women's Health Initiative Dietary Modification Trial," *JAMA,* 295 (2006): 39–49; Michael L. Dansigner and Ernst J. Schaefer, "Low-Fat Diets and Weight Change," *JAMA,* 295 (2006): 94–95; Women's Health Initiative, *Dietary Modification Trial,* 2006, http://www.nhlbi.nih.gov/whi/diet_mod.htm.

26. Ali H. Mokdad, James S. Marks, Donna F. Stroup, et al., "Correction: Actual Causes of Death in the United States, 2000," *JAMA,* 291 (2004): 1238 (admitting that the CDC overestimated the number of deaths caused by poor diet and physical inactivity through a computational error); Katherine M. Flegal, Barry I. Graubard, David F. Williamson, et al., "Excess Deaths Associated with Underweight, Overweight, and Obesity," *JAMA,* 293 (2005): 1861–67 (finding about 112,000 obesity-attributable deaths in 2000, far lower than the 414,000 estimated by Mokdad et al.); Daniel Henninger, "From Spin City to Fat City," *Wall Street Journal,* May 6, 2005 (attributing the CDC's error to overly zealous and careless advocacy); Linda Villeross, "New Fatness Guidelines Spur Debate on Fitness," *New York Times,* June 23, 1998.

27. *Compare* Stephen A. Feig, "Increased Benefit from Shorter Screening Mammography Intervals for Women Ages Forty to Forty-nine Years," *Cancer,* 80 (1997): 2091 (supporting screening of women age forty to forty-nine); *with* National Institutes of Health, "Breast Cancer Screening for Women Ages Forty to Forty-nine," *NIH Consensus Statement Online,* 15 (1997):1 (finding that evidence of effectiveness for screening women age forty to forty-nine is inconclusive).

28. Daniel Wikler and Dan E. Beauchamp, "Health Promotion and Health Education," in *Encyclopedia of Bioethics,* ed. Thomas Warren Reich (New York: Simon and Schuster Macmillan, 1995): 1126, 1128.

29. Campaigns are difficult to evaluate because of the diffuse nature of the target audience, the low salience of the campaign's subject matter, and the complexity of the causal relationship between the campaign and behavior change. Brian R. Flay and Thomas D. Cook, "Three Models for Summative Evaluation of Prevention Campaigns with a Mass Media Component," in *Public Communication Campaigns,* ed. R. Rice and C. Arkin (Beverly Hills, CA: Sage, 1989): 175. Moreover, researchers suggest that many of the campaigns that are evaluated appear to have limited effectiveness. See generally Charles K. Atkin and Vicki

Freimuth, "Formative Evaluation Research in Campaign Design," in *Public Communication Campaigns*, ed. Ronald E. Rice and Charles K. Atkins, 3d ed. (Thousand Oaks, CA: Sage, 2001): 131.

30. See, e.g., Thomas I. Emerson, *The System of Freedom of Expression* (New York: Random House, 1970): 697–716; Mark G. Yudof, "When Government Speaks: Politics, Law, and Government Expression in America," *Journal of Politics*, 46 (1983): 1291–93; Frederick Schauer, "Is Government Speech a Problem?" *Stanford Law Review*, 35 (1983): 373–86.

31. Tribe, *American Constitutional Law*.

32. The Supreme Court is quite prepared to defend government speech, even when government registers "official" disapproval of privately held ideas. For example, in *Meese v. Keene*, 481 U.S. 465 (1987), the Court upheld a Department of Justice classification of three foreign films as "political propaganda"—one concerning the environmental hazards of nuclear war and the other two concerning acid rain.

33. *Johanns v. Livestock Marketing Ass'n*, 544 U.S. 550 (2005) (stating that citizens have no First Amendment right not to fund government speech).

34. Kathleen Sullivan, "Unconstitutional Conditions," *Harvard Law Review*, 102 (1989): 1415–1506.

35. *Speiser v. Randall*, 357 U.S. 513, 517 (1958) ("To deny a [tax] exemption to claimants who engage in certain forms of speech is in effect to penalize them for such speech").

36. Professors Sullivan and Gunther offer the following distinction between an unconstitutional condition and a constitutionally permissible subsidy: A government may not use "a subsidy to induce recipients to refrain from speech they would otherwise engage in with their own resources, but it may refrain from paying for speech with which it disagrees." Kathleen M. Sullivan and Gerald Gunther, *First Amendment Law* (New York: Foundation Press, 1999): 310.

37. *Rust v. Sullivan*, 500 U.S. 173, 193–94 (1991).

38. *Velazquez v. Legal Services Corp.*, 531 US 533 (2001); but see *United States v. American Library Ass'n*, 539 U.S. 194 (2003) (upholding a federal statute denying public libraries federal funds for Internet access unless they install software to block pornographic images).

39. *Rumsfeld v. Forum for Academic and Institutional Rights, Inc*, 547 U.S. 4760 (2006).

40. Jon S. Vernick, Stephen P. Teret, and Daniel W. Webster, "Regulating Firearm Advertisements That Promise Home Protection," *JAMA*, 277 (1997): 1391 (regarding a *Ladies Home Journal* advertisement: "Self-protection is more than your right . . . it's your responsibility"); see also Garen J. Wintemute, *Advertising Firearms as Protection* (Sacramento, CA: Violence Prevention Research Program, 1995).

41. Stuart Elliot, "Liquor Industry Ends Its Ad Ban in Broadcasting," *New York Times*, November 8, 1996; Centers for Disease Control and Prevention, "Youth Exposure to Alcohol Advertising on Radio—United States, June–August 2004," *Morbidity and Mortality Weekly Revew*, 55 (2006): 937–40.

42. *Pearson v. Shalala*, 164 F.3d 650 (D.C. Cir. 1999), *denying petition for*

rehearing en banc, 172 F.3d 72 (D.C. Cir. 1999) (invalidating the same regulation because the FDA was required to consider whether inclusion of appropriate disclaimers would negate potentially misleading health claims); *Nat'l Council for Improved Health v. Shalala,* 122 F.3d 878 (10th Cir. 1997) (same); *National Council for Improved Health v. Shalala,* 122 F.3d 878 (10th Cir. 1997) (same); see David C. Vladeck, "Devaluing Truth—Unverified Health Claims in the Aftermath of *Pearson v. Shalala,*" *Food and Drug Law Journal,* 54 (1999): 535–53.

43. In a settlement between twelve attorneys general and SmithKline Beecham, the company agreed to cease using its misleading "the Power to Quit" slogan for antismoking products Nicorette and NicoDermCQ after evidence emerged that consumers start smoking again one year after they quit. Chemical Business NewsBase, December 22, 1998, available in WL 21881828. See also *Washington Legal Foundation v. Friedman,* 13 F. Supp. 2d 51 (D.D.C. 1998) (invalidating an FDA restriction on use of journal reprints and educational seminars to promote off-label prescription drug uses).

44. *Central Hudson Gas & Electric Corp. v. Public Service Commission,* 447 U.S. 557, 561 (1980).

45. *Virginia State Board of Pharmacy v. Virginia Citizens Consumer Council, Inc.,* 425 U.S. 748, 762 (1976).

46. In *Bad Frog Brewery, Inc. v. New York State Liquor Authority,* 134 F.3d 87 (2d Cir. 1998), the Second Circuit found that a beer label displaying a frog giving an insulting gesture was commercial speech but did not qualify as more fully protected speech, such as social commentary or political speech. Bad Frog labels met the three criteria for commercial speech. *Id.* at 97. The purported noncommercial message, however, was not "inextricably intertwined" enough to merit full First Amendment protection. *Id.*

47. *Bolger v. Youngs Drug Prods. Corp.,* 463 U.S. 60, 67 (1983).

48. In *New York Times Co. v. Sullivan,* 376 U.S. 254 (1964), the Court expressly rejected the argument that the First Amendment did not apply to "paid" commercial advertisements. Corporate speech can amount to fully protected political speech, such as when a company advocates its business interests in a political referendum campaign. See also *First National Bank of Boston v. Bellotti,* 435 U.S. 765 (1978) (invalidating a state statute prohibiting corporations from advertising designed to influence votes submitted to the electorate other than one materially affecting the corporation's business).

49. *New York Times,* September 26, 1995 (paid for by R.J. Reynolds and Philip Morris).

50. In 1985, R.J. Reynolds paid for editorial-style advertisements that appeared in twenty-five publications, including the *New York Times.* In the so-called advertorial "Of Cigarettes and Science," the company asserted that the Multiple Risk Factor Intervention Trial ("Mr. Fit") failed to find a relationship between smoking and heart disease. The FTC agreed to settle charges of false advertis ing, while the company pledged not to misrepresent scientific studies in the future. Barry Meier, "Selling or Advising? Dispute Settled on Tobacco Ads," *New York Times,* October 21, 1989.

51. For a discussion of the issue, see Peter S. Arno, Allan M. Brandt, Law-

rence O. Gostin, et al., "Tobacco Industry Strategies to Oppose Federal Regulation," *JAMA*, 275 (1996): 1258–62.

52. *Nike, Inc. v. Kasky*, 539 U.S. 654 (2003) (Stevens concurring); see *Riley v. National Federation of the Blind of North Carolina*, 487 U.S. 781 (1988) (declining to use a commercial speech test in striking down a statute mandating professional fundraisers to disclose the percentage of charitable contributions actually turned over to the charity). The Court stated that "even assuming that the mandated speech, in the abstract, is merely 'commercial,' it does not retain its commercial character when it is inextricably intertwined with the otherwise fully protected speech involved in charitable solicitations." *Id.* at 782.

53. *Kasky v. Nike*, 45 P.3d 243, 262 (Cal. 2002) (holding that "when a corporation, to maintain and increase its sales and profits, makes public statements defending labor practices and working conditions at factories where its products are made, those public statements are commercial speech that may be regulated to prevent consumer deception"), *cert. dismissed*, 539 U.S. 654 (2003).

54. David C. Vladeck, "Lessons from a Story Untold: *Nike v. Kasky* Reconsidered," *Case Western Reserve Law Review*, 54 (2004): 1049–89.

55. *Valentine v. Chrestensen*, 316 U.S. 52, 54 (1942).

56. *Bigelow v. Virginia*, 421 U.S. 809, 826 (1975) (invalidating a state statute making it a crime to sell or circulate any publication that encourages or prompts the procuring of an abortion).

57. *Bigelow*, 316 U.S. at 826 (1975).

58. *Carey v. Population Services International*, 431 U.S. 678 (1977) (invalidating a New York ban on advertising nonprescription contraceptives).

59. *Virginia State Board of Pharmacy v. Virginia Citizens Consumer Council, Inc.*, 425 U.S. 748 (1976).

60. *Id.* at 771–72 (stating that commercial speech enjoys no special procedural protections, such as the strict scrutiny of prior restraints or overly broad regulation); *Nutritional Health Alliance v. Shalala*, 144 F.3d 220 (2d Cir. 1998) (holding that the FDA requirement for prior approval of health claims on dietary supplement labels is not an unconstitutional prior restraint of commercial speech).

61. *Ohralik v. Ohio State Bar Assn.*, 436 U.S. 447, 455–56 (1978).

62. *Central Hudson Gas v. Public Serv. Comm'n*, 447 U.S. 557, 563 (1980).

63. Compare *Posadas de Puerto Rico Associates v. Tourism Co. of Puerto Rico*, 478 U.S. 328 (1986) (upholding a ban on advertising of legal gambling in Puerto Rico); with *Rubin v. Coors Brewing Co.*, 514 U.S. 476 (1995) (upholding a prohibition on beer labels displaying alcohol content).

64. But see *JR-MacDonald Inc. v. Canada (Attorney General)*, [1994] S.C.R. 311 (stating that the ban on tobacco advertising constituted an unreasonable limit on freedom of expression).

65. *Framework Convention on Tobacco Control*, art. 13(2), 42 I.L.M. 518 (2003); *European Parliament and European Council Directive 2003/33/EC of 26 May 2003 on the Approximation of the Laws, Regulations and Administrative Provisions of the Member States Relating to the Advertising and Sponsorship of Tobacco Products*, 2003 O.J. (L. 152) 16 (EC) (prohibiting tobacco ad-

vertising in print and radio and the sponsorship of events by tobacco companies in member states).

66. 447 U.S. 557 (1980).

67. *Greater New Orleans Broadcasting Ass'n v. United States,* 527 U.S. 173, 188 (1999).

68. *Florida Bar v. Went for It, Inc.,* 515 U.S. 618, 623 (1995).

69. *Edenfield v. Fane,* 507 U.S. 761, 770–71 (1993).

70. *Pittsburgh Press Co. v. Pittsburgh Commission on Human Relations,* 413 U.S. 376 (1973) (denying First Amendment protection to illegal gender-based classification in help wanted ads).

71. For example, the Supreme Court allows tort litigation by smokers based on claims that cigarette manufacturers engaged in fraudulent misrepresentation or conspiracy to misrepresent or conceal material facts. *Cipollone v. Liggett Group, Inc.,* 505 U.S. 504 (1992).

72. Sylvia Law, "Addiction, Autonomy and Advertising," *Iowa Law Review,* 77 (1992): 909–55.

73. *American Academy of Pain Management v. Joseph,* 353 F.3d 1099 (9th Cir. 2004) (upholding state regulation limiting physicians from advertising that they are "board certified" because the term is "inherently misleading").

74. On April 5, 2001, the European Union adopted a directive that bans "texts, names, trademarks and figurative or other signs suggesting that a particular tobacco product is less harmful than others." *Directive 2001/37/EC of the European Parliament and of the Council of 5 June 2001 on the Approximation of the Laws, Regulations and Administrative Provisions of the Member States Concerning the Manufacture, Presentation and Sale of Tobacco Products,* 2001 O.J. (L. 194) 26 (EC).

75. *Good v. Altria Group, Inc.,* 436 F. Supp. 2d 132 (D. Me. 2006) (refusing to even hear the argument on the basis that the Cigarette Labeling and Advertising Act preempted it).

76. *United States v. Philip Morris USA, Inc.,* 449 F. Supp. 2d 1 (D.D.C. 2006) (finding terms like *light* and *low tar* misleading); *Schwab v. Philip Morris USA, Inc.,* 449 F. Supp. 2d 992 (E.D.N.Y. 2006) (granting a class certification to smokers who had smoked "light" cigarettes, which were misleadingly marketed to them as less harmful).

77. Paul M. Fischer, John W. Richards, Jr., Earl J. Berman, et al., "Recall and Eye Tracking Study of Adolescents Viewing Tobacco Advertisements," *JAMA,* 261 (1989): 84–89; see also Kathleen J. Lester, "Cowboys, Camels, and Commercial Speech: Is the Tobacco Industry's Commodification of Childhood Protected by the First Amendment?" *Northern Kentucky Law Review,* 24 (1997): 615–72.

78. Daniel Dunaief, "AG Sends Kook Mixx Ads Up in Smoke," *New York Daily News,* June 18, 2004.

79. Marc T. Braverman and Leif Edvard Aar, "Adolescent Smoking and Exposure to Tobacco Marketing under a Tobacco Advertising Ban: Findings from Two Norwegian National Samples," *American Journal of Public Health,* 94 (2004): 1230–38.

80. The Federal Trade Commission, for example, regulates speech that is

"false or misleading." The FTC in 2004 punished as "misleading" KFC television advertisements comparing the nutritional value of KFC's "Original Recipe" fried chicken breasts to the Burger King Whopper. The FTC prohibited KFC from making health or diet-compatibility statements about its products "unless it substantiates the claim with competent and reliable evidence, including scientific evidence when appropriate." The FTC noted that KFC could make claims consistent with FDA food-labeling rules. Federal Trade Commission, "KFC's Claims That Fried Chicken Is a Better Way to 'Eat Better' Doesn't Fly," October 10, 2006, http://www.ftc.gov/opa/2004/06/kfccorp.htm.

81. In the mid-1950s, L & M Filters were advertised as the new "miracle product": the "alpha cellulose" filter is "just what the doctor ordered." R. J. Reynolds similarly advertised: "More doctors smoke Camels than any other cigarette." Thomas Whiteside, *Selling Death: Cigarette Advertising and Public Health* (New York: Liveright, 1971).

82. Institute of Medicine, *Clearing the Smoke: Assessing the Science Base for Tobacco Harm Reduction* (Washington, DC: National Academies Press, 2001).

83. *Ohralik v. Ohio State Bar Ass'n,* 436 U.S. 447, 462 (1978).

84. *Friedman v. Rogers,* 440 U.S. 1, 13 (1979) ("There is a significant possibility that trade names will be used to mislead the public").

85. *See Ohralik,* 436 U.S. at 465 (holding that face-to-face attorney solicitation inherently risks that clients will be deceived and pressured). However, in a contradictory ruling the Court found that personal solicitations by accountants are constitutionally protected. *Edenfield v. Fane,* 507 U.S. 761 (1993). In addition, attorneys may constitutionally engage in truthful, nondeceptive advertising of their services, provided it does not involve face-to-face solicitation. *Bates v. State Bar of Ariz.,* 433 U.S. 350 (1977); *Shapero v. Kentucky Bar Ass'n,* 486 U.S. 466 (1988); but see *Florida Bar v. Went for It, Inc.,* 515 U.S. 618 (1995) (upholding the prohibition of attorney mail solicitation for thirty days after an accident).

86. Vincent Blasi and Henry Paul Monaghan, "The First Amendment and Cigarette Advertising," *JAMA,* 256 (1986): 502–9.

87. *Metromedia, Inc. v. City of San Diego,* 453 U.S. 490 (1981) (upholding an ordinance prohibiting outdoor displays relating to commercial but not political speech because they pose a traffic hazard); but see *City of Cincinnati v. Discovery Network, Inc.,* 507 U.S. 410 (1993) (invalidating an ordinance prohibiting commercial newspapers from being distributed on news racks while allowing other kinds of newspapers to be sold).

88. *Rubin v. Coors Brewing Co.,* 514 U.S. 476, 485 (1995) (finding that the state has a significant interest in "preventing brewers from competing on the basis of alcohol strength, which could lead to greater alcoholism and its attendant social costs." The regulation, however, was found unconstitutional because it was more intrusive than necessary to achieve its goals).

89. *United States v. Edge Broadcasting Co.,* 509 U.S. 418 (1993) (upholding a federal law prohibiting lottery advertising by radio stations located in states that did not operate lotteries); *Posadas de Puerto Rico Associates v. Tourism Co. of Puerto Rico,* 478 U.S. 328, 341 (1986) (validating a ban on advertising casino gambling directed to residents when the Court had "no difficulty" finding that state interest in health constitutes a "substantial interest"). However, the Court

subsequently struck down this federal statute as applied to states where gambling was lawful. *Greater New Orleans Broadcasting Ass'n v. United States,* 527 U.S. 173 (1999).

90. *Oklahoma Telecasters Ass'n v. Crisp,* 699 F.2d 490, 501 (10th Cir. 1983), *rev'd on other grounds sub nom.*; *Capital Cities Cable v. Crisp,* 467 U.S. 691 (1984) (stating that it is not "constitutionally unreasonable for the State . . . to believe that advertising will increase sales . . . of alcoholic beverages").

91. 478 U.S. at 341–42. Chief Justice Rehnquist in *Posadas* made a now discredited argument that the greater power to completely ban a product necessarily includes the lesser power to regulate advertising of that product: "It would . . . surely be a strange constitutional doctrine which would concede to the legislature the authority to totally ban a product or activity, but deny to the legislature the authority to forbid the stimulation of demand for the product or activity." *Id.* at 346. This "greater includes the lesser" theory would give public health authorities virtually plenary authority to suppress advertising of tobacco, alcoholic beverages, and gambling. However, Rehnquist's argument wrongly assumes that speech restrictions *are* the lesser included power. Arguably, product prohibitions on health or safety grounds would be less offensive to the Constitution than speech prohibitions. See *Greater New Orleans Broadcasting,* 527 U.S. at 193 ("The power to prohibit or to regulate particular conduct does not necessarily include the power to prohibit or regulate speech about that conduct"); 44 *Liquormart, Inc. v. Rhode Island,* 517 U.S. 484, 513–14 (1996) (rejecting the argument that the power to restrict speech about certain socially harmful activities was as broad as the power to prohibit such conduct).

92. *Florida Bar v. Went for It, Inc.,* 515 US 618, 628 (1995) ("We do not read our case law to require that empirical data come to us accompanied by a surfeit of background information. . . . [W]e have permitted litigants to justify speech restrictions by reference to studies and anecdotes pertaining to different locales altogether, or even, in a case applying strict scrutiny, to justify restrictions based solely on history, consensus, and 'simple common sense'").

93. *Rubin v. Coors Brewing Co.,* 514 U.S. 476, 488–89 (1995).

94. 44 *Liquormart,* 517 U.S. at 505–7.

95. *Greater New Orleans Broadcasting,* 527 U.S. at 173 (finding that exemptions in the government's gambling policy prevent it from directly and materially advancing the asserted interests in reducing the social costs of casino gambling and assisting states that prohibit it within their own borders).

96. *Greater New Orleans Broadcasting,* 527 U.S. at 174.

97. *Id.* at 173.

98. After 44 *Liquormart,* the level of proof required to demonstrate that a commercial speech regulation directly advances the state's interest is unclear. No single standard has the support of the majority of the Court. Justice Stevens's plurality opinion in 44 *Liquormart* requires an evidentiary showing that the advertising regulation would significantly reduce demand for a hazardous product. However, Justice O'Connor, writing for four members of the Court, pointedly declined to adopt Justice Stevens's approach on the third prong of *Central Hudson Gas & Elec. Corp. v. Public Serv. Comm'n,* 447 U.S. 557, 530 (1980). 517 U.S. at 530. In *Greater New Orleans Broadcasting,* 527 U.S at 190, the Court

said it was not necessary on the facts of the case to resolve the evidentiary dispute within the Court because the flaw in the government's case is more fundamental.

99. *Edenfield v. Fane,* 507 U.S. 761, 770 (1993).

100. See, e.g., *Dunagin v. City of Oxford,* 718 F.2d 738, 751 (5th Cir. 1983) (en banc), *cert. denied,* 467 U.S. 1259 (1984); *Queensgate Investment Co. v. Liquor Control Commission,* 433 N.E.2d 138 (Ohio 1982), *cert. denied,* 459 U.S. 807 (1982).

101. 492 U.S. 469, 477 (1989) (upholding a university regulation restricting the operation of commercial enterprises on campus).

102. *Fox,* 492 U.S. at 480 (citations omitted).

103. In *Rubin v. Coors Brewing Co.,* the Court noted a number of alternative ways of preventing strength wars so the government's interest could be achieved "in a manner less intrusive to . . . First Amendment rights." 514 U.S. 476, 491. In 44 *Liquormart,* the plurality opinion concluded that "it is perfectly obvious that alternative forms of regulation that would not involve any restriction on speech would be more likely to achieve the State's goal of promoting temperance." 517 U.S. at 507. And in *Greater New Orleans Broadcasting,* the Court said, "There surely are practical and nonspeech-related forms of regulation . . . that could more directly and effectively alleviate some of the social costs of casino gambling." 527 U.S. at 192.

104. *Lorillard Tobacco Co. v. Reilly,* 533 U.S. 525 (2001).

105. *Id.* at 561 (quoting *Cincinnati v. Discovery Network, Inc.,* 507 U.S. 410, 417 [1993]).

106. *Thompson v. Western States Medical Center,* 535 U.S. 357 (2002).

107. 44 *Liquormart,* 517 U.S. at 501 (stating that not "*all* commercial speech regulations are subject to a similar form of constitutional review").

108. *Zauderer v. Office of Disciplinary Counsel,* 471 U.S. 626, 647 (1985). See also *Bad Frog Brewery, Inc. v. New York State Liquor Authority,* 134 F.3d 87, 96–97 (2d Cir. 1998) (holding that the label displaying a frog giving a well-known insulting gesture was reasonably understood as conveying the source of the product).

109. *Compare* David A. Strauss, "Persuasion, Autonomy and Freedom of Expression," *Columbia Law Review,* 91 (1991): 334–71, *with* Sylvia Law, "Addiction, Autonomy and Advertising," *Iowa Law Review,* 77 (1992): 909–55, 909.

110. 44 *Liquormart,* 517 U.S. at 501 ("When a State entirely prohibits the dissemination of truthful, nonmisleading commercial messages for reasons unrelated to the preservation of a fair bargaining process, there is far less reason to depart from the rigorous review that the First Amendment generally demands. . . . [C]omplete speech bans, unlike content-neutral restrictions on the time, place, or manner of expression, are particularly dangerous because they all but foreclose alternative means of disseminating certain information").

111. *Greater New Orleans Broadcasting Ass'n v. United States,* 527 U.S. 173 191 (1999) ("The government is committed to prohibiting accurate product information, not commercial enticements of all kinds, and then only conveyed over certain forms of media and for certain types of gambling").

112. *Anheuser-Busch, Inc. v. Schmoke,* 101 F.3d 325, 329 (4th Cir. 1996)

(upholding an ordinance prohibiting the placement of stationary outdoor alcohol beverage advertisements in certain areas where children walk to school or play because it merely restricts "time, place, and manner" and "does not foreclose the plethora of newspaper, magazine, radio, television, direct mail, Internet, and other media"); see *Penn Advertising, Inc. v. Mayor of Baltimore,* 101 F.3d 332 (4th Cir. 1996) (upholding an ordinance banning billboard advertisements for cigarettes in areas children frequent).

113. The *Schmoke* case, for example, distinguished between alcoholic beverage advertisements targeted to adults (as in 44 *Liquormart*) and those targeted to children.

114. Where advertising reaches both a lawful and an unlawful audience, the Court grants the commercial speech constitutional protection, but arguably at a lower level. *United States v. Edge Broadcasting Co.,* 509 U.S. 418, 428 (1993). The government's interest in protecting children does not justify an unnecessarily broad suppression of speech addressed to adults. *Reno v. American Civil Liberties Union,* 521 U.S. 844, 875 (1997) (invalidating a statute prohibiting transmission of obscene or indecent communications through the Internet to persons under age eighteen).

115. See, e.g., *Denver Area Educ. Telecomm. Consortium, Inc. v. FCC,* 518 U.S. 727, 744–45 (1996) (upholding cable television restrictions as a means of protecting children from indecent programming); *FCC v. Pacifica Found.,* 438 U.S. 726, 749 (1978) (upholding the FCC finding that indecent speech "in an afternoon broadcast when children are in the audience was patently offensive"); *Ginsberg v. New York,* 390 U.S. 629, 636 (1968) (rejecting the assertion that "the scope of the constitutional freedom of expression . . . cannot be made to depend on whether the citizen is an adult or a minor").

116. *Schmoke,* 101 F.3d at 329.

117. *Rubin v. Coors Brewing,* 514 U.S. 476, 482 (1995).

118. *Cincinnati v. Discovery Network, Inc.,* 507 U.S. 410, 424–30 (1993).

119. The United Kingdom has issued guidelines for labeling food with a color code (a red, amber, or green traffic light symbol) to inform consumers of the nutritional content in packaged foods. Felicity Lawrence, "Why Kellogg's Saw Red over Labeling Scheme," *Guardian,* December 28, 2006.

120. Related to warnings in the health context are compelled disclaimers in the consumer protection context. See *Borgner v. Brooks,* 284 F.3d 1204 (11th Cir. 2002), *cert. denied,* 123 S. Ct. 688 (2002) (upholding the requirement for a disclaimer that implant dentistry is not recognized in Florida).

121. William M. Sage, "Regulating through Information: Disclosure Laws and American Health Care," *Columbia Law Review,* 100 (1999): 1701–1829.

122. California Proposition 65, for example, requires businesses to provide a "clear and reasonable" warning before knowingly exposing anyone to a listed chemical carcinogen. *Safe Drinking Water and Toxic Enforcement Act of 1986,* Cal. Health & Safety Code §§ 25249.5–.13 (West 1992 & Supp. 1999). See Clifford Rechtschaffen, "The Warning Game: Evaluating Warnings under California's Proposition 65," *Ecology Law Quarterly,* 23 (1996): 303–68.

123. "Groups Petition FCC for Alcohol Counter-Ads, *Alcoholism and Drug Weekly,* May 26, 1997 (discussing counteradvertising proposals made by the Na-

tional Council on Alcoholism and Drug Dependence, Mothers against Drunk Driving, and twenty-two other organizations); Kathryn Murphy, "Can the Budweiser Frogs Be Forced to Sing a New Tune? Compelled Commercial Counter-Speech and the First Amendment," *Virginia Law Review*, 84 (1998): 1195–224.

124. *Vango Media, Inc. v. City of New York*, 829 F. Supp. 572 (S.D.N.Y. 1993) (finding that a New York City administrative law requiring the display of one public health message for every four tobacco advertisements on city property was preempted under the *Federal Cigarette Labeling and Advertising Act of 1965*, 15 U.S.C. §§ 1331–1340 [2000]).

125. The "fairness doctrine" (47 U.S.C. § 315 [1934]) required broadcasters to air public issues and give each side fair coverage. In 1972, Congress expanded the doctrine from political campaigns to "controversial matters of public importance." *Red Lion Broadcasting Co. v. FCC*, 395 U.S. 367 (1969) (validating the fairness doctrine under the First Amendment because government licenses broadcasters to use scarce resources).

126. *Larus & Brother Co. v. F.C.C.*, 447 F.2d 876 (4th Cir. 1971) (holding that tobacco is no longer a "controversial issue" for the purposes of the fairness doctrine); *Banzhaf v. F.C.C.*, 405 F.2d 1082 (D.C. Cir. 1968) (applying the fairness doctrine to tobacco advertising is constitutional); *cert. denied, sub nom. Tobacco Institute, Inc. v. F.C.C.*, 396 U.S. 842 (1969); *In re Television Station* WCBS-TV, *New York*, 9 F.C.C.2d 921 (1967) (applying the fairness doctrine to cigarette advertising, recognizing that tobacco is a controversial issue and emphasizing public health), aff'd *Banzhaf* 405 Fed. 876. The FCC abandoned the fairness doctrine in 1987. *In re Complaint of Syracuse Peace Council against Television Station* WTUH, 2 F.C.C.R. 5043 (1987).

127. *Wooley v. Maynard*, 430 U.S. 705, 714 (1977) ("The right of freedom of thought protected by the First Amendment against state action includes both the right to speak freely and the right to refrain from speaking at all"). As a corollary principle, government may not compel individuals to subsidize speech by private organizations such as trade unions and bar associations. See, e.g., *Abood v. Detroit Board of Education*, 431 U.S. 209 (1977) (pertaining to compelled contributions to union's agency shops); *Keller v. State Bar of Cal.*, 496 U.S. 1 (1990) (regarding state-compelled dues to an integrated bar association to advance political causes).

128. *West Virginia State Board of Education v. Barnette*, 319 U.S. 624 (1943).

129. *Wooley v. Maynard*, 430 U.S. 705 (1977).

130. *Talley v. California*, 362 U.S. 60 (1960).

131. *McIntyre v. Ohio Elections Comm.*, 514 U.S. 334 (1995).

132. Similarly, the Court has overturned state laws requiring groups to disclose their membership lists because they may discourage individuals from associating with an unpopular group. *Gibson v. Florida Legislative Investigation Committee*, 372 U.S. 539 (1963); *NAACP v. Alabama*, 357 U.S. 449 (1958). The Court has also invalidated state laws requiring parade organizers to include gay marchers, because it may discourage the organizers from holding the parade at all. *Hurley v. Irish-American Gay, Lesbian and Bisexual Group of Boston, Inc.*, 515 U.S. 557 (1995).

133. *Hurley v. Irish-American Gay, Lesbian and Bisexual Group of Boston,*

Inc., 515 U.S. 557 (1995) (upholding the right of parade organizers to exclude marchers who impart messages with which they do not agree).

134. *Boy Scouts of America v. Dale,* 530 U.S. 657 (2000) (upholding Boy Scouts' right to exclude a gay scoutmaster); but see *Rumsfeld v. Forum for Academic and Institutional Rights, Inc,* 547 U.S. 47 (2006) (finding that the Solomon Amendment, which requires law schools to host military recruiters as a condition of funding, does not compel speech).

135. *United States v. United Foods,* 533 U.S. 405 (2001).

136. *Id.* at 411.

137. *Glickman v. Wileman Brothers & Elliott, Inc.*, 521 U.S. 457 (1997) (upholding federal marketing orders requiring California fruit producers to fund a generic advertising program because it was ancillary to a comprehensive regulatory program).

138. *Johanns v. Livestock Marketing Association,* 544 U.S. 550 (2005) (holding that generic advertising funded by targeted assessment on beef producers was "government speech," and thus not susceptible to a First Amendment compelled-subsidy challenge).

139. See, e.g., 44 *Liquormart v. Rhode Island,* 517 U.S. 484, 501 (1996).

140. See, e.g., *United States v. Sullivan,* 332 U.S. 689, 693 (1948) (upholding a federal law requiring warning labels on "harmful foods, drugs and cosmetics").

141. *National Electrical Manufacturers Ass'n v. Sorrell,* 272 F.3d 104, 114 (2d Cir. 2001).

142. *Virginia State Board of Pharmacy v. Virginia Citizens Consumer Council, Inc.*, 425 U.S. 748, 772 (1976).

143. *Id.* at 772, n. 24 ("It is appropriate to require that a commercial message appear in such a form, or include such additional information, warnings and disclaimers as are necessary to prevent its being deceptive").

144. *Bates v. State Bar of Ariz.*, 433 U.S. 350, 384 (1977); see *In re R. M. J.*, 455 U.S. 191, 201 (1982) ("A warning or disclaimer might be appropriately required . . . in order to dissipate the possibility of consumer confusion or deception").

145. *Zauderer v. Office of Disciplinary Counsel,* 471 U.S. 626 (1985).

146. *Id.* at 651; but see *Ibanez v. Florida Department of Business and Professional Regulation,* 512 U.S. 136, 146–47 (1994) (finding the exhaustive disclaimer required in certain accountant advertisements overbroad).

147. 92 F.3d 67 (2d Cir. 1996); see *Cal-Almond, Inc. v. United States Dep't of Agriculture,* 14 F.3d 429 (9th Cir. 1993) (finding a marketing program requiring almond handlers to pay assessments toward advertising unconstitutional); *United States v. Frame,* 885 F.2d 119 (3d Cir. 1989), *cert. denied,* 493 U.S. 1094 (1990) (upholding a federal law requiring businesses to participate administratively and financially in the promotion of beef—"desirable, healthy, nutritious"—as constitutional).

148. *International Dairy Foods Ass'n v. Amestoy,* 92 F.3d 67, 73 (2d Cir. 1996).

149. *Id.* at 74 ("Were consumer interest alone sufficient, there is no end to the information that states could require manufacturers to disclose about their production methods"); but see the passionate dissent of Circuit Judge Leval, arguing that Vermont had legitimate concerns about human and animal health, novel biotechnology, and the survival of small dairy farms. *Id.* at 76.

150. Donna U. Vogt and Brian A. Jackson, *RS20507: Labeling of Genetically Modified Foods,* CRS Report for Congress, March 20, 2000.

151. Institute of Medicine, *Safety of Genetically Engineered Foods: Approaches to Assessing Unintended Health Effects* (Washington, DC: National Academies Press, 2004).

152. *Zauderer,* 471 U.S. at 651.

153. *Riley v. National Federation of the Blind,* 487 U.S. 781, 797–98 (1988).

154. *Glickman v. Wileman Bros. & Elliott, Inc.,* 521 U.S. 457, 471 (1997).

155. Susan Linn, *Beyond Commercials: Food Marketing to Children in the Twenty-first Century,* available at Informed Eating, "Special Report: Food Marketing to Children and the Law," October 13, 2006, http://www.informedeating.org/newsletters/051115.htm.

156. Jeffrey P. Koplan, Catharyn T. Liverman, and Vivica I. Kraak, eds., *Preventing Childhood Obesity: Health in the Balance* (Washington, DC: National Academies Press, 2005).

157. Wendy E. Parmet, "Free Speech and Public Health: A Population-Based Approach to the First Amendment," *Loyola of Los Angeles Law Review* 39 (2006): 363–446 (arguing that efforts to address the obesity epidemic must include an analysis of the role of commercial speech, as it is an important determinant of health).

158. McGinnis et al., *Food Marketing to Children and Youth.*

159. Linn, *Beyond Commercials.*

160. McGinnis et al., *Food Marketing to Children and Youth* (stating that the IOM could not, however, find conclusive evidence that advertising impacted the preferences, purchase requests, and beliefs of children twelve to eighteen years old).

161. Games featuring M&M candies can be found at the M&M Web site: http://us.mms.com/us/fungames/games/.

162. Linn, *Beyond Commercials.*

163. Institute of Medicine, *Food Marketing to Children and Youth: Threat or Opportunity* (Washington, DC: National Academies Press, 2006).

164. Amanda Spake, "Hey, Kids! We've Got Sugar and Toys," *US News,* November 17, 2003, http://www.usnews.com/usnews/health/articles/031117/17food.htm.

165. Center for Science in the Public Interest, *Junk Food in Schools Enjoys Bipartisan Support,* May 20, 2004, http://www.cspinet.org/new/200405201.html; Factiva, "Taste—Review and Outlook: Saving Us from Ourselves," *Wall Street Journal,* November 11, 2005 ("83% of American adults believe public schools need to do a better job of limiting children's access to unhealthy foods like snack foods, sugary soft drinks and fast food").

166. Lawrence O. Gostin, "Fast and Supersized: Is the Answer Diet by Fiat?" *Hastings Center Report,* 35 (2005): 11–12.

167. Institute of Medicine, *Nutrition Standards for Foods in Schools: Leading the Way toward Healthier Youth* (Washington, DC: National Academies Press, 2007).

168. USDA Food and Nutrition Service, "Healthy Schools," October 13, 2006, http://www.fns.usda.gov/tn/Healthy/wellnesspolicy_examples.html; USDA

Food and Nutrition Service, "School Breakfast Program," October 13, 2006, http://www.fns.usda.gov/cnd/breakfast/.

169. GAO, *School Lunch Program: Efforts Needed to Improve Nutrition and Encourage Healthy Eating* (2003), http://www.gao.gov/htext/d03506.html.

170. Institute of Medicine, *Food Marketing to Children and Youth: Threat or Opportunity.* There are indications that in the absence of government regulation, the snack food industry will voluntarily self-regulate, but the effects of these actions have yet to be seen. David B. Caruso, "Firms to Tout Healthy Snacks in Schools," *Boston Globe,* October 6, 2006 (discussing the decision by five snack food firms to stop supplying vending machines in schools); but see Centers for Disease Control and Prevention, "Youth Exposure to Advertising on Radio—United States, June–August 2004," *Morbidity and Mortality Weekly Report,* 55 (2006): 937–40 (describing how the beverage industry has ceased complying with a self-imposed ban on advertising to teenagers).

171. Tom Chornea, "Governor Signs Ban on Junk Food at California Schools," *San Francisco Chronicle,* September 16, 2005; Marian Burros, "Bottlers Agree to a School Ban on Sweet Drinks," *New York Times,* May 4, 2006.

172. Mark Vallianatos, *Healthy School Food Policies: A Checklist* (Los Angeles, CA: Center for Food and Justice, 2002).

173. Institute of Medicine, *Food Marketing to Children and Youth: Threat or Opportunity.*

174. *United States v. Jorgensen,* 144 F. 3d 550 (8th Cir. 1998).

175. *National Bakers Services, Inc. v. FTC,* 329 F.2d 365 (7th Cir. 1964).

176. 15 U.S.C. §§ 45(a)(1), 52(a)(1) (2002) (stating that the FTC is authorized to regulate "unfair or deceptive acts or practices in or affecting commerce" and, in particular, any "false advertisement . . . in or having an effect upon commerce, by any means, for the purpose of inducing, or which is likely to induce, directly or indirectly the purchase of food"); see FTC Policy Statement on Deception (1983), appended to *In re Cliffdale Associates, Inc.,* 103 F.T.C. 110, 174 (1984).

177. See FTC Policy Statement on Deception, available at http://www.ftc.gov/bcp/policystmt/ad-decept.htm.

178. In assessing product liability claims involving children, for example, courts often distinguish between what can be expected of a "reasonable child" and that expected of a "reasonable adult." See, e.g., *Swix v. Daisy Manufacturing Co.,* 373 F.3d 678 (6th Cir. 2004) (holding that in a product liability action the "reasonable child" and not the "reasonable adult" standard should apply when the typical user of the product is a child); *Bunch v. Hoffinger Industries, Inc.,* 329 F.3d 948 (2003).

179. Angela J. Campbell, "Restricting the Marketing of Junk Food to Children by Product Placement and Character Selling," *Loyola of Los Angeles Law Review,* 39 (2006): 447–505 (arguing that advertisements targeted to children are inherently misleading, making them unlawful under the first prong of *Central Hudson*).

180. Institute of Medicine, *Food Marketing to Children and Youth: Threat or Opportunity.*

181. Council of Better Business Bureaus, Children's Advertising Review Unit, "Self-Regulatory Program for Children's Advertising," 2006, http://www.caru.org

/guidelines/guidelines.pdf; John Schmeltzer, "Critics Sour on Rules for Kids' Food Ads," *Chicago Tribune,* November 15, 2006.

182. Merissa Marr and Janet Adamy, "Disney Pulls Its Characters from Junk Food," *Wall Street Journal,* October 17, 2006.

183. 16 C.F.R § 312.3 (2000) (stating that during the collection of information, privacy policies must be clearly displayed, parental permission must be obtained, and a child's participation in games or contests must not be conditioned "on the child disclosing more personal information than is reasonably necessary to participate in such activity").

184. Institute of Medicine, *Food Marketing to Children and Youth: Threat or Opportunity.*

185. *Video Software Dealers Ass'n v. Maleng,* 325 F. Supp. 2d 1180 (2004); *American Amusement Machine Ass'n v. Kendrick,* 244 F.3d 572 (2001).

186. Campbell, "Restricting the Marketing of Junk Food to Children."

187. See Gail H. Javitt, "Supersizing the Pint-Sized: The Need for FDA Mandated Child-Oriented Food Labeling," *Loyola of Los Angeles Law Review,* 39 (2006): 311–61 (arguing that the FDA needs to better implement the Nutrition Labeling and Education Act).

10. MEDICAL COUNTERMEASURES FOR EPIDEMIC DISEASE: BODILY INTEGRITY

SOURCES FOR CHAPTER EPIGRAPHS: Paul De Kruif, *Microbe Hunters* (New York: Harcourt, Brace, 1996): 115; Edward Jenner, *The Origin of the Vaccine Inoculation* (London: D. N. Shury, 1801); John Duffy, "School Vaccination: The Precursor to School Medical Inspection," *Journal of the History of Medicine and Allied Sciences,* 344 (1978): 344–55; Walter R. Dowdle, "The 1976 Experience," *Journal of Infectious Diseases,* 176 (1997): S69–S72; Institute of Medicine, *Reducing the Odds: Preventing Perinatal Transmission of HIV in the United States* (Washington, DC: National Academies Press, 1999): 37; *Union Pacific Ry. Co. v. Botsford,* 141 U.S. 250 (1891): 251.

1. The definition of *epidemic* is: "Of a disease: Prevalent among a people or a community at a special time, and produced by some special causes not generally present in the affected locality." It comes from the French *épidémique,* from *épidémie,* via late Latin from Greek *epidēmia* "prevalence of disease," from *epidēmios* "prevalent," from *epi* "upon" + *dēmos* "the people." *Oxford English Dictionary,* 2d ed. (Oxford: Oxford University Press, 1984). See Paul M. V. Martin and Estelle Martin-Granel, "2,500-Year Evolution of the Term *Epidemic,*" *Emerging Infectious Diseases,* 12 (2006): 976–80 ("The term epidemic already existed in 430 BC. The Greek word *epidemios* is constructed by combining the preposition *epi* [on] with the noun *demos* [people], but demos originally meant 'the country' [inhabited by its people] before taking the connotation 'the people' in classical Greek").

2. Joseph H. Bates and William W. Stead, "The History of Tuberculosis as a Global Epidemic," *Medical Clinics of North America,* 77 (1993): 1205–17 (stating that tuberculosis was initially a disease of lower mammals, and the etiologic agent probably preceded the development of man on earth).

3. George Rosen, *A History of Public Health* (Baltimore, MD: Johns Hopkins University Press, 1993).

4. Smallpox vaccination was preceded by the practice of variolation, believed to have originated in Central Asia in the early part of the second century. This technique, introduced to North America in 1721, consisted of an inoculation into the skin of a small amount of material taken from the pustule or scab of a smallpox patient. The intradermal transmission route induced a milder form of smallpox that afforded immunity against more serious infection acquired by the respiratory route. This benefit notwithstanding, variolation entailed a significant risk of the nonimmune person actually contracting and spreading the disease. John M. Barry, *The Great Influenza: The Epic Story of the Deadliest Plague in History* (New York: Penguin Books, 2005); Laura Gregario, "The Smallpox Legacy: A History of Pediatric Immunizations," *Pharos,* 7 (1996): 7–8.

5. Jenner's original work was self-published in 1798 under the title *An Inquiry into the causes and effects of the variolae vaccinae, a disease discovered in some of the western counties of England, particularly Gloucestershire, and known by the name of the Cow pox*. As a physician, Jenner had firsthand knowledge of the risks associated with variolation. His seminal innovation consisted of transferring a similar (and milder) agent—cowpox virus—instead of the smallpox virus, to a nonexposed individual. C. W. Dixon, *The History of Inoculation for the Smallpox* (London: Churchill, 1962); Donald A. Henderson, "Edward Jenner's Vaccine," *Public Health Reports,* 112 (1997): 116–21. The earliest European law on inoculation predated Jenner. Switzerland (Berne), Decree No. 119 of 21 March 1777 on Inoculation against Smallpox: "To prevent any further, uninterrupted spread of the epidemic of smallpox, it is hereby prescribed that inoculation against smallpox or children-pox should be made available to everyone, subject to the following restriction being observed namely that inoculation will not be carried out in towns but only in the countryside, and only during the spring and autumn."

6. Rosen, *A History of Public Health;* Barry, *The Great Influenza.*

7. In modern scientific terminology, vaccination is the administration of a vaccine or toxoid used to prevent, ameliorate, or treat infectious disease. A vaccine is a suspension of attenuated or noninfectious micro-organisms (bacteria, viruses, or rickettsiae), or derivative antigenic proteins. William Alexander Newman Dorland, *Dorland's Illustrated Medical Dictionary* (Philadelphia: W. B. Saunders, 2003). The terms *vaccination* and *immunization* are often used interchangeably. Immunization is the more inclusive term, denoting the process of inducing or providing immunity artificially by administering an immunobiologic. Immunization can be passive or active. Passive immunization involves the administration of antibodies produced by an immune animal or human, conferring short-term protection against infection. In active immunization (vaccination), the vaccine induces the host's own immune system to provide protection against the pathogen. W. Michael McDonnell and Frederick K. Askari, "Immunization," *JAMA,* 278 (1997): 2000–2007.

8. René Dubos and Thomas D. Brock, *Pasteur and Modern Science* (Washington, DC: American Society for Microbiology, 1998). The germ theory, of course, predated the pioneering microbiologists of the late nineteenth century.

Gerolamo Fracastoro, influenced by the syphilis epidemic, published his work *De Contagiounibus* in 1546. In 1675, Antoni van Leeuwenhoek was the first person to observe "animalcules" (protozoa) with a microscope. Abraham Schierbeek, *Measuring the Invisible World: The Life and Works of Antoni Van Leewenhoek* (London: Abelard-Schuman, 1959). Though Fracastoro and Leeuwenhoek both argued for the connection between microbes and disease, the doctrine of living contagion soon lost hold on the public and medicine, so that by the early nineteenth century the idea was discredited. John M. Eager, "Fighting Trim: The Importance of Right Living," *Public Health Reports,* 5 (1917).

9. Robert Koch, "A Further Communication on a Cure for Tuberculosis," in *From Consumption to Tuberculosis: A Documentary History,* ed. Barbara Gutmann Rosenkrantz (London: Garland, 1994).

10. Alexander Fleming, Howard H. Florey, and Ernst B. Chain, "On Antibacterial Action of Cultures of a Pencillium," *British Journal of Experimental Pathology,* 10 (1929).

11. Paul N. Zenker and Robert T. Rolfs, "Treatment of Syphilis, 1989," *Review of Infectious Diseases,* 12 (1990): S590–609.

12. Alexander Fleming, "Chemotherapy: Yesterday, To-day, To-morrow," Linacre Lectures, Cambridge University, Cambridge, May 6, 1946.

13. Centers for Disease Control and Prevention, "Ten Great Public Health Achievements, 1900–1999: Impact of Vaccines Universally Recommended for Children," *Morbidity and Mortality Weekly Report,* 48 (1999): 243–48.

14. Celia W. Dugger and Donald G. McNeil, Jr., "Rumor, Fear and Fatigue Hinder Final Push to End Polio," *New York Times,* March 20, 2006 ("The drive against polio threatens to become a costly display of all that can conspire against even the most ambitious efforts to eliminate a disease: cultural suspicions, logistical nightmares, competition for resources from many other afflictions, and simple exhaustion").

15. Jenifer Ehreth, "The Global Value of Vaccination," *Vaccine,* 21 (2003): 596–600.

16. Irina Serdobova and Marie-Paule Kieny, "Assembling a Global Vaccine Development Pipeline for Infectious Diseases in the Developing World," *American Journal of Public Health,* 96 (2006): 1554–59 (describing World Health Assembly Global Immunization Vision and Strategy 2006–2015); see Howard Markel, "The Search for Effective HIV Vaccines," *New Engl. J. Med.,* 353 (2005): 753–57; Susan Okie, "Betting on a Malaria Vaccine," *New Engl. J. Med.,* 353 (2005): 1877–81.

17. Centers for Disease Control and Prevention, "Update: Childhood Vaccine-Preventable Diseases: United States, 1994," *Morbidity and Mortality Weekly Report,* 43 (1994): 718–20. Smallpox was eradicated in 1979, and polio is on the verge of eradication (the last indigenous case in the United States occurred in 1979, and only fourteen countries are still reporting transmission as of mid-2006). World Health Organization, "The State of Polio Eradication," September 12, 2006, http://www.polioeradication.org/content/general/current_monthly_sitrep.asp. Moreover, diseases against which children routinely have been vaccinated have declined by 99 percent or more and are at all-time lows. Kevin M. Malone and Alan R. Hinman, "Vaccination Mandates: The Public Health Im-

perative and Individual Rights," in *Law in Public Health Practice,* ed. Richard A. Goodman, Marc A. Rothstein, R. E. Hoffman, et al. (New York: Oxford University Press, 2003): 262–84.

18. Daniel A. Salmon, Stephen P. Teret, C. Raina MacIntyre, et al., "Compulsory Vaccination and Conscientious or Philosophical Exemptions: Past, Present, and Future," *Lancet,* 367 (2006): 436–42. The first case discussing citizens' objections to vaccination requirements in the United States was *Hazen v. Strong,* 2 Vt. 427 (1830) (upholding the power of a town council to pay for vaccination of persons exposed even though there were no cases of smallpox).

19. Thomas Jefferson was an active supporter of Prof. Benjamin Waterhouse, an American disciple of Jenner, who actively practiced vaccination. Rosen, *A History of Public Health.*

20. These claims were evident as the Supreme Court struggled with the issue of vaccination in *Jacobson v. Massachusetts,* 197 U.S. 11 (1905): "Some physicians of great skill and repute do not believe that vaccination is a preventive" (quoting *Viemeister v. White,* 179 N.Y. 235, 239 [1904]). "Vaccination quite often caused serious and permanent injury to the health of the person vaccinated." *Id.* at 36 (quoting Henning Jacobson). "Compulsory vaccination is "hostile to the inherent right of every freeman to care for his own body and health." *Id.* at 15–16 (quoting Henning Jacobson).

21. James Colgrove, *State of Immunity: The Politics of Vaccination in Twentieth-Century America* (Berkeley: University of California Press, 2006); Steve P. Calandrillo, "Vanishing Vaccinations: Why Are So Many Americans Opting Out of Vaccinating Their Children?" *University of Michigan Journal of Law Reform,* 37 (2004): 353–439.

22. Kristine M. Severyn, " *Jacobson v. Massachusetts:* Impact on Informed Consent and Vaccine Policy," *Journal of Pharmacy and Law,* 5 (1996): 260–61; Charles L. Jackson, "State Laws on Compulsory Immunization in the United States," *Public Health Reports,* 84 (1969): 792–94.

23. Robert M. Wolfe, Lisa K. Sharp, and Martin S. Lipsky, "Content and Design Attributes of Antivaccination Websites," *JAMA,* 287 (2002): 3245–48.

24. Institute of Medicine, *Immunization Safety Review: Vaccines and Autism* (Washington, DC: National Academies Press, 2004).

25. California and Iowa ban thimerosal-containing vaccines, and bills are pending in other states. New York, effective in 2008, requires the commissioner to state annually that there are adequate supplies of thimerosal-free vaccines. Myron Levin, "Battle Lines Drawn over Mercury in Shots: States Push for Bans in Children's Vaccines; but Leading Medical Groups Are Pushing Back," *Los Angeles Times,* April 10, 2006.

26. British Medical Association Board of Science and Education, *Childhood Immunization: A Guide for Healthcare Professionals* (London: BMA, 2003) (concluding that compulsory vaccination was not appropriate for the United Kingdom, despite the decrease in vaccine coverage for measles, mumps, and rubella [MMR]).

27. Lawrence O. Gostin and Catherine D. DeAngelis, "Mandatory HPV Vaccination: Public Health vs. Private Wealth," *JAMA,* 297 (2007): 1921–23; James Colgrove, "The Ethics and Politics of Compulsory HPV Vaccination," *New Engl. J. Med.,* 355 (2007): 2389–91; Nancy Gibbs, "Defusing the War over the 'Pro-

miscuity' Vaccine," *Time,* June 21, 2006; Peter Sprigg, "Pro-Family, Pro-Vaccine: But Keep It Voluntary," *Washington Post,* July 15, 2006.

28. Institute of Medicine, *Risk Communication and Vaccination Workshop Summary* (Washington, DC: National Academies Press, 1997): 11.

29. Institute of Medicine, *Vaccines for the Twenty-first Century: A Tool for Decisionmaking* (Washington, DC: National Academies Press, 1999). In 1993, the World Bank stated that child immunization is one of the most cost-effective health interventions available. World Bank, *Investing in Health: The World Development Report 1993* (Washington, DC: World Bank, 1993).

30. Institute of Medicine, *Vaccine Safety Research, Data Access, and Public Trust* (Washington, DC: National Academies Press, 2005).

31. Angus Dawson, "The Determination of 'Best Interests' in Relation to Childhood Vaccinations," *Bioethics,* 19 (2005): 188–205.

32. The last case of poliomyelitis in the United States due to indigenously acquired wild poliovirus occurred in 1979. To reduce vaccine-associated paralytic polio (VAPP), national vaccine policy changed in 2000 from reliance on OPV to inactivated poliovirus vaccine (IPV). Lorraine Nino Alexander, Jane F. Seward, Tammy A. Santibanez, et al., "Vaccine Policy Changes and Epidemiology of Poliomyelitis in the United States," *JAMA,* 292 (2004): 1696–1701 (the change in vaccine policy from OPV to exclusive use of IPV led to elimination of VAPP in the United States).

33. Angus Dawson, "Herd Protection as a Public Good: Vaccination and Our Obligations to Others," in *Ethics, Prevention, and Public Health,* ed. Angus Dawson and Marcel Verweij (Oxford: Oxford University Press, 2007); Arthur Allen, "For the Good of the Herd," *New York Times,* January 25, 2007.

34. Under the principle of herd immunity, a population becomes resistant to attack by a disease if a large proportion of its members are immune. This concept explains why some members of a group can remain unvaccinated and the group can still remain protected against disease. Leon Gordis, *Epidemiology,* 3d ed. (Philadelphia: W. B. Saunders, 2004): 20.

35. Garrett Hardin, "The Tragedy of the Commons," *Science,* 162 (1968): 1243.

36. Although there were outbreaks of other diseases, Louis Pasteur had not yet developed the cholera vaccine, and the next major vaccine discoveries—Salk's discovery of the polio vaccine and Smith's discovery of a diphtheria toxin—did not occur until the early and middle twentieth century.

37. William Packer Prentice, *Police Powers Arising under the Law of Overruling Necessity* (Littleton, CO: Fred B. Rothman, 1993): 132 ("Compulsory vaccination has been instituted . . . by the laws of several States, in respect to minors. City ordinances regulate it, but the indirect methods of excluding children not vaccinated from schools and factories, or, in case of immigrants, insisting upon quarantine, and the offer of free vaccination . . . are more effective"); Charles L. Jackson, "State Laws on Compulsory Immunization in the United States," *Public Health Reports,* 84 (1969): 792–94 (stating that Massachusetts enacted the first mandatory vaccination law in 1809).

38. Duffy, "School Vaccination"; Malone and Hinman, "Vaccination Mandates."

39. *Jacobson v. Massachusetts,* 197 U.S. 11 (1905); *Viemeister v. White,* 179 N.Y. 235 (1904) (upholding a New York statute excluding from public schools all children who had not been vaccinated: "Nearly every state in the Union has statutes to encourage, or directly or indirectly to require, vaccination; and this is true of most nations of Europe" [*Id.* at 239–40]); William Fowler, "Principal Provisions of Smallpox Vaccination Laws and Regulations in the United States," *Public Health Reports,* 56 (1942): 325 (stating that only six states did not have a smallpox vaccination statute). It was not until the late 1930s that compulsory immunization laws pertaining to other diseases were enacted. William Fowler, "State Diphtheria Immunization Requirements," *Public Health Reports,* 57 (1942): 325.

40. In 1894, antivaccinationists in Rhode Island came within one vote of repealing an existing state school vaccination law. In Louisiana, a city physician showed high school girls a picture of a boy who had contracted erysipelas, a painful skin disease, as a result of smallpox vaccination. The girls naturally refused to be vaccinated despite a mandatory policy of the state board of health. In Chicago, active resistance contributed to recurring epidemics of smallpox in 1893–94, when less than 10 percent of schoolchildren were vaccinated despite a twelve-year old state law requiring vaccination. Duffy, "School Vaccination."

41. Centers for Disease Control and Prevention, "Measles and School Immunization Requirements—United States," *Morbidity and Mortality Weekly Reports,* 27 (1978): 303–4 (noting that states which strictly enforced vaccination laws had measles incidence rates more than 50 percent lower than in other states); Kenneth B. Robbins, David Brandling-Bennett, and Alan R. Hinman, "Low Measles Incidence: Association with Enforcement of School Immunization Laws," *American Journal of Public Health,* 71 (1981): 270–74 (noting that states with low incidence rates were significantly more likely to have and enforce laws requiring immunization of the entire school population).

42. In Alaska, 8.3 percent of the students failed to provide proof of vaccination and were excluded from school. In Los Angeles, approximately 4 percent of the students were excluded. The number of measles cases dropped significantly, demonstrating that the enforcement of mandatory vaccination was effective. Alan R. Hinman, Walter A. Orenstein, Don E. Williamson, et al., "Tools to Prevent Infectious Disease: Childhood Immunization: Laws That Work," *Journal of Law, Medicine, and Ethics,* 30 (2002): 122–27; John P. Middaugh and Lawrence D. Zyla, "Enforcement of School Immunization Law in Alaska," *JAMA,* 239 (1978): 2128.

43. Walter A. Orenstein and Alan R. Hinman, "The Immunization System in the United States: The Role of School Immunization Laws," *Vaccine,* 17 (1999): S19–S24.

44. Hinman, Orenstein, Williamson, et al., "Tools to Prevent Infectious Disease"; Malone and Hinman, "Vaccination Mandates."

45. National Network for Immunization Information, *Immunization Policy: Indications, Recommendations and Immunzation Mandates* (2005), http://www.immunizationinfo.org/immunization_policy_detail.cfv.

46. ACIP is a scientific advisory committee composed of fifteen experts selected by the director of the CDC and the Secretary of the Department of Health

and Human Services. The ACIP considers how the use of a new vaccine might fit into existing child and adult immunization programs. Advisory Committee on Immunization Practices, "Combination Vaccines for Childhood Immunization," *Morbidity and Mortality Weekly Report,* 48 (1999): 1–15; current CDC recommendations are available at http://www.cdc.gov.

47. National Network for Immunization Information, *Immunization Policy;* Kathryn M. Edwards, "State Mandates and Childhood Immunization," *JAMA,* 284 (2000): 3171–73. Some European countries are being criticized for failing to integrate hepatitis B vaccine into national immunization policies, as recommended by the WHO. One can argue, however, that the WHO's recommendation might not really apply to countries like Britain, which have hepatitis B virus carrier rates as low as 0.3% and report yearly incidences of acute infection of about 1/100,000. Philip P. Mortimer and Elizabeth Miller, "Commentary: Antenatal Screening and Targeting Should Be Sufficient in Some Countries," *British Medical Journal,* 314 (1997): 1036–37.

48. Marcel Verweij and Angus Dawson, "Ethical Principles for Collective Immunization Programmes," *Vaccine,* 22 (2004): 3122–26 (listing seven principles for collective vaccination programs: serious health threat, safety and effectiveness, small burden, favorable burden-benefit ratio, just distribution, voluntary if possible, and public trust).

49. As of 2000, all states require, as a condition of school entry, proof of vaccination against diphtheria, tetanus, measles, rubella, and polio; forty-two require mumps vaccine; thirty-nine require pertussis vaccine, thirty-one require hepatitis B vaccine, twenty-three require aemophilus influenza vaccine, and five require varicella (chicken pox) vaccine. James G. Hodge, Jr., and Lawrence O. Gostin, "School Vaccination Requirements: Historical, Social, and Legal Perspectives," *Kentucky Law Journal,* 90 (2002): 831–90.

50. Lawrence O. Gostin and Zita Lazzarini, "Childhood Immunization Registries: A National Review of Public Health Information Systems and the Protection of Privacy," *JAMA,* 274 (1995): 1793–99.

51. Daniel A. Salmon, Jason W. Sapsin, Stephen Teret, et al., "Public Health and the Politics of School Immunization Requirements," *American Journal of Public Health,* 94 (2005): 778–83.

52. *W. Va. Code* § 16–3-4 (1999); *Brown v. Stone,* 378 So.2d 218 (Miss. 1979), *cert. denied,* 449 U.S. 887 (1980) (holding religious exemption unconstitutional).

53. The language of religious exemptions varies from a strict standard ("recognized church or denomination whose teachings forbid vaccination," *Ark. Code Ann.* § 6–18–702 [2002]) to a more vague standard ("belief in relation to a Supreme being," *Del. Code Ann.,* Tit. 14, § 131 [2000]).

54. As of 2006–2007, twenty states had exemptions for nonreligious objections, such as moral, philosophical, or personal beliefs (Arkansas, Arizona, California, Colorado, Idaho, Louisiana, Maine, Michigan, Minnesota, New Mexico, North Dakota, Ohio, Oklahoma, Oregon, Pennsylvania, Texas, Utah, Vermont, Washington, and Wisconsin). Johns Hopkins Bloomberg School of Public Health, Institute of Vaccine Safety, http://www.vaccinesafety.edu/cc-exem.htm.

55. Jennifer S. Rota, Daniel A. Salmon, Lance E. Rodewald, et al., "The Process for Obtaining Nonmedical Exemptions to State Immunization Laws," *American Journal of Public Health,* 91 (2000): 645–48; Daniel A. Salmon, Saad B. Omer, Lawrence H. Moulton, et al., "The Role of School Policies and Implementation Procedures on School Immunization Requirements and Non-Medical Exemptions," *American Journal of Public Health,* 9 (2005): 436–40.

56. National Vaccine Advisory Committee, *Report of the NVAC Working Group on Philosophical Exemptions* (Atlanta, GA: Centers for Disease Control and Prevention, 1998) (noting that total exemptions in the 1994–95 school year were less than 1 percent of school entrants).

57. Thomas Novotny, Charles E. Jennings, Mary Doran, et al., "Measles Outbreaks in Religious Groups Exempt from Immunization Laws," *Public Health Reports,* 103 (1988): 49–54 (articulating that exemptors were between twenty-two and thirty-five times more likely to contract measles and 5.9 times more likely to acquire pertussis than vaccinated children). Moreover, when more people are exempted from immunization, the number of disease cases in the nonexempt population increases. Daniel R. Feikin, Dennis C. Lezotte, Richard F. Hamman, et al., "Individual and Community Risks of Measles and Pertussis Associated with Personal Exemptions to Immunization," *JAMA,* 284 (2000): 3145–50.

58. Daniel A. Salmon, Michael Haber, Eugene J. Gangarosa, et al., "Health Consequences of Religious and Philosophical Exemptions from Immunization Laws: Individual and Societal Risk of Measles," *JAMA,* 282 (1999): 47–53.

59. Saad B. Omer, William K. Y. Pan, Neal A. Halsey, et al., "Nonmedical Exemptions to School Immunization Requirements: Secular Trends and Association of State Policies with Pertussis Incidence," *JAMA,* 296 (2006): 1757–63 (from 2001 to 2004, states that offered personal belief exemptions had higher rates of nonmedical exemptions, and easier granting of exemptions and availability of personal belief exemptions were both associated with increased pertussis incidence).

60. 10 U.S.C. §1107 (1998).

61. *Doe v. Rumsfeld,* 297 F. Supp. 2d 119 (D.D.C. 2003) (finding that anthrax vaccine adsorbed [AVA] is an experimental drug unlicensed for its present use, and issuing a preliminary injunction against mandatory AVA).

62. Health officials, for example, may recommend immunizations for susceptible populations, such as the elderly (e.g., seasonal influenza and pneumonia), workers or hobbyists who work with animals (e.g., rabies), or individuals exposed to infection (e.g., rabies after an animal bite or tetanus after a puncture wound). For a collection of immunization laws, see Centers for Disease Control and Prevention, National Vaccine Program Office, "Immunization Laws," September 26, 2006, http://www.hhs.gov/nvpo/law.htm.

63. Vaccines needed for health care workers are hepatitis B, influenza, measles-mumps-rubella, and varicella (chicken pox). Centers for Disease Control and Prevention, "Adult Immunization Schedule," April 18, 2006, http://www.cdc.gov/nip/recs/adult-schedule.htm.

64. Following Hurricane Katrina, the CDC recommended certain vaccines for individuals providing assistance in the disaster area. Centers for Disease Control and Prevention, "Questions and Answers about Immunization Recommen-

dations following Hurricane Katrina," October 12, 2005, http://www.bt.cdc.gov/disasters/hurricanes/katrina/immunizationqa.asp.

65. Centers for Disease Control and Prevention, "Immunization Laws."

66. *Illegal Immigration Reform and Immigrant Responsibility Act of 1996,* Pub. L. No. 104–208, 110 Stat. 3009–546, § 341.

67. James A. Tobey, *Public Health Law: A Manual of Law for Sanitarians* (Baltimore, MD: Williams and Wilkins, 1926): 89–98 (assembling sixty-seven court cases, almost always upholding state power to vaccinate); James A. Tobey, "Vaccination and the Courts," *JAMA,* 83 (1924): 462.

68. *Wong Wai v. Williamson,* 103 F. 1 (C.C.N.D. Cal. 1900).

69. *Jacobson v. Massachusetts,* 197 U.S. 1 (1905).

70. See, e.g., *Maricopa County Health Department v. Harmon,* 750 P.2d 1364 (Ariz. Ct. App. 1987); *Cude v. State,* 377 S.W.2d 816 (Ark. 1964) (citing numerous precedents); *Brown v. Stone,* 378 So. 2d 218 (Miss. 1979), *cert. denied,* 449 U.S. 887 (1980).

71. *Zucht v. King,* 260 U.S. 174 (1922). State supreme courts also routinely upheld school vaccination requirements. See, e.g., *People ex rel. Hill v. Board of Education of the City of Lansing,* 195 N.W. 95 (Mich. 1923).

72. See, e.g., *Brown v. Stone,* 378 So.2d 218, 223 (Miss. 1979) ("The protection of the great body of school children . . . against the horrors of crippling and death resulting from [vaccine-preventable disease] demand that children who have not been immunized should be excluded from school. . . . To the extent that it may conflict with the religious beliefs of a parent, however sincerely entertained, the interests of the school children must prevail"); *Cude v. State,* 377 S.W.2d 816, 819 (Ark. 1964) ("According to the great weight of authority, it is within the police power of the State to require that school children be vaccinated . . . and that . . . it does not violate the constitutional rights of anyone, on religious grounds or otherwise").

73. *Employment Div. v. Smith,* 494 U.S. 872, 879 (1990); see *City of Boerne v. Flores,* 521 U.S. 507 (1997) (finding that Congress overstepped its authority in enacting the Religious Freedom Restoration Act of 1993, which attempted to legislatively override the ruling in *Smith*).

74. 321 U.S. 158, 166–67 (1944)

75. *Wright v. DeWitt School District No. 1,* 385 S.W.2d 644, 648 (Ark. 1965).

76. *Brown v. Stone,* 378 So. 2d 218 (Miss. 1979) (stating that the religious exemption violates equal protection of the laws because it "discriminates against the great majority of children whose parents have no such religious convictions. To give it effect would . . . expose [the great body of school children] . . . to the hazard of associating in school with children exempted . . . who had not been immunized").

77. See, e.g., *Mason v. General Brown Cent. School District,* 851 F.2d 47 (2d Cir. 1988); *Berg v. Glen Cove City School District,* 853 F. Supp. 651 (E.D.N.Y. 1994).

78. *Mason v. General Brown Cent. Sch. Dist.,* 851 F.2d 47 (2d Cir. 1988) (holding that parents' sincerely held belief that immunization was contrary to "genetic blueprint" was a secular, not religious, belief); *Hanzel v. Arter,* 625 F. Supp. 1259 (S.D. Ohio, 1985) (holding that parents with objections to vaccination based on

"chiropractic ethics" were not exempt); *McCartney v. Austin,* 293 N.Y.S.2d 188 (N.Y. Sup. Ct. 1968) (holding that a vaccination statute did not interfere with freedom of worship in the Roman Catholic faith, which does not have a proscription against vaccination); *In re Elwell,* 284 N.Y.S. 2d 924, 932 (Fam. Ct., Dutchess County 1967) (stating that though parents were members of a recognized religion, their objections to polio vaccine were not based on the tenets of their religion); but see *Berg v. Glen Cove City Sch. Dist.,* 853 F. Supp. 651, 655 (E.D.N.Y. 1994) (noting that although nothing in the Jewish religion prohibited vaccination, parents still had a sincere religious belief and were likely to succeed in their claim).

79. *Turner v. Liverpool Central School,* 186 F. Supp. 2d 187 (N.D.N.Y. 2002); *Jones ex rel. Jones v. State Department of Health,* 18 P.3d 1189 (Wyo. 2001) (finding that state law requires issuance of a religious waiver upon receipt of a written application and does not allow health officials to investigate the sincerity of the applicant's religious beliefs); *LePage v. State,* 18 P.3d 1177 (Wyo. 2001) (same).

80. Ross D. Silverman, "No More Kidding Around: Restructuring Non-Medical Childhood Immunization Exemptions to Ensure Public Health Protection," *Annals of Health Law,* 12 (2003): 277–94.

81. As a result of the conscientious objector cases arising out of the Vietnam War, most states have, however, removed such language from their statutes. Alicia Novak, "The Religious and Philosophical Exemptions to State-Compelled Vaccination: Constitutional and Other Challenges," *University of Pennsylvania Journal of Constitutional Law,* 7 (2005): 1101–29.

82. Compare *Sherr v. Northport-East Northport Union Free Sch. Dist.,* 672 F. Supp. 81, 91, 97 (E.D.N.Y. 1987) (upholding exemption for children of parents with "sincere religious beliefs," but finding that the provision requiring them to be "bona fide members of a recognized religious organization" violates the Establishment Clause); with *Kleid v. Board of Education,* 406 F. Supp. 902 (W.D. Ken. 1976) (exemption for a "nationally recognized and established church or religious denomination" does not violate the Establishment Clause).

83. *Dalli v. Board of Education,* 267 N.E.2d 219 (S. Jud. Ct. Mass. 1971) (articulating that an exemption for objectors who subscribe to the "tenets and practice of a recognized church or religious denomination" violates equal protection by extending preferred treatment to these groups while denying it to others with sincere religious objections).

84. *Boone v. Boozman,* 217 F. Supp. 2d 938 (E.D. Ark. 2002) (finding the state's requirement of a "recognized" religion violated the Establishment and Free Exercise Clauses as well as Equal Protection); *McCarthy v. Boozman,* 212 F. Supp. 2d 945 (W.D. Ark. 2002) (same); *In re Moses and Nagy v. Bayport Bluepoint Union Free School District,* No. 05-CV-3808 (E.D.N.Y. Feb. 13, 2007).

85. Arizona, Arkansas, California, Colorado, Idaho, Louisiana, Maine, Michigan, Minnesota, Missouri, Nebraska, New Mexico, North Dakota, Ohio, Oklahoma, Texas, Utah, Vermont, Washington, and Wisconsin. See Daniel A. Salmon and Andrew W. Siegel, "Religious and Philosophical Exemptions from Vaccination Requirements and Lessons Learned from Conscientious Objectors Conscription," *Public Health Reports,* 116 (2001): 289; Ross D. Silverman and Thomas May, "Private Choice versus Public Health: Religion, Morality, and Childhood Vaccination Law," *Margins,* 1 (2001): 505.

86. Daniel R. Feikin, Dennis C. Lezotte, Richard F. Hamman, et al., "Individual and Community Risks of Measles and Pertussis Associated with Personal Exemptions to Immunization," *JAMA,* 284 (2000): 3145–50 (stating that, overall, philosophical exemptions accounted for 87 percent of all exemptions); Donald G. McNeil, Jr., "When Parents Say No to Child Vaccination," *New York Times,* November 30, 2002.

87. Andrew Zoltan, "Jacobson Revisited: Mandatory Polio Vaccination as an Unconstitutional Condition," *George Mason Law Review,* 13 (2005): 735–64 (arguing that mandatory smallpox or polio vaccine would unacceptably increase the cost of exercising a constitutional right).

88. *Maricopa County Health Department v. Harmon,* 750 P.2d 1364 (Ariz. Ct. App. 1987).

89. *Cruzan v. Dir., Mo. Dep't of Health,* 497 U.S. 261, 278 (1990).

90. Lawrence O. Gostin, "*Jacobson v. Massachusetts* at One Hundred Years: Police Power and Civil Liberties in Tension," *American Journal of Public Health,* 95 (2005): 576–81; see also Wendy E. Parmet, "Informed Consent and Public Health: Are They Compatible When It Comes to Vaccines?" *Journal of Health Care Law and Policy,* 8 (2005): 71–110 (discussing the conflict between *Jacobson*'s recognition of the importance of public health and *Schloendorff's* respect for informed consent); D. George Joseph, "Uses of *Jacobson v. Massachusetts* in the Age of Bioterror," *JAMA,* 290 (2003): 2331 (discussing the Model State Emergency Health Powers Act in the historical context of *Jacobson*).

91. For a symposium on the "vaccine enterprise," see *Health Affairs,* 24 (2005): 594–769; see also David B. Rein, Amanda A. Honeycutt, Lucia Rojas-Smith, et al., "Impact of the CDC's Section 317 Immunization Grants Program Funding on Childhood Immunization," *American Journal of Public Health,* 96 (2006): 1548–53 (finding that federal funding of vaccination programs increases coverage rates).

92. Patricia M. Danzon, Nuno Sousa Pereira, and Sapna S. Tejwani, "Vaccine Supply: A Cross-National Perspective," *Health Affairs,* 24 (2005): 706–17.

93. Frank A. Sloan, Stephen Berman, Sara Rosenbaum, et al., "The Fragility of the U.S. Vaccine Supply," *New Engl. J. Med.,* 351 (2004): 2443–47.

94. Scott A. Harper, Keiji Fukuda, Timothy M. Uyeki, et al., "Prevention and Control of Influenza: Recommendations of the Advisory Committee on Immunization Practices," *Morbidity and Mortality Weekly Report,* 54 (2005): 1–40; Kathleen M. Neuzil and Marie R. Griffin, "Vaccine Safety: Achieving the Proper Balance," *JAMA,* 294 (2005): 2763–65.

95. Department of Health and Human Services, "Statement from the Department of Health and Human Services regarding Chiron Flu Vaccine," news release, October 5, 2004.

96. World Health Organization, Department of Communicable Disease Surveillance and Response, "Vaccines for Pandemic Influenza: Informal Meeting of WHO, Influenza Vaccine Manufacturers, National Licensing Agencies, and Government Representatives on Influenza Pandemic Vaccines," November 11–12, 2004, http://www.who.int/csr/resources/publications/influenza/WHO_CDS_CSR_GIP_2004_3/en/.

97. Although vaccines account only for a small percentage of pharmaceuti-

cal industry profits, development costs are high. Drug industry experts estimate that it costs nearly $900 million to bring a new vaccine to the market. The major costs are for clinical trials and for capital investments in new plants and infrastructure required to produce safe, reproducible, and effective vaccines. Furthermore, for new vaccines most of the investment must be made up front, before the vaccine's safety and efficacy are fully known and before the markets for the new product become clear. Tufts Center for the Study of Drug Development, "Total Cost to Develop a New Prescription Drug, Including Cost of Post-Approval Research, Is $897 Million," May 13, 2003, http://csdd.tufts.edu/NewsEvents/RecentNews.asp?newsid = 29.

98. In contrast to medications for chronic conditions that are taken repeatedly, the market for vaccines is limited. In most cases, individuals are injected just a few times in their lifetime, making demand for vaccines far smaller than the demand for medications taken repeatedly. Moreover, without government intervention, there is no ready market for vaccines developed for rare pathogens that could be used by a bioterrorist, or that may reemerge either by accident or due to changing environmental circumstances.

99. Under FDA regulations, vaccines, as biologics, are subject to particularly intense oversight and regulatory monitoring, adding to the cost of manufacture.

100. Institute of Medicine, *The Children's Vaccine Incentive: Achieving the Vision* (Washington, DC: National Academies Press, 1993) ("Because the private sector alone cannot sustain the costs and risks associated with the development of most vaccines, and because the successful development of vaccines requires an integrated process, the committee recommends that an entity, tentatively called the National Vaccine Authority, be organized to advance the development, production, and procurement of new and improved vaccines of limited commercial potential but of global public health need"); Institute of Medicine, Council on Vaccine Development, "Statement on Vaccine Development," November 5, 2001, http://www.iom.edu/CMS/5487.aspx.

101. Institute of Medicine, *Financing Vaccines in the Twenty-first Century: Assuring Access and Availability* (Washington, DC: National Academies Press, 2003) (recommending a government subsidy coupled with a requirement for insurers to cover vaccinations). Moreover, because the federal government is the largest purchaser of some vaccines, it has enormous market power, which it can use to reduce the price of vaccines. Parmet, "Informed Consent and Public Health."

102. The controversy over the safety of DPT (diphtheria-pertussis-tetanus) vaccines reached the U.S. public in 1982, when the television program "DPT: Vaccine Roulette" was first broadcast. The program portrayed children with severe neurological damage allegedly caused by the vaccines. In response, an advocacy group, Dissatisfied Parents Together, was formed and multiple Senate committee hearings were held. The number of lawsuits filed increased from 1 in 1979 to 255 in 1986. Vaccine manufacturers responded predictably to this avalanche of lawsuits; some ceased distribution of DPT and others raised prices (DPT vaccine cost 10,000 percent more in 1986 than it did in 1980). Geoffrey Evans, "Vaccine Liability and Safety Revisited," *Archives of Pediatrics and Adolescent Medicine,* 152 (1998): 7–10; Geoffrey Evans, Doug Harris, and Elliot Levine, "Legal

Issues," in *Vaccines,* ed. Samuel Plotkin and Walter Orenstein (Philadelphia: W. B. Saunders, 2003): 1591–1617; Geoffrey Evans, "Update on Vaccine Liability in the United States: Presentation at the National Vaccine Program Office Workshop on Strengthening the Supply of Routinely Recommended Vaccines in the United States, 12 February 2002," *Clinical Infectious Diseases,* 42 (2006): S130–37; Edward W. Kitch, "Vaccines and Product Liability: A Case of Contagious Litigation," *Regulation,* 9 (1985): 11–18; Martin H. Smith, "National Vaccine Injury Compensation Act," *Pediatrics,* 82 (1988): 264–69.

103. 42 U.S.C. §§ 300aa-10 through 34 (2003). On October 1, 1988, the National Childhood Vaccine Injury Act of 1986 created the National Vaccine Injury Program to ensure an adequate supply of vaccines, stabilize vaccine costs, and establish and maintain an accessible and efficient forum for individuals found to be injured by certain vaccines.

104. For example, it has been argued that the NVICP has become highly adversarial, that proving causation is extremely difficult, and that the limitations on attorneys' fees and expenses make experienced attorneys unwilling to represent claimants. Jaclyn S. Levine, "The National Vaccine Injury Compensation Program: Can It Still Protect Essential Technology?" *Boston University Journal of Science and Technology Law,* 4 (1998): 9–60; Julie Samia Mair and Michael Mair, "Vaccine Liability in the Era of Bioterrorism," *Biosecurity and Bioterrorism: Biodefense Strategy, Practice, and Science,* 1 (2003): 169–82. There have even been repeated efforts to amend the NVICP: see the *Vaccine Injured Children's Compensation Act of 2001,* H.R. 1287, 107th Cong., 1st Sess. (2001); *National Vaccine Injury Compensation Program Improvement Act of 2002,* H.R. 3741, 107th Cong., 2nd Sess. (2002).

105. Vaccines covered by the NVICP include diphtheria, tetanus, pertussis (DTP, DTaP, Tdap, DT, TT, or Td), measles, mumps, rubella (MMR or any components), polio (OPV or IPV), hepatitis A (HAV), hepatitis B (HBV), Haemophilus influenza type b (Hib), varicella (VZV), rotavirus (RV), pneumococcal conjugate (PCV), and trivalent influenza (TIV, LAIV) vaccines.

106. U.S. Department of Health and Human Services, Health Resources and Service Administration, "National Vaccine Injury Compensation Program," http://www.hrsa.gov/vaccinecompensation.

107. Theodore Eisenberg, Neil LaFountain, Brian Ostrom, et al., "Juries, Judges, and Punitive Damages," *Cornell Law Review,* 87 (2002): 743–45 (arguing that punitive damage awards against pharmaceutical manufacturers who complied with FDA requirements are rare, and when juries award damages they are often reduced by state caps or on appeal); Michelle M. Mello and Troyan A. Brennan, "Legal Concerns and the Influenza Vaccine Shortage," *JAMA,* 294 (2005): 1817–20; Bernard Wysocki, Jr., "Agency Chief Spurs Bioterror Research—and Controversy," *Wall Street Journal,* December 6, 2005; Public Broadcasting Service and Marcia Angell, "The Other Drug War: Interviews: Marcia Angell," *Frontline,* November 26, 2002, http://www.pbs.org/wgbh//pages/frontline/shows/other/interviews/angell.html (arguing that instead of developing vaccines, manufacturers choose to profit at a low cost by marketing drugs that are similar to an already proven "blockbuster" drug).

108. The Department of Defense passed the Public Readiness and Emergency

Preparedness Act as part of an appropriations bill for fiscal year 2006 (Division C of H. R. 2863; P.L. 109–148), and it was signed into law on December 30, 2005.

109. Connecticut General Assembly, Office of Legislative Research, "Federal Public Readiness and Emergency Preparedness Act," January 13, 2006, http://www.cga.ct.gov/2006/rpt/2006-R-0060.htm.

110. "Senate Provision Would Inoculate Vaccine Makers," *USA Today,* December 15, 2005 (citing Senator Kennedy saying, "They are trying to insert outrageous giveaways to the drug industry . . . without public scrutiny or debate. Congress should reject any backroom deal that gives a free pass to companies that act irresponsibly or denies fair compensation to injured patients"); Jeffrey H. Birnbaum, "Vaccine Funding Tied to Liability: Trial Lawyers Say Move Would Hurt Consumers," *Washington Post,* November 17, 2005.

111. Due to the substantial expense and risk of bringing a vaccine to the market, along with the infrequency with which these diseases occur naturally, manufacturers claim they have little incentive to invest. Philip K. Russell, "Vaccines in Civilian Defense against Bioterrorism," *Emerging Infectious Diseases,* 5 (1999).

112. U.S. Department of Defense, *Report on Biological Warfare Defense: Vaccine Research and Development Programs* (Washington, DC: Department of Defense, 2001). Current Department of Defense vaccine acquisition strategy focuses on eight vaccines: anthrax vaccine adsorbed (ava), smallpox, plague, tularemia, multivalent botulinum, next generation anthrax, ricin, and multivalent equine encephalitis.

113. Institute of Medicine, *Protecting Our Forces: Improving Vaccine Availability in the U.S. Military* (Washington, DC: National Academies Press, 2002); Jon Cohen and Eliot Marshall, "Vaccines for Biodefense: A System in Distress," *Science,* 294 (2001): 498–501.

114. Frank Gottron, *Project Bioshield* (Washington, DC: Congressional Research Service, 2003); Michael Greenberger, "Choking Bioshield: The Department of Homeland Security's Stranglehold on Biodefense Vaccine Development," *Microbe,* 1 (2006): 260–61.

115. George W. Bush, "Remarks by the President at the Signing of S.15—Project Bioshield Act of 2004," July 21, 2004.

116. Bioshield allows for $3.418 billion of the $5.6 billion Special Reserve Fund to be used during fiscal years 2004 to 2008. Michael Greenberger, "Choking Bioshield."

117. The legislation introduced in April 2005 as a corrective to the Bioshield Act (S.975 or the Bioshield II Act of 2005) places the major procurement responsibility principally in the hands of the Department of Homeland Security, reducing substantially the role of the Department of Health and Human Services.

118. Alex M. Azar II, "HHS Implementation of Project Bioshield: Testimony before the Subcommittee on Health, Committee on Energy and Commerce and the U.S. House of Representatives," April 6, 2006.

119. Eric Lipton, "Setbacks Stymie Bid to Stockpile Bioterror Drugs: Anthrax Vaccine Delayed," *New York Times,* September 18, 2006 ("'We will rally the great promise of American science and innovation to confront the greatest danger of our time,' President Bush said in starting [Bioshield]").

120. Mary Quirk, "Boost to U.S. National Security with Signing of Bioshield," *Lancet Infectious Diseases*, 4 (2004): 540; Bernard Wysocki, "U.S. Struggles for Drugs to Counter Biological Threats: As Bigger Firms Shun Effort, Small Ones Are Challenged," *Wall Street Journal*, July 11, 2005.

121. Lipton, "Setbacks Stymie Bid to Stockpile Bioterror Drugs" (reporting that the United States is moving slowly on contracts as suppliers battle each other).

122. Jocelyn Kaiser, "Bioshield Is Slow to Build U.S. Defenses against Bioweapons," *Science*, 313 (2006): 28–29 (the Biodefense and Pandemic Vaccine and Drug Development Act of 2005 [Bioshield II] would create a new federal agency, the Biomedical Advanced Research and Development Agency [BARDA], which would serve as a single point of authority for biodefense countermeasures); National Institutes of Health, Office of Legislative Policy and Analysis, "Protecting America in the War on Terror," October 3, 2006, http://olpa.od.nih.gov/legislation/109/pendinglegislation/bioterror.asp.

123. World Health Organization, *Advanced Market Commitments for Vaccines* (Geneva: World Health Organization, 2006). Infectious diseases account for less than 2 percent of deaths in developed countries, but are responsible for 21 percent of deaths in developing countries. About 80 percent of all deaths from yellow fever occur in Africa, as do 59 percent of deaths from measles, 58 percent of deaths from pertussis, and 41 percent of deaths from tetanus. More than 99 percent of maternal deaths occur in the developing world. In 2004, some 2.9 million deaths were attributed to HIV/AIDS in developing countries, compared with an estimated 22,000 in developed countries. East Asia and the Pacific are faced with 62 percent of all deaths from hepatitis B. Dean T. Jamison, Joel G. Breman, Anthony R. Measham, et al., *Disease Control Priorities in Developing Countries* (Washington, DC: World Bank Publications, 2006).

124. The eradication of smallpox, the success of the polio eradication initiative in reducing polio's global incidence by 99.9 percent, the achievements of the Expanded Program on Immunization, and the recent 39 percent decrease in the number of measles deaths worldwide all illustrate the benefits of vaccination. For example, the smallpox eradication campaign was completed at a total cost of $300 million, while its overall economic benefit has been roughly $1,000 million annually. Julie B. Milstein, Miloud Kaddar, and Marie Paule Kieny, "The Impact of Globalization on Vaccine Development and Availability," *Health Affairs*, 25 (2006): 1061–67; Leslie Roberts, "Polio: Health Workers Scramble to Contain African Epidemic," *Science*, 305 (2004): 24–25; World Health Organization, *The World Health Report 2005: Every Mother and Child Count* (Geneva: WHO, 2005).

125. The cost per fully immunized child for the six original EPI vaccines (TB, diphtheria, pertussis, tetanus, polio, and measles) is approximately $20. The cost per death averted from successfully vaccinating children against the six original EPI diseases is $250 per death averted in South Asia and sub-Saharan Africa, and $3,250 per death averted in Europe and Central Asia (this difference is largely due to the relatively high coverage rates in the latter region). Jamison, *Disease Control Priorities in Developing Countries.*

126. Owen Barder, Michael Kremer, and Heidi Williams, "Advance Market

Commitments: A Policy to Stimulate Investment in Vaccines for Neglected Diseases," *Economists' Voice,* 3 (2006): 1–6.

127. On average, immunization programs account for 6 percent of government health expenditures in developing countries. However, in the world's lowest-income countries, expanding coverage of vaccines could consume as much as 20 percent of a government's health budget. Jamison, *Disease Control Priorities in Developing Countries.*

128. G8 Summit 2006, "Fight against Infectious Diseases," *Official Website of the G8 Presidency of the Russian Federation 2006,* July 16, 2006, http://en.g8russia.ru/docs/10.html; Center for Global Development, "G8 Progress on Advance Market Commitments for Vaccines," July 17, 2006, http://blogs.cgdev.org/globalhealth/2006/07/g8_progress_on.php (noting that the World Bank and GAVI Alliance have led a significant effort on the technical details of implementing AMCs); International Finance Facility for Immunization, "About IFFIm," *Official Website for the International Finance Facility for Immunization,* http://www.iff-immunisation.org/01_about_iffim.html (describing how IFFIm has been designed to accelerate the availability of funds to be used for health and immunization programs, through the GAVI Alliance, in seventy of the poorest countries around the world).

129. World Health Organization, "Advanced Market Commitments for Vaccines," July 19, 2006, http://www.who.int/immunization/newsroom/amcs/en/index.html. Poor countries would decide whether to purchase a vaccine, and they (or the sponsors on their behalf) would pay a low price per person immunized. Sponsors would then top this low price to a higher, subsidized price, which would provide market returns to the vaccine developer comparable to those of other, average-revenue pharmaceutical products. Barder et al., "Advance Market Commitments."

130. G8 Summit 2006, "Fight against Infectious Diseases," "Center for Global Development," "G8 Progress on Advance Market Commitments for Vaccines" (reporting that Canada, Italy, the United Kingdom, the United States, and Russia support AMCs, particularly for pneumococcal infections). The first AMC became a reality in February 2007, when donors committed $1.5 billion for a pneumococcal vaccine. PneumoADIP, "U.S. $1.5 Billion Donor Commitment Launches Pilot Advanced Market Commitment for Pneumococcal Vaccine," February 9, 2007, http://www.preventpneumo.org/pdf/PneumoADIP_AMC_9Feb07.pdf.

131. Streptococcus pneumonia bacterium causes a variety of diseases, such as pneumonia, meningitis, and ear infections. "Acute respiratory infections, especially pneumonia, are the leading infectious cause of mortality world wide," according to Dr. Thomas Cherian, of the World Health Organization Department of Immunization, Vaccines and Biologicals. *GAVI Alliance,* "World Experts Unite in Urgent Effort to Fight Deadly Disease," news release, May 10, 2004, http://www.gavialliance.org/Media_Center/Press_Releases/pr_10may2004_isppd.php; see also Carlos G. Grijalva and Kathryn M. Edwards, "Promises and Challenges of Pneumococcal Conjugate Vaccines for the Developing World," *Clinical Infectious Diseases,* 43 (2006): 680–82.

132. World Health Organization, UNICEF, and the World Bank, *State of the World's Vaccines and Immunization* (Geneva: World Health Organization Department of Vaccines and Biologicals, 2002). Whereas in the late 1980s delivery of basic childhood vaccines, for example, had risen to achieve worldwide coverage of about 80 percent of infants, in 2000 less than 50 percent of children had access to basic immunization in sub-Saharan Africa. John Clemens and Luis Jodar, "Introducing New Vaccines into Developing Countries: Obstacles, Opportunities and Complexities," *Nature*, 11 (2005): S12–15; World Health Organization, "Low Investment in Immunization and Vaccines Threatens Global Health: Immunization Saves Three Million Lives Every Year, but Three Million More Could Be Saved," November 20, 2002, http://www.who.int/mediacentre/news/releases/pr87/en/index.html.

133. World Health Organization, "Low Investment in Immunization and Vaccines Threatens Global Health." The excess burdens of ill health in low- and middle-income countries are primarily associated with infectious diseases, reproductive health, and childhood illnesses. Just eight diseases and conditions account for 29 percent of all deaths in low- and middle-income countries: TB, HIV/AIDS, diarrheal diseases, vaccine-preventable childhood diseases, malaria, respiratory infections, maternal conditions, and neonatal deaths. If developing countries achieved the same rates of death from these eight diseases as do high-income countries, the number of deaths would fall from 17.6 million to 3.0 million per year. Dean T. Jamison, Joel G. Breman, and Anthony R. Measham, *Priorities in Health: Disease Control Priorities Companion Volume* (Washington, DC: World Bank Publications, 2006).

134. World Health Organization, *State of the World's Vaccines and Immunization* (Geneva: World Health Organization, 2002).

135. The facts for this case study were obtained from Richard E. Neustadt and Harvey Fineberg, *The Epidemic That Never Was: Policy-Making and the Swine Flu Affair* (New York: Vintage Books, 1983); Walter R. Dowdle, "The 1976 Experience."

136. Louis Weinstein, "Influenza, 1918: A Revisit?" *New Engl. J. Med.*, 294 (1976): 1058–60.

137. Cyril Wecht, "The Swine Flu Immunization Program: Scientific Venture or Political Folly?" *American Journal of Law and Medicine*, 3 (1977): 425; but see Nicholas Wade, "1976 Swine Flu Campaign Faulted, yet Principals Would Do It Again," *Science*, 202 (1978): 849, 851–52.

138. Richard E. Neustadt and Harvey V. Fineberg, *The Swine Flu Affair: Decision-Making on a Slippery Disease* (Washington, DC: U.S. Department of Health, Education, and Welfare, 1974).

139. Jonathan E. Fielding, "Managing Public Health Risks: The Swine Flu Immunization Program Revisited," *American Journal of Law and Medicine*, 4 (1978): 35–43.

140. Ronald Bayer, Carol Levine, and Susan Wolf, "HIV Antibody Screening: An Ethical Framework for Evaluating Proposed Programs," *JAMA*, 256 (1986): 1768–74.

141. William C. Black and H. Gilbert Welch, "Screening for Disease," *American Journal of Roentgenology*, 168 (1997): 3–11.

142. Stoto et al., *Reducing the Odds,* 22.

143. Martha A. Field, "Testing for AIDS: Uses and Abuses," *American Journal of Law and Medicine,* 16 (1990): 33–106, 34, 35; For a striking example of political controversy associated with AIDS screening, see Panos Institute and Norwegian Red Cross, *The Third Epidemic: Repercussions of the Fear of AIDS* (London: Panos Institute, 1990): 108 ("Irrespective of the cost of efficiency of [coercive] measures, significant political advantage can be gained from their implementation. The government is seen to be taking firm, decisive action and the epidemic appears to be under control. Those targeted for compulsory testing are often stigmatized by society and held responsible for spreading HIV, making the use of coercion seem more justifiable and acceptable. Yet the effect is ultimately to divide society and to discourage those at great risk from seeking advice and help").

144. For criteria to evaluate screening, see U.S. Preventive Services Task Force, *Guide to Clinical Preventive Services* (Washington, DC: Department of Health and Human Services, 1989). In the context of HIV screening, see Allan M. Brandt, Paul D. Cleary, and Lawrence O. Gostin, "Routine Hospital Testing for HIV: Health Policy Considerations," in *AIDS and the Health Care System,* ed. Lawrence O. Gostin (New Haven, CT: Yale University Press, 1990): 125; Lawrence O. Gostin, William J. Curran, and Mary E. Clark, "The Case against Compulsory Case Finding in Controlling AIDS: Testing, Screening and Reporting," *American Journal of Law and Medicine,* 12 (1986): 7–53; Richard Coker, "Migration, Public Health and Compulsory Screening for TB and HIV," Asylum and Migration Working Paper (London: Institute for Public Policy Research, 2003).

145. Judith S. Mausner and Shira Kramer, *Mausner and Bahn Epidemiology: An Introductory Text,* 2d ed. (Philadelphia: W. B. Saunders, 1985): 217.

146. For example, a study recently showed that a widely used diagnostic test for genetic breast-cancer risk misses 10 to 12 percent of women who are at high risk, making them think their chance of getting cancer is low when in fact it remains substantial. Thomas M. Burton, "Test for Breast-Cancer Risk Could Miss Mark: As Many as 12 Percent of Women with Strong Family History Get Inaccurate Reading," *Wall Street Journal,* March 22, 2006.

147. Litjen Tan, Roy Altman, and Nancy H. Nielsen, "Screening Nonimmigrant Visitors to the United States for Tuberculosis: Report of the Council on Scientific Affairs," *Archives of Internal Medicine,* 161 (2001): 334–40 (concluding that overseas TB screening of nonimmigrant visitors, who are unlikely to have active TB, will be of extremely low yield and therefore not justified).

148. Conversely, negative PV is the proportion of those who are healthy among those with a negative test. NPV is mostly determined by a test's sensitivity and the disease's prevalence.

149. A test's sensitivity is relevant to PPV, but for diseases with low prevalence, even fairly large differences in sensitivity will have little effect on PPV.

150. Only two states have passed legislation requiring HIV testing before marriage, but those laws did not last long, in part because of very low detection rates. A growing number of states are abolishing all blood tests as a marriage requirement. Nevertheless, six states (Connecticut, Georgia, Indiana, Mississippi, Mon-

tana, and Oklahoma) and the District of Columbia still require a syphilis or rubella test before issuing a marriage license. Robert H. Schmerling, "The Truth about Premarital Blood Testing," *Aetna InteliHealth,* Nov. 29, 2004; Steve LeBlanc, "Bay State Abolishes Blood Tests for Marriage Licenses," *Standard Times,* February 3, 2005.

151. Bernard J. Turnock and Chester J. Kelly, "Mandatory Premarital Testing for Human Immunodeficiency Virus: The Illinois Experience," *JAMA,* 261 (1989): 3415–18 (the Illinois program was later repealed); see Paul D. Cleary, Michael J. Barry, Kenneth H. Mayer, et al., "Compulsory Premarital Screening for the Human Immunodeficiency Virus: Technical and Public Health Considerations," *JAMA,* 258 (1987): 1757–62.

152. Lawrence O. Gostin, *The AIDS Pandemic: Complacency, Injustice, and Unfulfilled Expectations* (Chapel Hill: University of North Carolina Press, 2004).

153. John Maxwell Glover Wilson and Gunnar Jungner, *Principles and Practice of Screening for Disease* (Geneva: WHO, 1968).

154. Timothy F. Brewer, S. Jody Heymann, Susan M. Krumplitsch, et al., "Strategies to Decrease Tuberculosis in U.S. Homeless Populations: A Computer Simulation Model," *JAMA,* 287 (2001): 834–42 (the rate of TB among homeless persons is about twenty times that of the general adult population); Centers for Disease Control and Prevention, "Tuberculosis Transmission in a Homeless Shelter Population—New York, 2000–2003," *Morbidity and Mortality Weekly Report,* 54 (2005): 149–52 (stating that in 2003, 6.3 percent of reported TB cases in the United States were among homeless persons); Centers for Disease Control and Prevention, *HIV/AIDS among Men Who Have Sex with Men,* July 2006, http://www.cdc.gov/hiv/resources/factsheets/PDF/msm.pdf (stating that gay males accounted for 70 percent of all estimated HIV infections among male adults in 2004); Centers for Disease Control and Prevention, "HIV/AIDS and African Americans," August 31, 2006, http://www.cdc.gov/hiv/topics/aa/affecting.htm (noting that even though African Americans account for less than a quarter of the U.S. population, they account for about half of the people with HIV/AIDS).

155. Howard Markel, "Scientific Advances and Social Risks: Historical Perspectives of Genetic Screening Programs for Sickle Cell Disease, Tay-Sachs Disease, Neural Tube," in *Promoting Safe and Effective Genetic Testing in the United States,* ed. Neil A. Holtzman and Michael S. Watson (Bethesda, MD: National Institutes of Health, 2006); *Genetic Information Nondiscrimination Act of 2003,* S. Rep. No. 108–22 (2003).

156. Though screening small high-risk groups is cost-effective and can advance the welfare of the public, it often leads to targeting of welfare dependents, homosexuals, and persons of a particular gender or ethnicity. There is a real threat that new, insidious forms of surveillance and control over "problem populations" may be introduced under the guise of public health. Some have even expressed their concerns about the potential for compulsory screening to operate as a new eugenics. Alan Petersen, "The New Genetics and the Politics of Public Health," *Critical Public Health,* 8 (1998): 59–71.

157. Testing measures are usually both overinclusive and underinclusive in scope. For example, in *People of the State of Illinois v. Henrietta Adams et al.,*

the defendants challenged the constitutionality of an Illinois statute requiring all persons convicted for prostitution, soliciting prostitution, keeping a place of prostitution, pimping, and criminal sexual assault or abuse to submit to a court-ordered test to determine whether they had any sexually transmissible disease. The defendants argued that the statute was overinclusive because it included within its scope offenses having no risk of AIDS transmission and underinclusive because it failed to require HIV testing for people who engaged in other criminal sexual activities, such as sexual misconduct or bigamy, or who engaged in promiscuous noncriminal sexual activity. The Supreme Court of Illinois stated, however, that in deciding which offenses to include in the statutory requirement and which ones to omit, the legislature may discretionally consider the costs and utility of testing. *People v. Adams,* 597 N.E.2d 574 (Ill. 1992).

158. Ronald Bayer, *Private Acts, Social Consequences: AIDS and the Politics of Public Health* (New Brunswick, NJ: Rutgers University Press, 1991); UN Program on HIV/AIDS and World Health Organization, "UNAIDS and WHO Policy Statement on HIV Testing," June 2004, http://data.unaids.org/unadocs/hivtestingpolicy_en.pdf; Terje J. Anderson, David Atkins, Catherine Baker-Cirac, et al., "Revised Guidelines for HIV Counseling, Testing, and Referral," *Morbidity and Mortality Weekly Report,* 50 (2001): 1–58.

159. Ruth R. Faden, Nancy E. Kass, and Madison Powers, "Warrants for Screening Programs: Public Health, Legal and Ethical Frameworks," in *AIDS, Women, and the Next Generation,* ed. Ruth R. Faden, Gail Geller, and Madison Powers (New York: Oxford University Press, 1991).

160. See, e.g., *Hill v. Evans,* 1993 U.S. Dist. LEXIS 1997 (M.D. Ala.) (finding mandatory HIV testing of "high risk" individuals unconstitutional because it is not rationally related to the state's interest in public health).

161. Soju Chang, Lani S. M. Wheeler, and Katherine P. Farrell, "Public Health Impact of Targeted Tuberculosis Screening in Public Schools," *American Journal of Public Health,* 92 (2002): 1942–45.

162. Katherine L. Acuff and Ruth R. Faden, "A History of Prenatal and Newborn Screening Programs: Lessons for the Future," in *AIDS, Women, and the Next Generation;* see also National Conference of State Legislatures, *Sexually Transmitted Diseases: A Policymaker's Guide and Summary of State Laws* (Denver, CO: National Conference of State Legislatures, 1998).

163. David L. Saunders, Dona M. Olive, Susan B. Wallace, et al., "Tuberculosis Screening in the Federal Prison System: An Opportunity to Treat and Prevent Tuberculosis in Foreign-Born Populations," *Public Health Reports,* 116 (2001): 210–18; Audrey A. Reichard, Mark N. Lobato, Cheryl A. Roberts, et al., "Assessment of Tuberculosis Screening and Management Practices of Large Jail Systems," *Public Health Reports,* 118 (2003): 500–507; Centers for Disease Control, "Routine HIV Testing of Inmates in Correctional Facilities," August 23, 2006, http://www.cdc.gov/Hiv/topics/prev_prog/AHP/resources/guidelines/Interim_RoutineTest.htm.

164. The reasonable suspicion standard, for example, is often used for alcohol and drug testing in schools and workplace settings. U.S. Department of Health and Human Services, Substance Abuse and Mental Health Services Administration, "Mandatory Guidelines for Federal Workplace Drug Testing Programs,"

November 2004, http://dwp.samhsa.gov/FedPgms/Pages/HHS_Mand_Guid_Effective_Nov_04.aspx; see *Vt. Stat. Ann.*, Tit. 18, §1092 (1982) (authorizing testing of persons reasonably suspected of being infected with a venereal disease).

165. E.g., *N.C. Gen. Stat.* § 15A-615 (1997) (authorizing STI testing of sex offenders who are alleged to have had sexual contact with a minor).

166. U.S. Citizenship and Immigration Services, *Medical Examinations*, January 2006, http://www.uscis.gov/graphics/Medical_Examd.htm#needed; e.g., *N.J. Stat. Ann.* § 26:4–49.6 (West 1996) (requiring migrant laborers to submit to syphilis and gonorrhea testing).

167. As of 1999, at least eleven states mandated HIV testing of persons convicted of prostitution. National Conference of State Legislatures, *Sexually Transmitted Diseases*, 78.

168. E.g., *Ohio Rev. Code Ann.* § 3701.49 (1997) (requiring syphilis and gonorrhea testing of specimens taken from pregnant women).

169. E.g., *N.Y. Pub Health* § 2500-f (1999) (mandating HIV testing of newborns and notification of parent of the results).

170. E.g., *Va. Code* § 32.1–59 (1997) (requiring venereal disease testing for any person admitted to a state correctional institution or state hospital).

171. See, e.g., *R.I. Gen. Laws* § 23–6-14 (1989) (permitting involuntary HIV testing when "a person [complainant] can document significant exposure to the blood or other bodily fluids of another person" in the course of performing occupational duties). As of 1999, twenty-one states permitted mandatory testing of patients who exposed a health care worker, emergency personnel, or law enforcement officer to HIV. National Conference of State Legislatures, *Sexually Transmitted Diseases*, 62.

172. E.g., *N.Y. Public Health Law* § 2301 (McKinney 1993) (authorizing a health officer to apply to a court for an order to test for an STI).

173. Centers for Disease Control and Prevention, "Targeted Tuberculin Testing and Treatment of Latent Tuberculosis Infection," *Morbidity and Mortality Weekly Report*, 49 (2000): 1–54 (stating that tuberculin testing should be conducted only among groups at high risk, including employees of high-risk congregate settings such as health care workers and adults working with children); see Lawrence O. Gostin, "Controlling the Resurgent Tuberculosis Epidemic: A Fifty State Survey of Tuberculosis Statutes and Proposals for Reform," *JAMA*, 269 (1993): 255–61.

174. Certain immigrants are required to be tested for HIV, including refugees, asylum seekers, certain nonimmigrant visa applicants, and anyone applying for an adjustment of status in the United States or for an immigrant visa at a U.S. consular post abroad. Waivers for HIV-positive immigrants and visitors may be granted. U.S. Citizenship and Immigration Services, "Medical Examinations," October 17, 2006, http://www.uscis.gov/graphics/Medical_Exam.htm#needed; see Lawrence O. Gostin, Paul Cleary, Kenneth Mayer, et al., "Screening and Exclusion of International Travelers and Immigrants for Public Health Purposes: An Evaluation of United States Policy," *New Eng. J. Med.*, 322 (1990): 1743–46.

175. U.S. Department of State, Bureau of Consular Affairs, "Human Immunodeficiency Virus (HIV) Testing Requirements for Entry into Foreign Coun-

tries," March 2006, http://travel.state.gov/travel/tips/brochures/brochures_1230.html (listing countries requiring HIV testing for foreigners, usually long-term visitors such as students and workers). See *O'Brien v. Cunard Steamship Company,* 28 N.E. 266 (Mass. 1891) (finding no battery or negligence when physician vaccinated plaintiff pursuant to quarantine regulations requiring vaccination of steerage passengers arriving from overseas).

176. Prakash Khanal, "Emerging Diseases Fuel Health Screening," *Bulletin of the World Health Organization,* 83 (2005): 725–26.

177. Richard Coker, "Compulsory Screening of Immigrants for Tuberculosis and HIV," *British Medical Journal,* 328 (2004): 298–300 (concluding that screening of immigrants for TB and HIV is not based on evidence and has practical and ethical problems).

178. Disability discrimination law also regulates screening programs if there is a potential for unequal treatment. See *School Board of Nassau County v. Arline,* 480 U.S. 273 (1987) (finding that the exclusion from school of a teacher with Mycobacterium tuberculosis violated the federal Rehabilitation Act). The *Americans with Disabilities Act of 1990,* 42 U.S.C. §12101 *et seq.* (1992), specifically regulates medical screening, physical examinations, and inquiries: *pre-offer,* an employer is not permitted to screen applicants before offering a job; *post-offer,* an employer is permitted to screen after a job offer is made, provided that all entering employees are screened and the medical information is kept confidential; and *current employees,* an employer may screen only if job-related and consistent with business necessity.

179. *Schmerber v. California,* 384 U.S. 757, 767–68 (1966).

180. *Illinois v. Lidster,* 540 U.S. 419, 429 (2004) ("In judging reasonableness, we look to the gravity of the public concerns served by seizure, the degree to which the seizure advances the public interest, and the severity of the interference with individual liberty").

181. *Maryland v. Pringle,* 540 U.S. 366, 371 (2003) (holding that the standard is "incapable of precise definition or quantification into percentages because it deals with probabilities and depends on the totality of circumstances"); *Ornelas v. United States,* 517 U.S. 690, 696 (1996) (stating that "reasonable suspicion" exists where the known facts and circumstances are sufficient to justify the belief that contraband will be found).

182. *Skinner v. Railway Labor Executives Assn.,* 489 U.S. 602, 613–14 (1989) (upholding drug tests following major train accidents for employees who violate safety rules, even without reasonable suspicion of impairment); *National Treasury Employees Union v. Von Raab,* 489 U.S. 656 (1989) (upholding suspicionless drug testing by U.S. Customs Service due to government's "compelling" interest in safeguarding borders and public safety). The special needs doctrine extends beyond medical screening. See *MacWade v. Kelly,* 460 F.3d 260 (9th Cir. 2006) (holding that preventing a terrorist attack on the subway is a "special" need within the meaning of the special needs doctrine).

183. Compare *United States v. Sczubelek,* 402 F.3d 175 (3d Cir. 2005) (upholding DNA testing of a person on probation based on the more rigorous "totality of circumstances" established in *United States v. Knights,* 534 U.S. 112, 118 (2001), rather than the "special needs" standard); with *United States v. Kim-*

ler, 335 F.3d 1132 (10th Cir. 2003) (upholding DNA testing using the "special needs" standard).

184. *In re Juveniles A, B, C, D, E*, 847 P.2d 455 (Wash. 1993).

185. Lawrence O. Gostin, Zita Lazzarini, Dianne D. Alexander, et al., "HIV Testing, Counseling, and Prophylaxis after Sexual Assault," *JAMA*, 271(1994): 1436–44.

186. *Board of Education v. Earls*, 536 U.S. 822, 829 (2002) ("When special needs, beyond the normal need for law enforcement, make the warrant and probable cause requirement impractical . . . the reasonableness of the search [is determined] by balancing the nature of the intrusion on the individual's privacy against the promotion of legitimate governmental interests"). In *Earls*, the court found that drug testing of high school participants in extracurricular activities is a reasonable means of protecting schoolchildren given the students' reduced expectations of privacy interests, the negligible intrusion associated with urine tests, and important state interests in students' health and safety.

187. *Skinner v. Railway Labor Executives Assn.*, 489 U.S. 602, 625 (1989).

188. See, e.g., *Veronia School District 47J v. Acton*, 515 U.S. 646 (1995) (upholding random urinalysis for participation in interscholastic athletics).

189. *Anonymous Fireman v. City of Willoughby*, 779 F. Supp. 402 (N.D. Ohio 1991) (upholding mandatory HIV testing for firefighters and paramedics because they are "high-risk" employees).

190. *Plowman v. United States Department of Army*, 698 F. Supp. 627 (E.D. Va. 1988) (upholding HIV testing of federal civilian employees).

191. *Local 1812, American Federation of Government Employees v. United States Department of State*, 662 F. Supp. 50 (D.D.C. 1987) (upholding HIV testing of foreign service employees).

192. *Haitian Centers Council Co. v. Sale*, 823 F. Supp. 1028 (E.D.N.Y. 1993).

193. *In re Juveniles A, B, C, D, E*, 847 P.2d 455 (Wash. 1993) (upholding mandatory HIV testing for juveniles convicted of sexual offenses).

194. *Ferguson v. City of Charleston*, 532 U.S. 67 (2001).

195. *Id.* at 81 (quoting *Indianapolis v. Edmond*, 531 U.S. 32, 44 [2000]).

196. But see *Glover v. Eastern Nebraska Cmty. Office of Retardation*, 686 F. Supp. 243 (D. Neb. 1988), *aff'd*, 867 F.2d 461 (9th Cir. 1989) (invalidating on Fourth Amendment grounds chronic infectious disease policy mandating HIV and HBV screening of employees).

197. Centers for Disease Control and Prevention, "Revised Guidelines for HIV Counseling, Testing, and Referral," *Morbidity and Mortality Weekly Report*, 50 (2001): 1–62.

198. Zita Lazzarini and Lorilyn Rosales, "Legal Issues concerning Public Health Efforts to Reduce Perinatal HIV Transmission," *Yale Journal of Health Policy Law and Ethics*, 3 (2002–3): 67–98.

199. Nicola M. Zetola, Jeffrey D. Klausner, Barbara Haller, et al., "Association between Rates of HIV Testing and Elimination of Written Consents in San Francisco," *JAMA*, 297 (2007): 1061–62.

200. Bernard M. Branson, H. Hunter Handsfield, Margaret A. Lampe, et al., "Revised Recommendations for HIV Testing of Adults, Adolescents, and Preg-

nant Women in Health-Care Settings," *Morbidity and Mortality Weekly Report,* 55 (2006): 1–17.

201. Margaret A. Chesney and Ashley W. Smith, "Critical Delays in HIV Testing and Care: The Potential Role of Stigma," *American Behavioral Scientist,* 42 (1999): 1162–74.

202. Gary Marks, Nicole Crepaz, Walton J. Senterfitt, et al., "Meta-Analysis of High-Risk Sexual Behavior in Persons Unaware They Are Infected with HIV in the United States: Implications for HIV Prevention Programs," *Journal of Acquired Immune Deficiency Syndromes,* 39 (2005): 446–53 (estimating that untested HIV-infected individuals are twice as likely to engage in high-risk sexual behavior).

203. A. David Paltiel, Milton C. Weinstein, April D. Kimmel, et al., "Expanded Screening for HIV in the United States—An Analysis of Cost-Effectiveness," *New Engl. J. Med.,* 352 (2005): 586–95; Gillian D. Sanders, Ahmed M. Bayoumi, Vandana Sundaram, et al., "Cost-Effectiveness of Screening for HIV in the Era of Highly Active Antiretroviral Therapy," *New Engl. J. Med.,* 352 (2005): 570–85.

204. Thomas R. Frieden, Moupali Das-Douglas, Scott E. Kellerman, et al., "Applying Public Health Principles to the HIV Epidemic," *New Engl. J. Med.,* 353 (2005): 2397–2402; Institute of Medicine, *No Time to Lose: Getting More from HIV Prevention* (Washington, DC: National Academies Press, 2001); U.S. Preventive Services Task Force, "Screening for HIV: Recommendation Statement," *Annals of Internal Medicine,* 143 (2005): 32–37.

205. Gary Marks, Nicole Crepaz, and Robert S. Janssen, "Estimating Sexual Transmission of HIV from Persons Aware and Unaware That They Are Infected with the Virus in the USA," *AIDS,* 20 (2006): 1447–50.

206. Frank J. Palella, Jr., Maria Deloria-Knoll, Joan S. Chmiel, et al., "Survival Benefit of Initiating Antiretroviral Therapy in HIV-Infected Persons in Different CD4+ Cell Strata," *Annals of Internal Medicine,* 138 (2003): 620–26.

207. Kevin M. DeCock, Mary Glenn Fowler, Eric Mercier, et al., "Prevention of Mother-to-Child HIV Transmission in Resource-Poor Countries," *JAMA,* 283 (2000): 1175–82.

208. Catherine Pechkam and Diana Gibb, "Mother-to-Child Transmission of the Human Immunodeficiency Virus," *New Engl. J. Med.,* 333 (1995): 289–303; Lazzarini and Rosales, "Legal Issues concerning Public Health Efforts to Reduce Perinatal HIV Transmission."

209. Ellen R. Cooper, Manhattan Charurat, Lynne Mofenson, et al., "Combination Antiretroviral Strategies for the Treatment of Pregnant HIV-1-Infected Women and Prevention of Perinatal HIV-1 Transmission," *Journal of Acquired Immune Deficiency Syndromes,* 29 (2002): 484–94.

210. Centers for Disease Control and Prevention, "Recommendations of the U.S. Public Health Service Task Force on the Use of Zidovudine to Reduce Perinatal Transmission of Human Immunodeficiency Virus," *Morbidity and Mortality Weekly Report,* 43 (1994): 1–20.

211. Centers for Disease Control and Prevention, "U.S. Public Health Service Recommendations for Human Immunodeficiency Virus Counseling and Vol-

untary Testing for Pregnant Women," *Morbidity and Mortality Weekly Report,* 44 (1995): 1–10.

212. *Ryan White Comprehensive AIDS Resources Emergency (CARE) Act Amendments,* Pub. L. No. 104–146 (codified at 42 U.S.C. §300ff [1996]) (requiring HHS Secretary to determine whether HIV screening of infants was "routine practice"; if so, Ryan White Treatment funds would become contingent upon the states demonstrating that perinatal transmission had declined by half, 95 percent of woman are screened during prenatal care visits, or a program of mandatory newborn screening had been instituted).

213. *N.Y. Pub. Health* § 2500-f (Consol. 1996).

214. Institute of Medicine, *Reducing the Odds: Preventing Perinatal Transmission of HIV in the United States* (Washington, DC: National Academies Press, 1999).

215. Centers for Disease Control and Prevention, "Revised Guidelines for HIV Counseling, Testing, and Referral and Revised Recommendations for HIV Screening of Pregnant Women," *Morbidity and Mortality Weekly Report,* 50 (2001): 59–86.

216. Lawrence O. Gostin, "Public Health Strategies for Confronting AIDS. Legislative and Regulatory Policy in the United States," *JAMA,* 261 (1989): 1621–30.

217. Health Research and Educational Trust, *Map to HIV Testing Laws of All U.S. States* (Chicago: American Hospital Association, 2006); National HIV/AIDS Clinicians' Consultation Center, *State HIV Testing Laws Compendium,* http://ucsf.edu/hivcntr/PDFs/WEB2006State%20Laws.pdf; James G. Hodge, Jr., *Advancing HIV Prevention Initiative: A Limited Legal Analysis of State HIV Statutes* (Washington, DC: Center for Law and the Public's Health, 2004).

218. Lawrence O. Gostin, John W. Ward, and A. Cornelius Baker, "National HIV Case Reporting for the United States: A Defining Moment in the History of the Epidemic," *New Engl. J. Med.,* 337 (1997): 1162–67.

219. Ronald Bayer and Amy L. Fairchild, "Changing the Paradigm for HIV Testing: The End of Exceptionalism?" *New Engl. J. Med.,* 355 (2006): 647–49; Ronald Bayer, "Public Health Policy and the AIDS Epidemic: An End to HIV Exceptionalism?" *New Engl. J. Med.,* 324 (1991): 1500–1504.

220. Sewell Chan, "Rifts Emerge on Push to End Written Consent for HIV Tests," *New York Times,* December 25, 2006.

221. *Riggins v. Nevada,* 504 U.S. 127, 127 (1992) (requiring an "overriding justification and a determination of medical appropriateness"). For a discussion of the general justifications for regulation, see chapter 4.

222. For good discussions of informed consent, see *Hales v. Pitman,* 576 P.2d 493 (1978) (holding that physicians must disclose the risks of a procedure to the patient for consent to be informed); *Cobbs v. Grant,* 8 Cal. 3d 229 (1972) (same); *O'Brien v. Cunard Steamship Company,* 28 N.E. 266 (Mass. 1891) (finding no battery or negligence when a physician vaccinated the plaintiff, who did not register an objection); see also Ruth R. Faden, Tom L. Beauchamp, and Nancy M. P. King, *A History and Theory of Informed Consent* (New York: Oxford University Press, 1986); Marjorie M. Schultz, "From Informed Consent to Patient

Choice: A New Protected Interest," *Yale Law Journal,* 95 (1985): 219–99; Peter H. Schuck, "Rethinking Informed Consent," *Yale Law Journal,* 103 (1994): 889–960.

223. Unless there is no consent at all (e.g., a person gives permission for procedure X and the physician administers procedure Y), the doctrine of informed consent is usually based on negligence rather than on battery. William Lloyd Prosser, W. Page Keeton, Dan B. Dobbs, et al., *Prosser and Keeton on Torts,* 5th ed. (St. Paul, MN: West Publishing, 1984): secs. 15 and 30.

224. Approximately half the states adopt a "patient-centered" standard of disclosure—the information that a reasonable patient would want to know. See e.g., *Canterbury v. Spence,* 464 F. 2d 772 (D.C. Cir.), *cert denied,* 409 U.S. 1064 (1972). The remaining states adopt a "physician-centered" standard—the information a reasonable physician would disclose in the circumstances. See, e.g., *Chapel v. Allison,* 785 P.2d 204 (Mont. 1990).

225. Thomas L. Beauchamp, "Methods and Principles in Biomedical Ethics," *Journal of Medical Ethics,* 29 (2003): 269–74.

226. *Restatement (Second) of Torts* § 892B (1965) (regarding consent under mistake, misrepresentation, or duress).

227. National Conference of State Legislatures, *Sexually Transmitted Diseases,* 85–91, 123–27.

228. Advisory Council for the Elimination of Tuberculosis, "Tuberculosis Control Laws—United States, 1993," *Morbidity and Mortality Weekly Reports,* 42 (1993): 7–8; Lawrence O. Gostin, "Controlling the Resurgent Tuberculosis Epidemic: A Fifty-State Survey of TB Statutes and Proposals for Reform," *JAMA,* 269 (1993): 256–58.

229. Mandatory treatment powers are also found in mental health and substance abuse statutes. See, e.g., Stefanie Klag, Frances O'Callaghan, and Peter Creed, "The Use of Legal Coercion in the Treatment of Substance Abusers: An Overview and Critical Analysis of Thirty Years of Research," *Substance Use and Misuse,* 40 (2005): 1777–95; Phil Fennell, *Treatment without Consent: Law, Psychiatry and Treatment of Mentally Disordered People since 1845* (London: Routledge, 1996).

230. *City of New York v. Antoinette R.,* 630 N.Y.S.2d 1008 (1995) (finding that the patient was consistently uncooperative with TB treatment).

231. The right to refuse treatment is also protected under state constitutions. See, e.g., *Rivers v. Katz,* 495 N.E.2d 337, 343 (N.Y. 1986) (finding that persons of "adult years and sound mind" have the right to "control the course of [their] medical treatment").

232. See, e.g., *Stenberg v. Carhart,* 530 U.S. 914 (2000) (striking down a Nebraska late-term abortion prohibition); *Planned Parenthood of Southeastern Pennsylvania v. Casey,* 505 U.S. 833 (1992).

233. *Cruzan v. Director, Mo. Dep't of Health,* 497 U.S. 261 (1990) (upholding a state requirement of clear and convincing evidence of the patient's wishes to withdraw treatment from a patient in a persistently vegetative state); *Washington v. Glucksberg,* 521 U.S. 702 (1997) (upholding a ban on doctor-assisted suicide); *Vacco v. Quill,* 521 U.S. 793 (1997) (same); see also *Abigail Alliance for Better Access to Development Drugs v. von Eschenbach,* 445 F.3d 470 (D.C. Cir.

2006) (holding that the FDA must present a compelling interest in order to maintain its present policy of denying terminally ill patients access to drugs that are not yet approved but had cleared phase I trials); Lawrence O. Gostin, "Deciding Life and Death in the Courtroom," *JAMA*, 279 (1998): 1259–60; Rob McStay, "Terminal Sedation: Palliative Care for Intractable Pain, Post *Glucksberg* and *Quill*," *American Journal of Law and Medicine*, 29 (2003): 45–76.

234. *Washington v. Harper*, 494 U.S. 210, 221–22 (1990) (holding that mentally ill prisoners possess "a significant liberty interest in avoiding the unwanted administration of antipsychotic drugs under the Due Process Clause"). But see *Hydrick v. Hunter*, 500 F. 3d 978, 995–96 (9th Cir. 2007) (holding that civilly committed sexually violent predators lack a "clearly established" liberty interest in not being force-medicated and that, therefore, defendants were entitled to qualified immunity).

235. *Casey*, 505 U.S. at 851.

236. *Mills v. Rogers*, 457 U.S. 291, 299 (1982) ("The substantive issue involves a definition of that protected constitutional [liberty] interest, as well as identification of the conditions under which competing state interests might outweigh it").

237. See, e.g., *Cruzan*, 497 U.S. at 261 (finding that preservation of life outweighs refusal of life-sustaining treatment); *Harper*, 494 U.S. at 210 (preventing danger outweighs refusal of antipsychotic drugs); *Nat'l Treasury Employees Union v. Von Raab*, 489 U.S. 656 (1989) (holding that national security outweighs refusal of drug tests).

238. *Harper*, 494 U.S. 210.

239. *Riggins v. Nevada*, 504 U.S. 127, 133–35 (1992).

240. *Sell v. United States*, 539 US 166 (2003).

241. Lawrence O. Gostin, "Compulsory Medical Treatment: The Limits of Bodily Integrity," *Hastings Center Report*, 33 (2003): 11–12.

242. The state interests that are often identified in "right to die" cases include preserving life, preventing suicide, maintaining the integrity of the medical profession, and protecting innocent third parties. See, e.g., *Thor v. Superior Court of Solano County*, 855 P.2d 375, 383 (Cal. 1993).

243. *Schloendorff v. Society of New York Hospital*, 105 N.E. 92, 93 (N.Y. 1914) (Justice Cardozo) ("Every human being of adult years and sound mind has a right to determine what shall be done with his own body").

244. *In re M.B. Mental Hygiene Legal Service*, 846 N.E. 2d 794 (N.Y. 2006) (holding that a guardian is entitled to withdraw lifesaving treatment for an incompetent person); *Shine v. Vega*, 709 N.E.2d 58 (Mass. 1999) (reviewing extensive state case law upholding the right of competent adults to refuse treatment).

245. See, e.g., *Rogers v. Commissioner of Department of Mental Health*, 458 N.E.2d 308 (Mass. 1983) (finding that an institutionalized mental patient is competent to make treatment decisions unless adjudicated incompetent).

246. *Jolly v. Coughlin*, 76 F.3d 468 (2d Cir. 1996) (permitting a competent prisoner to sue for imposing a TB test over his religious objections).

247. See, e.g., *Public Health Trust of Dade County v. Wons*, 541 So. 2d 96 (Fla. 1989) (permitting a Jehovah's Witness to refuse a blood transfusion); but see *Application of President & Dirs. of Georgetown College, Inc.*, 331 F.2d 1000

(D.C. Cir. 1964) (upholding an order authorizing a hospital to administer a blood transfusion to a Jehovah's Witness).

248. *A.D.H. v. State Department of Human Resources,* 640 So.2d 969 (Ala. Civ. App. 1994) (ordering a parent to permit treatment of an HIV-infected child); *People ex rel. Wallace v. Labrenz,* 104 N.E.2d 769 (Ill. 1952) (authorizing a blood transfusion over the parents' religious objections).

249. See, e.g., *In re M.B. Mental Hygiene Legal Service,* 846 N.E. 2d 794 (N.Y. 2006) (explaining that a "best interest" standard is statutorily required to be applied when making medical decisions about people who are not competent to make decisions for themselves). The doctrine and cases are discussed in Lawrence O. Gostin and Robert F. Weir, "Life and Death Choices after Cruzan: Case Law and Standards of Professional Conduct," *Milbank Quarterly,* 69 (1991): 143–73.

250. *Washington v. Harper,* 494 U.S. 210, 227 (1990) (upholding forced administration of antipsychotic medication if the inmate is dangerous to himself or others and the treatment is in the inmate's medical interest); see *McCormick v. Stalder,* 105 F.3d 1059, 1061 (5th Cir. 1997) (finding that the state's compelling interest in reducing the spread of tuberculosis justifies involuntary treatment); *United States v. Bechara,* 935 F. Supp. 892, 894 (S.D. Tex. 1996) (upholding involuntary sedation of a deportee to ensure public safety).

251. *Reynolds v. McNichols,* 488 F.2d 1378 (10th Cir. 1973) (upholding mandatory physical examination, treatment, and detention of a person suspected of having venereal disease); *People ex rel. Baker v. Strautz,* 54 N.E.2d 441 (Ill. 1944) (same); *Rock v. Carney,* 185 N.W. 798 (Mich. 1921) (upholding physical examination, but only upon reasonable grounds). For an investigation of the constitutionality of mandatory HIV screening of pregnant women, see Dorian L. Eden, "Is It Constitutional and Is It Effective? An Analysis of Mandatory HIV Testing of Pregnant Women," *Health Matrix,* 11 (2001): 659–86.

252. *City of New York v. Doe,* 614 N.Y.S.2d 8 (N.Y. App. Div. 1994) (upholding continued detention for tuberculosis treatment based on the fact that public health could not be protected by less restrictive means).

253. *Riggins v. Nevada,* 504 U.S. 127, 135 (1992) (invalidating forced administration of antipsychotic medication during the course of a trial without findings that there were no less intrusive alternatives, that the medication was medically appropriate, and that it was essential for the defendant's safety or the safety of others).

254. *Irwin v. Arrendale,* 159 S.E.2d 719 (Ga. Ct. App. 1967) (finding that requiring a prisoner to be x-rayed had no medical reason, was wholly capricious, and was done solely to exercise power).

255. See, e.g., Rick A. Bright, David K. Shay, Bo Shu, et al., "Adamantane Resistance among Influenza A Viruses Isolated Early during the 2005–2006 Influenza Season in the United States," *JAMA,* 295 (2006): 891–94; Dan I. Andersson, "Persistence of Antibiotic Resistant Bacteria," *Current Opinion in Microbiology,* 6 (2003): 452–56; Douglas D. Richman, ed., *Antiviral Drug Resistance* (Chichester, UK: John Wiley and Sons, 1996); see, generally, Enrico Mihich, ed., *Drug Resistance and Selectivity: Biochemical and Cellular Basis* (New York: Academic Press, 1973).

256. Sophia V. Kazakova, Jeffrey C. Hageman, and Matthew Matava, "A Clone of Methicillin-Resistant Staphylococcus Aureus among Professional Football Players," *New Engl. J. Med.,* 52 (2005): 68–475 (during the 2003 football season, eight MRSA infections occurred among five of the fifty-eight Rams players, all of which developed at turf-abrasion sites; MRSA infection was significantly associated with the lineman or linebacker position); Franz Josef Schmitz, Elke Lindenlauf, Basia Hofmann, et al., "The Prevalence of Low- and High-Level Mupirocin Resistance in Staphylococci from Nineteen European Hospitals," *Journal of Antimicrobial Chemotherapy,* 42 (1998): 489–95. For example, see the 2006 outbreak of MRSA in Scotland. Richard Gray, "MRSA Scheme Is £15 Million Failure," *Scotsman,* July 16, 2006.

257. See, e.g., Alan B. Bloch, Ida M. Onorato, Kenneth G. Castro, et al., "Nationwide Survey of Drug-Resistant Tuberculosis in the United States," *JAMA,* 271 (1994): 665–71; Barry R. Bloom and Christopher J. L. Murray, "Tuberculosis: Commentary on a Reemergent Killer," *Science,* 257 (1992): 1055–62; Centers for Disease Control and Prevention, "Emergence of Mycobacterium Tuberculosis with Extensive Resistance to Second-Line Drugs—Worldwide, 2000–2004," *Morbidity and Mortality Weekly Report,* 55 (2006): 301–5; see also Carlos A. Ball and Mark Barnes, "Public Health and Individual Rights: Tuberculosis Control and Detention Procedures in New York City," *Yale Law and Policy Review,* 12 (1994): 38–67; Josephine Gittler, "Controlling Resurgent Tuberculosis: Public Health Agencies, Public Health Policy, and Law," *Journal of Health Politics, Policy and Law,* 19 (1994): 107–47; Rosemary G. Reilly, "Combating the Tuberculosis Epidemic: The Legality of Coercive Measures," *Columbia Journal of Law and Social Problems,* 27 (1993): 101–49.

258. See, e.g., Centers for Disease Control and Prevention, "Investigation of a New Diagnosis of Multidrug-Resistant, Dual-Tropic HIV-1 Infection—New York City, 2005," *Morbidity and Mortality Weekly Report,* 55 (2006): 793–96; Douglas L. Mayer, "Prevalence and Incidence of Resistance to Zidovudine and Other Antiretroviral Drugs," *American Journal of Medicine,* 102 (1997): 70–75.

259. See, e.g., Michael D. Iseman, "Treatment of Multidrug-Resistant Tuberculosis," *New Eng. J. Med.,* 329 (1993): 784–91.

260. The overuse of antibiotics in animals is also thought to contribute to the problem of drug resistance. See Henrik C. Wegener, "The Consequences for Food Safety of the Use of Fluoroquinolones in Food Animals," *New Engl. J. Med.,* 340 (1999): 1581–82.

261. Ronald Bayer and David Wilkinson, "Directly Observed Therapy for Tuberculosis: History of an Idea," *Lancet,* 345 (1995): 1545–48.

262. Office of Technology Assessment, *The Continuing Challenge of Tuberculosis,* Pub. No. OTA-H-574 (Sept. 1993), http://www.wws.princeton.edu/ota/disk1/1993/9347_n.html.

263. Marcos A. Espinal and Cristopher Dye, "Can DOTS Control Multidrug-Resistant Tuberculosis?" *Lancet,* 365 (2005): 1206–9 (stating that DOT is a broader public health strategy, including diagnosis, support over six to eight months of treatment, and systems for maintenance of drug supplies and for recording and reporting); Jimmy Volmink, Patrice Matchaba, and Paul Garner, "Directly Observed Therapy and Treatment Adherence," *Lancet,* 355 (2000):

1345–49 (stating that DOT programs consist of more than supervised treatment, including incentives, tracing defaulters, legal sanctions, patient-centered approaches, staff motivation, and supervision).

264. C. Patrick Chaulk and Vahe A. Kazandjian, "Directly Observed Therapy for Treatment Completion of Pulmonary Tuberculosis: Consensus Statement of the Public Health Tuberculosis Guidelines Panel," *JAMA,* 279 (1998): 943–48 (noting that treatment completion rates for traditional self-administered therapy [SAT] ranged from 41.9 to 82 percent); Bruce L. Davidson, "A Controlled Comparison of Directly Observed Therapy vs. Self-Administered Therapy for Active Tuberculosis in the Urban United States," *Chest,* 114 (1998): 1239–43 (stating that nearly two-thirds of patients who started SAT had not completed therapy within eight months).

265. Jimmy Volmink and Paul Garner, "Directly Observed Therapy," *Lancet,* 349 (1997): 1399–1400 (noting that evidence for the effectiveness of DOT is not reliable).

266. See, e.g., Chaulk and Kazandjian, "Directly Observed Therapy" (recognizing that treatment completion rates for DOT ranged from 86 to 96.5 percent); Centers for Disease Control and Prevention, "Approaches to Improving Adherence to Anti-Tuberculosis Therapy—South Carolina and New York, 1986–1991," *Morbidity and Mortality Weekly Report,* 42 (1993): 74–75, 81 (providing a 93.9 percent completion rate).

267. Stephen E. Weiss, Philip C. Slocum, Francis X. Blais, et al., "The Effect of Directly Observed Therapy on the Rates of Drug Resistance and Relapse in Tuberculosis," *New Engl. J. Med.,* 330 (1994): 1179–84.

268. S. K. Sharma and J. J. Liu, "Progress of DOTS in Global Tuberculosis Control," *Lancet,* 367 (2006): 951–52 (noting that DOT has been implemented in 182 countries).

269. Kelly Morris, "WHO Sees DOTS," *Lancet,* 349 (1997): 855.

270. Centers for Disease Control and Prevention, *Improving Patient Adherence to Tuberculosis Treatment,* rev. ed. (Atlanta, GA: Centers for Disease Control and Prevention, 1994) (stating that CDC supports DOT); Centers for Disease Control and Prevention, "Initial Therapy for Tuberculosis in the Era of Multidrug Resistance," *Morbidity and Mortality Weekly Report,* 42 (1993): 1 (same).

271. See, e.g., American Thoracic Society, "Treatment of Tuberculosis and Tuberculosis Infection in Adults and Children," *American Journal of Respiratory and Critical Care Medicine,* 149 (1994): 1359–74 (supporting DOT); Chaulk and Kazandjian, "Directly Observed Therapy" (remarking that the Tuberculosis Guidelines Panel supports DOT).

272. Lawrence O. Gostin, Scott Burris, Zita Lazzarini, "The Law and the Public's Health: A Study of Infectious Disease Law in the United States," *Columbia Law Review,* 99 (1999): 59–128.

273. Ronald Bayer, Catherine Stayton, Moïse Desvarieux, et al., "Directly Observed Therapy and Treatment Completion for Tuberculosis in the United States: Is Universal Supervised Therapy Necessary?" *American Journal of Public Health,* 88 (1998): 1052–58 (noting that many locales with high treatment completion rates do not rely on DOT).

274. Thomas R. Frieden, Paula I. Fujiwara, Rita M. Washko, et al., "Tuberculosis in New York City: Turning the Tide," *New Engl. J. Med.,* 333 (1995): 229–33; M. Rose Gasner, Khin Lay Maw, Gabriel E. Feldman, et al., "The Use of Legal Action in New York City to Ensure Treatment of Tuberculosis," *New Engl. J. Med.,* 340 (1999): 359–66 (stating that for most patients treatment completion can usually be achieved without regulatory intervention).

275. Centers for Disease Control and Prevention, "Sexually Transmitted Diseases Treatment Guidelines, 2006," *Morbidity and Mortality Weekly Report,* 55 (2006): 1–94; James G. Hodge, Jr., Amy Pulver, Matthew Hogben, et al., "Expedited Partner Therapy: Assessing the Legal Environment," *American Journal of Public Health* (forthcoming 2007).

276. Centers for Disease Control and Prevention, *Expedited Partner Therapy in the Management of Sexually Transmitted Diseases* (Atlanta, GA: U.S. Department of Health and Human Services, 2006).

277. Jeffrey D. Klausner and Janice K. Chaw, "Patient-Delivered Therapy for Chlamydia: Putting Research into Practice," *Sexually Transmitted Diseases,* 30 (2003): 509–11.

278. Matthew R. Golden, William L. H. Whittington, H. Hunter Handsfield, et al., "Effect of Expedited Treatment of Sex Partners on Recurrent or Persistent Gonorrhea or Chlamydial Infection," *New Engl. J. Med.,* 352 (2005): 676–85.

279. James G. Hodge, Jr., *Expedited Partner Therapies for Sexually Transmitted Diseases: Assessing the Legal Environment* (Washington, DC: Center for Law and the Public's Health, 2006) (reporting that EPT is permissible or possible in thirty-nine jurisdictions and prohibited in thirteen jurisdictions), http://www.cdc.gov/std/ept/legal/default.htm.

280. Institute of Medicine, *The Hidden Epidemic: Confronting Sexually Transmitted Diseases* (Washington, DC: National Academies Press, 1997).

11. PUBLIC HEALTH STRATEGIES FOR EPIDEMIC DISEASE: ASSOCIATION, TRAVEL, AND LIBERTY

SOURCES FOR CHAPTER EPIGRAPHS: Albert Camus, *The Plague,* trans. Stuart Gilbert (New York: A. A. Knopf, 1948): 34. See Charles E. Rosenberg, "What Is an Epidemic? AIDS in Historical Perspective," in *Explaining Epidemics and Other Studies in the History of Medicine* (New York: Cambridge University Press, 1992): 278–92 (adapting Camus's *The Plague* to characterize an epidemic as a dramaturgic event in four acts: progressive revelation, managing randomness, negotiating public response, and subsidence and retrospection); State of Maine, Department of Human Services, quoted in Ronald Bayer and Amy Fairchild-Carrino, "AIDS and the Limits of Control: Public Health Orders, Quarantine, and Recalcitrant Behavior," *American Journal of Public Health,* 83 (1993): 1471–76; Institute of Medicine, *Microbial Threats to Health: Emergence, Detection and Response* (Washington, DC: National Academies Press, 2003): xvii.

1. Prevailing theories of disease ranged from foul air or soil to hereditary causes; scientists sometimes flatly rejected theories of contagion. Christopher J. Duncan and Susan Scott, "What Caused the Black Death," *Postgraduate Medical Journal,* 81 (2005): 315–20; Erwin H. Ackerknecht, "Anti-Contagionism between

1821 and 1867," *Bulletin of the History of Medicine,* 22 (1948): 562–93; John M. Eager, *The Early History of Quarantine: Origin of Sanitary Measures Directed against Yellow Fever* (Washington, DC: Government Printing Office, 1903): 5–15.

2. David P. Fidler and Lawrence O. Gostin, *Biosecurity in the Global Age: Biological Weapons, Public Health, and the Rule of Law* (Palo Alto, CA: Stanford University Press, 2007).

3. White House, Homeland Security Council, *National Strategy for Pandemic Influenza,* November 2005, http://www.whitehouse.gov/homeland/nspi.pdf; World Health Organization, *Global Influenza Preparedness Plan* (Geneva: World Health Organization, 2005).

4. Criminal prosecution for risking or causing the transmission of infectious disease is discussed on the *Reader* Web site.

5. A pest is any deadly epidemic disease or a pestilence, notably bubonic plague, derived from the French *peste,* from the Old French *pestilence* or the Latin *pestis. Oxford English Dictionary,* 2d ed., 1989. For a general history of the use of quarantine, see Gian Franco Gensini, Magdi H. Yacoub, and Andrea A. Conti, "The Concept of Quarantine in History: From Plague to SARS," *Journal of Infection,* 49 (2004): 257–61.

6. The Bible states: "All days wherein the Plague shall be in him he shall be defiled; he is unclean; he shall dwell alone; outside the camp shall his habitation be." Leviticus 13:46 (King James).

7. *Oxford English Dictionary,* 2d ed., 1989; see also "Lazar-house": a house for lazars, or diseased persons; "Lazar: a poor and diseased person, usually one afflicted with a loathsome disease." *Id.* (quoting Byron [1820]: "Thou must be cleansed of the black blood which makes thee / A lazar-house of tyranny"; and G. Meredith [1880]: "Their house would be a lazar-house, they would be condemned to seclusion").

8. Eager, *Early History of Quarantine,* 4–5.

9. Oleg P. Schepin and Waldemar V. Yermakov, *International Quarantine,* trans. Boris Meerovich and Vladimir Bobrov (Madison, CT: International Universities Press, 1991): 11; George Rosen, *A History of Public Health* (Baltimore, MD: Johns Hopkins University Press, 1993): 40.

10. Rosen, *History of Public Health,* 41–43; Eager, *Early History of Quarantine,* 5–6; Schepin and Yermakov, *International Quarantine,* 10.

11. Eager, *Early History of Quarantine,* 16–18; Rosen, *History of Public Health,* 43–44.

12. Frank Gerard Clemow, "Origin of Quarantine," *British Medical Journal,* 1 (1929): 122–23.

13. Eager, *Early History of Quarantine,* 18, 20–21.

14. Elizabeth C. Tandy, "Local Quarantine and Inoculation for Smallpox in the American Colonies (1620–1775)," *American Journal of Public Health,* 13 (1923): 203–7.

15. Donald Hopkins, *Princes and Peasants: Smallpox in History* (Chicago: University of Chicago Press, 1983): 238–39; James A. Tobey, "Public Health and the Police Power," *New York University Law Review,* 4 (1927): 126–33; Schepin and Yermakov, *International Quarantine,* 17–18.

16. *Acts and Resolves of the Province of Mass. Bay,* vol. 1, ch. 9 (1701–1702).

17. *Colonial Laws of N.Y.,* vol. 3, ch. 9973 (1755).

18. Wendy E. Parmet, "AIDS and Quarantine: The Revival of an Archaic Doctrine," *Hofstra Law Review,* 14 (1985): 53–90.

19. Sandeep Jauhar, "Leper Home to Fade but Not Memories of Prejudice," *Houston Chronicle,* June 29, 1998 (reporting on the transfer of the Gillis W. Long Hansen's Disease Center, called the "Louisiana Leper Home" or "Carville," from the United States to the state, which plans to close the hospital).

20. 1 Stat. 474 (1796); see *Annals of Congress* (1796): 1349–59 (debating whether to authorize the president to impose quarantines at ports of entry, with opponents arguing that the authority belonged to the states); Kathleen S. Swendiman and Jennifer K. Elsea, *Federal and State Quarantine and Isolation Authority* (Washington, DC: Congressional Research Service, 2006). See also Alfred J. Sciarrino, "The Grapes of Wrath and the Speckled Monster (Epidemics, Biological Terrorism and the Early Legal History of Two Major Defenses—Quarantine and Vaccination)," *Journal of Medicine and Law,* 7 (2003): 117–76; Edwin Maxey, "Federal Quarantine Law," *American Law Review,* 43 (1909): 382.

21. *Act of Feb. 25, 1799,* ch. 12, 1 Stat. 619.

22. *Federal Quarantine Act,* 20 Stat. L. 37 (1878) (see National Institutes of Health, "The NIH Almanac—Historical Chronology," *National Institutes of Health,* March 16, 2006, http://www.nih.gov/about/almanac/historical/legislative_chronology.htm).

23. "An Act Granting Additional Quarantine Powers and Imposing Additional Duties upon the Marine Hospital Service." See *Compagnie Française de Navigation à Vapeur v. Board of Health,* 186 U.S. 380, 395–96 (1902).

24. Ernest Freund, *The Police Power: Public Policy and Constitutional Rights* (Chicago: Callaghan, 1904): 124–30; Blewett H. Lee, "Limitations Imposed by the Federal Constitution on the Right of the States to Enact Quarantine Laws," *Harvard Law Review,* 2 (1889): 267–82. A conflict regarding quarantine, of course, can also ensue among different states. See *Louisiana v. Texas,* 176 U.S. 1 (1900) (upholding a Texas quarantine on goods from New Orleans, where yellow fever had been reported, against a complaint by Louisiana).

25. *Hennington v. Georgia,* 163 U.S. 299 (1896) (holding that state police power regulation affecting commerce is valid until superseded by Congress); see also William H. Cowles, "State Quarantine Laws and the Federal Constitution," *American Law Review,* 25 (1891): 45–73.

26. *Gibbons v. Ogden,* 22 U.S. 1, 205–6 (1824) ("Congress may control the state [quarantine] laws . . . for the regulation of commerce"); *Compagnie Française de Navigation à Vapeur,* 186 U.S. 380; *United States ex rel. Siegel v. Shinnick,* 219 F. Supp. 789 (1963).

27. See generally Irwin W. Sherman, *The Power of Plagues* (Washington, DC: American Society for Microbiology Press, 2006); William H. McNeill, *Plagues and Peoples,* 2d ed. (New York: Anchor Books, 1977).

28. Jared M. Diamond, *Guns, Germs, and Steel,* rev. ed. (New York: Norton, 2005); Barry S. Levy and Victor W. Sidel, eds., *War and Public Health* (New York: Oxford University Press, 1997).

29. Rosen, *History of Public Health*, 41; see also Saul N. Brody, *The Disease of the Soul: Leprosy in Medieval Literature* (Ithaca, NY: Cornell University Press, 1974).

30. See generally Howard Markel, *When Germs Travel: Six Major Epidemics That Have Invaded America and the Fears They Have Unleashed* (New York: Vintage Books, 2005); Thomas B. Stoddard and Walter Rieman, "AIDS and the Rights of the Individual: Toward a More Sophisticated Understanding and Discrimination," *Milbank Quarterly*, 68, supp. 1 (1990): 143–74; Paul J. Edelson, "Quarantine and Social Inequity," *JAMA*, 290 (2003): 2874.

31. David Musto, "Quarantine and the Problem of AIDS," *Milbank Quarterly*, 64, supp. 1 (1986): 97–117.

32. Guenter B. Risse, "Epidemics and History: Ecological Perspectives and Social Burdens," in *AIDS: The Burdens of History*, ed. Elizabeth Fee and Daniel M. Fox (Berkeley: University of California Press, 1988): 33–66.

33. Philip K. Wilson, "Bad Habits and Bad Genes: Early Twentieth Century Eugenic Attempts to Eliminate Syphilis and Associated 'Defects' from the United States," *Canadian Bulletin of Medical History*, 20 (2003): 11–41; Allan M. Brandt, *No Magic Bullet: A Social History of Venereal Disease in the United States since 1880* (New York: Oxford University Press, 1987).

34. Guenter B. Risse, "Revolt against Quarantine: Community Responses to the 1916 Polio Epidemic, Oyster Bay, New York," *Transactions and Studies of the College of Physicians of Philadelphia*, 14 (1992): 23–50.

35. Public health officials of San Francisco were convinced that Asian people were more susceptible to plagues as a result of their dietary reliance on rice rather than animal protein. Edelson, "Quarantine and Social Inequity," 2874.

36. Sheila M. Rothman, *Living in the Shadow of Death: Tuberculosis and the Social Experience of Illness in American History* (New York: Basic Books, 1994): 192–93; see Barron H. Lerner, "New York City's Tuberculosis Control Efforts: The Historical Limitations of War on Consumption," *American Journal of Public Health*, 83 (1993): 758–66 (stating that health departments detained TB patients after 1903, principally patients from socially disadvantaged groups).

37. Charles E. A. Winslow, *The Life of Hermann M. Biggs* (Philadelphia: Lea and Febiger, 1929): 158; Charles V. Chapin, "Pleasures and Hopes of the Health Officer," in *Papers of Charles V. Chapin, M.D.*, ed. Frederick P. Gorham (New York: Commonwealth Fund, 1934): 6.

38. John M. Grange, Matthew Gandy, Paul Farmer, et al., "Historical Declines in Tuberculosis: Nature, Nurture, and the Biosocial Model," *International Journal of Tuberculosis and Lung Disease*, 5 (2001): 208–12 (arguing that the decline in TB resulted from social improvements, a range of public health measures, and ecological changes in the disease); René Dubos and Jean Dubos, *The White Plague: Tuberculosis, Man and Society*, 2d ed. (New Brunswick, NJ: Rutgers University Press, 1987) (attributing the decline in mortality to vastly improved social conditions).

39. Though the United States did not adopt severe restrictions on the activities of people with HIV, some other countries did. Cuba, for example, engaged from 1986 to 1994 in widespread HIV screening and mandatory detention of HIV-positive people at sanitaria, where they were required to undergo treatment.

Though the detention policy is no longer in effect, about half of Cuba's HIV patients still live in the facilities. Though proponents argue that such restrictions are responsible for Cuba's low HIV rates, others give more credit to Cuba's political and geographical isolation, relatively strong health care system, and other aggressive public health measures. Helena Hansen and Nora Groce, "Human Immunodeficiency Virus and Quarantine in Cuba," *JAMA,* 290 (2003): 2875. See also Helena Hansen and Nora Groce, "From Quarantine to Condoms: Shifting Policies and Problems of HIV Control in Cuba," *Medical Anthropology,* 19 (2001): 259–92; Ronald Bayer and Cheryl Healton, "Controlling AIDS in Cuba: The Logic of Quarantine," *New Engl. J. Med.,* 320 (1989): 1022–24.

40. Ryan White and Ann Marie Cunningham, *Ryan White: My Own Story* (New York: Dial Books for Young Readers, 1991); see also David L. Kirp, *Learning by Heart: AIDS and School Children in America's Communities* (New Brunswick, NJ: Rutgers University Press, 1990); Lawrence O. Gostin and David W. Webber, "The AIDS Litigation Project: HIV/AIDS in the Courts in the 1990s, Part 2," *AIDS and Public Policy Journal,* 13 (1998): 3–19.

41. Robin Marantz Henig, "AIDS: A New Disease's Deadly Odyssey," *New York Times Magazine,* February 6, 1983 ("Innocent bystanders caught in the path of a new disease, they can make no behavioral decisions to minimize their risk: hemophiliacs cannot stop taking bloodclotting medication; surgery patients cannot stop getting transfusions; women cannot control the drug habits of their mates; babies cannot choose their mothers").

42. Allan M. Brandt, "AIDS: From Social History to Social Policy," *Law, Medicine and Health Care,* 14 (1986): 231–42.

43. William F. Buckley, Jr., "Identify All the Carriers," *New York Times,* March 18, 1986 (recommending that persons with HIV infection be tattooed on their forearms and buttocks).

44. See, e.g., Nola M. Ries, "Public Health Law and Ethics: Lessons from SARS and Quarantine," *Health Law Review,* 13 (2004): 3–6 (reporting on public opinion surveys in the 1980s that found one-third to one-half of the American public supporting quarantine of AIDS patients); James F. Grutsch and A. D. J. Robertson, "The Coming of AIDS: It Didn't Start with the Homosexuals and It Won't End with Them," *American Spectator,* 19 (1986): 12–15; "Florida Considering Locking Up Some Carriers of the AIDS Virus," *New York Times,* January 27, 1988 (reporting on a state proposal of "special lock-up" wards); Tamar Lewin, "Rights of Citizens and Society Raise Legal Muddle on AIDS," *New York Times,* October 14, 1987 (reporting that Senator Helms and Pat Robertson suggest "quarantine may be necessary").

45. David J. Rothman, "The Single Disease Hospital: Why Tuberculosis Justifies a Departure that AIDS Does Not," *Journal of Law, Medicine, and Ethics,* 21 (1993): 296–302.

46. Francis M. Pottenger, "Is Another Chapter in Public Phthisiophobia About to Be Written?" *California State Journal of Medicine,* 1 (1903): 81.

47. See generally Randy Shilts, *And the Band Played On* (New York: St. Martin's Press, 1987); David Altman, *AIDS in the Mind of America* (Garden City, NY: Anchor Press, 1986).

48. Lawrence O. Gostin, Ronald Bayer, and Amy L. Fairchild, "Ethical and

Legal Challenges Posed by Severe Acute Respiratory Syndrome: Implications for the Control of Severe Infectious Disease Threats," *JAMA,* 290 (2003): 3229–37.

49. Especially vigorous quarantine policies—and unfair stigma for diseases they were perceived to bring—were often levied against immigrants in the nineteenth and early twentieth centuries. Katherine Stephenson, "The Quarantine War: The Burning of the New York Marine Hospital in 1858," *Public Health Reports,* 119 (2004): 79–92; Howard Markel, *Quarantine! East European Jewish Immigrants and the New York City Epidemics of 1892* (Baltimore, MD: Johns Hopkins University Press, 1997).

50. Though health departments have the power to confine, they may not have an affirmative duty to provide inpatient care to persons with infectious disease. See *County of Cook v. City of Chicago,* 593 N.E.2d 928 (Ill. App. Ct. 1992) (finding that the county had no duty to provide inpatient treatment for persons with TB).

51. Cease and desist orders are issued on the administrative authority of the health department. An order typically specifies that the individual has failed to modify his behavior despite counseling, and warns of further legal action, including criminal prosecution, if the individual persists in specified behaviors, such as unprotected sex or needle sharing.

52. *Oxford English Dictionary,* 2d ed., 1989.

53. *Id.* (quoting *Pepys's Diary,* November 26, 1663: "Making of all ships coming from thence . . . to perform their quarantine for thirty days . . . contrary to the import of the word . . . it signifies now the thing, not the time spent in doing it"; and Jephson [1859]: "The lepers often sought a voluntary death as the only escape from their perpetual quarantine").

54. Paul S. Sehdev, "The Origin of Quarantine," *Clinical Infectious Diseases,* 35 (2002): 1071–72.

55. David L Heymann, ed., *Control of Communicable Diseases Manual,* 18th ed. (Washington, DC: American Public Health Association, 2004): 621 (describing two forms of quarantine: absolute and modified).

56. *Id.,* 617–19 (describing six forms of isolation: strict, contact, respiratory, tuberculosis, enteric precautions, and drainage/secretion precautions). See also Marguerite M. Jackson and Patricia Lynch, "Isolation Practices: A Historical Perspective," *American Journal of Infection Control,* 13 (1985): 21–31.

57. Richard Coker, "Just Coercion? Detention of Nonadherent Tuberculosis Patients," *Annals of the New York Academy of Science,* 953 (2001): 216–23; Barron H. Lerner, "Catching Patients: Tuberculosis and Detention in the 1990s," *Chest,* 115 (1999): 236–41.

58. Gostin, Bayer, and Fairchild, "Ethical and Legal Challenges Posed by Severe Acute Respiratory Syndrome," 3229–37.

59. GlobalSecurity.org, "Flu Pandemic Mitigation—Quarantine and Isolation," http://www.globalsecurity.org/security/ops/hsc-scen-3_flu-pandemic-quarantine.htm (advising quarantined individuals to "minimize contact with other household members by sleeping and eating in a separate room, using a separate bathroom, and using protective equipment such as masks").

60. City of Toronto, "Work Quarantine," May 27, 2003, http://www.toronto.ca/health/sars/pdf/sars_workers.pdf.

61. Markel, *Quarantine!*

62. *Oxford English Dictionary,* 2d ed. (1989).

63. *Jew Ho v. Williamson,* 103 F.10 (C.C.N.D. Cal. 1900).

64. Joseph Barbera, Anthony Macintyre, Lawrence O. Gostin, et al., "Large-Scale Quarantine following Biological Terrorism in the United States: Scientific Examination, Logistic and Legal Limits, and Possible Consequences," *JAMA,* 286 (2001): 2711–17.

65. Robert J. Blendon, Catherine M. DesRoches, Martin S. Cetron, et al., "Attitudes toward the Use of Quarantine in a Public Health Emergency in Four Countries," *Health Affairs,* 25 (2006): w15–25.

66. Centers for Disease Control and Prevention, "Efficiency of Quarantine during an Epidemic of Severe Acute Respiratory Syndrome—Beijing, China, 2003," *Morbidity and Mortality Weekly Report,* 52 (2003): 1037–40.

67. *Gibbons v. Ogden,* 22 U.S. 1, 25 (1824); *Hennington v. Georgia,* 163 U.S. 299 (1896).

68. National Conference of State Legislatures, *Sexually Transmitted Diseases: A Policymaker's Guide and Summary of State Laws* (Denver, CO: National Conference of State Legislatures, 1998): 85–91 (cataloguing quarantine in the fifty states); see Lewis W. Petteway, "Compulsory Quarantine and Treatment of Persons Infected with Venereal Diseases," *Florida Law Journal,* 18 (1944): 13.

69. Howard Markel, *When Germs Travel,* 13–46; Lawrence O. Gostin, "Controlling the Resurgent Tuberculosis Epidemic: A Fifty State Survey of Tuberculosis Statutes and Proposals for Reform," *JAMA*, 269 (1993): 256–61 (cataloguing civil commitment in the fifty states); Advisory Council for the Elimination of Tuberculosis (ACET), "Tuberculosis Control Laws—United States, 1993," *Morbidity and Mortality Weekly Report,* 42 (1993): 7–9.

70. Lawrence O. Gostin, Scott Burris, and Zita Lazzarini, "The Law and the Public's Health: A Study of Infectious Disease Law in the United States," *Columbia Law Review,* 99 (1999): 59–128. See also Bayer and Fairchild-Carrino, "AIDS and the Limits of Control," 1471–76 (in the first decade of the epidemic, twenty-five states enacted statutes for isolation of persons with HIV, usually based on risk behavior); Paul Barron, "State Statutes Dealing with HIV and AIDS: A Comprehensive State-by-State Summary," *Law and Sexuality: A Review of Lesbian, Gay, Bisexual, and Transgender Legal Issues,* 13 (2004): 1–603 (providing a comprehensive overview of laws pertaining to HIV in each state).

71. National Conference of State Legislatures, "Overview of State Public Health Preparedness," January 28, 2002, http://www.ncsl.org/programs/press/2002/snapshot.htm#quarantine.

72. Gostin, Burris, and Lazzarini, "The Law and the Public's Health"; Daniel S. Reich, "Modernizing Local Responses to Public Health Emergencies: Bioterrorism, Epidemics, and the Model State Emergency Health Powers Act," *Journal of Contemporary Health Law and Policy,* 19 (2003): 379–414.

73. White House, Office of Homeland Security, *National Strategy for Homeland Security,* July 2002, http://www.whitehouse.gov/homeland/book/nat_strat_hls.pdf. See also Institute of Medicine, *The Future of the Public's Health in the Twenty-first Century* (Washington, DC: National Academies Press, 2002) (urging reform of outdated public health statutes).

74. Center for Law and the Public's Health at Georgetown and Johns Hopkins Universities, "Model State Health Powers Act Legislative Surveillance Table," July 15 2006, http://www.publichealthlaw.net/MSEHPA/MSEHPA%20Surveillance.pdf (thirty-seven states have passed legislation based on the MSEHPA).

75. Lawrence O. Gostin, Jason W. Sapsin, Stephen P. Teret, et al., "The Model State Emergency Health Powers Act: Planning for and Response to Bioterrorism and Naturally Occurring Infectious Diseases," *JAMA,* 288 (2002): 622–28.

76. James G. Hodge, Lawrence O. Gostin, Kristine Gebbie, et al., "Transforming Public Health Law: The Turning Point Model State Public Health Act," *Journal of Law, Medicine, and Ethics,* 34 (2006): 77–84.

77. *Public Health Service Act* §§ 361–68, 42 U.S.C. §§ 264–72.

78. 42 U.S.C. § 264.

79. 42 U.S.C. § 271; 28 U.S.C § 1331.

80. Department of Health and Human Services, Control of Communicable Diseases (Proposed Rule), 42 CFR Parts 70 and 71 (November 30, 2005). The current federal regulations are found in 42 CFR parts 70 and 71 (part 71 deals with foreign arrivals, and part 70 deals with interstate matters).

81. U.S. Const. Art. I, § 10, cl. 2. See *Brown v. Maryland,* 25 U.S. (12 Wheat.) 419 (1827); Cowles, "State Quarantine Laws," 50–52.

82. *Gibbons,* 22 U.S. (9 Wheat.) at 205.

83. Deborah Jones Merritt, "The Constitutional Balance between Health and Liberty," *Hastings Center Report,* 16 (1986): supp. 2–10; Deborah Jones Merritt, "Communicable Disease and Constitutional Law: Controlling AIDS," *New York University Law Review,* 61 (1986): 739–99; Parmet, "AIDS and Quarantine," 62–66.

84. See, e.g., *Mugler v. Kansas,* 123 U.S. 623 (1887) (holding that the state could exercise police powers to prohibit manufacture or sale of liquor); *Staples v. Plymouth County,* 17 N.W. 569 (Iowa 1883) (holding that the provider of lumber to build a pest house during a smallpox epidemic could proceed with an action to recoup costs from the county); *Haverty v. Bass,* 66 Me. 71 (1875) (upholding removal to a separate facility of a child believed to have smallpox).

85. See, e.g., *Smith v. St. Louis & Southwestern Railway Co.,* 181 U.S. 248 (1901) (upholding a quarantine of cattle that affected interstate commerce); *People ex rel. Barmore v. Robertson,* 134 N.E. 815 (Ill. 1922) (upholding quarantine and other restrictions of a typhoid carrier); *Ex parte Culver,* 202 P. 661 (1921) (upholding imprisonment of a woman who removed a quarantine placard after being placed in quarantine when she came into contact with a diphtheria carrier); *Ex parte McGee,* 185 P. 14 (Kan. 1919) (upholding detention of men with venereal diseases in a prison); *Daniel v. Putnam County,* 38 S.E. 980 (Ga. 1901) (holding that a county did not have the authority to tax for the purchase of smallpox vaccine); *Board of Health v. Ward,* 54 S.W. 725 (Ky. 1900) (granting a county health board the entitlement to sue to regain control of a pest house from fiscal court); *Brown v. Manning,* 172 N.W. 522 (Neb. 1919) (holding that people detained to prevent transmission of venereal disease are not entitled to a writ of habeas corpus); *White v. City of San Antonio,* 60 S.W. 426 (Tex. 1901) (denying a claim by a hotel owner for loss of business when the city quarantined people with yellow

fever in the hotel); *Highland v. Schlute,* 82 N.W. 62 (Mich. 1900) (upholding quarantine of a man whose coresident was ill with smallpox).

86. See, e.g., *Varholy v. Sweat,* 15 So. 2d 267 (Fla. 1943) (denying the assertion of a woman held in quarantine for venereal disease that she had a right to be released on bond); *State v. Rackowski,* 86 A. 606 (Conn. 1913) (and cases cited therein); *Allison v. Cash,* 137 S.W. 245 (Ky. 1911) (holding that closure of the plaintiff's store during a smallpox investigation was not a taking, and destruction of goods by necessary fumigation was not illegal); *Highland,* 82 N.W. at 63–64.

87. Most courts held that such delegations were constitutional and the powers exercised were not *ultra vires*. See, e.g., *People v. Tait,* 103 N.E. 750 (Ill. 1913) (upholding a conviction for violating a quarantine order for scarlet fever); *Rock v. Carney,* 185 N.W. 798 (Mich. 1921) (upholding the forced examination and quarantine of a woman with venereal disease); but see *State ex rel. Adams v. Burdge,* 70 N.W. 347 (Wis. 1879) (overturning removal of children from school for lack of smallpox vaccinations when there was no present health emergency). The cases are collected in *General Delegation of Power to Guard against Spread of Contagious Disease,* 8 A.L.R. 836 (1920).

88. *White,* 60 S.W. at 426; but see *Haag v. Board of Commissioners,* 60 Ind. 511 (1878) (allowing a nuisance case to go forward against a pesthouse for smallpox).

89. *Spring v. Hyde Park,* 137 Mass. 554 (1884) (holding that the city was not liable for expenses from using an apartment building as a hospital because the health board was not acting as agent of the city when it took possession of the building).

90. *Pinkham v. Dorothy,* 55 Me. 135 (1868) (holding that the municipality did not have specific authority to impress a carriage stagecoach to transport smallpox patients).

91. A good overview of early American quarantine cases can be found in Sciarrino, "The Grapes of Wrath," 117–76.

92. *In re Martin,* 188 P.2d 287 (Cal. Ct. App. 1948) (holding that quarantine was reasonable because prostitutes are likely to have venereal diseases); *State ex rel. Kennedy v. Head,* 185 S.W.2d 530 (Tenn. 1945) (upholding a fine for escaping from quarantine); *Varholy,* 15 So. 2d at 267; *City of Little Rock v. Smith,* 163 S.W.2d 705 (Ark. 1942) (upholding detention of a woman with venereal disease); *Ex parte Company,* 139 N.E. 204 (Ohio 1922) (same); *Ex parte Arata,* 198 P. 814 (Cal. Ct. App. 2nd Dist. 1921) (upholding presumption of venereal disease and quarantine of prostitutes but granting the defendant's habeas petition because government had not proven she was a prostitute); *Ex parto Shepard,* 195 P. 1077 (Cal. Ct. App. 1921) (holding that a health officer had to assert more than mere suspicion of venereal disease to detain); *McGee,* 184 P. at 14; *State ex rel. McBride v. Superior Court,* 174 P. 973 (Wash. 1918) (holding that the legislature can make the finding of a health officer final and binding on the courts).

93. *Greene v. Edwards,* 263 S.E.2d 661 (W. Va. 1980) (requiring the same due process for TB detention as for civil commitment for mental illness); *In re Halko,* 54 Cal. Rptr. 661 (Cal. Ct. App. 1966) (upholding detention for TB); *Jones v. Czapkay,* 6 Cal. Rptr. 182 (Cal. Ct. App. 1960) (refusing to find county health officials liable for a secondary case of TB after the initial case left quar-

antine); *White v. Seattle Local Union No. 81,* 337 P.2d 289 (Wash. 1959) (holding that a union did not wrongfully remove an officer who was confined for TB).

94. *Crayton v. Larabee,* 116 N.E. 355 (N.Y. 1917), aff'g 147 N.Y.S. 1105 (N.Y. App. Div. 1914) (overturning a quarantine decision where it was unlikely that the plaintiff was exposed to smallpox); *Allison,* 137 S.W. at 245; *Hengehold v. City of Covington,* 57 S.W. 495 (Ky. 1900) (upholding removal of smallpox patients to pesthouse); *Henderson County Board of Health,* 54 S.W. at 725; *Highland,* 82 N.W. at 62; *Smith v. Emery,* 42 N.Y.S. 258 (N. Y. App. Div. 1896) (reversing judgment in favor of smallpox detainee for false imprisonment); *In re Smith,* 40 N.E. 497 (N.Y. 1895) (refusing a health commission power to quarantine anyone who refuses smallpox vaccination); *Spring,* 137 Mass. at 554; *Beckwith v. Sturdevant,* 42 Conn. 158 (1875) (holding that a family with smallpox could not be placed in unoccupied house without the consent of the owner).

95. *Tait,* 103 N.E. at 750; *Rackowski,* 86 A. at 606.

96. *Kirk v. Wyman,* 65 S.E. 387 (S. C. 1909) (enjoining an order to place an elderly woman with leprosy in a pesthouse).

97. *Rudolphe v. City of New Orleans,* 11 La. Ann. 242 (1854) (upholding quarantine of a ship carrying passengers with cholera).

98. *Jew Ho,* 103 F. 10 (forbidding quarantine of an area that was directed entirely against Chinese).

99. See, e.g., *McBride,* 174 P. at 979.

100. *Kirk,* 65 S.E. at 392.

101. See, e.g., *McGee,* 185 P. at 14.

102. See, e.g., *Mugler,* 123 U.S. at 660–61 (1887) (the power to quarantine "so as to bind us all must exist somewhere; else, society will be at the mercy of the few, who, regarding only their appetites or passions, may be willing to imperil the security of the many, provided only they are permitted to do as they please"); *Irwin v. Arrendale,* 159 S.E.2d 441 (Ga. Ct. App. 1967) (holding that individuals must submit to reasonable public health measures for the common good); *City of Little Rock v. Smith,* 163 S.W.2d 697–99 (Ark. 1942) ("Private rights . . . if any, must yield in the interest of security"; venereal disease "affects the public health so intimately and so insidiously that considerations of delicacy and privacy may not be permitted to thwart measures necessary to avert the public peril").

103. *Tait,* 103 N.E. at 752.

104. See, e.g., *Huffman v. District of Columbia,* 39 A.2d 558, 560 (D.C. App. 1944); *Ex parte Dillon,* 186 P. 170 (Cal. 1919) (ordering the discharge of people held in jail, for lack of evidence that they had a venereal disease).

105. *Viemeister v. White,* 72 N.E. 97 (N.Y. 1904) (upholding mandatory vaccination of schoolchildren).

106. *Smith v. Emery,* 42 N.Y. Supp. 258, 260 (1896) ("The mere possibility that persons may have been exposed to disease is not sufficient. . . . They must have been exposed to it, and the conditions actually exist for a communication of the contagion"); *Ex parte Shepard,* 195 P.2d 1077 (Cal. 1921) (holding that mere suspicion of VD is insufficient to uphold a quarantine order); *Arata,* 198 P. at 816 ("Mere suspicion unsupported by facts . . . will afford no jurisdiction at all for depriving people of their liberty"); *State v. Snow,* 324 S.W.2d 532

(Ark. 1959) (holding that commitment for TB treatment requires a finding that the patient is a danger to the public health).

107. See e.g, *Dillon,* 186 P. at 170 (holding that marital status, in the absence of prostitution, cannot provide reasonable cause for suspicion of STI); *Wragg v. Griffin,* 170 N.W. 400 (Iowa 1919) (holding that health authorities could not detain a man "suspected" of having gonorrhea); *Snow,* 324 S.W.2d at 533 (officials have to provide evidence of active TB [chest x-ray, sputum tests, or other approved diagnostic procedures] to justify involuntary commitment); see Parmet, "AIDS and Quarantine," 67–68.

108. *Ex Parte Mason,* 22 Ohio N.P. (n.s.) 21 (Ohio Ct. Com. Pl. 1919); *Ex parte Company,* 139 N.E. at 205–6 (Ohio 1922); see also *Ex parte Johnson,* 180 P. 644 (Cal. Ct. App. 1919).

109. *People ex rel. Baker v. Strautz,* 54 N.E. 2d 441, 444 (Ill. 1944). As late as 1973, a federal court of appeals said: "It is not illogical or unreasonable, and on the contrary it is reasonable, to suspect that known prostitutes are a prime source of infectious venereal disease. Prostitution and venereal disease are no strangers." *Reynolds v. McNichols,* 488 F. 2d 1378, 1382 (10th Cir. 1973); see also *Head,* 185 S.W.2d at 530; *In re Caselli,* 204 P. 364 (Mont. 1922) (denying habeas claim to a woman with gonorrhea).

110. The court in *Kirk v. Wyman,* 65 S.E. 387, 391 (S.C. 1909), would not subject Mary Kirk to an unsafe environment. She was to have been isolated in a pesthouse—a "structure of four small rooms in a row, with no piazzas, used heretofore for the isolation of negroes with smallpox, situated within a hundred yards of the place where the trash of the city . . . is collected and burned." The court concluded that "even temporary isolation in such a place would be a serious affliction and peril to an elderly lady, enfeebled by disease, and accustomed to the comforts of life." See *Jew Ho,* 103 F. 10 at 22 (confining large groups of people in an area where bubonic plague was suspected placed them at increased risk). The court was less rigorous, however, in reviewing the conditions of isolation in *Ex parte Martin,* 188 P.2d 287, 291 (Cal. Ct. App. 1948). The court supported giving health officers discretion as to the place of isolation. The county jail was designated as a quarantine area for people with STIs despite uncontested evidence that it was overcrowded and had been condemned by a legislative investigating committee. The court supported the attorney general's position that "while jails, as public institutions, were established for purposes other than confinement of diseased persons, occasions of emergency or lack of other public facilities for quarantine require that jails be used."

111. The theory of habitable and healthful conditions is found mostly in mental health cases, but courts have extended it to infectious disease control. *Neimes v. Ta,* 985 S.W.2d 132, 141–42 (Tex. Ct. App. 1998) (reading *Youngberg* to extend to civil confinement of persons with TB); *Souvannarath v. Hadden,* 116 Cal. Rptr. 2d 7 (Cal. Ct. App. 2002) (holding that state law forbids detainment of a noncompliant multidrug-resistant TB patient in a jail); *Benton v. Reid,* 231 F.2d 780 (D.C. Cir. 1956) (persons with infectious disease are not criminals and should not be detained in jails); *State v. Hutchinson,* 18 S. 2d 723 (Ala. 1944) (same); but see *Ex parte Martin,* 188 P.2d 287 (Cal. Ct. App. 1948) (upholding quarantine in a county jail although it was overcrowded and had been condemned).

112. 457 U.S. 307, 315, 319, 324 (1982) (finding entitlement to "such minimally adequate or reasonable training to ensure safety and freedom from undue restraint").

113. *Jew Ho*, 103 F.10. The quarantine in *Jew Ho* followed directly after another public health initiative designed to harass Chinese residents of San Francisco. In *Wong Wai v. Willliamson*, 103 F. 1 (C.C.N.D. Cal. 1900), the court struck down as discriminatory an order that required all Chinese residents to be vaccinated against bubonic plague prior to leaving the city.

114. *Jew Ho*, 103 F. 10 at 24.

115. David Markovits, "Quarantines and Distributive Justice," *Journal of Law, Medicine and Ethics*, 33 (2005): 323–44.

116. *Shapiro v. Thompson*, 394 U.S. 618 (1969) (holding unconstitutional a one-year residency requirement to receive welfare benefits); *Korematsu v. United States*, 323 U.S. 214, 218 (1944) ("Nothing short of . . . the gravest imminent danger to the public safety can constitutionally justify" either "exclusion from the area in which one's home is located" or "constant confinement to the home" during certain hours); *Kansas v. Hendricks*, 521 U.S. 346, 356 (1997) (noting that while freedom from physical restraint is at the core of the liberty protected by the Due Process Clause, that liberty interest is not absolute); *Snow*, 324 S.W.2d at 532 (holding that civil commitment law is not penal, but is to be strictly construed to protect rights of citizens).

117. *Vitek v. Jones*, 445 U.S. 480, 491 (1980) (holding that an inmate was entitled to due process before transfer to a mental institution); see *Addington v. Texas*, 441 U.S. 418, 425 (1979) (holding that civil commitment is a "significant deprivation of liberty").

118. *Greene v. Edwards*, 263 S.E. 2d 661, 663 (W. Va. 1980).

119. *City of Cleburne v. Cleburne Living Center*, 473 U.S. 432, 440 (1985). But see *Seling v. Young*, 531 U.S. 250 (2001) (stating that civil commitment of violent sexual predators need only bear a rational relationship to state goals of treatment and incapacitation).

120. Scott Burris, "Fear Itself: AIDS, Herpes and Public Health Decisions," *Yale Law and Policy Review*, 3 (1985): 479–518. See *Kansas v. Crane*, 534 U.S. 407 (2002) (holding that, in order to commit repeat sex offenders, the state must demonstrate "proof of serious difficulty in controlling behavior," which can distinguish a committable offender from a typical recidivist).

121. 422 U.S. 563 (1975).

122. See, e.g., *Suzuki v. Yuen*, 617 F.2d 173, 178 (9th Cir. 1980) (holding that Hawaii law allowing civil commitment on threat of harm to any property was unconstitutionally overbroad).

123. Although courts defer to the professional judgment of health officials, they do require a finding of dangerousness. See *Souvannarath*, 116 Cal. Rptr. 2d at 11–12 (discussing a California statute requiring a finding that a tuberculosis patient is both a danger to the public health and substantially unlikely to complete treatment before the patient can be confined for treatment); *Snow*, 324 S.W.2d at 534 (Ark. 1959) (basing the rationale for commitment on "the theory that the public has an interest to be protected"); *In re Halko*, 54 Cal. Rptr. 661 (Cal. Ct. App. 1966) (holding that isolation of a person with TB does

not deprive a person of due process if the health officer has reasonable grounds to believe he is dangerous); *Moore v. Draper,* 57 So. 2d 648, 650 (Fla. 1952) (holding that, when a person's disease is arrested to the point where he is no longer a danger, he may seek release); *Moore v. Armstrong,* 149 So. 2d 36 (Fla. 1963) (same).

124. 614 N.Y.S.2d 8, 9 (App. Div. 1994); see *City of New York v. Antoinette R.,* 630 N.Y.S.2d 1008 (N.Y. Sup. Ct. 1995) (upholding detention for TB treatment upon clear and convincing evidence that less restrictive means would not result in successful treatment).

125. *Souvannarath,* 116 Cal. Rptr. 2d at 11–12 (discussing a California statute that requires health officers to list what less restrictive options were considered and why they were rejected in detention orders); *City of New York v. Doe,* 614 N.Y.S.2d 8 (App. Div. 1994). The most developed expression of the right to less restrictive alternatives occurs in mental health cases. See, e.g., *Covington v. Harris,* 419 F.2d 617 (D.C. 1969) (requiring a finding that there are no less restrictive alternatives to hold a patient in the maximum security section of a psychiatric hospital); *Lessard v. Schmidt,* 349 F. Supp. 1078 (E.D. Wis. 1972) (requiring consideration of less restrictive alternatives prior to civil commitment). See also *Model State Public Health Act* § 5–108(b)(1) (Pub. Health Statute Modernization Nat'l Excellence Collaborative 2003) (requiring that isolation and quarantine be used only when they are the least restrictive means necessary).

126. Lawrence O. Gostin, "The Resurgent Tuberculosis Epidemic in the Era of AIDS: Reflections on Public Health, Law, and Society," *Maryland Law Review,* 54 (1995): 1–131.

127. Response to Public Comments concerning Proposed Amendments to Section 11.47 of the Health Code 7 (March 2, 1993).

128. *O'Connor v. Donaldson,* 422 U.S. 563, 580 (1975) (Berger, C.J., concurring) (holding that the involuntary commitment of a patient who was not a danger to self or others in a psychiatric hospital violated his constitutional rights). See *Vitek v. Jones,* 445 U.S. 480 (1980) (requiring procedural due process before transfer of a patient from prison to psychiatric hospital); *Project Release v. Prevost,* 722 F.2d 960 (2d Cir. 1983) (upholding civil commitment under a law that adequately protected procedural and substantive due process); *Addington v. Texas,* 441 U.S. 418 (1979) (holding that civil commitment requires a finding that the patient was a risk to self or others by more than a preponderance of the evidence).

129. *Washington v. Harper,* 494 U.S. 210 (1990) (holding that prisoners' right to refuse medication must be balanced against the state's interest in treating mentally ill prisoners and maintaining a safe prison).

130. See, e.g., *In re Ballay,* 482 F. 2d 648, 563–66 (D.C. Cir. 1973) (requiring proof beyond a reasonable doubt of dangerousness for a long-term civil commitment); but see *Morales v. Turman,* 562 F.2d 993, 998 (5th Cir. 1977) ("[The] state should not be required to provide the procedural safeguards of a criminal trial when imposing a quarantine to protect the public against a highly communicable disease").

131. *Addington,* 441 U.S. at 425. See *Jackson v. Indiana,* 406 U.S. 715 (1972)

(holding that due process requires that the duration of commitment bear some reasonable relation to the purpose for which the individual is committed).

132. *Addington,* 441 U.S. at 426 (requiring that the standard of proof in commitments for mental illness must be greater than the preponderance of evidence standard, but the reasonable doubt standard is not constitutionally required).

133. *Greene v. Edwards,* 263 S.E.2d 661 (W. Va. 1980).

134. However, the Supreme Court has ruled that incurability of a dangerous condition alone, which entails a high likelihood that the detained person will never be released, is not grounds to invalidate that person's civil confinement. *Seling,* 531 U.S. at 262.

135. Centers for Disease Control and Prevention, *Interim Pre-Pandemic Planning Guidance: Community Strategy for Pandemic Influenza Mitigation in the United States* (Atlanta: CDC, 2007); Institute of Medicine, *Modeling Community Containment for Pandemic Influenza* (Washington, DC: National Academies Press, 2006); Trust for America's Health, *Ready or Not? Protecting the Public's Health from Diseases, Disasters and Bioterrorism* (Washington, DC: Trust for America's Health, 2006); World Health Organization Writing Group, "Nonpharmaceutical Interventions for Pandemic Influenza, National and International Measures," *Emerging Infectious Diseases,* 12 (2006): 81–94 (evaluating the empirical evidence for NPI); Julia E. Aledort, Sam Bozzette, Nicole Lurie, et al., *Nonpharmacological Public Health Interventions for Pandemic Influenza: Proceedings of an Expert Panel Meeting,* WR-408-DHHS (Washington, DC: Rand, 2006) (recommending community hygiene, hospital infection control, limited mandatory segregation, and sheltering at home); David Heyman, *Model Operational Guidelines for Disease Exposure Control* (Washington, DC: Center for Strategic and International Studies, 2005); Thomas V. Inglesby, Jennifer B. Nuzzo, Tara O'Toole, and D. A. Henderson, "Disease Mitigation Measures in the Control of Pandemic Influenza," *Biosecurity and Bioterrorism: Biodefense Strategy, Practice, and Science,* 4 (2006): 1–10.

136. Howard Markel, Alexandra M. Stern, J. Alexander Navarro, et al., *A Historical Assessment of Nonpharmaceutical Disease Containment Strategies Employed by Selected U.S. Communities during the Second Wave of the 1918–1920 Influenza Pandemic* (Fort Belvoir, VA: Defense Threat Reduction Agency, 2006) (finding that protective sequestration—if enacted early enough, crafted to encourage community compliance, and continued for the lengthy period of time during which the area is at risk—stands the best chance of success).

137. American Public Health Association, "Influenza: A Report of APHA," *JAMA,* 71 (1918): 2068–73.

138. World Health Organization. "Hospital Infection Control Guidance for Severe Acute Respiratory Syndrome (SARS)," April 24, 2003, http://www.who.int/csr/sars/infectioncontrol/en/; Centers for Disease Control and Prevention, "Public Health Guidance for Community-Level Preparedness and Response to Severe Acute Respiratory Syndrome (SARS), Version 2/3," May 3, 2005, http://www.cdc.gov/ncidod/sars/guidance/index.htm.

139. World Health Organization Writing Group, "Controlled Studies of the Effect of Hand Washing on Transmitting Respiratory Infections," *Emerging Infectious Diseases,* 12 (2006): 88–94.

140. Centers for Disease Control and Prevention, "Public Health Guidance for Community-Level Preparedness."

141. Anna Balazy, Mika Toivola, Atin Adhikari, et al., "Do N95 Respirators Provide 95 Percent Protection Level against Airborne Viruses, and How Adequate Are Surgical Masks?" *American Journal of Infection Control,* 34 (2006): 51–57.

142. American Society for Microbiology. "Hand Washing Survey Fact Sheet," http://www.washup.org/assets/fact_sheet.pdf.

143. World Health Organization, *Avian Influenza: Assessing the Pandemic Threat* (Geneva: World Health Organization, 2005); Alexandra M. Stern and Howard Markel, "International Efforts to Control Infectious Diseases, 1851–present," *JAMA,* 292 (2004): 1474–79.

144. James Hodge, Dru Bhattacharya, and Jennifer Gray, "Assessing Legal Preparedness for School Closures in Response to Pandemic Flu or Other Emergencies," *Center for Law and the Public's Health,* http://www.publichealthlaw.net/Research/Affprojects.htm#SC.

145. Neil M. Ferguson, Derek A. T. Cummings, Christophe Fraser, et al., "Strategies for Mitigating an Influenza Pandemic," *Nature,* 442 (2006): 448–52.

146. National Ethics Advisory Committee, *Getting Through Together: Ethical Values for a Pandemic* (NEAC: Auckland, 2006) (good decisions are based on minimizing harm, respect, fairness, neighborliness, reciprocity, and unity).

147. *Shapiro v. Thompson,* 394 U.S. 618 (1969).

148. Centers for Disease Control and Prevention, "Imported Lassa Fever—New Jersey, 2004," *Morbidity and Morality Weekly Report,* 53 (2004): 894–97.

149. Centers for Disease Control and Prevention, "Multistate Outbreak of Monkeypox—Illinois, Indiana, Kansas, Missouri, Ohio, and Wisconsin, 2003," *Morbidity and Morality Weekly Report,* 52 (2003): 642–46.

150. *Public Health Service Act,* §361, 42 U.S.C. §264 (1946).

151. In fiscal 2003, Congress began to allocate funds for seventeen additional quarantine states at U.S. ports of entry. Institute of Medicine, *Quarantine Stations at Ports of Entry Protecting the Public's Health* (Washington, DC: National Academies Press, 2006): 1.

152. *Id.* For a history of medical inspection and quarantine of immigrants at entry points to the United States, see Amy L. Fairchild, *Science at the Borders* (Baltimore, MD: Johns Hopkins University Press, 2003).

153. World Health Organization, *WHO SARS Risk Assessment and Preparedness Framework* (Geneva: World Health Organization, 2004).

154. David M. Bell, World Health Organization Working Group, "Public Health Interventions and SARS Spread, 2003," *Emerging Infectious Diseases,* 10 (2004): 1900–1906; Ron K. St. John, Arlene King, Dick deJong, et al., "Border Screening for SARS," *Emerging Infectious Diseases,* 11 (2005): 6–10.

155. Milan Brahmbhatt, *Avian and Human Pandemic Influenza: Economic and Social Impacts* (Washington, DC: World Bank, 2005).

156. Human Rights Committee, *General Comment No. 27 to Article 12 of the International Covenant on Civil and Political Rights* (New York: United Nations, 1999).

157. Appellate Body Report, *European Communities—Measures Affecting Asbestos and Asbestos-Containing Products,* ¶ 172, WT/DS135/AB/R (Mar. 12, 2001).

158. Writing Committee of the World Health Organization, "Avian Influenza A (H5N1) Infection in Humans," *New Engl. J. Med.,* 353 (2005): 1374–85.

159. Jeffrey K. Taubenberger, Ann H. Reid, Raina M. Lourens, et al., "Characterization of the 1918 Influenza Virus Polymerase Genes," *Nature,* 437 (2005): 889–93; Terrence M. Tumpey, Christopher F. Basler, Patricia V. Aguilar, et al., "Characterization of the Reconstructed 1918 Spanish Influenza Pandemic Virus," *Science,* 310 (2005): 77–80.

160. Michael T. Osterholm, "Preparing for the Next Pandemic," *Foreign Affairs,* 84 (2005): 24–28.

161. Department of Health and Human Services, *HHS Pandemic Influenza Plan,* November 2005, http://www.hhs.gov/pandemicflu/plan/; White House, *National Strategy for Pandemic Influenza.*

162. World Health Organization, *Global Influenza Preparedness Plan.*

163. Klaus Stöhr and Marja Esveld, "Will Vaccines Be Available for the Next Influenza Pandemic?" *Science,* 306 (2004): 2195–96.

164. Food and Drug Administration, "FDA Approves First U.S. Vaccine for Humans against the Avian Influenza Virus H5N1," *FDA News,* April 19, 2007, http://www.fda.gov/bbs/topics/NEWS/2007/NEW01611.html.

165. Scott A. Harper, Keiji Fukuda, Timothy M. Uyeki, et al., "Prevention and Control of Influenza: Recommendations of the Advisory Committee on Immunization Practices," *Morbidity and Mortality Weekly Report,* 54 (2005): 1–40.

166. World Health Organization, *Vaccines for Pandemic Influenza* (Geneva: World Health Organization, 2004) (referring to the "unique risks and constraints" of manufacturing vaccines).

167. Patricia M. Danzon, Nuno Sousa Pereira, and Sapna S. Tejwani, "Vaccine Supply: A Cross-National Perspective," *Health Affairs,* 24 (2005): 706–17.

168. Institute of Medicine Council, "Statement on Vaccine Development," in Institute of Medicine, *Biological Threats and Terrorism: Assessing the Science and Response Capabilities: Workshop Summary* (Washington, DC: National Academies Press, 2002).

169. Center for Global Development, "G-7 to Pilot Advanced Market Commitments," December 3, 2005, http://blogs.cgdev.org/vaccine/archive/2005/12/g7_to_pilot_adv.php.

170. Gigi Kwik Gronvall and Luciana L. Borio, "Removing Barriers to Global Pandemic Influenza Vaccination," *Biosecurity and Bioterrorism: Biodefense Strategy, Practice, and Science* 4 (2006): 168–75.

171. Lisa Schnirring, "Roche Cuts Tamiflu Production as Demand Cools," *CIDRAP,* April 26, 2007, http://www.cidrap.umn.edu?cidrap/content/influenza/panflu/news/apr2607tamiflu.html.

172. Jane Zhang, "Politics and Economics: Vaccine Firms Get Immunity from the U.S.," *Wall Street Journal,* February 2, 2007.

173. Michelle M. Mello and Troyen A. Brennan, "Legal Concerns and the Influenza Vaccine Shortage," *JAMA,* 294 (2005): 1817–20.

174. John D. Arras, "Rationing Vaccine during an Avian Influenza Pandemic: Why It Won't Be Easy," *Yale Journal of Biology and Medicine,* 78 (2005): 287–300.

175. Lois Uscher-Pines, Saad B. Omer, Daniel J. Barnett, et al., "Priority Setting for Pandemic Influenza: An Analysis of National Preparedness Plans," *PLoS Medicine,* 3 (2006): e436 (finding that allocation decisions varied across countries, with health care workers consistently ranked the top priority and then a wide variation in who would be next in line: the elderly, children, or essential service workers).

176. Ezekiel J. Emanuel and Alan Wertheimer, "Who Should Get Influenza Vaccine When Not All Can?" *Science,* 312 (2006): 854–55 (discussing the "life-cycle" principle, based on the idea that each person should have an opportunity to live through all life stages).

177. Robin P. Silverstein, Harvey S. Frey, Alison P. Galvani, et al., "The Ethics of Influenza Vaccination (Letter)," *Science,* 313 (2006): 758–60 (arguing that the value of a life depends on age: a sixty-year-old has invested a lot in his life but has also reaped the most returns).

178. World Health Organization Writing Group, "Nonpharmaceutical Interventions for Pandemic Influenza, International Measures," *Emerging Infectious Diseases,* 12 (2006): 81–87.

179. World Health Organization Writing Group, "Nonpharmaceutical Interventions for Pandemic Influenza, National and Community Measures," *Emerging Infectious Diseases,* 12 (2006): 88–94.

180. Lesley Rosling and Mark Rosling, "Pneumonia Causes Panic in Guangdong Province," *British Medical Journal,* 326 (2003): 416.

181. Lauran Neergaard, "Survey: In Flu Pandemic, Staying Home Raises Paycheck, Care Questions," *CNN.com,* October 27, 2006, http://www.cnn.com/2006/HEALTH/10/25/flu.pandemic.ap/.

182. Sherry Cooper, "The Avian Flu Crisis: An Economic Update," *BMO Nesbitt Burns,* March 13, 2006, http://www.bmonesbittburns.com/economics/reports/20060313/report.pdf.

183. Joseph T. Wu, Steven Rile, Christophe Fraser, et al., "Reducing the Impact of the Next Influenza Pandemic Using Household-Based Public Health Interventions," *PLoS Medicine,* 3 (2006): e361.

12. ECONOMIC LIBERTY AND THE PURSUIT OF PUBLIC HEALTH

SOURCES FOR CHAPTER EPIGRAPHS: *Commonwealth of Massachusetts v. Alger,* 61 Mass. 53, 84–85 (Mass. 1851) (upholding a local law forbidding the construction of permanent structures beyond a certain distance into Boston harbor); *Vanderbilt v. Adams,* 7 Cow. 349, 351–52 (N.Y. 1827) (upholding a fine imposed on a ship commander for failure to move a vessel when ordered to do so to allow another boat to enter a wharf); H. Wood, *A Practical Treatise on the Law of Nuisances in Their Various Forms,* 3d ed. (Albany, NY: J. D. Parsons, Jr., 1893): 1–3; Joel Bishop, *Commentaries on Non-Contract Law and Especially as to Common Affairs Not of Contract or the Every-Day Rights and Torts* (Chicago: T. H. Flood, 1889): sec. 411, n. 1; Charles Fried, *Order and Law: Arguing the Rea-*

gan Revolution, a Firsthand Account (New York: Simon and Schuster, 1991): 183; Douglas T. Kendall and Charles P. Lord, "The Takings Project: A Critical Analysis and Assessment of the Progress So Far," *Boston College Environmental Affairs Law Review,* 25 (1998): 509–88, 510 (referring to Richard A. Epstein, *Takings, Private Property and the Power of Eminent Domain* [Cambridge, MA: Harvard University Press, 1985]); *Berman v. Parker,* 348 U.S. 26, 33 (1954) (holding that the District of Columbia could take private property for urban development); James Madison, "Property," *National Gazette,* March 29, 1792; Heinrich Von Staden, *Herophilus: The Art of Medicine in Early Alexandria* (Cambridge: Cambridge University Press, 1989): 407.

1. Perhaps the most important proponent of laissez-faire economics was the Scotsman Adam Smith. *An Inquiry into the Nature and Causes of the Wealth of Nations,* ed. Malcolm Graham (Nashville, TN: Parthenon Press, 1937) (stating that except for limited functions such as defense, justice, and certain public works, the state should refrain from interfering with economic life).

2. Milton Friedman and Anna J. Schwartz, *A Monetary History of the United States, 1867–1960* (Princeton, NJ: Princeton University Press, 1963).

3. Lawrence O. Gostin and M. Gregg Bloche, "The Politics of Public Health: A Reply to Richard Epstein," *Perspectives in Biology and Medicine,* 46, supp. 3 (Summer 2003): S160–75; Ronald Bayer, Lawrence Gostin, and Devon C. McGraw, "Trades, AIDS, and the Public's Health: The Limits of Economic Analysis," *Georgetown Law Review,* 83 (1995): 79–107.

4. Although the terms *license* and *permit* are often used interchangeably, they are historically different. "A license was thought of as a special privilege, granted by the sovereign, to do what otherwise would be unlawful such as selling liquor or running a lottery; a permit was thought of as official leave to carry on an activity or to perform an act that, although not morally questionable, was not allowable without such authority such as practicing medicine or driving a car." Frank Grad, *Public Health Law Manual,* 3d ed. (Washington, DC: American Public Health Association, 2005): 121, n. 3. I use the term *license* to refer both to licenses and permits.

5. *Dent v. West Virginia,* 129 U.S. 114 (1889) (upholding the licensing of physicians on public health grounds, thus becoming one of the most important licensing precedents).

6. Individuals may be required to record information as a condition of engaging in certain conduct, but unlike licenses and permits, registration does not impose standards or qualifications for pursuing the occupation. Through registration, public health officials are informed of the persons engaging in activities, but the agency does not actively supervise the conduct.

7. *Oxford English Dictionary,* 2d ed., 1989 ("c1400 *Rom. Rose* 7692, 'I am licenced boldely / In divinitee to rede'").

8. Grad, *Public Health Law Manual,* 121.

9. Local government has no inherent power to require licenses for the pursuit of professions or activities; licenses are void if the local government does not have power under state law to impose them. *Arnold v. City of Chicago,* 56 N.E.2d 795 (Ill. 1944) (finding a city ordinance that regulated businesses facially invalid because the state had delegated no such authority); *Nugent v. City*

of East Providence, 238 A.2d 758 (R.I. 1968) (holding that a municipality had no power to license television transmission when such a power had never been delegated to it).

10. *Gibson v. Berryhill,* 411 U.S. 564 (1973) (holding that professional licensing board members' pecuniary bias disqualified them from passing on the issues).

11. *Gaudiya Vaishnava Society v. San Francisco,* 952 F.2d 1059 (9th Cir. 1990) (granting of the power to license without providing public servants with standards is an unconstitutional delegation of legislative power); *State ex rel. Bennett v. Stow,* 399 P.2d 221 (Mont. 1965) (allowing an administrative officer to ascertain whether qualifications, facts, or conditions exist for a license).

12. *Dolan v. City of Tigard,* 512 U.S. 374 (1994) (holding that the city's conditions on issuance of a permit must be reasonably related to legitimate state interests); *Craigmiles v. Giles,* 312 F.3d 220 (6th Cir. 2002) (invalidating a requirement that caskets only be sold by licensed funeral directors because it bears no rational relationship to public health or safety). Licenses can also be denied under a quota system if quotas are reasonably necessary to protect the public's health. See also *Strub v. Village of Deerfield,* 167 N.E.2d 178 (Ill. 1960) (upholding limitation of the number of trash collectors because it advanced the public's health).

13. American Medical Association, *State Medical Licensure Requirements and Statistics* (Chicago: American Medical Association, 2006).

14. *Restivo v. City of Shreveport,* 566 So. 2d 669 (La. Ct. App. 1990) (holding that licensing plumbers is the duty of the state).

15. Clark Havighurst and Nancy M.P. King, "Private Credentialing of Health Care Personnel: An Antitrust Perspective, Parts 1 and 2," *American Journal of Law and Medicine,* 9 (1983): 131–204, 263–334.

16. *Florida v. Mathews,* 526 F.2d 319 (5th Cir. 1976) (affirming that regulation of public health institutions is within state agency jurisdiction).

17. *United Beverage Co. of South Bend v. Indiana Alcoholic Beverage Commission,* 760 F.2d 155 (7th Cir. 1985) ("A state has power to delegate licensing authority to agencies independent of federal constraint").

18. *Belleville Chamber of Commerce v. Town of Belleville,* 238 A.2d 181 (N.J. 1968) (upholding licensing fees not found to be "unreasonable or discriminatory as to any individual plaintiff").

19. *City of Laconia v. Gordon,* 219 A.2d 701, 703 (N.H. 1966) ("To be valid charges made as license fees must bear a relation to and approximate the expense of issuing the licenses and of inspecting and regulating the business licensed").

20. *City of Prichard v. Richardson,* 17 So. 2d 451, 454 (Ala. 1944) ("It seems well settled by authority that the power to license if granted as a police power, must be exercised as a means of regulation only, and cannot be used as a source of revenue").

21. *Lewis v. City of Grand Rapids,* 356 F.2d 276 (6th Cir.), *cert. denied,* 385 U.S. 838 (1966) (finding racial discrimination in licensing to be unconstitutional).

22. *People ex rel. Nechamcus v. Warden,* 39 N.E. 686 (N.Y. 1895) (alleging that Jews, immigrants, and those who did not belong to a union were discriminated against in obtaining a plumber's license).

23. *Steele v. FCC,* 770 F.2d 1192 (D.C. Cir. 1985) (holding that FCC preference for female-owned radio stations in licensing decisions was improper).

24. *Goodridge v. Department of Public Health*, 798 N.E.2d 941 (Mass. 2003) (striking down a state law that allowed marriage licenses to be issued only to heterosexual couples, on state constitution equal protection grounds).

25. *Yick Wo v. Hopkins*, 118 U.S. 356 (1886). The White owners of steam laundries who competed with Chinese hand laundries provided the motivating force behind the laundry ordinance. *In re Wo Lee*, 26 F. 471, 474 (C.C.D. Cal. 1886), *rev'd sub nom*, *Yick Wo*, 118 N.S. 356.

26. See David E. Bernstein, "Licensing Laws: A Historical Example of the Use of Government Regulatory Power against African Americans," *San Diego Law Review*, 31 (1994): 89–104 (arguing that certain groups could not satisfy licensing standards despite their practical experience because unions did not admit certain minorities or women into their apprenticeship training programs and because the public education system offered little formal training).

27. Reuben A. Kessel, "The A.M.A. and the Supply of Physicians," *Law and Contemporary Problems*, 35 (1970): 267–83; Todd L. Savitt, "The Education of Black Physicians at Shaw University, 1882–1918," in *Black Americans in North Carolina and the South*, ed. Jeffrey J. Crow and Flora J. Hatley (Chapel Hill: University of North Carolina Press, 1984): 160–88.

28. Lawrence M. Friedman, "Freedom of Contract and Occupational Licensing 1890–1910: A Legal and Social Study," *California Law Review*, 53 (1965): 487–534 (arguing that, even if the licensing system originated in the public interest, the licensed group quickly gained control of the process and used it to benefit its members by limiting the number of new entrants, thus assuring those already in the field of higher incomes).

29. Richard A. Epstein, *Forbidden Grounds: The Case against Employment Discrimination Laws* (Cambridge, MA: Harvard University Press, 1992): 91–129.

30. Timothy S. Jost, Linda Mulcahy, Stephen Strasser, et al., "Consumers, Complaints, and Professional Discipline: A Look at Medical Licensure Boards," *Health Matrix*, 3 (1993): 309–38.

31. Stanley J. Gross, *Of Foxes and Hen Houses: Licensing and the Health Professions* (Westport, CT: Quorum Books, 1977).

32. *Nguyen v. State Department of Health Medical Quality Assurance Comission*, 29 P.3d 689 (Wash. 2001) (requiring a heightened standard of proof to strip a physician of a license to practice).

33. *Bird v. State of Minn. Department of Public Safety*, 375 N.W.2d 36 (Minn. Ct. App. 1985) (holding that a hearing is required to revoke an automobile dealer's license); *Perry v. Sindermann*, 408 U.S. 593 (1972) (holding that a college teacher is entitled to a hearing when a contract is not renewed).

34. *Watchtower Bible and Tract Society of New York v. Village of Stratton*, 536 U.S. 150 (2002) (holding that requiring a permit to engage in door-to-door canvassing unconstitutionally burdened the right to both religious and political expression); *Cox v. New Hampshire*, 312 U.S. 569 (1941) (finding that a license for a religious parade is constitutional only where no censorship or prohibitory fee is imposed and the license is necessary for public safety).

35. *City of Littleton v. Z.J Gifts D-4, L.L.C.*, 541 U.S. 774 (2004) (holding that licensing decisions that burden First Amendment rights must be made promptly, but that Colorado's normal judicial review process is sufficient);

FW/PBS, Inc. v. City of Dallas, 493 U.S. 215 (1990) (finding a licensing provision unconstitutional due to lack of procedural safeguards).

36. *New York v. New St. Mark's Baths,* 497 N.Y.S.2d 979 (Sup. Ct. 1986) (holding that closure of bathhouse on nuisance grounds due to high-risk sexual activity is constitutional even though it burdens right of assembly).

37. *City of Lakewood v. Plain Dealer Publishing Co.,* 486 U.S. 750 (1988) (finding unconstitutional the portion of an ordinance giving the mayor unfettered discretion to deny a permit and unbounded authority to condition a permit on any additional terms).

38. U.S. Const. art. I, § 10, cl. 2 (permitting states to lay imposts or duties on imports or exports, without the consent of Congress, where "absolutely necessary for executing its inspections Laws"). See *Oxford English Dictionary,* 2d ed., 1989 ("1753 *in Maryland Hist. Mag.* [1908] III. 366 'Which made me apprehend they intended some Opposition to the Inspection Law'").

39. *City of Smyrna v. Parks,* 242 S.E.2d 73 (Ga. 1978) (upholding an ordinance regulating fence design and construction to minimize injury as a valid exercise of police powers).

40. *Food, Drug, and Cosmetic Act,* 21 U.S.C. § 374(a) (2006) (authorizing FDA inspectors to enter and inspect a food, drug, or cosmetic factory or warehouse).

41. *Patapsco Guano Co. v. North Carolina Board of Agric.,* 171 U.S. 345 (1898) (allowing tax to be spent to appoint officials to enforce agricultural inspection laws).

42. *Contreras v. City of Chicago,* 119 F.3d 1286, 1291 (7th Cir. 1997) (upholding restaurant inspection that was reasonable in time, place, and scope); *Johnson's Markets Inc. v. New Carlisle Department of Health,* 567 N.E.2d 1018 (Utah 1991) (commenting on the constitutionality of inspection of food service establishments).

43. *Occupational Safety and Health Act,* 29 U.S.C. §§ 651–78 (2005) (describing inspection of a workplace).

44. *Federal Environmental Pesticide Control Act,* 7 U.S.C. §§ 136 (e)–(q) (2006) (establishing an investigation program for pesticide manufacture and use).

45. *Resource Conservation and Recovery Act,* 42 U.S.C. §§ 6900–6907 (2006) (describing inspection programs for generators of hazardous waste).

46. The Fourth Amendment safeguards an individual's "reasonable expectation of privacy." *Wilson v. Health & Hospital Corp. of Marion County,* 620 F.2d 1201 (7th Cir. 1980) (finding that health officials' warrantless, consentless searches violated a reasonable expectation of privacy).

47. *Ohio ex rel. Eaton v. Price,* 364 U.S. 263 (1960) (upholding conviction of a home owner who refused to permit health inspectors to enter and inspect his residence with a warrant); *Frank v. Maryland,* 359 U.S. 360 (1959) (similar holding).

48. 387 U.S. 523 (1967) (finding the Fourth Amendment to be violated when a housing inspector entered an apartment to make a routine inspection without consent or a warrant).

49. 387 U.S. 541, 543 (1967) (finding the Fourth Amendment to be violated when a fire inspector sought to inspect a business without consent or warrant: "The businessman, like the occupant of a residence, has a constitutional right to go about his business free from unreasonable official entries upon his private commercial property").

50. The cases are collected in the "Thirty-Fourth Annual Review of Criminal Procedure," *Georgetown Law Journal Annual Review of Criminal Procedure,* 34 (2005): 111–16 (2005); Judy E. Zelin, Annotation, *Propriety of State or Local Government Health Officer's Warrantless Search-Post-Camara Cases,* 53 A.L.R. Fed. 1168 (1998); see also Grad, *Public Health Law Manual,* 157–79.

51. *Michigan v. Clifford,* 464 U.S. 287 (1984) (requiring a warrant for administrative search of a residence to investigate the cause of a fire).

52. *Marshall v. Barlow's, Inc.,* 436 U.S. 307, 310 (1978) (finding that warrantless searches of businesses to investigate occupational safety violations are presumptively unreasonable: "The Warrant Clause of the Fourth Amendment protects commercial buildings as well as private homes"); *In re Establishment Inspection of Caterpillar, Inc.,* 55 F.3d 334 (7th Cir. 1995) (requiring a warrant for an administrative search of a business for occupational safety inspection).

53. *Lenz v. Winburn,* 51 F.3d 1540 (11th Cir. 1995) (finding that a minor's consent conferred valid third-party consent to the entry of a social worker); *J. L. Foti Construction Co. v. Donovan,* 786 F.2d 714 (6th Cir. 1986) (finding that consent by a general contractor with "common authority" over the work site conferred valid third-party consent to OSHA inspection); *Pollard v. Cockrell,* 578 F.2d 1002 (5th Cir. 1978) (finding the administrative search of a massage parlor valid with consent).

54. *Camara v. Municipal Court,* 387 U.S. 523, 539 (1967) ("Warrants should normally be sought only after entry is refused"); *People v. Cacciola,* 315 N.Y.S.2d 586 (N.Y. Dist. Ct. 1970) (upholding a search as having implied consent when a baker did not explicitly refuse to allow inspection). Consent should normally be given by the person who has the greatest privacy interest, such as a tenant. *Village of Palatine v. Reinke,* 454 N.E.2d 1099 (Ill. App. Ct. 1983) (upholding a warrantless search following consent of the tenant, even though the owner did not consent).

55. *North American Cold Storage Co. v. City of Chicago,* 211 U.S. 306 (1908) (justifying entry to seize unwholesome food intended for human consumption); *Clifford,* 464 U.S. at 293 (justifying entry without a warrant by the immediate threat that a fire might rekindle); *McCabe v. Life-Line Ambulance Service,* 77 F.3d 540, 545 (1st Cir. 1996) (justifying entry to protect a suicidal mentally ill resident); *Camuglia v. City of Albuquerque,* 375 F.Supp.2d 1299 (D.N.M. 2005) (finding that restaurant inspection provides adequate due process for restaurant closing).

56. *L. R. Willson & Sons, Inc. v. Occupational Safety & Health Review Commission,* 134 F.3d 1235 (4th Cir. 1998) (finding surveillance of a workplace for safety violations from the upper story of a nearby hotel to be reasonable without a warrant because there was no expectation of privacy in what could be seen by hotel occupants). See also *Katz v. United States,* 389 U.S. 347 (1967) (describing reasonable expectation of privacy).

57. *Donovan v. Lone Steer, Inc.,* 464 U.S. 408 (1984) (finding that entering the public lobby of a motel restaurant does not violate the Fourth Amendment).

58. *Air Pollution Variance Board v. Western Alfalfa Corp.,* 416 U.S. 861 (1974) (upholding visual pollution tests of smoke being emitted from a business's chimney); *Ehlers v. Bogue,* 626 F.2d 1314 (5th Cir. 1980) (upholding visual inspection by a county health officer of the exterior of an apartment and a refuse dump-

ster); *Department of Transp. v. Armacost,* 474 A.2d 191 (Md. 1984), *rev'd on other grounds,* 532 A.2d 1056 (Md. 1987) (testing automobile exhaust for pollutants held valid).

59. *Coolidge v. New Hampshire,* 403 U.S. 443 (1971) (holding that a search is not reasonable when a warrant is issued by the attorney general instead of a neutral magistrate).

60. *Marshall v. Barlow's, Inc.,* 436 U.S. 307, 320–21 (1978) (holding that an OSHA inspector's entitlement to search does not depend on his demonstrating probable cause); *Tri-State Steel Construction, Inc. v. Occupational Safety & Health Review Commission,* 26 F.3d 173 (D.C. Cir. 1994) (holding that the court may issue a warrant on showing specific evidence of an existing OSHA violation).

61. *Barlow's, Inc.,* 436 U.S. at 320–21; *Camara v. Municipal Court,* 387 U.S. 523, 535–39 (1967); *United States v. Two Units,* 49 F.3d 479 (9th Cir. 1995) (finding a report that demonstrated the company sold a fraudulent cure for AIDS sufficient for FDA inspection); *Martin v. International Matex Tank Terminals-Bayonne,* 928 F.2d 614 (3d Cir. 1991) (finding that written complaints from employees and an investigation to confirm the complaint provided OSHA with specific evidence).

62. *Barlow's, Inc.,* 436 U.S. at 320–21; *In re Trinity Industries, Inc.,* 876 F.2d 1485 (11th Cir. 1989) (finding an OSHA search reasonable when based on neutral criteria and a detailed inspection plan); *Board of County Commissioners v. Grant,* 954 P.2d 695 (Kan. 1998) (finding that valid public interest justifies a warrant for inspection of drains connected to sewer line); *City of Chicago v. Pudlo,* 462 N.E.2d 494 (Ill. App. Ct. 1983) (regarding inspection of a food facility); *Commonwealth v. Frodyma,* 436 N.E.2d 925 (Mass. 1982) (regarding inspection of a pharmacy).

63. *Michigan v. Clifford,* 464 U.S. 287 (1984) (holding that search of a home by fire inspectors to collect evidence of arson was unreasonable without exigent circumstances); *Abel v. United States,* 362 U.S. 217 (1960) (holding that an inspection warrant may not be used as a pretext for obtaining criminal evidence); *Swint v. City of Wadley,* 51 F.3d 988 (11th Cir. 1995) (finding an inspection unlawful when directed at finding illicit drugs rather than a violation of liquor laws).

64. *Clifford,* 464 U.S. at 294; *City of Indianapolis v. Edmond,* 531 U.S. 32 (2000) (invalidating vehicle checkpoints on public roads in an effort to interdict unlawful drugs because the program's primary purpose is indistinguishable from the general interest in crime control).

65. *New York v. Burger,* 482 U.S. 691 (1987) (holding that the discovery of criminal evidence during an otherwise lawful inspection did not render the search illegal). As to the role of police in an administrative search, compare *United States v. Nechy,* 827 F.2d 1161 (7th Cir. 1987) (holding that police participation does not invalidate a search), with *Alexander v. City & County of San Francisco,* 29 F.3d 1355, 1360 (9th Cir. 1994) (plurality opinion) (holding that police participation invalidates an inspection if their primary purpose was to arrest the house owner, not assist the health department).

66. *Clifford,* 464 U.S. at 294 (holding that criminal evidence revealed during a valid inspection may be seized under the "plain view" doctrine); *United States v. Doe,* 61 F.3d 107 (1st Cir. 1995) (finding that public officials properly

seized contraband inadvertently discovered during a routine airline security search); contra *United States v. Bulacan,* 156 F.3d 963 (9th Cir. 1998) (holding that drug paraphernalia was improperly seized in Social Security offices following the Oklahoma City bombing because the search for items other than weapons was an unconstitutional expansion of administrative search).

67. *Burger,* 482 U.S. at 708 (permitting warrantless inspection of a junkyard, which was extensively regulated under New York law); *United States ex rel. Terraciano v. Montanye,* 493 F.2d 682 (2d Cir. 1974) (permitting the health department to audit pharmacy narcotic records).

68. *Burger,* 482 U.S. at 702–3; *Contreras v. City of Chicago,* 119 F.3d 1286 (7th Cir. 1997) (requiring no warrant to inspect a restaurant where necessary to further a regulatory scheme); *Hroch v. City of Omaha,* 4 F.3d 693 (8th Cir. 1993) (requiring no warrant to implement an order to condemn buildings); but see *People v. Scott,* 593 N.E.2d 1328 (N.Y. 1992) (rejecting the "closely regulated industry" exception on state constitutional grounds); *Commonwealth v. Waltz,* 749 A.2d 1058 (Pa. Commw. Ct. 2000), petition for allowance of appeal denied, 764 A.2d 1072 (2000) (holding that the *Burger* criteria did not apply to an administrative search of a private home).

69. *Donovan v. Dewey,* 452 U.S. 594 (1981) (permitting a warrantless administrative search of mining facilities as required by the Mine Safety and Health Act).

70. *United States v. Biswell,* 406 U.S. 311 (1972) (upholding warrantless searches of a licensed gun dealer because of diminished expectation of privacy).

71. *Colonnade Catering Corp. v. United States,* 397 U.S. 72 (1970) (upholding a fine for refusal to allow health officials to inspect a liquor storeroom).

72. *United States v. V-1 Oil Co.,* 63 F.3d 909 (9th Cir. 1995) (upholding a warrantless search of a propane retailer due to reduced expectation of privacy in a heavily regulated industry).

73. *Condon v. Reno,* 155 F.3d 453 (4th Cir. 1998) *rev'd on other grounds, Reno v. Condon* 528 U.S. 141 (2000) (finding that there is no reasonable expectation of privacy in motor vehicle records); *United States v. Cardona-Sandoval,* 6 F.3d 15 (1st Cir. 1993) (holding that a search of a vessel that caused significant damage required probable cause, though acknowledging the Coast Guard has broad authority to conduct warrantless and suspicionless searches on the high seas).

74. *Blue v. Koren,* 72 F. 3d 1075, 1080–81 (2d Cir. 1995) (justifying extensive warrantless inspections by a strong state interest in the highly regulated nursing industry); *Uzzillia v. Comm'r of Health,* 367 N.Y.S.2d 795 (N.Y. App. Div. 1975) (holding that the nature of nursing homes makes them always subject to inspection).

75. *People v. Firstenberg,* 155 Cal. Rptr. 80 (Cal. Ct. App. 1979) (holding that warrantless search of a nursing home's premises and business records was constitutional due to the need for heavy regulation of the industry). In theory, operators of licensed businesses give their implied consent to searches. *People v. White,* 65 Cal. Rptr. 923 (Cal. App. Dep't Super. Ct. 1968) (finding that the license to operate a hospital provided implied consent to inspection).

76. *People v. Curco Drugs, Inc.,* 350 N.Y.S.2d 74 (N.Y. Crim. Ct. 1973) (holding that a search of pharmacy records pursuant to state law was constitutional).

77. See *Burger,* 482 U.S. at 691 (upholding warrantless search of a vehicle dismantler's junkyard because of diminished expectation of privacy and an important state interest in controlling automobile theft); *Donovan v. Dewey,* 452 U.S. 594 (1981) (upholding warrantless inspection of underground mines); *Marshall v. Texoline Co.,* 612 F.2d 935 (5th Cir. 1980) (upholding warrantless search of a gravel mine pit).

78. See *Burger,* 482 U.S. at 704–7; *Dewey,* 452 U.S. at 598–600.

79. *United States v. Biswell,* 406 U.S. 311, 315 (1972) (holding that a search must be "carefully limited in time, place and scope"); *United States ex rel. Terraciano,* 493 F.2d 682 (2d Cir. 1974) (permitting a search during normal business hours); *People v. Hedges,* 447 N.Y.S.2d 1007 (N.Y. Dist. Ct. 1982) (requiring a statute authorizing warrantless search for untagged shellfish to be restricted in time and purpose).

80. *Finn's Liquor Shop Inc. v. State Liquor Authority,* 31 A.D. 2d 15 (N.Y. App. Div. 1968) (applying the exclusionary rule to suspension of a liquor license for selling liquor on credit). Courts that apply the exclusionary rule in administrative proceedings also apply a "good faith" exception that permits use of illegal evidence if the agency acted in good faith. *Donovan v. Federal Clearing Die Casting Co.,* 695 F.2d 1020 (7th Cir. 1982) (admitting evidence obtained pursuant to an OSHA warrant subsequently declared invalid).

81. *United States v. Article of Food Consisting of Twelve Barrels,* 477 F. Supp. 1185, 1191 (S.D.N.Y. 1979) (rejecting application of the exclusionary rule to FDA condemnation proceedings).

82. *Oxford English Dictionary,* 2d ed., 1989 ("13th Cent., Anglo-Norman hurt, injury, annoyance").

83. Nuisance originated with the common law action of the assize of nuisance, dealing with interferences with rights in enjoyment of land, including private easements like a neighbor's right of way. By a natural process, interference with a public easement, like a public right of way over private land, also came to be known as a nuisance. F. H Newark, "The Boundaries of Nuisance," *Law Quarterly Review,* 65 (1949): 480–90; see also John R. Spencer, "Public Nuisance: A Critical Examination," *Cambridge Law Journal,* 48 (1989): 55–84.

84. The cases on public nuisance are collected in William Lloyd Prosser, W. Page Keeton, Dan B. Dobbs, et al., *Prosser and Keeton on Torts,* 5th ed. (St. Paul, MN: West Publishing, 1984): sec. 90; J. D. Lee, *Modern Tort Law: Liability and Litigation* (Deerfield, IL: Clark Boardman Callaghan, 1998): sec. 35.03; Sandra M. Stevenson and Chester James Antieau, *Antieau on Local Government Law* (New York: M. Bender, 1997): sec. 29.02. For a comparison to English law, see *R. v. Goldstein & Rimmington* (2005) U.K.H.L. 63 [2006] A.C. 459 (U.K.) (holding that common law nuisances not currently covered by statutes remained actionable, and that common law nuisances were sufficiently clear to be valid under Article 7 of the European Convention on Human Rights).

85. Louise A. Halper, "Untangling the Nuisance Knot," *Boston College Environmental Affairs Law Review,* 26 (1998): 89–130.

86. *Kitsap County v. Kev, Inc.,* 720 P.2d 818 (Wash. 1986) (declaring an erotic dance studio sufficiently offensive to be deemed a public nuisance).

87. *Restatement (Second) of Torts* § 821C (1965).

88. John G. Culhane and Jean Macchiaroli Eggen, "Defining a Proper Role for Public Nuisance Law in Municipal Suits against Gun Sellers: Beyond Rhetoric and Expedience," *South Carolina Law Review*, 52 (2001): 287–329.

89. Eric L. Kintner, "Bad Apples and Smoking Barrels: Private Actions for Public Nuisance against the Gun Industry," *Iowa Law Review*, 90 (2004): 1163–1240.

90. *City of Chicago v. Beretta U.S.A. Corp.*, 821 N.E.2d 1099, 1138 (Ill. 2004) (rejecting handgun sales as a public nuisance where the city could not meet the requisite pleading of a right common to the general public, a substantial and unreasonable interference with that right, proximate cause, or injury).

91. *Protection of Lawful Commerce in Arms Act*, 15 U.S.C. § 7901 (2005). The act precludes public nuisance suits brought in civil court against gun manufacturers or sellers for the criminal use of firearms by third parties. However, the legislation does not immunize the gun industry against public nuisance claims brought in criminal court or claims that fall into several other exceptions to the act, including negligence per se, negligent entrustment, or products liability. See chapter 6 for more on the PLCAA.

92. Culhane and Eggen, "Defining a Proper Role for Public Nuisance Law," 289 (explaining that public nuisance law is variously described as a "wilderness of law," a "mystery," a "legal garbage can," and "the least satisfactory department of [tort law]").

93. James Stephen, *A General View of the Criminal Law of England* (London: Macmillan, 1890): 105; see *McKee v. City of Mt. Pleasant*, 328 S.W.2d 224, 229 (Tex. Civ. App. 1959) (holding public nuisance to be "anything that worketh hurt, inconvenience or damage to the subjects of the Crown").

94. *State v. Excelsior Powder Manufacturing Co.* 169 S.W. 267 (Mo. 1914) (finding that storage of large amount of gunpowder at a powder mill near homes was a public nuisance); *Landau v. City of New York*, 72 N.E. 631 (N.Y. 1904) (finding that setting off fireworks in town is a public nuisance).

95. *Seacord v. People*, 13 N.E. 194 (Ill. 1887) (finding the operation of hog rendering tanks to be a public nuisance); *Board of Health v. Vink*, 151 N.W. 672 (Mich. 1915) (holding unlicensed trash collection to be a public nuisance).

96. *Durand v. Dyson*, 111 N.E. 143 (Ill. 1915) (allowing destruction of diseased cattle).

97. *Bearcreek Tp. v. De Hoff*, 49 N.E.2d 391 (Ind. 1943) (holding that a nuisance was created by improper discharge of sewage).

98. *Gay v. State*, 18 S.W. 260 (Tenn. 1891) (holding the smell of a hog farm to be a nuisance).

99. 65 *Ill. Comp. Stat.* § 5/11–20–5 (West 2006); see *Tex. Local Gov't Code Ann.* § 217.042 (West 2005) ("Each city shall have the power to define all nuisances and prohibit the same within the city and outside the city limits for a distance of 5000 feet"); *Board of Commissioners v. Elm Grove Mining Co.*, 9 S.E.2d 813 (W.Va. 1940) (holding that "the health officer shall inquire into all nuisances affecting public's health").

100. *Cal. Civ. Code* § 3479 (West 2006); see *Ga. Code Ann.* § 41–1-1 (2006) (defining a public nuisance to be anything that "causes hurt, inconvenience, or damage to another"); *Pottawattamie County v. Iowa Department of Environmental*

Quality, 272 N.W.2d 448, 453 (Iowa 1978) (defining public nuisance to be "antisocial conduct that injures a substantial number of people"); *New York Trap Rock Corp. v. Town of Clarkstown*, 85 N.E.2d 873 (N.Y. 1949) (defining a public nuisance as an act or omission that obstructs or causes damage to the public in exercise of rights common to all).

101. *Ariz. Rev. Stat.* § 36–601(A)(1)(2005); *Spur Industries, Inc. v. Del E. Webb Development Co.*, 494 P.2d 700, 705 (Ariz. 1972) (entitling a developer to enjoin a cattle feeding operation as a nuisance).

102. *N.Y. Comp. Codes R. & Regs.*, Tit. 10, § 24–2.2 (2005).

103. *Greater Chicago Combine & Center, Inc. v. City of Chicago*, 431 F.3d 1065 (7th Cir. 2005) (holding that the city could regulate the keeping of pigeons to protect the public's health and to promote enjoyment of private residential property).

104. *Gacke v. Pork Xtra, L.L.C.*, 684 N.W.2d 168 (Iowa 2004), *reh'g denied* (July 30, 2004); see *Boremann v. Board of Supervisors*, 584 N.W.2d 309 (Iowa 1998). *Gacke* and *Boremann* are fairly adventurous decisions not followed in most jurisdictions. See *Moon v. North Idaho Farmers Ass'n*, 96 P.3d 637 (Idaho 2004).

105. *Mitchell v. Commission on Adult Entertainment Establishments*, 10 F.3d 123 (3d Cir. 1993) (finding that the constitutional rights of an adult video store were not infringed by an "open booth" regulation that sought to reduce high-risk sexual activity).

106. *City of Nokomis v. Sullivan*, 153 N.E.2d 48 (Ill. 1958) (finding that "the cases have turned, in the last analysis, upon the court's appraisal of the reasonableness of the municipal action").

107. *City of Corsicana v. Wilson*, 249 S.W.2d 290 (Tex. Civ. App. 1952) (upholding the designation of a livestock facility within city limits as a nuisance, even though the facility predated the nuisance law).

108. *Ozark Poultry Products, Inc. v. Garman*, 472 S.W.2d 714 (Ark. 1971) (holding odors that prevented neighbors from sleeping or eating meals without nausea to be a nuisance).

109. *Skinner v. Coy*, 90 P.2d 296 (Cal. 1939) (holding that diseased peach trees are an agricultural nuisance).

110. *State v. Charpentier*, 489 A.2d 594 (N.H. 1985) (finding that dumping hazardous waste constitutes a nuisance); *Commonwealth ex rel. Shumaker v. New York & Pennsylvania Co.*, 79 A.2d 439 (Pa. 1951) (finding that discharge of industrial waste into a river can constitute a nuisance).

111. *Shaw v. Salt Lake County*, 224 P.2d 1037 (Utah 1950) (holding that smoke, dust, noise, and odors from an asphalt plant constitute a nuisance).

112. *Polsgrove v. Moss*, 157 S.W. 1133 (Ky. 1913) (allowing a city to condemn an unsafe house); *City of Honolulu v. Cavness*, 364 P.2d 646 (Haw. 1961) (similar holding).

113. *Springfield v. City and County of Little Rock*, 290 S.W.2d 620 (Ark. 1956) (allowing removal as a nuisance of a building that constituted a fire hazard).

114. Peter B. Lord, "Three Companies Found Liable in Lead-Paint Nuisance Suit," *Providence Journal*, February 23, 2006 (reporting on a Rhode Island trial court finding public nuisance liability against three manufacturers of lead paint and ordering abatement).

115. *Ritholz v. Arkansas State Bd. of Optometry,* 177 S.W.2d 410 (Ark. 1944) (regarding optometry); *Attorney Gen. ex rel. Michigan Board of Optometry v. Peterson,* 164 N.W.2d 43 (Mich. 1969) (regarding optometry); *State v. Red Owl Stores, Inc.* 115 N.W.2d 643 (Minn. 1962) (regarding a pharmacy); *State ex rel. Marron v. Compere,* 103 P.2d 273 (N.M. 1940) (regarding medicine).

116. *Doe v. City of Minneapolis,* 898 F.2d 612 (8th Cir. 1990).

117. *Hirsh v. City of Atlanta,* 401 S.E.2d 530 (Ga. 1991) (upholding narrowly tailored restrictions on protests that disrupted traffic and endangered public safety).

118. *New York v. New St. Mark's Baths,* 497 N.Y.S.2d 979 (N.Y. Sup. Ct. 1986); but see Ralph Bolton, John Vincke, and Rudolf Mak, "Gay Baths Revisited: An Empirical Analysis," *GLQ: A Journal of Lesbian and Gay Studies,* 1 (1994): 255–74 (arguing that bathhouses could serve as a focal point in which gay men could be educated about AIDS); Rong Gong Lin II, "Bathhouses Not Sex Venues, Suit Says," *Los Angeles Times,* March 12, 2006 (describing suit filed by bathhouse owners to stop closure on public nuisance grounds).

119. *State Fire Marshal v. Schaneman,* 279 N.W.2d 101 (Neb. 1979) (allowing demolition of a building after owners neglected to make repairs).

120. *City of Philadelphia v. Watt,* 57 A.2d 591, 594 (Pa. Super. Ct. 1948) (holding that a city's paving of a driveway was appropriate under circumstances where defective paving created a public nuisance).

121. The Fifth and Fourteenth Amendments, respectively, provide that neither the federal government nor the states shall deprive any person of "life, liberty, or property without due process of law." U.S. Const. amend. V; U.S. Const. amend. XIV, § 1.

122. U.S. Const. art. I, § 10 ("No State shall . . . pass any . . . law impairing the obligations of Contracts").

123. U.S. Const. amend. V ("Nor shall private property be taken for public use without just compensation").

124. For early conservative scholarship, see Herbert Spencer, *Social Statics* (London: John Chapman, 1851) (advocating laissez-faire, unregulated economy); Christopher Tiedeman, *A Treatise on the Limitations of the Police Power in the United States* (Clark, NJ: Lawbook Exchange, 2001) (stating that government regulations unduly interfere with the natural rights of people to own and use property). For more recent accounts, see Bernard Siegan, *Economic Liberties and the Constitution,* 2d ed. (New Brunswick, NJ: Transaction Publishers, 2006).

125. Randy Barnett, *The Structure of Liberty: Justice and the Rule of Law* (Oxford: Clarendon Press, 1998).

126. Courts have long treated corporations as "persons" for due process purposes. *Santa Clara County v. Southern Pacific Railroad,* 118 U.S. 394, 396 (1886) (holding that a railroad is to be treated as a person for Fourteenth Amendment purposes in an action to recover unpaid taxes).

127. *Terrett v. Taylor,* 13 U.S. 43 (1815) (holding that a legislature could not repeal a law allowing corporations to exist without the consent of those with an interest in the corporation); *Fletcher v. Peck,* 10 U.S. 87 (1810) (holding that a contract for the sale of land cannot be impeded by state law); *Calder v. Bull,* 3

U.S. (3 Dall.) 386 (1798) (holding that the ex post facto provisions of the Constitution only apply to criminal actions).

128. *Slaughter-House Cases,* 83 U.S. (16 Wall.) 36, 81 (1873) ("Under no construction of [due process] . . . can the restraint . . . upon the exercise of their trade be held to be a deprivation of property"); see also Wendy E. Parmet, "From Slaughter-House to Lochner: The Rise and Fall of the Constitutionalization of Public Health," *American Journal of Legal History,* 40 (1996): 476–505.

129. *Mugler v. Kansas,* 123 U.S. 623 (1887) (upholding a state prohibition on the sale of alcoholic beverages).

130. *Jacobson v. Massachusetts,* 197 U.S. 11 (1905).

131. *Lochner v. New York,* 198 U.S. at 75 (1905) (Holmes, J., dissenting).

132. Robert G. McCloskey, "Economic Due Process and the Supreme Court: An Exhumation and Reburial," *Supreme Court Review,* 1962 (1962): 34–62 (arguing that there are strong reasons for reviving economic due process, but that the Supreme Court should not do so for reasons of judicial economy).

133. Richard Posner, *The Federal Courts: Crisis and Reform* (Cambridge, MA: Harvard University Press, 1985): 209 n. 25.

134. Michael J. Phillips, "Another Look at Economic Substantive Due Process," *Wisconsin Law Review,* 1987 (1987): 265–324; David A. Strauss, "Why Was *Lochner* Wrong?" *University of Chicago Law Review,* 70 (2003): 373–86.

135. U.S. Const. art. I, § 10.

136. Breach of contracts between the federal government and private parties, however, are frequently litigated in the U.S. Court of Federal Claims. See *United States v. Winstar Corp.,* 518 U.S. 839 (1996).

137. *Ogden v. Saunders,* 25 U.S. 213 (1827) (holding that a bankruptcy law does not violate the Contract Clause because it operates prospectively).

138. *Manigault v. Springs,* 199 U.S. 473, 480 (1905) (holding that the construction of a dam that impaired a contract to keep a creek open did not violate the Contract Clause because it is limited by the police powers).

139. A more stringent test is used for interference with government contracts. *United States Trust Co. of New York v. New Jersey,* 431 U.S. 1 (1977).

140. *Energy Reserves Group, Inc. v. Kansas Power & Light Co.,* 459 U.S. 400, 411–13 (1983) (holding that price controls for natural gas are not a violation of the Contract Clause because the market is heavily regulated).

141. *RUI One Corp. v. City of Berkeley,* 371 F.3d 1137, 1150 (9th Cir. 2004).

142. Richard Epstein, "Toward a Revitalization of the Contract Clause," *University of Chicago Law Review,* 51 (1984): 703–51, 734.

143. "A Process-Oriented Approach to the Contract Clause," *Yale Law Journal,* 89 (1979–80): 1623–51.

144. The Fifth Amendment's restraint on "taking" private property for public use without just compensation was the first clause in the Bill of Rights to be applied to the states. *Chicago, Burlington & Quincy Railroad v. City of Chicago,* 166 U.S. 226 (1897) (holding that condemnation of land under public safety law is not a taking requiring more than nominal compensation).

145. See generally Steven J. Eagle, *Regulatory Takings* (Charlottesville, VA: Michie, 1996); Robert Meltz, Dwight H. Merriam, and Richard M. Frank, *The*

Takings Issue Constitutional Limits on Land-Use Control and Environmental Regulation (Washington, DC: Island Press, 1999); Jed Rubenfeld, "Usings," *Yale Law Journal,* 102 (1993): 1077–1164.

146. *Calder v. Bull,* 3 U.S. (3 Dall.) 386, 388, 1 L.Ed. 648 (1798) ("An act of the Legislature [for I cannot call it a law] contrary to the great first principles of the social compact, cannot be considered a rightful exercise of legislative authority. . . . A law that takes property from A. and gives it to B: It is against all reason and justice, for a people to entrust a Legislature with such powers").

147. *Eastern Enters. v. Apfel,* 524 U.S. 498, 537 (1998) ("When . . . that solution singles out certain employers to bear a burden that is . . . unrelated to any commitment that the employers made or to any injury they caused, the governmental action implicates fundamental principles of fairness underlying the Takings Clause"); *Armstrong v. United States,* 364 U.S. 40, 49 (1960) ("A primary purpose of the Takings Clause is "to bar the Government from forcing some people alone to bear public burdens which, in all fairness and justice, should be borne by the public as a whole"); Frank I. Michelman, "Property, Utility and Fairness: Comments on the Ethical Foundations of 'Just Compensation Law,'" *Harvard Law Review,* 80 (1967): 1165–1258.

148. *Berman v. Parker,* 348 U.S. 26, 36 (1954) (upholding the taking of an area of land to remove slum conditions).

149. Wilfredo Lopez, General Counsel for Health, New York City, e-mail message to author, June 20, 2006 (explaining NYC settlement of a just compensation issue—power to take was not an issue—of taking two animal shelters, after a contract with the ASPCA fell apart, to maintain the level of animal control necessary to protect the public's health).

150. Lawrence O. Gostin, Jason W. Sapsin, Stephen P. Teret, et al., "The Model State Emergency Health Powers Act," *JAMA,* 288 (2002): 622–28 (outlining the power to procure facilities during a public health emergency under the proposed model act); but see *Davidson v. Massachusetts,* 395 N.E.2d 1314, 1318 (1979) (ruling that the takeover of a nursing home by the state after the governor declared a public health emergency to be an exercise of the police powers and not the power of eminent domain, for which no compensation was due). The taking of a private hospital during an emergency does, however, raise important logistical questions. A modern hospital cannot be run without a wide variety of staff—both medical and support—and it is unlikely that they could be compelled to remain at work.

151. Epstein, *Takings.*

152. *Pennsylvania Coal Co. v. Mahon,* 260 U.S. 393, 413 (1922) (holding a law that forbids subsurface mining of coal when there are buildings on the surface to be an unconstitutional taking).

153. *Id.*

154. *Id.* ("As long recognized, some values are enjoyed under an implied limitation and must yield to the police power"); see Catherine Connors, "Back to the Future: The 'Nuisance Exception' to the Just Compensation Clause," *Capital University Law Review,* 19 (1990): 139–86; Joseph Sax, "Takings and the Police Power," *Yale Law Journal,* 74 (1964): 36–77.

155. *Lucas v. South Carolina Coastal Council,* 505 U.S. 1003 (1992); see Richard J. Lazarus, "Putting the Correct 'Spin' on Lucas," *Stanford Law Review,* 45 (1993): 1411–32.

156. Regulatory takings doctrine applies principally to real property (real estate or land) rather than personal property (e.g., commercial activities such as manufacture or sale): "By reason of the State's traditionally high degree of control over commercial dealings, he [the regulatory subject] ought to be aware of the possibility that new regulation might even render his property worthless." *Lucas,* 505 U.S. at 1029. The state has wider authority to regulate personal property than real property without falling afoul of the Takings Clause.

157. *Id.* at 1029. The Court has also said that police power regulation becomes a taking if the burden imposed is not roughly proportionate to the government's justification for regulating. *Dolan v. City of Tigard,* 512 U.S. 374 (1994).

158. *Tahoe-Sierra Preservation Council, Inc. v. Tahoe Regional Planning Agency,* 535 U.S. 302 (2002) (holding that a moratorium on building along Lake Tahoe while suitable environmental regulations were created did not constitute a taking).

159. The Supreme Court has, in recent years, largely backed away from Scalia's intended expansion of per se taking rules in regulatory takings cases. Richard J. Lazarus, "The Measure of a Justice: Justice Scalia and the Faltering of the Property Rights Movement within the Supreme Court," *Hastings Law Journal,* 57 (2006): 759–825.

160. *Palazzolo v. Rhode Island,* 533 U.S. 606 (2001). The Court, however, said there was no per se taking because there were still economically valuable uses of the land, but remanded for a balancing analysis under *Penn Central. Lucas* and *Palazzolo* are quite complex. In *Lucas,* the regulation was imposed after the claimant purchased the property, which undoubtedly influenced the Court. But Justice Scalia stated that where the regulation denies the owner all economically viable use of the property, it would be irrelevant whether she knew abou the restrictions at the time of purchase (although such expectations might be relevant in a *Penn Central* case). The Court in *Palazzolo* essentially reaffirmed that a lack of investment-backed expectations (as opposed to background principles) cannot bar a *Lucas* claim. What was new in *Palazzolo* was that the Court held that advance notice was not a complete bar to a *Penn Central* claim.

161. *Lucas,* 505 U.S. at 1055 (Blackman, J., dissenting) ("One searches in vain . . . for anything resembling a principle in the common law of nuisance"); William Prosser, "Nuisance without Fault," *Texas Law Review,* 20 (1942): 399–426 (describing common law nuisance as "an "impenetrable jungle," "legal garbage," and full of "vagueness, uncertainty and confusion").

162. *Tahoe-Sierra,* 535 U.S. 302 at 324.

163. In the vast majority of cases, courts find that there was no categorical taking. Courts usually find that the regulation did not strip a land of all economically valuable uses, that the complete deprivation was only temporary, or that complete deprivation only extended to part of the land. In any of these instances, courts will not find a categorical taking. See, e.g., *Sartori v. United States,* 67 Fed. Cl. 263 (2005) (finding no per se taking when the EPA proscribed agricultural production for nine years under the Clean Waters Act); *Rose Acre Farms, Inc. v.*

United States, 373 F.3d 1177 (Fed. Cir. 2004) (finding no per se taking when the USDA confiscated and destroyed—for tissue testing—hens from a farm that had flocks infected with salmonella); *Norman v. United States,* 63 Fed. Cl. 231 (2004) (finding no complete deprivation of land value when the Army Corps of Engineers required a developer to set aside 220 out of 2,280 acres as wetlands in exchange for a permit to fill other wetlands). Note that in several of these cases, courts did not dismiss claims that compensation is due under the *Penn Central* test. *Coast Range Conifers v. Board of Forestry,* 76 P.3d 1148 (Or. 2003) (ruling that regulation protecting threatened or endangered species does not result in a taking).

164. William P. Barr, Henry Weismann, and John P. Frantz, "The Gild That Is Killing the Lily: How Confusion over Regulatory Takings Doctrine Is Undermining the Core Protections of the Takings Clause," *George Washington Law Review,* 73 (2005): 429–520.

165. *State ex rel. R.T.G., Inc. v. State,* 780 N.E.2d 998 (Ohio 2002) (finding a categorical taking when the state prohibited mining on 883 acres of land in order to protect a municipal drinking water source).

166. *MacPherson v. Department of Administrative Services,* 130 P.3d 308 (Or. 2006) (upholding the constitutionality of Ballot Measure 37, requiring the state to either compensate landowners for reductions of fair market value due to land use regulations or modify, remove, or not apply such regulations).

167. John D. Echeverria, "Making Sense of Penn Central," *Journal of Environmental Law,* 23 (2006): 101–40 (arguing that *Penn Central* is not a balancing test because the factors are incommensurate).

168. *Penn Central Transportation Co. v. City of New York City,* 438 U.S. 104 (1978) (holding that restrictions on the development of a site designated as a landmark are not a taking).

169. *Rose Acre Farms, Inc. v. United States,* 373 F.3d 1177 (Fed. Cir. 2004) (involving destruction by the USDA of flocks infected with salmonella; the court found some of the prongs of the *Penn Central* test were met and remanded to determine how to balance the various prongs of the test); *Yancey v. United States,* 915 F.2d 1534 (Fed. Cir. 1990) (finding a taking for the quarantine of a turkey flock when nearby farms had been infected with highly pathogenic avian influenza).

170. *Philip Morris Inc. v. Reilly,* 312 F.3d 24 (1st Cir. 2002) (ruling that the Disclosure Act was an unconstitutional taking because it did not advance the public's health, which is probably no longer good law after *Lingle*); *Ruckelshaus v. Monsanto Co.,* 467 U.S. 986 (1984) (upholding, in part, a pesticide manufacturer's claim that compelled disclosure of trade secrets constituted a regulatory taking).

171. The four consistent votes in the Rehnquist Court favoring an expansive reading of the Takings Clause were the Chief Justice and Justices Scalia, Thomas, and O'Connor. The views of the new Justices (Chief Justice Roberts and Justice Alito) are unknown. See Lazarus, "Putting the Correct Spin," 109–21; Douglas T. Kendall and Charles P. Lord, "The Takings Project: A Critical Analysis and Assessment of the Progress So Far," *Boston College Environmental Affairs Law Review,* 25 (1998): 509–88.

172. *Thompson v. Consolidated Gas Utilities Corp.,* 300 U.S. 55, 80 (1937)

(holding that "one person's property may not be taken for the benefit of another person without a justifying public purpose, even though compensation be paid").

173. *Hawaii Housing Authority v. Midkiff,* 467 U.S. 229, 245 (1984) (holding that "purely private taking could not withstand the scrutiny of the public use requirement; it would serve no legitimate purpose of government and would thus be void").

174. *Midkiff,* 467 U.S. at 240 ("The public use requirement is thus coterminous with the scope of a sovereign's police powers"); Joseph Sax, "Takings and the Police Power," *Yale Law Journal,* 74 (1964): 36–77.

175. *Midkiff,* 467 U.S. at 241; *Kelo v. City of New London,* 545 U.S. 469 (2005) (Kennedy, J., concurring) (stating, "This deferential standard of review echoes the rational-basis test used to review economic regulation under the Due Process and Equal Protection Clauses").

176. *Berman v. Parker,* 348 U.S. 26 (1954).

177. *Kelo,* 545 U.S. 469. See *A Condemnation Proceeding,* 891 A.2d 820 (Pa. Commw. Ct. 2006) (invalidating an exercise of eminent domain in which land was to be condemned and transferred to a religious organization to be used for a school). Unlike *Kelo,* the transfer was for private benefit and not "comprehensive economic development." *Id.* at 825.

178. *Kelo* (O'Connor, J., dissenting), 545 U.S. 469.

179. *Kelo* (Thomas, J., dissenting), 545 U.S. 469.

180. Elizabeth Mehren, "Political Lightning Rod Planted on New Hampshire Farmhouse," *Los Angeles Times,* August 1, 2005 (reporting on an opinion poll in New Hampshire that found 93 percent opposition to *Kelo*).

181. H.R. 4128, 109th Cong., 1st Sess. (2005). See Kenneth R. Harney, "On Capitol Hill, a Move to Curb Eminent Domain," *Washington Post,* November 5, 2005.

182. National Conference of State Legislatures, *Eminent Domain 2006 State Legislation,* June 1, 2006, http://www.ncls.org/programs/natres/eminentdomain leg06.htm (reporting legislation in response to *Kelo* considered in forty-three states and passed in twenty-four states; of these, legislation in sixteen states has the force of law due to pending approval by the governor or by referendum); John M. Broder, "States Curbing Right to Seize Private Homes," *New York Times,* February 21, 2006 ("In a rare display of unanimity that cuts across partisan and geographic lines, lawmakers in virtually every statehouse across the country are advancing bills and constitutional amendments to limit use of the government's power of eminent domain to seize private property for economic development purposes"); see *City of Norwood v. Horney,* 853 N.E. 2d 1115 (Ohio 2006) (the prospect of economic benefit to a community is not enough to support government appropriation of private property under the Ohio Constitution).

183. John Tierney, "Supreme Home Makeover," *New York Times,* March 14, 2006.

184. Prof. Echeverria argues convincingly that *Kelo* did not actually expand the power of eminent domain at all, but was rather the logical extension of a long line of expansive takings cases. John D. Echeverria, "The Myth That *Kelo* Has Expanded the Scope of Eminent Domain," *Georgetown Law and Policy In-*

stitute, July 18, 2005, http://www.law.georgetown.edu/gelpi/news/documents/KeloMythFinalLetterHead.pdf. But see Tim Sandefur, *Cornerstone of Liberty: Property Rights in Twenty-first Century America* (Washington: Cato Institute, 2006) (describing property rights as a "cornerstone of liberty" and discussing how the Constitution's protections have been eroded); Ilya Somin, "Controlling the Grasping Hand: Economic Development Takings after *Kelo,*" *Supreme Court Economic Review,* forthcoming (arguing that the courts should forbid most if not all uses of the economic development rationale as inconsistent with the Public Use Clauses of the federal and state constitutions).

185. Charles Cohen, "Eminent Domain after *Kelo v. City of New London:* An Argument for Banning Economic Development Takings," *Harvard Journal of Law and Public Policy,* 29 (2006): 491–568; Donald E. Sanders, "The Aftermath of *Kelo,*" *Real Estate Law Journal,* 34 (2005): 157–71.

186. National Association for the Advancement of Colored People, "Statement of Mr. Hilary O. Shelton Director NAACP Washington Bureau before the Senate Judiciary Committee," *National Association for the Advancement of Colored People,* September 20, 2005, http://www.naacp.org/inc/washington/109/109_aa-2005–09–20.pdf.

187. Diane Cardwell, "Bloomberg Says Power to Seize Private Land Is Vital to Cities," *New York Times,* May 3, 2006 (quoting Mayor Bloomberg: "You would never build any big thing any place in any big city if you didn't have the power of eminent domain . . . you wouldn't have a job, neither would anybody else. . . . Albany and Washington do not appreciate the crucial importance of eminent domain to our ability to shape our own future. They mistakenly equate it with an abuse of government power, and ignore the benefits that come to us all from responsible development of formerly blighted areas").

188. Richard A. Epstein, "Supreme Folly," *Wall Street Journal,* June 27, 2005.

189. Linda Greenhouse, "Justices Uphold Taking Property for Development," *New York Times,* June 23, 2005.

190. Institute for Justice, Castle Coalition Web site, http://www.castlecoalition.org.

191. Property Rights Alliance, "Fifty-three Organizations Request Senate Action on Eminent Domain Abuse," *Property Rights Alliance,* May 2, 2006, http://www.propertyrightsalliance.org/index.php?content=PRA (a group of fifty-three conservative organizations actively campaigning against eminent domain claiming that government will "snap up a family's home or church").

192. George F. Will, "Damaging Deference," *Washington Post,* June 24, 2005 (arguing that the conservative movement's emphasis on judicial restraint and deference to elected officials limits the courts' ability to ensure limited government).

193. "Eminent Latitude," *Washington Post,* June 24, 2005.

194. Georgetown Environmental Law and Policy Institute, "Introduction to the Takings Issue," *Georgetown Environmental Law and Policy Institute,* http://www.law.georgetown.edu/gelpi/takings/index.htm; Robert G. Dreher and John D. Echeverria, *Kelo's Unanswered Questions* (Washington, DC: Georgetown Environmental Law and Policy Institute, 2006).

195. *Miller v. Schone,* 276 U.S. 272, 279 (1928) ("When forced to make a choice the state does not exceed its constitutional powers by deciding upon the

destruction of one class of property to save another which, in the judgment of the legislature, is the greater value to the public").

13. CONCLUDING REFLECTIONS ON THE FIELD

SOURCES FOR CHAPTER EPIGRAPHS: Charles-Edward A. Winslow, "The Untilled Fields of Public Health," *Science,* 51 (1920): 23–33, 30; William Roper, "Why the Problem of Leadership in Public Health?" in *Leadership in Public Health* (New York: Milbank Memorial Fund, 1994); "Tony Blair's Speech on Healthy Living," *Guardian Unlimited,* July 26, 2006; "Victors and Victims: Self-Regulation, Not Regulation: A Healthy Alternative," *London Times,* June 12, 2004.

1. Lawrence O. Gostin, Scott Burris, and Zita Lazzarini, "The Law and the Public's Health: A Study of Infectious Disease Law in the United States, *Columbia Law Review,* 99 (1999): 59–128.

2. For a fascinating explanation of the relationship between politics and scientific knowledge, see Daniel M. Fox, "The Determinants of Policy for Population Health," *Health Economics* 1 (2006): 395–407 (making a distinction between "general" and "specialized" government).

3. Barbara Gutmann Rosenkrantz, *Public Health and the State: Changing Views in Massachusetts, 1842–1936* (Cambridge, MA: Harvard University Press, 1972), citing N.Y. in City Health Department, *Monthly Bull.* (October 1911): 5.

4. See, e.g., Daniel M. Fox, "Accretion, Reform, and Crisis: A Theory of Public Health Politics in New York City," *Yale Journal of Biology and Medicine,* 64 (1991): 455–56 (describing the politics of public health in New York City and proposing three descriptive models: accretion, reform, and crisis).

5. Under Geoffrey Rose's "prevention paradox," measures that have the greatest potential for improving the public's health (like seat-belt use) offer little benefit to any individual, while measures that heroically save individual lives (like heart transplants) make no significant contribution to the population's health. Public health, in other words, has as its chief duties the unenviable tasks of providing common goods and controlling negative externalities, both difficult at best. Telling individuals and businesses to change what they do (and profit by) in order to achieve the absence of illness in others is a hard sell in the marketplace of social resources. Geoffrey Rose, "Sick Individuals and Sick Populations," *International Journal of Epidemiology,* 14 (1985): 32–38.

6. Kay W. Eilbert, Mike Barry, Ron Bialek, et al., *Measuring Expenditures for Essential Public Health Services* (Washington, DC: Public Health Foundation, 1996): 17 (noting that, overall, the proportion of national health expenditures allocated to population-based initiatives is approximately 1 percent).

7. Richard H. Morrow and John H. Bryant, "Health Policy Approaches to Measuring and Valuing Human Life: Conceptual and Ethical Issues," *American Journal of Public Health,* 85 (1995): 1356–60.

8. Roper, "Why the Problem of Leadership in Public Health?"

9. Carol Graham and Andrew Felton, "Variance in Obesity across Cohorts and Countries: A Norms-Based Explanation Using Happiness Surveys," CSED

Working Paper 42 (Washington, DC: Brookings Institution, 2005) (stating that obesity is largely a problem of poor people, who suffer higher well-being and happiness costs).

10. U.S. Department of Health and Human Services, *Healthy People 2010* (Washington, DC: Department of Health and Human Services, 2000) (setting the objective of reducing to 15 percent the prevalence of obesity among adults).

11. Kenneth F. Adams, Arthur Schatzkin, Tamara B. Harris, et al., "Overweight, Obesity, and Mortality in a Large Prospective Cohort of Persons Fifty to Seventy-one Years Old," *New Eng. J. Med.,* 355 (2006): 763–78 (finding that obesity and overweight are strongly associated with risk of death).

12. Overweight is defined by body-mass index (BMI) (weight in kilograms divided by the square of the height in meters) of twenty-five or more, obesity by a BMI of thirty or more, and extreme obesity by a BMI of forty or more.

13. Centers for Disease Control, "State-Specific Prevalence of Obesity among Adults—United States, 2005," *Morbidity and Mortality Weekly Report,* 55 (2006): 985–88.

14. Trust for America's Health, *F as in Fat: How Obesity Policies Are Failing in America* (Washington, DC: Trust for America's Health, 2004).

15. Allison A. Hedley, Cynthia L. Ogden, Clifford L. Johnson, et al., "Overweight and Obesity among US Children, Adolescents, and Adults, 1999–2002," *JAMA,* 291 (2004): 2847–50 (reporting a 16 percent prevalence of overweight in ages six to nineteen from 1999 to 2002, representing a 45 percent increase from 1988 to 1994).

16. S. Jay Olshansky, Douglas J. Passaro, Ronald C. Hershow, et al., "A Potential Decline in Life Expectancy in the United States in the Twenty-first Century," *New Eng. J. Med.,* 352 (2005): 1138–45; Samuel H. Preston, "Deadweight? The Influence of Obesity on Longevity," *New Eng. J. Med.,* 352 (2005): 1135–37.

17. World Health Organization, "Obesity and Overweight," *World Health Organization,* 2003, http://www.who.int/dietphysicalactivity/publications/facts/obesity/en/; Mickey Chopra, Sarah Galbraith, and Ian Darnton-Hill, "A Global Response to a Global Problem: The Epidemic of Overnutrition," *Bulletin of the World Health Organization,* 80 (2002). The global dimensions of obesity have become so apparent that, under the auspices of WHO, Europe adopted a regional Charter on Counteracting Obesity. Maria Cheng, "Europeans OK Anti-Obesity Charter," *Washington Post,* November 16, 2006; WHO Ministerial Conference on Counteracting Obesity, "European Charter on Counteracting Obesity," *World Health Organization Europe,* November 16, 2006, http://www.euro.who.int/Document/E89567.pdf.

18. Daniel Henninger, "From Spin City to Fat City," *Wall Street Journal,* May 6, 2005.

19. Ali H. Mokdad, James S. Marks, Donna F. Stroup, et al., "Correction: Actual Causes of Death in the United States, 2000," *JAMA,* 293 (2005): 293–94; see Betsy McKay, "Admitting Errors, Agency Experts to Revise Findings: Big Health Concerns Remain," *Wall Street Journal,* November 23, 2004.

20. Katherine M. Flegal, Barry I. Graubard, David F. Williamson, et al., "Ex-

cess Deaths Associated with Underweight, Overweight, and Obesity," *JAMA,* 293 (2005): 1861–67.

21. David H. Mark, "Deaths Attributable to Obesity," *JAMA,* 293 (2005): 1918–19.

22. Flegal et al., "Excess Deaths Associated with Underweight."

23. U.S. Department of Health and Human Services, "Foreword from the Surgeon General," November 13, 2006, http://www.surgeongeneral.gov/topics/obesity/calltoaction/foreward.htm ("Left unabated, overweight and obesity may soon cause as much preventable disease and death as cigarette smoking").

24. Ali H. Mokdad, "Correction: Actual Causes of Death in the United States, 2000," *JAMA,* 293 (2005): 293–94.

25. *Random House Webster's Dictionary* (New York: Random House, 1991): 449.

26. Richard Epstein, "What (Not) to Do about Obesity: A Moderate Aristotelian Answer," *Georgetown Law Journal,* 93 (2005): 1361–86, 1368.

27. M. Gregg Bloche, "Obesity and the Struggle within Ourselves," *Georgetown Law Journal,* 93 (2005):1335–59; Kathryn Foxhall, "Beginning to Begin: Reports from the Battle on Obesity," *American Journal of Public Health,* 96 (2006): 2106–12.

28. Eric A. Finkelstein, Ian C. Fiebelkorn, and Guijing Wang, "State-Level Estimates of Annual Medical Expenditures Attributable to Obesity," *Obesity Research,* 12 (2004): 18–24.

29. Kenneth Thorpe, Curtis S. Florence, David H. Howard, et al., "The Impact of Obesity on Rising Medical Spending," *Health Affairs,* 25 (2004): 378–88.

30. Marc Suhrcke, Rachel A. Nugent, David Stuckler, et al., *Chronic Disease: An Economic Perspective* (London: Oxford Health Alliance, 2006), http://www.oxha.org/initiatives/economics/chronic-disease-an-economic-perspective (noting four market failures for risk factors that give rise to chronic diseases: externalities [costs borne by society], nonrational behavior [children and others who cannot make informed choices], insufficient and asymmetric information [consumers with unequal information and bargaining power vis-à-vis corporations], and time-inconsistent preferences [causing serious self-control problems]).

31. Epstein, "What (Not) to Do about Obesity."

32. Geoffrey Rose, "Sick Individuals and Sick Populations," *International Journal of Epidemiology,* 14 (1985): 32–38.

33. Charles-Edward A. Winslow, *The Life of Hermann Biggs* (New York: Lea and Febiger, 1915) (quoting a speech delivered at the British Medical Association's annual meeting in Montreal, Canada, September 3, 1897).

34. Amy Fairchild and James Colgrove, "Father Mike," *New York Times,* October 22, 2006 (supporting Mayor Michael Bloomberg's paternalistic campaign to combat tobacco and obesity).

35. Albert J. Stunkard and Thorkild I. A. Sorensen, "Obesity and Socioeconomic Status—A Complex Relation," *New Engl. J. Med.,* 329 (1993): 1036–37; Virginia W. Chang and Diane S. Lauderdale, "Income Disparities in Body Mass Index and Obesity in the United States, 1971–2002," *Archives of Internal Medicine,* 165 (2005): 2122–28; Parke E. Wilde and Jerusha N. Peterman, "Indi-

vidual Weight Change Is Associated with Household Food Security Status," *Community and International Nutrition,* 136 (2006): 1395–1400.

36. Madison Powers and Ruth Faden, *Social Justice: The Moral Foundations of Public Health and Health Policy* (New York: Oxford University Press, 2006); Lawrence O. Gostin and Madison Powers, "What Does Justice Require for the Public's Health? Public Health Ethics and Policy Imperatives of Social Justice," *Health Affairs,* 25 (2006): 1053–60.

37. Federal Trade Commission, *Perspectives on Marketing, Self-Regulation, and Childhood Obesity* (Washington, DC: Federal Trade Commission, 2006).

38. Kelly D. Brownell and Katherine Battle Horgen, *Food Fight: The Inside Story of the Food Industry, America's Obesity Crisis, and What We Can Do about It* (New York: McGraw Hill, 2003); Greg Critser, *Fat Land: How Americans Became the Fattest People in the World* (New York: Houghton Mifflin, 2003); Marion Nestle, *Food Politics: How the Food Industry Influences Nutrition and Health* (Berkeley: University of California Press, 2002).

39. "Fast Food as Addictive as Heroin," *BBC News,* January 30, 2003.

40. McDonald's USA, "McDonald's USA Nutrition Facts for Popular Menu Items," June 20, 2006, http://www.mcdonalds.com/app_controller.nutrition.index1.html. For a popular account, see the movie *Supersize Me* (Morgan Spurlock, 2004).

41. Paul Campos, *The Obesity Myth: Why America's Obsession with Weight Is Hazardous to Your Health* (New York: Gotham Books, 2004).

42. Michelle M. Mello, David M. Studdert, and Troyen A. Brennan, "Obesity—The New Frontier of Public Health Law," *New Eng. J. Med.,* 354 (2006): 2601–9.

43. Department of Health and Human Services, "HHS Announces Revised Medicare Obesity Coverage Policy: Policy Opens Door to Coverage Based on Evidence," July 15, 2004, http://www.dhhs.gov/news/press/2004pres/20040715.html.

44. Alan Zale, "Products Promoted as Nutritious Get a Second Opinion," *New York Times,* November 6, 2006 (stating that products marketed as healthy—such as low fat, high fiber, or high in vitamins—often contain trans fats, saturated fats, cholesterol, or added salt and sugar); Tara Parker-Pope, "A Fat-Free Product That's 100% Fat: How Food Labels Legally Mislead," *Wall Street Journal,* July 15, 2003 (discussing highly misleading labeling of foods based on serving size, percentage of ingredients, and inaccurate weights).

45. Scot Burton, Elizabeth H. Creyer, Jeremy Kees, et al., "Attacking the Obesity Epidemic: The Potential Health Benefits of Providing Nutrition Information in Restaurants," *American Journal of Public Health,* 96 (2006): 1669–75 (arguing that nutrition information on restaurant menus could have a positive impact on public health); Kim Severson, "New York Gets Ready to Count Calories," *New York Times,* December 13, 2006 (describing the New York policy that requires some restaurants to include calorie information on their menus).

46. Health Canada, "TRANSforming the Food Supply," June 27, 2006, http://www.hc-sc.gc.ca/fn-an/nutrition/gras-trans-fats/tf-ge/tf-gt_rep-rap_e.html; U.S. Food and Drug Administration, "Trans Fat Nutrition Labeling," January 1, 2006, http://www.cfsan.fda.gov/~dms/qatrans2.html.

47. Andrew Martin, "The Colonel Is Phasing Out Trans Fat from the Menu," *New York Times,* October 31, 2006 (noting that while trans fat will be eliminated from KFC chicken, it will remain in biscuits, pot pies, and some desserts).

48. Robert Clarke and Sarah Lewington, "Trans Fatty Acids and Coronary Heart Disease," *British Medical Journal,* 333 (2006): 214; *BBC News,* "Call to Label Hidden Fats in Food," July 27, 2006, http://news.bbc.co.uk/2/hi/health/5218240.stm.

49. Alan Zale, "Products Promoted as Nutritious Get a Second Opinion," *New York Times,* November 6, 2006.

50. Statement of Commissioner Pamela Jones Harbour, *In the Matter of KFC Corporation,* FTC Dkt. No. C-4118, available at http://www.ftc.gov/os/caselist/0423033/0423033.htm. (pertaining to a consent agreement with KFC to settle allegations that the company deceptively advertised its fried chicken as being compatible with a low-carbohydrate diet and other claims).

51. Jess Alderman and Richard A. Daynard, "Obesity Lawsuits—Lessons Learned from Tobacco Litigation," *American Journal of Preventive Medicine,* 30 (2006): 82–88; Theodore H. Frank, "A Taxonomy of Obesity Litigation," *University of Arkansas at Little Rock Law Review,* 28 (2006): 427–41; Michelle M. Mello, Eric B. Rimm, and David M. Studdert, "The McLawsuit: The Fast-Food Industry and Legal Accountability for Obesity," *Health Affairs,* 22 (2003): 207–16.

52. *Pelman v. McDonald's,* 396 F.3d 508 (2005) (holding that the plaintiff's allegations stated a claim against the defendant for its violation of the deceptive trade practices provision of the New York Consumer Protection Act).

53. National Restaurant Association, "State Frivolous-Lawsuit Legislation," *Restaurant.org,* August 16, 2006, http://www.restaurant.org/government/state/nutrition/bills_lawsuits.cfm (illustrating that as of October 2006, twenty-one states had enacted "commonsense consumption" or "personal responsibility" laws that, with slight variations, prevent lawsuits seeking personal injury damages for obesity-related diseases).

54. Advergaming includes interactive games on company Web sites, games that use product mascots or symbols, and advertising within a game.

55. Mello et al., "Obesity—The New Frontier of Public Health Law."

56. Institute of Medicine, *Food Marketing to Children and Youth: Threat or Opportunity?* (Washington, DC: National Academies Press, 2006).

57. Dale Kunkel, Brian L. Wilcox, Joanne Cantor, et al., *Report of the APA Task Force on Advertising and Children* (Washington, DC: American Psychological Association, 2004).

58. Michael F. Jacobson and Kelly D. Brownell, "Small Taxes on Soft Drinks and Snack Foods to Promote Health," *American Journal of Public Health,* 90 (2000): 854–57 (providing that nineteen states taxed food such as soft drinks and candy); Forbes.com, "The Fat Tax: A Controversial Tool in War against Obesity," January 11, 2006, http://www.forbes.com/lifestyle/health/feeds/hscout/2006/01/11/hscout530229.html.

59. World Health Organization, "Global Strategy on Diet, Physical Activity and Health," November 13, 2006, http://www.who.int/dietphysicalactivity/faq/en/index.html; "WHO Wants Twinkie Tax to Discourage Junk Foods," *Post-Gazette,* December 6, 2003.

60. Forbes.com, "The Fat Tax"; but see Jacobson and Brownell, "Small Taxes on Soft Drinks and Snack Foods to Promote Health" (noting that 45 percent of adults surveyed supported a one-cent per pound tax on soft drinks, chips, and butter, with the revenues used to fund health education programs).

61. U.S. Government Accountability Office, *School Lunch Program: Efforts Needed to Improve Nutrition and Encourage Healthy Eating,* GAO-03-506 (Washington, DC: U.S. Government Accountability Office, 2003).

62. Paul J. Veugelers and Angela L. Fitzgerald, "Effectiveness of School Programs in Preventing Childhood Obesity: A Multilevel Comparison," *American Journal of Public Health,* 95 (2005): 432–35 (remarking that school programs are effective in preventing childhood obesity).

63. Sheila Fleischhacker, "Food Fight: The Battle over Redefining Competitive Foods," *Journal of School Health,* 77 (2007): 147–52 (arguing that there is a need to federally regulate foods of minimal nutritional value in schools); Karen Pallarito, "Reviewing the School Cupcake Ban," *Washington Post,* January 30, 2007 (discussing the National School Lunch and School Breakfast Program requirement that every school district write a "wellness policy"); Institute of Medicine, *Nutritional Standards for Foods in Schools: Leading the Way toward Healthier Youth* (Washington, DC: National Academies Press, 2007).

64. Marian Burros, "Producers Agree to Send Healthier Foods to School: Effort to Fight Rising Childhood Obesity," *New York Times,* October 7, 2006 (regarding pronouncement by five large snack food producers that they would provide more nutritious foods to schools, replacing sugary, fat-laden products in vending machines and cafeterias); Marian Burros and Melanie Warner, "Bottlers Agree to a School Ban on Sweet Drinks," *New York Times,* May 4, 2006 (reporting that three top soft-drink companies announced removal of sweetened drinks from school cafeterias and vending machines in response to a growing threat of lawsuits and legislation).

65. However, some school policies have become unexpectedly controversial, such as the practice of sending children home with body mass "report cards." Jodi Kantor, "As Obesity Fight Hits Cafeteria, Many Fear a Note from School," *New York Times,* January 8, 2007.

66. Steven C. J. Cummins, Laura McKay, and Sally MacIntyre, "McDonald's Restaurants and Neighborhood Deprivation in Scotland and England," *American Journal of Preventive Medicine,* 29 (2005): 308–10 (noting that poor, minority neighborhoods have more fast-food restaurants and fewer supermarkets than do rich, White neighborhoods); Jason Block, Richard A. Scribner, and Karen B. DeSalvo, "Fast Food, Race/Ethnicity, and Income: A Geographic Analysis," *American Journal of Preventive Medicine,* 27 (2004): 211–17 (same); Elizabeth A. Baker, Mario Schootman, Ellen Barnidge, et al., "The Role of Race and Poverty in Access to Foods That Enable Individuals to Adhere to Dietary Guidelines," *Preventing Chronic Disease* (July 2006), http://www.cdc.gov/pcd/issues/2006/jul/05_0217.htm (demonstrating that the spatial distribution of fast-food restaurants and supermarkets that provide options for meeting recommended dietary intake differed according to racial distribution and poverty rates).

67. Javier Lopez-Zetina, Howard Lee, and Robert Friis, "The Link between Obesity and the Built Environment: Evidence from an Ecological Analysis of Obe-

sity and Vehicle Miles of Travel in California," *Health and Place,* 12 (2006): 656–64; Kim Krisberg, "Built Environment Adding to Burden of Childhood Obesity: Designing Healthier Communities for Kids," *Nation's Health* (October 2006).

68. James G. Hodge, "The Use of Zoning to Restrict Fast Food Outlets: A Potential Strategy to Combat Obesity," *Center for the Law and the Public's Health at Georgetown and Johns Hopkins Universities,* November 13, 2006, http://www.publichealthlaw.net/Research/Affprojects.htm#Zoning.

69. Manny Fernandez, "Pros and Cons of a Zoning Diet: Fighting Obesity by Limiting Fast-Food Restaurants," *New York Times,* September 24, 2006 (reporting the adoption of "formula restaurant" zoning in Calistoga, California, and a similar proposal in New York City).

70. Wendy C. Perdue, Lawrence O. Gostin, and Lesley A. Stone, "Public Health and the Built Environment: Historical, Empirical, and Theoretical Foundations for an Expanded Role," *Journal of Law, Medicine and Ethics,* 31 (2003): 557–66; Wendy C. Perdue, Lesley A. Stone, and Lawrence O. Gostin, "The Built Environment and Its Relationship to the Public's Health: The Legal Framework," *American Journal of Public Health,* 93 (2003): 1390–94.

71. Virginia Postrel, "The Pleasantville Solution: The War on 'Sprawl' Promises 'Livability' but Delivers Repression, Intolerance—and More Traffic," *Reason,* 30 (1999): 4–11.

72. Ruth Colagiuri, Stephen Colagiuri, and Derek Yach, "The Answer to Diabetes Prevention: Science, Surgery, Service Delivery, or Social Policy," *American Journal of Public Health,* 96 (2006): 1562–69 (stressing that social policy is the key to achieving and sustaining social and physical environments required to achieve widespread reductions in diabetes); Russell P. Lopez and H. Patricia Hynes, "Obesity, Physical Activity, and the Urban Environment: Public Health Research Needs," *Environmental Health: A Global Access Science Source,* 5 (2006): 25–35.

73. Institute of Medicine, *Dietary Reference Intakes for Energy, Carbohydrate, Fiber, Fat, Fatty Acids, Cholesterol, Protein, and Amino Acids* (Washington, DC: National Academies Press, 2005).

74. Dariush Mozaffarian, Martijn B. Katan, Alberto Ascherio, et al., "Trans Fatty Acids and Cardiovascular Disease," *New Eng. J. Med.,* 354 (2006): 1601–13 ("From a nutritional standpoint, the consumption of trans fatty acids results in considerable potential harm but no apparent benefit").

75. "Denmark: Lower Trans Fat or Go to Jail: Two Years After Artery-Clogging Oils Made Illegal, Pastries Are Still Tasty," *Associated Press,* October 17, 2006 (noting that Danish law limits trans fats from sources other than meats and dairy products to a maximum of 2 percent of total fat in each food item).

76. Ban Trans Fats, "Project Tiburon: America's First Trans Fat–Free City," November 13, 2006, http://www.bantransfats.com/projecttiburon.html.

77. Thomas J. Leuck, "New York Health Board Hears Comments on Restaurant Proposals," *New York Times,* October 30, 2006; Thomas J. Leuck, "New York City Plans Limits on Restaurants' Use of Trans Fats," *New York Times,* September 27, 2006; Thomas J. Lueck and Kim Severson, "New York Bans Most Trans Fats in Restaurants," *New York Times,* December 6, 2006.

78. Institute of Medicine, *Dietary Reference Intakes,* 424 ("Trans fatty acid consumption should be as low as possible while consuming a nutritionally adequate diet"); Health Canada, "TRANSforming the Food Supply," http://www.hc-sc.gc.ca/fn-an/nutrition/gras-trans-fats/tf-ge/tf-gt_rep-rap_e.html (recommending trans fats be limited to less than 1 percent of overall energy intake).

79. Susan Okie, "New York to Trans Fats: You're Out," *New Engl. J. Med.,* 356 (2007): 2017–21.

80. John Tierney, "One Cook Too Many," *New York Times,* September 30, 2006 ("But if New Yorkers consume trans fat, . . . it's because they ordered it themselves. Telling them what kind of fat they're buying might be useful. But they're perfectly capable of figuring out what to eat").

81. Parker-Pope, "A Fat-Free Product That's 100% Fat."

82. John Ruskin, *Unto This Last and Other Writings* (London: Penguin, 1997): 222.

Selected Bibliography

This is a selective listing of books and articles on public health, ethics, and the law arranged by topic and listed in reverse chronological order. Each work is listed only once, even if it covers more than one topic.

C. HIV/AIDS
D. Tuberculosis
E. Sexually Transmitted Infections
F. Tobacco
G. Firearms
H. Public Health Genetics
I. Obesity

I. PUBLIC HEALTH LAW IN THE UNITED STATES

Goodman, Richard A., Mark A. Rothstein, Richard E. Hoffman, et al. *Law in Public Health Practice.* 2d ed. New York: Oxford University Press, 2007.

Hodge, James G., Jr., Lawrence O. Gostin, Kristine Gebbie, et al. "Transforming Public Health Law: The Turning Point Model State Public Health Act." *Journal of Law, Medicine, and Ethics,* 34 (2006): 77–84.

Bailey, Tracey M., Timothy Caulfield, and Nola M. Ries, eds. *Public Health Law and Policy in Canada.* Markham, ON: Butterworths, 2005.

Gostin, Lawrence O., and Peter D. Jacobson. *Law and the Health System.* New York: Foundation Press, 2005.

Grad, Frank P. *The Public Health Law Manual.* 3d ed. Washington, DC: American Public Health Association, 2005.

Reynolds, Christopher (with Genevieve Howse). *Public Health: Law and Regulation.* Sydney: Federation Press, 2004.

Wing, Kenneth R. *The Law and the Public's Health.* 6th ed. Chicago: Health Administration Press, 2003.

Martin, Robyn, and Linda Johnson, eds. *Law and the Public Dimension of Health.* London: Cavendish Publishing, 2001.

Christoffel, Tom, and Stephen P. Teret. *Protecting the Public: Legal Issues in Injury Prevention.* New York: Oxford University Press, 1993.

Gostin, Lawrence O. "The Future of Public Health Law." *American Journal of Law and Medicine,* 12 (1986): 461–90.

Tobey, James A. *Public Health Law: A Manual of Law for Sanitarians.* Baltimore, MD: Williams and Wilkins, 1926.

Parker, Leroy, and Robert H. Worthington. *The Law of Public Health and Safety, and the Powers and Duties of Boards of Health.* Albany, NY: Bender, 1892.

II. GLOBAL HEALTH LAW

Gostin, Lawrence O. "Meeting Basic Survival Needs for the World's Least Healthy People: Toward a Framework Convention on Global Health." *Georgetown Law Journal* (forthcoming, 2008).

Fidler, David P., and Lawrence O. Gostin. *Biosecurity in the Global Age: Biological Weapons, Public Health, and the Rule of Law.* Palo Alto, CA: Stanford University Press, 2007.

Fidler, David M., and Lawrence O. Gostin. "The New International Health Regulations: An Historic Development for International Law and Public Health." *Journal of Law, Medicine, and Ethics,* 34 (2006): 85–94.

Aginam, Obijiofor. *Global Health Governance: International Law and Public Health in a Divided World.* Toronto: University of Toronto Press, 2005.
Fidler, David P. "From International Sanitary Conventions to Global Health." *Chinese Journal of International Law,* 4 (2005): 325–92.
Garrett, Laurie, and Scott Rosenstein. "Missed Opportunities: Governance of Global Infectious Diseases." *Harvard International Review,* 27 (2005): 64–69.
Burci, Gian Luca, and Claude-Henri Vignes. *World Health Organization.* Frederick, MD: Aspen Publishers, 2004.
Taylor, Allyn L. "Governing the Globalization of Public Health." *Journal of Law, Medicine, and Ethics,* 32 (2004): 500–502.
Fidler, David P. "Emerging Trends in International Law concerning Global Infectious Disease Control." *Emerging Infectious Diseases,* 9 (2003): 285–90.
Taylor, Allyn L., Douglas W. Bettcher, Sev S. Fluss, et al. "International Health Instruments: An Overview." In *Oxford Textbook of Public Health,* edited by Roger Detels et al., 359–86. Oxford: Oxford University Press, 2002.
Fidler, David P. *International Law and Public Health.* Ardsley, NY: Transnational Publishers, 2000.
Garrett, Laurie. *Betrayal of Trust: The Collapse of Global Public Health.* New York: Hyperion, 2000.
Fidler, David P. *International Law and Infectious Diseases.* Oxford: Clarendon Press, 1999.

III. PUBLIC HEALTH HISTORY

Markel, Howard. *When Germs Travel: Six Major Epidemics That Have Invaded America and the Fears They Have Unleashed.* New York: Vintage, 2005.
Bashford, Alison. *Imperial Hygiene: A Critical History of Colonialism, Nationalism and Public Health.* New York: Palgrave Macmillan, 2004.
Porter, Dorothy. *Health, Civilization and the State: A History of Public Health from Ancient to Modern Times.* New York: Routledge, 1999.
Hays, J. N. *The Burdens of Disease: Epidemics and Human Response in Western History.* New Brunswick, NJ: Rutgers University Press, 1998.
McNeill, William H. *Plagues and Peoples.* New York: Anchor Books, 1998.
Novak, William J. *The People's Welfare: Law and Regulation in Nineteenth-Century America.* Chapel Hill: University of North Carolina Press, 1996.
Porter, Dorothy, ed. *The History of Public Health and the Modern State.* Amsterdam: Rodopi, 1994.
Rosen, George. *A History of Public Health.* Expanded edition. Baltimore, MD: Johns Hopkins University Press, 1993.
Duffy, John. *The Sanitarians: A History of American Public Health.* Urbana: University of Illinois Press, 1990.
Dubos, René, and Jean Dubos. *The White Plague: Tuberculosis, Man and Society.* New Brunswick, NJ: Rutgers University Press, 1987.
Rosenburg, Charles. *The Cholera Years: The United States in 1832, 1849, and 1866.* Chicago: University of Chicago Press, 1987.
Duffy, John. *A History of Public Health in New York City, 1625–1866.* New York: Russell Sage Foundation, 1968.

———. *Epidemics in Colonial America.* Baton Rouge: Louisiana State University Press, 1953.

Williams, R. C. *The United States Public Health Service, 1798–1950.* Washington, DC: Commissioned Officers Association of the U.S. Public Health Service, 1951.

Shattuck, Lemuel. *Report of a General Plan for the Promotion of Public and Personal Health, Devised, Prepared, and Recommended by the Commissioners Appointed under a Resolve of the Legislature of Massachusetts, Relating to a Sanitary Survey of the State.* Boston: Dutton and Wentworth, 1850. Reprint, Cambridge, MA: Harvard University Press, 1948.

Winslow, Charles-Edward. *A Life of Hermann Biggs.* Philadelphia: Lea and Febiger, 1929.

Farr, William. *Vital Statistics: A Memorial Volume of Selections from the Reports and Writing, with a Biographical Sketch.* Edited by Noel A. Humphreys. London: Sanitary Institute, 1885.

IV. PUBLIC HEALTH THEORY AND POLITICS

Daniels, Norman. *Just Health: A Population View.* New York: Cambridge University Press, 2007.

Bloche, Gregg M., and Lawrence O. Gostin. "Health Law and the Broken Promise of Equity." In *Law and Class America: Trends since the Cold War,* edited by Paul Carrington and Trina Jones. New York: New York University Press, 2006.

Gostin, Lawrence O., and Madison Powers. "What Does Justice Require for the Public's Health? Public Health Ethics and Policy Imperatives of Social Justice." *Health Affairs,* 25 (2006): 1053–60.

Epstein, Richard A. "Let the Shoemaker Stick to His Last: A Defense of the 'Old' Public Health." *Perspectives in Biology and Medicine,* 46 (2003): S138–59.

Gostin, Lawrence O., and M. Gregg Bloche. "The Politics of Public Health: A Reply to Richard Epstein." *Perspectives in Biology and Medicine,* 46, supplement 3 (Summer 2003): S160–75.

Hofrichter, Richard. *Health and Social Justice. Politics, Ideology, and Inequity in the Distribution of Disease.* San Francisco, CA: John Wiley and Sons, 2003.

"The Determinants of Health" (symposium). *Health Affairs* 21 (2002): 7–318.

Malmot, Michael, and Richard G. Wilkinson, eds. *Social Determinants of Health.* New York: Oxford University Press, 1999.

Burris, Scott. "The Invisibility of Public Health: Population-Level Measures in a Politics of Market Individualism." *American Journal of Public Health,* 87 (1997): 1607–10.

———. "Rationality Review and the Politics of Public Health." *Villanova Law Review,* 34 (1989): 933–82.

Beauchamp, Dan E. *The Health of the Republic: Epidemics, Medicine, and Moralism as Challenges to Democracy.* Philadelphia: Temple University Press, 1988.

———. "Community: The Neglected Tradition of Public Health." *Hastings Center Report,* 15 (1985): 28–36.
Beauchamp, Dan E. "What Is Public about Public Health?" *Health Affairs,* 2 (1983): 76–87.
Walzer, Michael. *Spheres of Justice: A Defense of Pluralism and Equality.* New York: Basic Books, 1983.
Beauchamp, Dan E. "Public Health as Social Justice." *Inquiry,* 13 (1976): 3–14.
Hardin, Garrett. "The Tragedy of the Commons." *Science,* 162 (1968): 1243–48

V. PUBLIC HEALTH SYSTEMS AND PRACTICE

Novick, Lloyd F., Cynthia B. Morrow, and Glen P. Mays, eds. *Public Health Administration Principles for Population-Based Management.* 2d ed. Sudbury, MA: Jones and Bartlett, 2007.
"The State of Public Health" (symposium). *Health Affairs,* 25 (2006): 898–1190.
Gostin, Lawrence O., Jo Ivey Boufford, and Rose Marie Martinez. "The Future of the Public's Health: Vision, Values, and Strategies." *Health Affairs,* 23 (2004): 96–107.
Turnock, Bernard J. *Public Health: What It Is and How It Works.* 3d ed. Sudbury, MA: Jones and Bartlett, 2004.
Baum, Fran. *The New Public Health.* 2d ed. New York: Oxford University Press, 2003.
Institute of Medicine. *The Future of the Public's Health in the Twenty-first Century.* Washington, DC: National Academies Press, 2002.
Gebbie, Kristine M. "State Public Health Laws: An Expression of Constituency Expectations." *Journal of Public Health Management Practice,* 6 (2000): 46–54.
Mays, Glen P., C. Arden Miller, and Paul K. Halverson, eds. *Local Public Health Practice: Trends and Models.* Washington, DC: American Public Health Association, 2000.
Bowser, René, and Lawrence O. Gostin. "Managed Care and the Health of a Nation." *Southern California Law Review,* 72 (1999): 1209–95.
Centers for Disease Control and Prevention. "Ten Great Public Health Achievements—United States, 1900–1999" (series). *Morbidity and Mortality Weekly Report,* 48 (1999): 241–48.
Gebbie, Kristine M., and Inseon Hwang. *Identification of Health Paradigms in Use in State Public Health Agencies.* New York: Columbia University School of Nursing, 1997.
Holland, Walter W., and Susie Stewart. *Public Health: The Vision and the Challenge.* London: Nuffield Trust, 1997.
Lasker, Roz D. *Medicine and Public Health: The Power of Collaboration.* Chicago: Health Administration Press, 1997.
Roper, William. "Why the Problem of Leadership in Public Health?" In *Leadership in Public Health.* New York: Milbank Memorial Fund, 1994.
Rose, Geoffrey. *The Strategy of Preventive Medicine.* Oxford: Oxford University Press, 1992.

Institute of Medicine. *The Future of Public Health*. Washington, DC: National Academies Press, 1988.

Rose, Geoffrey. "Sick Individuals and Sick Populations." *International Journal of Epidemiology*, 14 (1985): 32–38.

Winslow, Charles-Edward A. *The Evolution and Significance of the Modern Public Health Campaign*. New Haven, CT: Yale University Press, 1923.

———. "The Untilled Fields of Public Health." *Science*, 51 (1920): 23–33.

VI. PUBLIC HEALTH ETHICS

Bayer, Ronald, Lawrence O. Gostin, Bruce Jennings, et al. *Public Health Ethics: Theory, Policy and Practice*. New York: Oxford University Press, 2007.

Kahn, Jeffery, and Anna Mastroianni. "Bioethics and Public Health: Trends for the New Millennium." In *Annual Review of Public Health*. Palo Alto, CA: Annual Reviews, 2007.

Anand, Sudhir, Fabienne Peter, and Amartya Sen. *Public Health, Ethics, and Equity*. New York: Oxford University Press, 2004.

Kass, Nancy. "Public Health Ethics: From Foundations and Frameworks to Justice and Global Public Health." *Journal of Law, Medicine, and Ethics*, 32 (2004): 232–42.

Childress, James F., Ruth R. Faden, Ruth D. Gaare, et al. "Public Health Ethics: Mapping the Terrain." *Journal of Law, Medicine, and Ethics*, 30 (2002): 170–81.

Beauchamp, Tom L., and James F. Childress. *Principles of Biomedical Ethics*. 5th ed. New York: Oxford University Press, 2001.

Kass, Nancy. "An Ethics Framework for Public Health." *American Journal of Public Health*, 91 (2001): 1776–82.

Bradley, Peter, and Amanda Burls, eds. *Ethics in Public and Community Health*. New York: Routledge, 2000.

Coughlin, Steven S., ed. *Ethics in Epidemiology and Public Health Practice: Collected Works*. Columbus, GA: Quill Publications, 1997.

Coughlin, Steven S., and Tom L. Beauchamp. *Ethics and Epidemiology*. New York: Oxford University Press, 1996.

VII. HEALTH AND HUMAN RIGHTS

Ruger, Jennifer Prah. "Democracy and Health." *Quarterly Journal of Medicine*, 98 (2006): 299–304.

Gruskin, Sofia, Michael A. Grodin, George J. Annas, et al., eds. *Perspectives on Health and Human Rights: A Reader*. New York: Routledge, 2005.

Hunt, Paul. "Report of Paul Hunt, Special Rapporteur on the Right of Everyone to the Enjoyment of the Highest Attainable Standard of Physical and Mental Health." UN Doc. E/CN.4/2005/51 (February 11, 2005).

Meier, Benjamin Mason. "Breathing Life into the Framework Convention on Tobacco Control: Smoking Cessation and the Right to Health." *Yale Journal of Health, Policy, Law, and Ethics*, 5 (2005): 137–92.

Yamin, Alicia Ely. "The Right to Health under International Law and Its Relevance to the United States." *American Journal of Public Health*, 95 (2005): 1156–61.
Gostin, Lawrence O., and Lance Gable. "The Human Rights of Persons with Mental Disabilities: A Global Perspective on the Application of Human Rights Principles to Mental Health." *Maryland Law Review*, 63 (2004): 120–21.
Kinney, Eleanor D., and Brian Alexander Clark. "Provisions for Health and Health Care in the Constitutions of the Countries around the World." *Cornell International Law Journal*, 37 (2004): 285–355.
Cook, Rebecca, B. M. Dickens, and M. F. Fathalla. *Reproductive Health and Human Rights: Integrating Medicine, Ethics and Law.* Oxford: Oxford University Press, 2003.
Herr, Stanley S., Lawrence O. Gostin, and Harold Hongju Koh, eds. *The Human Rights of Persons with Intellectual Disabilities: Different but Equal.* Oxford: Oxford University Press, 2003.
Gostin, Lawrence O. "Public Health, Ethics, and Human Rights: A Tribute to the Late Jonathan Mann." *Journal of Law, Medicine, and Ethics*, 29 (2001): 121–30.
Toebes, Brigit C. A. "Towards an Improved Understanding of the International Human Right to Health." *Human Rights Quarterly*, 21 (1999): 661–79.
Gostin, Lawrence O., and Zita Lazzarini. *Human Rights and Public Health in the AIDS Pandemic.* New York: Oxford University Press, 1997.
Mann, Jonathan M. "Medicine and Public Health, Ethics and Human Rights." *Hastings Center Report*, 27 (May 15, 1997): 6–13.
Cook, Rebecca J. *Women's Health and Human Rights: The Promotion and Protection of Women's Health through International Human Rights Law.* Geneva: World Health Organization, 1994.
Gostin, Lawrence O., and Jonathan M. Mann. "Towards the Development of a Human Rights Impact Assessment for the Formulation and Evaluation of Health Policies." *Health and Human Rights*, 1 (1994): 58–81.
Jamar, Steven D. "The International Human Right to Health." *Southern University Law Review*, 22 (1994): 1–68.
Mann, Jonathan, Lawrence Gostin, Sofia Gruskin, et al. "Health and Human Rights." *Health and Human Rights*, 1 (1994): 6–23.

VIII. PUBLIC HEALTH POWERS: CONSTITUTIONAL STRUCTURE AND PRINCIPLES

Gostin, Lawrence O. "The Supreme Court's Impact on Medicine and Health: The Rehnquist Court, 1986–2005." *JAMA*, 294 (2005): 1685–87.
Parmet, Wendy, Richard Goodman, and Amy Farber. "Individual Rights versus the Public's Health—One Hundred Years after *Jacobson v. Massachusetts*." *New England Journal of Medicine*, 352 (2005): 652–54.
"Symposium on the Legacy of *Jacobson v. Massachusetts*." *American Journal of Public Health*, 95 (2005): 571–90.
Tiedeman, Christopher. *A Treatise on the Limitations of the Police Power in the United States.* Clark, NJ: Lawbook Exchange, 2001.

Hodge, James G., Jr. "The Role of New Federalism and Public Health Law." *Journal of Law and Health*, 12 (1998): 309–57.

Parmet, Wendy E. "From Slaughter-House to Lochner: The Rise and Fall of the Constitutionalization of Public Health." *American Journal of Legal History*, 40 (1996): 476–505.

Prentice, William Packer. *Police Powers Arising under the Law of Overruling Necessity.* Littleton, CO: Fred B. Rothman, 1993.

Parmet, Wendy E. "Health Care and the Constitution: Public Health and the Role of the State in the Framing Era." *Hastings Constitutional Law Quarterly*, 20 (Winter 1992): 267–334.

Merritt, Deborah Jones. "Communicable Disease and Constitutional Law: Controlling AIDS." *New York University Law Review*, 61 (1986): 739–99.

———. "The Constitutional Balance between Health and Liberty." *Hastings Center Report*, 16 (1986): supp. 2–10.

Mustard, Harry. *Government in Public Health.* New York: Commonwealth Fund, 1945.

Tobey, James A. "Public Health and the Police Power." *New York University Law Review*, 4 (1927): 126–33.

Freund, Ernst. *The Police Power: Public Policy, and Constitutional Rights.* Chicago: Callaghan, 1904.

IX. LAW AND ECONOMICS: RISKS, BENEFITS, AND COSTS

Viscusi, Kip. "Regulation of Health, Safety, and Environmental Risks." NBER Working Paper 11934. Cambridge, MA: National Bureau of Economic Research, 2006.

Ackerman, Frank, and Lisa Heinzerling. *Priceless: On Knowing the Price of Everything and the Value of Nothing.* New York: New Press, 2004.

Bloche, M. Gregg, and Elizabeth R. Jungman. "Health Policy and the WTO." *Journal of Law, Medicine, and Ethics*, 31 (2003): 529–45.

Sapsin, Jason W., Theresa M. Thompson, Lesley Stone, et al. "International Trade, Law, and Public Health Advocacy." *Journal of Law, Medicine, and Ethics*, 31 (2003): 546–56.

Sunstein, Cass R. *Risk and Reason: Safety, Law, and the Environment.* Cambridge: Cambridge University Press, 2002.

Bennett, Peter, and Kenneth Calman, eds. *Risk Communication and Public Health.* Oxford: Oxford University Press, 2001.

Jacobson, Peter D., and Matthew L. Kanna. "Cost-Effectiveness Analysis in the Courts: Recent Trends and Future Prospects." *Journal of Health Politics, Policy, and Law*, 26 (2001): 291–326.

Heinzerling, Lisa. "Regulatory Costs of Mythic Proportions." *Yale Law Journal*, 107 (1998): 1981–2070.

Arrow, Kenneth J. *Benefit-Cost Analysis in Environmental, Health, and Safety Regulations: A Statement of Principles.* Washington, DC: AEI, 1996.

Arrow, Kenneth J., Maureen L. Cropper, George C. Eads, et al. "Is There a Role for Benefit-Cost Analysis in Environmental, Health, and Safety Regulation?" *Science*, 272 (1996): 221–22.

National Research Council. *Understanding Risk: Informing Decisions in a Democratic Society.* Washington, DC: National Academies Press, 1996.
Sunstein, Cass R. "Health-Health Tradeoffs." *University of Chicago Law Review,* 63 (1996): 1533–71.
Bayer, Ronald, Lawrence O. Gostin, and Devon C. McGraw. "Trades, AIDS, and the Public's Health: The Limits of Economic Analysis." *Georgetown Law Journal,* 83 (1994): 79–107.
Breyer, Stephen. *Breaking the Vicious Circle: Toward Effective Risk Regulation.* Cambridge, MA: Harvard University Press, 1993.
Philipson, Thomas J., and Richard A. Posner. *Private Choices and Public Health: The AIDS Epidemic in an Economic Perspective.* Cambridge, MA: Harvard University Press, 1993.

X. SURVEILLANCE AND PRIVACY

Fairchild, Amy L., Ronald Bayer, James Colgrove, et al. *Searching Eyes: Privacy, the State, and Disease Surveillance in America.* Berkeley: University of California Press, 2007.
Fairchild, Amy L., Lance Gable, Lawrence O. Gostin, et al. "Public Goods, Private Data: HIV and the History, Ethics, and Uses of Personally Identifiable Public Health Information." *Public Health Reports,* supplement 1 (2007): 7–15.
Baker, Michael G., and David P. Fidler. "Global Public Health Surveillance under New International Health Regulations." *Emerging Infectious Diseases,* 12 (2006): 1058–65.
Hodge, James G., Jr. "An Enhanced Approach to Distinguishing Public Health Practice and Human Subjects Research." *Journal of Law, Medicine, and Ethics,* 33 (2005): 125–40.
Rothstein, Mark A. "Currents in Contemporary Ethics: Research Privacy under HIPAA and the Common Rule." *Journal of Law, Medicine, and Ethics,* 33 (2005): 154–58.
Fairchild, Amy L., and Ronald Bayer. "Ethics and the Conduct of Public Health Surveillance." *Science,* 303 (2004): 631–32.
Mokdad, Ali H., James S. Marks, Donna F. Stroup, et al. "Actual Causes of Death in the United States, 2000." *JAMA,* 291 (2003): 1238–45.
Gostin, Lawrence O., and James G. Hodge, Jr. "Personal Privacy and Common Goods: A Framework for Balancing under the National Health Information Privacy Rule." *Minnesota Law Review,* 86 (2002): 1439–79.
Lumpkin, John R., and Margaret S. Richards. "Transforming the Public Health Information Infrastructure." *Health Affairs,* 21 (2002): 45–56.
Bayer, Ronald, and Amy L. Fairchild. *The Role of Name-Based Notification in Public Health and HIV Surveillance.* Geneva: UNAIDS, 2000.
Teutsch, Steven M., and R. Elliott Churchill, eds. *Principles and Practice of Public Health Surveillance.* 2d ed. New York: Oxford University Press, 2000.
National Research Council. *For the Record: Protecting Electronic Health Information.* Washington, DC: National Academies Press, 1997.
Gostin, Lawrence O., Zita Lazzarini, Verla S. Neslund, et al. "The Public Health

Information Infrastructure: A National Review of the Law on Health Information Privacy." *JAMA,* 275 (1996): 1921–27.
Gostin, Lawrence O. "Health Information Privacy." *Cornell Law Review,* 80 (1995): 451–528.
McGinnis, Michael J., and William H. Foege. "Actual Causes of Death in the United States." *JAMA,* 270 (1993): 2207–12.
Langmuir, Alexander D. "The Surveillance of Communicable Diseases of National Importance." *New England Journal of Medicine,* 268 (1963): 182–92.

XI. HEALTH PROMOTION AND HEALTH COMMUNICATION: FREE EXPRESSION

Buchanan, David R. *An Ethic for Health Promotion: Rethinking the Sources of Human Well-Being.* New York: Oxford University Press, 2000.
Callahan, Daniel, ed. *Promoting Health Behavior: How Much Freedom? Whose Responsibility?* Washington, DC: Georgetown University Press, 2000.
Sage, William M. "Regulating through Information: Disclosure Laws and American Health Care." *Columbia Law Review,* 99 (1999): 1701–1829.
Faden, Ruth R. "Ethical Issues in Government Sponsored Public Health Campaigns." *Health Education Quarterly,* 14 (1987): 27–37.
Bayer, Ronald, and Jonathan Moreno. "Health Promotion: Ethical and Social Dimensions of Government Policy." *Health Affairs,* 5 (1986): 72–85.

XII. PUBLIC HEALTH POWERS: LIBERTY INTERESTS

A. Isolation and Quarantine

Institute of Medicine. *Quarantine Stations at Ports of Entry.* Washington, DC: National Academies Press, 2006.
Markel, Howard, Alexandra M. Stern, J. Alexander Navarro, et al. *A Historical Assessment of Nonpharmaceutical Disease Containment Strategies Employed by Selected U.S. Communities during the Second Wave of the 1918–1920 Influenza Pandemic.* Fort Belvoir, VA: Defense Threat Reduction Agency, 2006.
Heyman, David. *Model Operational Guidelines for Disease Exposure Control.* Washington, DC: Center for Strategic and International Studies, 2005.
Markovits, David. "Quarantines and Distributive Justice." *Journal of Law, Medicine, and Ethics,* 33 (2005): 323–44.
Heymann, David L., ed. *Control of Communicable Diseases Manual.* 18th ed. Washington, DC: American Public Health Association, 2004.
Parmet, Wendy E. "Quarantine Redux: Bioterrorism, AIDS, and the Curtailment of Individual Liberty in the Name of Public Health." *Health Matrix,* 13 (2003): 85–116.
Rothstein, Mark A., M. Gabriela Alcalde, and Nanette R. Elster. "Quarantine and Isolation: Lessons Learned from SARS." CDC Report, 2003.
Barbera, Joseph, Anthony Macintyre, Lawrence O. Gostin, et al. "Large-Scale

Quarantine following Biological Terrorism in the United States: Scientific Examination, Logistic and Legal Limits, and Possible Consequences." *JAMA,* 286 (2001): 2711–17.
Bayer, Ronald, and Amy Fairchild-Carrino. "AIDS and the Limits of Control: Public Health Orders, Quarantine, and Recalcitrant Behavior." *American Journal of Public Health,* 83 (1993): 1471–76.
Shepin, Oleg P., and Waldemar V. Yermakov. *International Quarantine.* Translated by Boris Meerovich and Vladimir Bobrov. Madison, CT: International Universities Press, 1991.
Gostin, Lawrence O. "The Politics of AIDS: Compulsory State Powers, Public Health, and Civil Liberties." *Ohio State Law Journal,* 49 (1989): 1017–58.
Sullivan, Kathleen M., and Martha A. Field. "AIDS and the Coercive Power of the State." *Harvard Civil Rights–Civil Liberties Law Review,* 23 (1988): 139–97.
Musto, David. "Quarantine and the Problem of AIDS." *Milbank Quarterly,* 64 (1986): 97–117.
Parmet, Wendy. "AIDS and Quarantine: The Revival of an Archaic Doctrine." *Hofstra Law Review,* 14 (1985): 53–90.
Clemons, F. G. "Origin of Quarantine." *British Medical Journal* (1929): 122–23.
Tandy, Elizabeth C. "Local Quarantine and Inoculation for Smallpox in the American Colonies (1620–1775)." *American Journal of Public Health,* 13 (1923): 203–7.
Eager, John M. *The Early History of Quarantine: Origin of Sanitary Measures Directed against Yellow Fever.* Washington, DC: U.S. Government Printing Office, 1903.

B. Immunization

Dawson, Angus, and Marcel Verweij, eds. *Ethics, Prevention, and Public Health.* Oxford: Oxford University Press, 2007.
Colgrove, James. *State of Immunity: The Politics of Vaccination in Twentieth-Century America.* Berkeley: University of California Press, 2006.
World Health Organization. *Advanced Market Commitments for Vaccines.* Geneva: World Health Organization, 2006.
Danzon, Patricia M., Nuno Sousa Pereira, and Sapna S. Tejwani. "Vaccine Supply: A Cross-National Perspective." *Health Affairs,* 24 (2005): 706–17.
Dawson, Angus. "The Determination of 'Best Interests' in Relation to Childhood Vaccinations." *Bioethics,* 19 (2005): 188–205.
Institute of Medicine. *The Smallpox Vaccination Program: Public Health in an Age of Terrorism.* Washington, DC: National Academies Press, 2005.
———. *Vaccine Safety Research, Data Access, and Public Trust.* Washington, DC: National Academies Press, 2005.
"The Vaccine Enterprise" (symposium). *Health Affairs* 24 (2005): 594–769.
Calandrillo, Steve P. "Vanishing Vaccinations: Why Are So Many Americans Opting Out of Vaccinating Their Children?" *University of Michigan Journal of Law Reform,* 37 (2004): 353–440.

Institute of Medicine. *Immunization Safety Review: Vaccines and Autism.* Washington, DC: National Academies Press, 2004.

Verweij, Marcel, and Angus Dawson. "Ethical Principles for Collective Immunization Programmes." *Vaccine,* 22 (2004): 3122–26.

Institute of Medicine. *Financing Vaccines in the Twenty-first Century: Assuring Access and Availability.* Washington, DC: National Academies Press, 2003.

Silverman, Ross D. "No More Kidding Around: Restructuring Non-Medical Childhood Immunization Exemptions to Ensure Public Health Protection." *Annals of Health Law,* 12 (2003): 277–94.

Hinman, Alan R., Walter A. Orenstein, Don E. Williamson, et al. "Tools to Prevent Infectious Disease: Childhood Immunization: Laws That Work." *Journal of Law, Medicine, and Ethics,* 30 (2002): 122–27.

Hodge, James G., Jr., and Lawrence O. Gostin. "School Vaccination Requirements: Historical, Social, and Legal Perspectives." *Kentucky Law Journal,* 90 (2002): 831–90.

Institute of Medicine. *Protecting Our Forces: Improving Vaccine Availability in the U.S. Military.* Washington, DC: National Academies Press, 2002.

World Health Organization. *State of the World's Vaccines and Immunization.* Geneva: World Health Organization, 2002.

Cohen, Jon, and Eliot Marshall. "Vaccines for Biodefense: A System in Distress." *Science,* 294 (2001): 498–501.

Salmon, Daniel A., Michael Harbor, Eugene J. Gangarosa, et al. "Health Consequences of Religious and Philosophical Exemptions from Immunization Laws: Individual and Societal Risk of Measles." *JAMA,* 282 (1999): 47–53.

Gostin, Lawrence O., and Zita Lazzarini. "Childhood Immunization Registries: A National Review of Public Health Information Systems and the Protection of Privacy." *JAMA,* 274 (1995): 1793–99.

National Vaccine Advisory Committee. *Developing a National Childhood Immunization System: Registries, Reminders, and Recall.* Washington, DC: U.S. Department of Health and Human Services, 1994.

Neustadt, Richard E., and Harvey Fineberg. *The Epidemic That Never Was: Policy-Making and the Swine Flu Affair.* New York: Vintage Books, 1983.

C. *Testing and Screening*

Faden, Ruth R., Nancy E. Kass, and Madison Powers. "Warrants for Screening Programs: Public Health, Legal and Ethical Frameworks." In *AIDS, Women, and the Next Generation: Towards a Morally Acceptable Public Policy for HIV Testing of Pregnant Women and Newborns,* edited by Ruth R. Faden, Gail Geller, and Madison Powers, 3–26. New York: Oxford University Press, 1991.

Bayer, Ronald, Carol Levine, and Susan Wolf. "HIV Antibody Screening: An Ethical Framework for Evaluating Proposed Programs." *JAMA,* 256 (1986): 1768–74.

Gostin, Lawrence O., William J. Curran, and Mary E. Clark. "The Case against Compulsory Casefinding in Controlling AIDS: Testing, Screening and Reporting." *American Journal of Law and Medicine,* 12 (1986): 7–53.

D. Reporting

Roush, Sandra, Guthrie Birkhead, Denise Koo, et al. "Mandatory Reporting of Diseases and Conditions by Health Care Providers and Laboratories." *JAMA*, 282 (1999): 164–70.
American Civil Liberties Union. *HIV Surveillance and Name Reporting*. New York: ACLU, 1998.
Gostin, Lawrence O., and James G. Hodge, Jr. "The 'Names Debate': The Case for National HIV Reporting in the United States." *Albany Law Review*, 61 (1998): 679–743.
Gostin, Lawrence O., John W. Ward, and A. Cornelius Baker. "National HIV Case Reporting for the United States: A Defining Moment in the History of the Epidemic." *New England Journal of Medicine*, 337 (1997): 1162–67.
Fox, Daniel M. "From TB to AIDS: Value Conflicts in Reporting Disease." *Hastings Center Report*, 11 (1986): 11–16.

E. Partner Notification

Webber, David W. "Self-Incrimination, Partner Notification, and the Criminal Law: Negatives for the CDC's 'Prevention for Positives' Initiative." *AIDS and Public Policy Journal*, 19 (2004): 54–66.
Dolbear, Gail L., and Linda T. Newell. "Consent for Prenatal Testing: A Preliminary Examination of the Effects of Named HIV Reporting and Mandatory Partner Notification." *Journal of Public Health Management Practice*, 8 (2002): 69–72.
Gostin, Lawrence O., and James G. Hodge, Jr. "Piercing the Veil of Secrecy in HIV/AIDS and Other Sexually Transmitted Diseases: Theories of Privacy and Disclosure in Partner Notification." *Duke Journal on Gender Law and Policy*, 5 (1998): 28–32.
Rothenburg, Karen H., and Stephen J. Paskey. "The Risk of Domestic Violence and Women with HIV Infection: Implications for Partner Notification, Public Policy, and the Law." *American Journal of Public Health*, 85 (1995): 1569–76.
Bayer, Ronald, and Kathleen E. Toomey. "HIV Prevention and the Two Faces of Partner Notification." *American Journal of Public Health*, 82 (1992): 1158–64.

F. Physical Examination and Treatment

Lucas, Gregory M. "Directly Observed Therapy for the Treatment of HIV: Promises and Pitfalls." *Hopkins HIV Report*, 13 (2001): 12–15.
Volmink, Jimmy, Patrice Matchaba, and Paul Garner. "Directly Observed Therapy and Treatment Adherence." *Lancet*, 355 (2000).
Bayer, Ronald. "Directly Observed Therapy and Treatment Completion for Tuberculosis in the United States: Is Universal Supervised Therapy Necessary?" *American Journal of Public Health*, 88 (1998): 1052–58.
Bayer, Ronald, and David Wilkinson. "Directly Observed Therapy for Tuberculosis: History of an Idea." *Lancet*, 345 (1995): 1545–48.

XIII. PUBLIC HEALTH POWERS: PROPERTY INTERESTS

Epstein, Richard. *Takings: Private Property and the Power of Eminent Domain.* Cambridge, MA: Harvard University Press, 1985.
Tandy, Elizabeth C. "The Regulation of Nuisances in the American Colonies." *American Journal of Public Health,* 13 (1923): 810–13.

XIV. TORT LAW AND THE PUBLIC'S HEALTH

Jacobson, Peter D., and Soheil Soliman. "Litigation as Public Health Policy: Theory or Reality?" *Journal of Law, Medicine, and Ethics,* 30 (2002): 224–38.
Institute of Medicine. *Reducing the Burden of Injury: Advancing Prevention and Treatment.* Washington, DC: National Academies Press, 1999.
Jacobson, Peter, and Kenneth E. Warner. "Litigation and Public Health Policy Making: The Case of Tobacco Control." *Journal of Health Politics, Policy, and Law,* 24 (1999): 769–804.
Margaret G. Farrell. "*Daubert v. Merrell Dow Pharmaceuticals, Inc.*: Epistemology and Legal Process." *Cardozo Law Review,* 15 (1994): 2183–17.
Cristoffel, Tom, and Stephen P. Teret. "Epidemiology and the Law: Courts and Confidence Intervals." *American Journal of Public Health,* 81 (1991): 1661–66.
Huber, Peter W. *Galileo's Revenge: Junk Science in the Courtroom.* New York: Basic Books, 1991.

XV. PUBLIC HEALTH: ISSUES AND CONCERNS

A. Emerging Infectious Diseases

Sherman, Irwin W. *The Power of Plagues.* Washington, DC: American Society for Microbiology Press, 2006.
World Health Organization Writing Group. "Nonpharmaceutical Interventions for Pandemic Influenza, National and International Measures." *Emerging Infectious Diseases,* 12 (2006): 81–94.
Barry, John M. *The Great Influenza: The Epic Story of the Deadliest Plague in History.* New York: Penguin Books, 2005.
Diamond, Jared M. *Guns, Germs, and Steel.* Rev. ed. New York: Norton, 2005.
World Health Organization. *Avian Influenza: Assessing the Pandemic Threat.* Geneva: World Health Organization, 2005.
Gostin, Lawrence O., Ronald Bayer, and Amy L. Fairchild. "Ethical and Legal Challenges Posed by Severe Acute Respiratory Syndrome: Implications for the Control of Severe Infectious Disease Threats." *JAMA,* 290 (2003): 3229–37.
Institute of Medicine. *Microbial Threats to Health: Emergence, Detection and Response.* Washington, DC: National Academies Press, 2003.
Koplow, David A. *Smallpox: The Fight to Eradicate a Global Scourge.* Berkeley: University of California Press, 2003.
Public Health Agency of Canada. *Learning from SARS—Renewal of Public Health*

in Canada: A Report of the National Advisory Committee on SARS and Public Health. Public Health Agency of Canada, October 2003.
Gostin, Lawrence O., Scott Burris, and Zita Lazzarini. "The Law and the Public's Health: A Study of Infectious Disease Law in the United States." *Columbia Law Review,* 99 (1999): 59–128.
Gostin, Lawrence O. "The Law and Commmunicable Diseases: The Role of Law in an Era of Microbial Threats." *International Digest of Health Legislation,* 49 (1998): 221–33.
Gostin, Lawrence O., Scott Burris, Zita Lazzarini, et al. *Improving State Law to Prevent and Treat Infectious Disease.* New York: Milbank Memorial Fund, 1998.
Fidler, David P. "Return of the Fourth Horseman: Emerging Infectious Diseases and International Law." *Minnesota Law Review,* 81 (1997): 771–868.
Lederberg, Joshua. "Infectious Diseases as an Evolutionary Paradigm." *Emerging Infectious Diseases,* 3 (1997): 417–23.
Centers for Disease Control and Prevention. *Addressing Emerging Infectious Disease Threats: A Prevention Strategy for the United States.* Washington, DC: U.S. Department of Health and Human Services, 1994.
Garrett, Laurie. *The Coming Plague: Newly Emerging Diseases in a World Out of Balance.* New York: Farrar, Straus and Giroux, 1994.
Institute of Medicine. *Emerging Infections: Microbial Threats in the United States.* Washington, DC: National Academies Press, 1992.

B. Bioterrorism

Fidler, David P., and Lawrence O. Gostin. *Biosecurity in the Global Age: Biological Weapons, Public Health, and the Rule of Law.* Palo Alto, CA: Stanford University Press, 2007.
Gostin, Lawrence O. "When Terrorism Threatens Health: How Far Are Limitations on Personal and Economic Liberties Justified?" *Florida Law Review,* 55 (2003): 1105–70.
Levy, Barry S., and Victor W. Sidel, eds. *Terrorism and Public Health.* Oxford: Oxford University Press, 2003.
Moreno, Jonathan D. *In the Wake of Terror: Medicine and Morality in a Time of Crisis.* Cambridge, MA: Massachusetts Institute of Technology Press, 2003.
Sutton, Victoria. *Law and Bioterrorism.* Durham, NC: Carolina Academic Press, 2003.
Fidler, David P. "Bioterrorism, Public Health, and International Law." *Chicago Journal of International Law,* 3 (2002): 7–26.
Gostin, Lawrence O. "Public Health Law in an Age of Terrorism: Rethinking Individual Rights and Common Goods." *Health Affairs,* 21 (2002): 79–93.
Inglesby, Thomas V., David T. Dennis, Donald A. Henderson, et al. "Plague as a Biological Weapon: Medical and Public Health Management." *JAMA,* 283 (2000): 2281–90.
Henderson, Donald A. "The Looming Threat of Bioterrorism." *Science,* 283 (1999): 1279–82.

C. HIV/AIDS

Gostin, Lawrence O. *The AIDS Pandemic: Complacency, Injustice, and Unfulfilled Expectations.* Chapel Hill: University of North Carolina Press, 2004.
Institute of Medicine. *No Time to Lose: Getting More from HIV Prevention.* Washington, DC: National Academies Press, 2001.
Feldman, Eric, and Ronald Bayer, eds. *Blood Feuds: AIDS, Blood, and the Politics of Medical Disaster.* New York: Oxford University Press, 1999.
Institute of Medicine. *Reducing the Odds: Preventing Perinatal Transmission of HIV in the United States.* Washington, DC: National Academies Press, 1999.
Gostin, Lawrence O., and David W. Webber. "The AIDS Litigation Project: HIV/AIDS in the Courts in the 1990s, Part 2." *AIDS and Public Policy Journal,* 13 (1998): 3–19.
———. "The AIDS Litigation Project: HIV/AIDS in the Courts in the 1990s, Part 1." *AIDS and Public Policy Journal,* 12 (1997): 105–21.
Webber, David W., ed. *AIDS and the Law.* 4th ed. New York: Wiley Law Publications, 1997.
Bayer, Ronald. "AIDS Prevention—Sexual Ethics and Responsibility." *New England Journal of Medicine,* 334 (1996): 1540–42.
Gostin, Lawrence O., Zita Lazzarini, Diane Alexander, et al. "HIV Testing, Counseling, and Prophylaxis after Sexual Assault." *JAMA,* 271 (1994): 1436–44.
Burris, Scott, Harlon L. Dalton, and Judith Leonie Miller, eds. *AIDS Law Today: A New Guide for the Public.* New Haven, CT: Yale University Press, 1993.
Bayer, Ronald. *Private Acts, Social Consequences: AIDS and the Politics of Public Health.* New Brunswick, NJ: Rutgers University Press, 1991.
Gostin, Lawrence O., Paul Cleary, Kenneth Mayer, et al. "Screening and Exclusion of International Travelers and Immigrants for Public Health Purposes: An Evaluation of United States Policy." *New England Journal of Medicine,* 332 (1990): 1743–46.
Stoddard, Thomas B., and Walter Rieman. "AIDS and the Rights of the Individual: Toward a More Sophisticated Understanding of Discrimination." *Milbank Quarterly,* 68, supplement 1 (1990): 143–74.
Curran, William, Lawrence O. Gostin, and Mary Clark. *AIDS: Legal, Regulatory, and Policy Analysis.* Washington, DC: U.S. Department of Health and Human Services, 1986. Republished, Frederick, MD: University Publishing Group, 1988.
Burris, Scott. "Fear Itself: AIDS, Herpes and Public Health Decisions." *Yale Law and Policy Review,* 3 (1985): 479–518.

D. Tuberculosis

Gostin, Lawrence O. "The Resurgent Tuberculosis Epidemic in the Era of AIDS: Reflections on Public Health, Law, and Society." *Maryland Law Review,* 54 (1995): 1–131.
Ball, Carlos A., and Mark Barnes. "Public Health and Individual Rights: Tu-

berculosis Control and Detention Procedures in New York City." *Yale Law and Policy Review,* 12 (1994): 38–67.
Gittler, Josephine. "Controlling Resurgent Tuberculosis: Public Health Agencies, Public Health Policy, and Law." *Journal of Health Politics, Policy and Law,* 19 (1994): 107–46.
Rothman, Sheila M. *Living in the Shadow of Death: Tuberculosis and the Social Experience of Illness in American History.* New York: Basic Books, 1994.
Reilly, Rosemary G. "Combating the Tuberculosis Epidemic: The Legality of Coercive Measures." *Columbia Journal of Law and Social Problems,* 27 (1993): 101–49.
Dubler, Nancy N., Ronald Bayer, et al. *The Tuberculosis Revival: Individual Rights and Societal Obligations in a Time of AIDS.* New York: United Hospital Fund, 1992.

E. Sexually Transmitted Infections

Centers for Disease Control and Prevention. *Expedited Partner Therapy in the Management of Sexually Transmitted Diseases.* Atlanta, GA: U.S. Department of Health and Human Services, 2006.
———. "Sexually Transmitted Diseases Treatment Guidelines, 2006." *Morbidity and Mortality Weekly Report,* 55 (2006): 1–94.
Hodge, James G., Jr. *Expedited Partner Therapies for Sexually Transmitted Diseases: Assessing the Legal Environment.* Washington, DC: Center for Law and the Public's Health, 2006.
National Conference of State Legislatures. *Sexually Transmitted Diseases: A Policymaker's Guide and Summary of State Laws.* Denver, CO: National Conference of State Legislatures, 1998.
Institute of Medicine. *The Hidden Epidemic: Confronting Sexually Transmitted Diseases.* Washington, DC: National Academies Press, 1997.
Brandt, Allan M. *No Magic Bullet: A Social History of Venereal Disease in the United States since 1880.* New York: Oxford University Press, 1987.

F. Tobacco

Brandt, Allan M. *The Cigarette Century: The Rise and Fall of the Drug That Defined America.* New York: Basic Books, 2007.
Feldman, Eric A., and Ronald Bayer. *Conflicts over Tobacco Policy and Public Health.* Cambridge, MA: Harvard University Press, 2004.
Taylor, Allyn L., Douglas W. Bettcher, and Richard Pect. "International Law and the International Legislative Process: The WHO Framework Convention on Tobacco Control." In *Global Public Health Goods for Health: Health Economic and Public Health Perspectives,* edited by Richard Smith et al., 212–29. Oxford: Oxford University Press, 2003.
Institute of Medicine. *Clearing the Smoke: Assessing the Science Base for Tobacco Harm Reduction.* Washington, DC: National Academies Press, 2001.
Jha, Prabhat, and Frank Chaloupka, eds. *Tobacco Control in Developing Countries.* New York: Oxford University Press, 2000.

Pope, Thaddeas Mason. "Balancing Public Health against Individual Liberty: The Ethics of Smoking Regulations." *University of Pittsburgh Law Review*, 61 (2000): 419–98.

Jacobson, Peter D., Jeffrey Wasserman, and John Anderson. "Historical Overview of Tobacco Legislation and Regulation." *Journal of Social Issues*, 53 (1997): 75–95.

Rabin, Robert. "A Sociolegal History of the Tobacco Tort Litigation." *Stanford Law Review*, 44 (1992): 853–78.

Warner, Kenneth E. *Selling Smoke: Cigarette Advertising and Public Health*. Washington, DC: American Public Health Institute, 1986.

G. Firearms

Lytton, Timothy, ed. *Suing the Gun Industry: A Battle at the Crossroads of Gun Control and Mass Torts*. Ann Arbor: University of Michigan Press, 2005.

National Research Council. *Firearms and Violence*. Washington, DC: National Academies Press, 2005.

Hemenway, David. *Private Guns, Public Health*. Ann Arbor: University of Michigan Press, 2004.

Vernick, Jon S., Jason W. Sapsin, Stephen P. Teret, et al. "How Litigation Can Promote Product Safety." *Journal of Law, Medicine, and Ethics*, 32 (2004): 551–55.

Vernick, Jon S., and Julie Samia Mair. "How the Law Affects Gun Policy in the United States: Law as Intervention or Obstacle to Prevention." *Journal of Law, Medicine, and Ethics*, 30 (2002): 692–704.

Culhane, John G., and Jean Macchiaroli Eggen. "Defining a Proper Role for Public Nuisance Law in Municipal Suits against Gun Sellers: Beyond Rhetoric and Expedience." *South Carolina Law Review*, 52 (2001): 287–329.

Vernick, Jon S., and Stephen P. Teret. "New Courtroom Strategies regarding Firearms: Tort Litigation against Firearm Manufacturers and Constitutional Challenges to Gun Laws." *Houston Law Review*, 36 (1999): 1713–54.

Teret, Stephen P., Daniel W. Webster, and Jon S. Vernick. "Support for New Policies to Regulate Firearms: Results of Two National Surveys." *New England Journal of Medicine*, 339 (1998): 813–18.

Polston, Mark D., and Douglas S. Weil. "Unsafe by Design: Using Tort Actions to Reduce Firearm-Related Injuries." *Stanford Law and Policy Review*, 8 (1997): 13–24.

Vernick, Jon S., Stephen P. Teret, and Daniel W. Webster. "Regulating Firearm Advertisements That Promise Home Protection." *JAMA*, 277 (1997): 1391–97.

H. Public Health Genetics

Holtzman, Neil A., and Michael S. Watson, eds. *Promoting Safe and Effective Genetic Testing in the United States*. Bethesda, MD: National Institutes of Health, 2006.

Institute of Medicine. *Implications of Genomics for Public Health*. Washington, DC: National Academies Press, 2005.

Institute of Medicine. *Safety of Genetically Engineered Foods: Approaches to Assessing Unintended Health Effects.* Washington, DC: National Academies Press, 2004.

Hodge, James G., Jr., and Mark E. Harris. "International Genetics Research and Issues of Group Privacy." *Journal of Biolaw and Business,* special supplement (2001): 15–21.

Khoury, Muin J., Wylie Burke, and Elizabeth J. Thomson, eds. *Genetics and Public Health in the Twenty-first Century: Using Genetic Information to Improve Health and Prevent Disease.* New York: Oxford University Press, 2000.

I. Obesity

Mello, Michelle M., David M. Studdert, and Troyen A. Brennan. "Obesity—The New Frontier of Public Health Law." *New England Journal of Medicine,* 354 (2006): 2601–9.

Gostin, Lawrence O. "Fast and Supersized: Is the Answer Diet by Fiat?" *Hastings Center Report,* 35 (2005): 11–12.

Kersh, Rogan, and James A. Morone. "Obesity, Courts, and the New Politics of Public Health." *Journal of Health Politics, Policy, and Law,* 30 (2005): 839–68.

Table of Cases

Index

Text: 10/13 Sabon
Display: Sabon
Compositor: Integrated Composition Systems
Printer and binder: Maple-Vail Manufacturing Group

About the Author

LAWRENCE GOSTIN, an internationally acclaimed scholar, is Associate Dean and the Linda D. and Timothy J. O'Neill Professor of Global Health Law at the Georgetown University Law Center, where he directs the O'Neill Institute for National and Global Health Law. Dean Gostin is also Professor of Public Health at the Johns Hopkins University and Director of the Center for Law and the Public's Health at Georgetown and Johns Hopkins Universities—a Collaborating Center of the World Health Organization and the Centers for Disease Control and Prevention. Dean Gostin is Visiting Professor of Public Health (Faculty of Medical Sciences) and Research Fellow (Centre for Socio-Legal Studies) at Oxford University.

Dean Gostin has honorary degrees from the State University of New York and Cardiff University, Wales. He is an elected lifetime Member of the Institute of Medicine, serves on the Board on Health Science Policy, and has chaired IOM Committees on public health genomics, prisoner research, and health informational privacy. The IOM awarded Dean Gostin the Adam Yarmolinsky Medal for distinguished service to further the IOM mission of science and health. He received the Public Health Law Association's Distinguished Lifetime Achievement Award "in recognition of a career devoted to using law to improve the public's health." Internationally, Dean Gostin received the Rosemary Delbridge Memorial Award from the National Consumer Council (United Kingdom) for the person "who has most influenced Parliament and government to act for the welfare of society." He also received the Key to Tohoko University (Japan) for distinguished contributions to human rights in mental health.